Polycystic Ovary Syndrome

Polycystic Ovary Syndrome

Basic Science to Clinical Advances Across the Lifespan

Edited by

Rehana Rehman, MBBS, MPhil, PhD, FHEA, MHPE

Associate Professor and Director Graduate Studies
Department of Biological & Biomedical Sciences
Aga Khan University, Karachi
Sindh
Pakistan

Aisha Sheikh, MBBS, FCPS, FACE, PGDipDiab, PGDipEndocrine

Lecturer & Consultant Endocrinologist
Medicine
The Aga Khan University Hospital, Karachi
Sindh
Pakistan
Tutor, University of South Wales, Cardiff, United Kingdom

ELSEVIER

Elsevier
1600 John F. Kennedy Blvd.
Ste 1800
Philadelphia, PA 19103-2899

POLYCYSTIC OVARY SYNDROME

ISBN: 978-0-323-87932-3

Content Strategist: Humayra Khan
Content Development Specialist: Shilpa Kumar
Content Development Manager: Somodatta Roy Choudhury
Publishing Services Manager: Shereen Jameel
Project Manager: Haritha Dharmarajan
Design Direction: Bridget Hoette

Printed in India

Last digit is the print number: 9 8 7 6 5 4 3 2 1

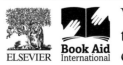

Contributors

Tauseef Ahmad, MSc, PhD
Researcher
Department of Epidemiology and Health Statistics
School of Public Health
Southeast University
Nanjing, China

Intisar Ahmed, MBBS
Fellow
Aga Khan University
Medicine
Aga Khan University, Karachi
Sindh
Pakistan

Faiza Alam, MBBS, MPHIL, PHD
Assistant Professor Clinical Academia
Medicine
PAPRSB Institute of Health Sciences
Muara, Bandar Seri Begawan
Brunei Darussalam

Sobia Sabir Ali, MBBS, FCPS, MRCP(UK), FRCP(Edin), MHPE
Professor
Diabetes & Endocrinology
Peshawar Medical College, Peshawar
KPK
Pakistan

Azra Amerjee, MBBS, FCPS, MCPS(HPE)
Doctor, Assistant Professor
Obstetrics & Gynecology
The Aga Khan University Hospital, Karachi
Sindh
Pakistan

Muzna Arif, MBBS, FCPS Pediatrics
Fellow
Pediatrics and Child Health
Aga Khan University, Karachi
Sindh
Pakistan

Nargis Asad
Chair, Associate Professor
Department of Psychiatry
Aga Khan University Hospital, Karachi
Sindh
Pakistan

Mukhtiar Baig, MBBS, MPhil, PhD
Professor
Clinical Biochemistry
King Abdulaziz University
Jeddah
Saudi Arabia

Sumera Batool, MBBS, FCPS (Medicine), FCPS (Endocrinology & Diabetes)
Consultant Endocrinologist & Diabetologist
Department of Medicine
Dr. Ziauddin University Hospital, Karachi
Sindh
Pakistan

Amna Subhan Butt, MBBS, FCPS (Medicine), FCPS (Gastroenterology), MSc Clinical Researcher, WGO Fellow in ERCP
Associate Professor
Medicine
The Aga Khan University Hospital, Karachi
Sindh
Pakistan

Bhagwan Das, MBBS, FCPS (Medicine), FCPS (Endocrinology), SCE-Endocrine and Diabetes, Diabetes, Endocrine, and Metabolism Fellow
Consultant Physician and Endocrinologist
Medicine and Endocrine
Aster Sanad Hospital
Riyadh
KSA

Jalpa Devi, MBBS
Postgraduate Trainee
Gastroenterology
Liaquat University of Medical and Health Sciences
Hyderabad
Pakistan

Raj HT Dodia, MBChB, MMEd, MRCOG
Obstetrics & Gynecology
MPShah Hospital
Nairobi
Kenya

Rubia Farid, MBBS, FCPS
PCOS Phenotypes
Family Medicine
Aga Khan University Hospital, Karachi
Sindh
Pakistan

Mahwish Fatima, Pharm-D, MPhil (Pharmacology), PhD Scholar (Pharmacology)
Program Coordinator (Diabetes and Hypertension)
The Indus Hospital and Health Network
Karachi
Pakistan

Tehseen Fatima, MBBS, FCPS (Medicine)
Assistant Professor and consultant
Endocrinologist, Hamdard University, Karachi
Sindh
Pakistan

Shayana Rukhsar Hashmani, MBBS
Resident
Dermatology
Aga Khan Hospital, Karachi
Sindh
Pakistan

Muhammad Faisal Hashmi, MBBS
Clinical Fellow
Internal Medicine
The Royal Wolverhampton NHS Trust
Wolverhampton
United Kingdom

Khadija Nuzhat Humayun, MBBS, FCPS, Adv. DHPE
Paediatrics Endocrinologist
Associate Professor
Paediatrics and Child Health
Aga Khan University, Karachi
Sindh
Pakistan

Zaheena Islam, MBBS, FCPS
Assistant Professor
Obstetrics & Gynecology
Aga Khan University Hospital, Karachi
Sindh
Pakistan

Sumerah Jabeen, FCPS(Medicine), FCPS(Endocrinology)
Consultant Endocrinologist
Medicine Department
Patel Hospital, Karachi
Sindh
Pakistan

Muhammad Abdullah Javed
Medical Student
Medical College
Aga Khan University, Karachi
Sindh
Pakistan

Hafiz S. Kamran, MBBS, FCPS, MRCP
Registrar
Acute Medicine
Royal Preston Hospital
Dudley
United Kingdom

Rakhshaan Khan, MBBS, MPH, MBA
MEd Hearing Impairment
Doctor
Public Health
ICAT, Karachi
Sindh
Pakistan

Unab I. Khan, MBBS, MS
Associate Professor
Family Medicine
Aga Khan University, Karachi
Sindh
Pakistan

Kimmee Khan, MBBS, BSc, MRCOG
Doctor
Obstetrics & Gynaecology
St Georges Hospital NHS Trust
London
United Kingdom

Zareen Kiran, MBBS, FCPS (Med), MRCP (UK), FCPS (Endo)
Assistant Professor Endocrinology
Endocrinology, Medicine
National Institute of Diabetes and Endocrinology
Dow University of Health Sciences, Karachi
Sindh
Pakistan
Consultant Endocrinologist
Endocrinology, Medicine
Aga Khan University Hospital, Karachi
Sindh
Pakistan

Sadia Masood, MBBS, FCPS, MHPE
Assistant Professor
Medicine
Aga Khan University, Karachi
Sindh
Pakistan

Malik Hassan H. Mehmood, BPharm, MPhil, PhD
Associate Professor and Chairperson
Department of Pharmacology
Government College University,
Faisalabad, Faisalabad
Punjab
Pakistan

Fozia Memon, MBBS, FCPS
Instructor Pediatric Endocrinology
Pediatrics and Child Health
Aga Khan University, Karachi
Sindh
Pakistan

Asma Altaf Hussain Merchant, MBBS
Research Fellow, Dean's Office
Aga Khan Medical College
Karachi
Pakistan

Ahmed Sayed Mohammed Sayed Mettawi, MSc, DIP, MB ChB
Clinical Nutrition Specialist
Clinical Nutrition & Endocrine Service
CareZone Clinics, Giza
Egypt
Interim Clinical Director & Chief Physician Nutrition
    Specialist
Clinical Nutrition Department
Al Haram Hospital, Giza
Egypt

Sarah Nadeem, MD, FACE
Director, CCBP, Assistant Professor
Section of Endocrinology
Department of Medicine
Aga Khan University, Karachi
Sindh
Pakistan

Tania Nadeem, MBBS
Clinical Associate Professor
Psychiatry
Aga Khan University, Karachi
Sindh
Pakistan

Nida Najmi, MRCOG, FCPS, MHPE, MSc. Clinical Research
Assistant Professor
Obstetrics & Gynaecology
Aga Khan University, Karachi
Sindh
Pakistan

Sumaira Naz, MBBS, FCPS
Senior Instructor
Obstetrics & Gynecology
Aga Khan University Hospital, Karachi
Sindh
Pakistan

Aisha Noorullah, MBBS, FCPS
Senior Instructor
Department Of Psychiatry
Aga Khan University Hospital, Karachi
Sindh
Pakistan

Kamal Ojha, MD FRCOG
Obstetrics & Gynaecology
St Georges Hospital
London
United Kingdom

Ouma Pillay
Doctor
St George's University Hospitals NHS Foundation Trust
Blackshaw Road
Tooting
London
SW17 0QT

Rahat Najam Qureshi, MBBS, FRCOG
Consultant
Obstetrics & Gynecology
Aga Khan University, Karachi
Sindh
Pakistan

Muhammad Hassan Raza Raja
Medical Student
Medical College
Aga Khan University, Karachi
Sindh
Pakistan

Muhammad Owais Rashid, MBBS, FCPS(Medicine), FCPS(Endocrinology)
Assistant Professor
Diabetes & Endocrinology
Liaquat National Hospital, Karachi
Sindh
Pakistan
Consultant Endocrinologist
Department of Medicine (Section of Endocrinology)
Aga Khan University Hospital, Karachi
Sindh
Pakistan

Rehana Rehman, MBBS, MPhil, PhD, FHEA, MHPE
Associate Professor and Director Graduate Studies
Department of Biological & Biomedical Sciences
Aga Khan University, Karachi
Sindh
Pakistan

Tamar Saeed, MBBS, MRCP(UK), MRCP(Endocrine & Diabetes)
CCT Endocrine & Diabetes (UK), FRCP(Glasg)
RCP(London)
Consultant in Endocrinology and Diabetes Mellitus
Foundation Training Programme Director
MTI Lead in Department of Medicine
Diabetes and Endocrine Centre, North Wing
The Dudley Group NHS Foundation Trust
Russells Hall Hospital
Dudley
United Kingdom

Zainab Samad, MBBS, MHS
Professor & Chair
Department of Medicine
Aga Khan University, Karachi
Sindh
Pakistan

Maheen Shahid, MBBS
Research Scholar & Teaching Assistant
Department of Biological & Biomedical Sciences
Aga Khan University, Karachi
Sindh
Pakistan

Pirbhat Shams, MBBS
Resident Cardiology
Department of Medicine
Aga Khan University, Karachi
Sindh
Pakistan

Aisha Sheikh, MBBS, FCPS, FACE, PGDipDiab, PGDipEndocrine
Lecturer & Consultant Endocrinologist
Department of Medicine
The Aga Khan University Hospital, Karachi
Sindh
Pakistan
Tutor, University of South Wales, Cardiff,
   United Kingdom

Lumaan Sheikh
Associate Professor & Chair
Department of Obstetrics & Gynecology
Aga Khan University Hospital, Karachi
Sindh
Pakistan

Rida Siddique Pharm D, MPhil and PhD (Pharmacology)
Department of Pharmacology
Faculty of Pharmaceutical Sciences
Government College University
Faisalabad
Punjab
Pakistan

Sairabanu Mohamed Rashid Sokwala, MBBS, MMed(Internal Medicine)
PGDip(Diabetes), PGDip(Endocrinology)
Consultant
Diabetes and Endocrinology
Aga Khan University Hospital
Nairobi
Kenya

Saba Tariq, MBBS, MPhil, PhD
Professor/ Head of Department
Pharmacology & Therapeutics
University Medical and Dental College
The University of Faisalabad, Faisalabad
Punjab
Pakistan

Syeda Muneela Wajid, MBBS, MAIUM, MCPS
Gynecologist, Obstetrician
Marium General Hospital, Karachi
Sindh
Pakistan

Farheen Yousuf, FRCOG, FCPS, MCPS(HPE), MCPS(OBGYN)
Assistant Professor
Obstetrics & Gynecology
Aga Khan University, Karachi
Sindh
Pakistan

Nadeem Zuberi, MBBS, FCPS
Associate Professor
Department of Obstetrics & Gynecology
The Aga Khan University, Karachi
Sindh
Pakistan

Foreword

This first edition of *Polycystic Ovary Syndrome: Basic Science to Clinical Advances Across the Lifespan* is impressive in both the depth and breadth of its coverage of the common yet complex entity of polycystic ovary syndrome (PCOS). Beyond being contemporaneous and comprehensive in the coverage of epidemiology, the spectrum of clinical presentations (involving the *soma* and the *psyche*), and the gamut of intersecting pathways of pathophysiologic relevance (genetics, insulin resistance, inflammation, endocrinopathy, epigenetics) and in presenting a targeted approach to symptom burden, this body of work is unique in its prioritization of global nuances in the prevalence and presentation of PCOS. The revisitation of the plausibility of a male equivalent of PCOS, consideration of complementary and alternative therapeutic options, and reflections on unaddressed needs of the present and the future are thought provoking. The editor and contributors are to be commended on the thoughtful approach to context and the thoroughness of content of this text, which is sure to serve a broad range of readership, from trainees to clinicians to researchers and policymakers. It is my hope that this effort will serve as a *call for action* toward collaborative endeavors that would allow for the garnering of population-based data toward gaining clarity on the prevalence, presentation, and burden of PCOS in South Asian women. I am privileged at the opportunity of offering my endorsement of this impressive effort and wish the team much success.

Lubna Pal, MBBS, FRCOG, MS
Professor of Obstetrics Gynecology
& Reproductive Sciences
Director, Program for PCOS, Yale Reproductive
Endocrinology & Infertility
Yale School of Medicine
New Haven, CT, USA

Preface

Polycystic ovary syndrome, or PCOS, is the most common endocrine disorder among females of reproductive age, persisting from menarche to menopause. The prevalence of PCOS in different regions of the world, its causes, diagnosis, clinical practices, treatment regimes, and the impact on psychosocial heath are perplexing and need intervention. Associated comorbidities, such as obesity, impaired glucose tolerance, acne, hirsutism, anovulatory cycles, and genetics, may occur simultaneously and may draw the focus of healthcare away to interrelated health-related complications rather than the disease itself. The exact prevalence of PCOS is still unclear because of inconsistencies in the diagnostic criteria being used; however, the proportion of patients has increased in the past decade. The high prevalence, unrevealed of the disease, and ethnic and geographic disparity limit the lifetime management of PCOS to the "International Evidence-Based PCOS Guidelines."

We have made a tremendous effort to review and compile comprehensive information to create a better understanding of PCOS, especially regarding its etiology, prevalence, diagnosis, trends, and management in different parts of the world, and have summarized the findings in four sections. The first section presents an overview of PCOS, focusing on its prevalence, classification, and phenotypes as they appear in adolescence and present through adult life. The second section discusses in detail the pathogenesis and clinical presentation of the disease, the interplay of various associated comorbidities, and the issues of fertility. The third section goes into detail about the management of PCOS, including general health and fertility concerns along with associated comorbidities. Because the prevalence and characteristics vary geographically and appear to be linked to divergent genetic and environmental tendencies that affect the response to management protocols, the fourth section presents a comprehensive situation analysis of PCOS as it prevails in different regions of the world and the factors that affect the trend of the disease. These may include the healthcare systems of a particular state, the health and cultural beliefs of its people, the health-seeking and lifestyle behaviors, the traditional healing practices, the trends of the disease, women's health in the region and the focus of public health initiatives, genetic predisposition of the problem, and the interplay of various factors that impact the psychosocial health of the people in the region. The availability of diagnostic screening, fertility tests, and fertility management is a cross-cutting feature across the sections.

We hope that this book delivers the desired comprehensive knowledge of the global situation of the disease, emphasizing the burden of disease on the healthcare budget and the need for early identification and prevention to deal with the increasing prevalence of PCOS.

We are extremely thankful to Dr. Lubna Pal, who accepted our request to write the Foreword for this book. Our sincere thanks to all the contributors for their efforts to provide explicit details about the topics assigned to them.

Dr. Rehana Rehman
Associate Professor & Director-Graduate Studies
Department of Biological & Biomedical Sciences
Aga Khan University
Dr. Aisha Sheikh
Lecturer & Consultant Endocrinologist
Department of Medicine
Aga Khan University Hospital
Tutor, University of South Wales, Cardiff,
United Kingdom

Acknowledgment

Our humblest thanks to the omnipresent Allah Almighty, the one above all of us, for answering our prayers and for giving us the strength to plod on. We want to continue by thanking our parents, husbands, and children, without the support of whom, this would not have been possible.

Our special thanks to:

- The departments of Biological & Biomedical Sciences and Medicine (Endocrinology), Aga Khan University, and respective chairs; Dr Kulsoom Ghias and Dr Zainab Samad for their motivation and absolute support.
- Dr. Rakhshaan Khan for correction of write up, illustration of figures, and steadfast encouragement to complete this study.
- Dr. Saira Sokawala for review of selected chapters of the manuscript.
- Our colleagues and friends who made our work as pleasant and relaxing as possible.

We would also like to extend our thanks to all authors and others who directly or indirectly extended their help during this research work.

Thank you,

Dr. Rehana Rehman
Dr. Aisha Sheikh

Contents

Polycystic Ovary Syndrome

1

Introduction to Polycystic Ovary Syndrome

MUHAMMAD FAISAL HASHMI

Introduction

Polycystic ovary syndrome (PCOS) is an endocrinopathy that occurs worldwide in 5% to 15% of females in the reproductive age group.[1,2] It is a leading cause of infertility and pregnancy-related complications. Around 70% to 80% of females with PCOS are infertile and present with various forms of menstrual irregularities and anovulatory problems. PCOS draws much attention because of its considerable prevalence and possible reproductive, cardiovascular, and metabolic associations.[3]

Interestingly, PCOS is inherited as a complex genetic trait.[4] More so, the diversity was apparent in the first narrative by Stein and Leventhal, who delineated seven people with varying phenotypic features (i.e., hirsutism, acne, obesity, and amenorrhea) related to bilateral polycystic ovaries.[5,6]

The disparity in knowledge and absence of agreement gives rise to a lack of correct diagnosis. Failure to diagnose or delayed diagnosis often result in distressful and distrustful patients, while depriving the healthcare system of opportunities for early deterrence, patient education, and intervention.[7] The number of females who are affected by delayed diagnosis or underdiagnosis emphasizes the significance of deterring such an unfortunate circumstance by providing patients with an insight into their complaints and concerns. Studies also reveal that it is not the diagnosis that distresses a patient the most; rather, it is the lack of understanding and anticipation of the associated comorbidities that concern them to a very great degree.

On the other hand, overdiagnosis may incite unnecessary dismay among females who are not actually suffering from the syndrome. It may also encourage an uncalled for anticipation and distress regarding potential consequences of diabetes, infertility, cardiovascular compromise, and obesity.[8] The other point of concern associated with misdiagnosis is having to deal with unnecessary exposure of females to the possible adverse effects of the drugs that are commonly used in the management of PCOS, such as oral contraceptives, metformin, or spironolactone. Lastly, another detrimental result of misdiagnosis is wrongful cataloging of health insurance that could hamper the approach to coverage by health insurance.

The presentation of PCOS at the outset in terms of menstrual irregularity, acne, and polycystic morphology of ovaries may develop during adolescent years. Nevertheless, these manifestations are also distinctive of physiologic pubertal development and may lead to wrong interpretations. Therefore providers should be on the lookout for thoughtful prospects to discourse accompanying diseases as quite often they may be missed.[9]

Understanding of several deep-rooted problems in the interpretation and management of PCOS in the adolescent age group encouraged a pediatric endocrinology international signal to increase the attentiveness to PCOS.[10] It was recognized that there was a need to establish guidance on PCOS in a holistic manner that is spread across the lifespan. Subsequently, an international endeavor involving a number of societies by 71 countries emerged with the International Evidence-Based Guideline for both evaluation and management of PCOS over different stages of life. Multidisciplinary groups for guideline development were designed to analytically approach accessible data and formulate practice recommendations. Thus consequent robust scrutiny inspires evidence-based consistent guidance encompassing the following comprehensive topics in relation to PCOS[11]:

1. Investigations, identification, and appraisal of potential risks during the reproductive age
2. Approaches to addressing the emotional perspectives of the patient for effective management
3. Modifications in standards of living
4. Therapeutic management of issues other than fertility
5. Extensive diagnosis and management plan for fertility issues

These recommendations reiterate the importance of precise identification and the deterrence, screening, diagnosis, and management of the illnesses linked with PCOS (Fig. 1.1).

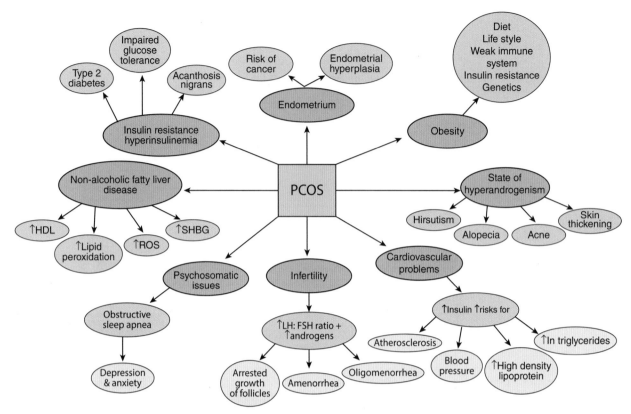

• **Fig. 1.1** An Overview of the Impact of Polycystic Ovary Syndrome. *FSH*, Follicle-stimulating hormone; *HDL*, high density lipoprotein; *LH*, luteinizing hormone; *PCOS*, polycystic ovary syndrome; *ROS*, reactive oxygen species; *SHBG*, sex hormone–binding globulin.

Health Issues of Polycystic Ovary Syndrome

The impact on health can be broadly explained in terms of effects on reproduction, metabolism, and psychosomatic effects on the PCOS patient, as given in Fig. 1.2.[12] The cost associated with PCOS in dealing with the medical and emotional burdens of patients having these comorbidities is substantial.[13] There are many international recommendations available that advocate good medical practice standards and extend detailed information resources not only for health professionals but also for females in general. Having established the significant impact of PCOS on a patient's health, it is crucial to emphasize the diagnosis, clinical presentation, patient education, and deterrence of the complications accompanying these patients across their life cycle.[14]

History of Polycystic Ovary Syndrome

Since the description put forward by Stein and Leventhal in 1935, the definition and diagnosis of PCOS have been in a constant state of evolution. Although considerable progress was made in characterizing the syndrome between the late 1950s and the late 1980s, on the basis of scarcity of consensus in the "diagnostic criteria," significant confusion persisted in defining the syndrome in a holistic manner. In April 1990, a conference was convened at the National Institutes of Health (NIH), which aimed to resolve this ambiguity

through a survey of joining participants. On that occasion, the current definition known as "classic" PCOS came into existence.[5]

In May 2003, European colleagues held a second conference in Rotterdam to redefine and review the definition of PCOS. They further expanded the diagnostic criteria to make the definition all-inclusive.

Lastly, in November 2006, recommendations for diagnosis were published by the Androgen Excess and PCOS Society that principally rooted in the existence of a relationship between the criteria for PCOS and the related health hazards like metabolic instabilities.

A step forward in the understanding of PCOS was when it appeared that PCOS could be divided into four phenotypes based on three main clinical and/or biochemical features:

• Hyperandrogenism
• Chronic anovulation
• Polycystic morphology of ovaries on ultrasound

The realization that the Rotterdam Criteria 2003 and the recommendations of the Androgen Excess Society in 2006 were simply extensions of the NIH 1990 criteria also developed our understanding of the syndrome. Establishing a comprehensive definition of PCOS has helped us recognize the global prevalence of PCOS. Nevertheless, it is crucial to understand that "consensus science" played a critical role in wading through mud and coming up with globally acceptable criteria and definitions of PCOS. There is excessive

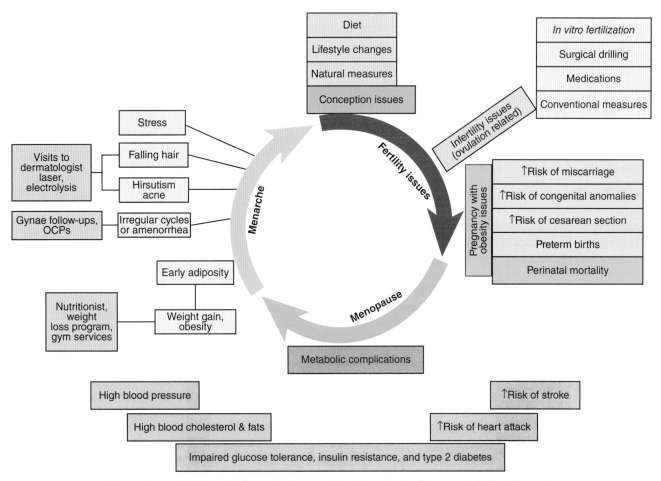

• **Fig. 1.2** Impact of Polycystic Ovary Syndrome. A "health and budget" concern in the health paradigm of a woman (from menarche to menopause).

variability in the clinical presentation and underlying pathophysiology of PCOS; thus scientific dialogue and debate were rightly exercised in understanding the syndrome. Despite having made substantial progress over the past 50 years, there is still a great deal of understanding to be made in diagnosing various phenotypes of PCOS and managing patients who are suffering from the syndrome.

Definition

There has been a great deal of debate over the definition of PCOS. Currently, it is understood as a syndrome that presents with ovarian dysfunction and endocrinopathies with the cardinal features of androgen excess, hyperinsulinemia, and metabolic disease. The joint European Society of Human Reproduction and Embryology (ESHRE)/American Society for Reproductive Health (ASRM) conference that convened in Rotterdam in 2003 submitted that it is a clinical condition that is based on the presence of two out of the three criteria recommended, after having excluded other possible causes of androgen excess and menstrual irregularities[15,16]:

1. Oligo- and/or anovulation manifested as oligo- and/or amenorrhea

2. Clinical or biochemical hyperandrogenism
3. Sonographic evidence of polycystic ovaries

Oligo or anovulation are menstrual cycles of fewer than 21 or more than 35 days, and the morphology of polycystic ovaries is labeled diagnostically significant when there are at least 12 follicles with a diameter between 2 and 9 mm or an inclusive ovarian volume greater than 10 mL. Nevertheless, these diagnostic criteria become irrelevant in adolescents because an overlap exists between puberty-related physiologic changes and the pathologic changes of PCOS.[17]

The Discourse on the Definition of Polycystic Ovary Syndrome

At present, the emergence of new definitions taking into account ovarian morphology, besides chronic anovulation and hyperandrogenism, as a basis of diagnosis has made the phenotypic form of PCOS more varied. The NIH Experts Panel maintains the more inclusive diagnostic criteria of Rotterdam[15] but emphasizes that there is a continuing demand for the documentation of the exact phenotype of all patients suffering from the syndrome. The possible combinations of these standards identify the following phenotypic presentations of PCOS:

1	H-CA	Clinical or biochemical and chronic anovulation
2	H-PCOM	Hyperandrogenism and polycystic ovaries on ultrasound but with ovulatory cycles
3	CA-PCOM	Chronic anovulation and polycystic ovaries on ultrasound without hyperandrogenism
4	H-CA-PCOM	Hyperandrogenism, chronic anovulation, and polycystic ovaries on ultrasound

Prevalence of Polycystic Ovary Syndrome

PCOS affects females of premenopausal ages, and often the age of onset has been found to be perimenarchal. Nevertheless, there is often a delay in the recognition of the clinical signs of the syndrome because the irregularity of menstruation, hirsutism, and other such symptoms can be missed by patients because of an overlap between the findings associated with PCOS and physiologic maturation 2 years after menarche. Lean females who have a genetic predilection to PCOS may manifest the syndrome when they gain weight subsequently.[18]

The occurrence differs among different countries. The prevalence of PCOS in the United States is between 4% and 12% among reproductive age females.[19] Some studies conducted in Europe show a different prevalence of PCOS, such as between 6.5% and 8%.[20] Iran and China observed a prevalence of 3% and 2.2%, respectively. A prevalence ranging between 5% and 10% was found in countries such as Brazil, Sri Lanka, Beijing, Palestine, the UK, Greece, and Spain. High incidence was reported in Denmark, Turkey, and Australia (15%–20%).[21] A study was conducted in 2017 in Bhopal, India. It observed the prevalence of PCOS in 500 college-going girls aged between 17 and 24 and published a prevalence rate of 8.2.[22] A high prevalence of PCOS, 28.9% according to NIH criteria and 34.3% by AE-PCOS criteria, was reported in Kashmiri females, which is likely the maximum broadcasted globally.[23]

The variability that has been often observed in the prevalence of PCOS is a multifactorial phenomenon. First, the location of data collection can impart a great deal of heterogeneity in the ethnic, racial, and age distribution of the selected population. These factors may influence the presentation of androgen excess and the sonographic appearance of ovarian follicles gradually. In many cases worldwide, females do not receive a formal diagnosis of PCOS or if/when they do, it may take several different doctors and years before a formal diagnosis is established. This may be because of a lack of educational material provided at the correct level for healthcare providers and individuals. It could also be attributable to the lack of awareness.

References

1. Azziz R, Carmina E, Dewailly D, et al. The Androgen Excess and PCOS Society criteria for the polycystic ovary syndrome: the complete task force report. *Fertil Steril*. 2009;91(2):456-488. Available at: https://doi.org/10.1016/j.fertnstert.2008.06.035.

2. Franks S. Diagnosis of polycystic ovarian syndrome: in defense of the Rotterdam criteria. *J Clin Endocrinol Metab*. 2006;91(3):786-789. Available at: https://doi.org/10.1210/jc.2005-2501.

3. Wild S, Pierpoint T, McKeigue P, Jacobs H. Cardiovascular disease in women with polycystic ovary syndrome at long-term follow-up: a retrospective cohort study. *Clin Endocrinol*. 2000;52(5):595-600.

4. Legro RS. The genetics of obesity Lessons for polycystic ovary syndrome. *Ann N Y Acad Sci*. 2000;l900(1):193-202.

5. Azziz R. How polycystic ovary syndrome came into its own. *F S Sci*. 2021;2(1):2-10. Available at: https://doi.org/10.1016/j.xfss.2020.12.007.

6. Stein IF, Leventhal ML. Amenorrhea associated with bilateral polycystic ovaries. *Am J Obstet Gynecol*. 1935;29(2):181-191. Available at: https://doi.org/10.1016/S0002-9378(15)30642-6.

7. Gibson-Helm M, Teede H, Dunaif A, Dokras A. Delayed diagnosis and a lack of information associated with dissatisfaction in women with polycystic ovary syndrome. *J Clin Endocrinol Metab*. 2017;102(2):604-612. Available at: https://doi.org/10.1210/jc.2016-2963.

8. Rowlands IJ, Teede H, Lucke J, Dobson AJ, Mishra GD. Young women's psychological distress after a diagnosis of polycystic ovary syndrome or endometriosis. *Hum Reprod*. 2016;31(9):2072-2081. Available at: https://doi.org/10.1093/humrep/dew174.

9. Dokras A, Witchel SF. Are young adult women with polycystic ovary syndrome slipping through the healthcare cracks? *J Clin Endocrinol Metab*. 2014;99(5):1583-1585. Available at: https://doi.org/10.1210/jc.2013-4190.

10. Ibáñez L, Oberfield SE, Witchel S, et al. An international consortium update: pathophysiology, diagnosis, and treatment of polycystic ovarian syndrome in adolescence. *Horm Res Paediatr*. 2017;88(6):371-395. Available at: https://doi.org/10.1159/000479371.

11. Teede HJ, Misso ML, Costello MF, et al. Recommendations from the international evidence-based guideline for the assessment and management of polycystic ovary syndrome. *Hum Reprod*. 2018;33(9):1602-1618. Available at: https://doi.org/10.1093/humrep/dey256.

12. Cooney LG, Lee I, Sammel MD, Dokras A. High prevalence of moderate and severe depressive and anxiety symptoms in polycystic ovary syndrome: a systematic review and meta-analysis. *Hum Reprod*. 2017;32(5):1075-1091. Available at: https://doi.org/10.1093/humrep/dex044.

13. Ding T, Hardiman PJ, Petersen I, Baio G. Incidence and prevalence of diabetes and cost of illness analysis of polycystic ovary syndrome: a Bayesian modelling study. *Hum Reprod*. 2018;33(7):1299-1306. Available at: https://doi.org/10.1093/humrep/dey093.

14. Gilbert EW, Tay CT, Hiam DS, Teede HJ, Moran LJ. Comorbidities and complications of polycystic ovary syndrome: an overview of systematic reviews. *Clin Endocrinol (Oxf)*. 2018;89(6):683-699. Available at: https://doi.org/10.1111/cen.13828.

15. Rotterdam ESHRE/ASRM-Sponsored PCOS Consensus Workshop Group. Revised 2003 consensus on diagnostic criteria and long-term health risks related to polycystic ovary syndrome (PCOS). *Hum Reprod*. 2004;19(1):41-47. Available at: https://doi.org/10.1093/humrep/deh098.

16. Varanasi LC, Subasinghe A, Jayasinghe YL, et al. Polycystic ovarian syndrome: prevalence and impact on the wellbeing of Australian women aged 16-29 years. *Aust N Z J Obstet Gynaecol*. 2018;58(2):222-233. Available at: https://doi.org/10.1111/ajo.12730.

17. Fauser BC, Tarlatzis BC, Rebar RW, et al. Consensus on women's health aspects of polycystic ovary syndrome (PCOS): the Amsterdam ESHRE/ASRM-Sponsored 3rd PCOS Consensus Workshop Group. *Fertil Steril.* 2012;97(1):28-38.e25. Available at: https://doi.org/10.1016/j.fertnstert.2011.09.024.

18. Barber TM, Hanson P, Weickert MO, Franks S. Obesity and polycystic ovary syndrome: implications for pathogenesis and novel management strategies. *Clin Med Insights Reprod Health.* 2019;13:1179558119874042. Available at: https://doi.org/10.1177/1179558119874042.

19. Azziz R, Woods KS, Reyna R, Key TJ, Knochenhauer ES, Yildiz BO. The prevalence and features of the polycystic ovary syndrome in an unselected population. *J Clin Endocrinol Metab.* 2004;89(6):2745-2749. Available at: https://doi.org/10.1210/jc.2003-032046.

20. Asunción M, Calvo RM, San Millán JL, Sancho J, Avila S, Escobar-Morreale HCF. A prospective study of the prevalence of the polycystic ovary syndrome in unselected Caucasian women from Spain. *J Clin Endocrinol Metab.* 2000;85(7):2434-2438. Available at: https://doi.org/10.1210/jcem.85.7.6682.

21. Ding T, Hardiman PJ, Petersen I, Wang FF, Qu F, Baio G. The prevalence of polycystic ovary syndrome in reproductive-aged women of different ethnicity: a systematic review and meta-analysis. *Oncotarget.* 2017;8(56):96351-96358. Available at: https://doi.org/10.18632/oncotarget.19180.

22. Gupta M, Singh D, Toppo M, Priya A, Sethia S, Gupta P. A cross sectional study of polycystic ovarian syndrome among young women in Bhopal, Central India. *Int J Community Med Public Health.* 2018;5(1):95-100.

23. Ganie MA, Rashid A, Sahu D, Nisar S, Wani IA, Khan J. Prevalence of polycystic ovary syndrome (PCOS) among reproductive age women from Kashmir valley: a cross-sectional study. *Int J Gynecol Obstet.* 2020;149(2):231-236. Available at: https://doi.org/10.1002/ijgo.13125.

2

Polycystic Ovary Syndrome Phenotypes

UNAB I. KHAN AND RUBIA FARID

Introduction

Polycystic ovary syndrome (PCOS) remains the most common endocrinopathy, affecting 5% to 8% of females of reproductive age.[1] The pathophysiology of PCOS is multifactorial and polygenic. In addition, lifestyle-influenced epigenetic alterations[2] at the ovarian level leading to disturbances in folliculogenesis and ovulatory dysfunction[3,4] and at the adipose tissue level leading to insulin resistance[5] also play a role in the pathogenesis.

The clinical manifestations of PCOS are also a collection of diverse metabolic and reproductive abnormalities. Although ovarian dysfunction, hyperandrogenism, and polycystic ovarian morphology remain key characteristics, insulin resistance and hyperinsulinism manifesting as overweight and increased abdominal adiposity are linked to the adverse long-term cardiometabolic outcomes such as development of type 2 diabetes mellitus (DM), hypertension, dyslipidemia, and cardiovascular disease.[6] This diversity in clinical presentations makes it challenging to define unequivocal criteria for the diagnosis of PCOS, leading to inconsistencies not only in assessment and management but also in epidemiologic and clinical research.

In this chapter, we will discuss how diverse clinical manifestations have been incorporated in the diagnostic criteria, with the evolution toward a phenotypic definition. We will then discuss the important differences among PCOS phenotypes, the recognition of which can not only allow for more effective clinical care and improved health outcomes but also provide a standardized platform for global research.

Ethnic Variations in PCOS Prevalence and Clinical Presentation

Regardless of the definition used, the prevalence of PCOS varies widely with ethnicity.[7,8] Although prospective studies from Europe and the United States report a prevalence of 4% to 8% in females of reproductive age,[9-11] a cross-sectional study in Pakistan estimates a prevalence of 20% in females presenting for infertility treatments.[12] In addition, the prevalence is higher among females from underdeveloped countries who have immigrated to developed countries. The prevalence in Mexican American females is estimated at 13%;[13] and a study in UK reported a prevalence of 52% in South Asian females compared with 20% in white females.[14]

Clinical presentation also varies by race and ethnicity with differences in the frequency of hirsutism, acne, polycystic-appearing ovaries, obesity, and insulin resistance.[15] South Asians have a higher prevalence of metabolic syndrome and a high risk of type 2 DM,[16] whereas menstrual irregularity and polycystic ovaries without hyperandrogenism are more prevalent among Korean patients.[16]

Understanding the diverse clinical presentations will not only allow for more accurate estimation of the health impacts of the disorder but also shed light on the underlying environmental or ethnic factors that may affect the prevalence, severity, and complications of PCOS.[17]

Evolution of Diagnostic Criteria

The diagnostic criteria for PCOS have evolved since it was first described as "Stein-Leventhal syndrome" in 1935. Irving Stein and Michael Leventhal described the syndrome as "characterized by secondary amenorrhea, sterility, bilateral polycystic ovaries and hirsutism occurring in young women in the second or third decades of life."[18] Clinicians and scientists started reporting variances in patient characteristics almost immediately after the defined criteria were introduced.[19-21] Since then, diagnostic criteria have been revised based on scientific progress, such as the ability to quantify hormone levels,[22] and use of ultrasounds for noninvasive examination of ovarian morphology.[23] Regardless of the definition used, the key features of PCOS include (1) ovulatory dysfunction; (2) biochemical/clinical hyperandrogenism; and (3) polycystic ovaries.[24]

The 1990 National Institutes of Health (NIH) criteria characterized PCOS as a disorder of hyperandrogenemia and required the presence of both oligo- or anovulation

(ANOV) and biochemical or clinical manifestation of hyperandrogenism (HA), in the absence of known endocrinologic disorders.

In 2003, an expert conference convened in Rotterdam by the European Society for Human Reproduction and Embryology (ESHRE) and the American Society for Reproductive Medicine (ASRM) recommended that the definition include presence of polycystic ovaries (PCO) as the third criteria. Hence, according to the 2003 Rotterdam criteria, PCOS is diagnosed when at least two of the three criteria (ANOV, HA, and PCO) are present in the absence of other endocrinologic abnormalities that could explain the hyperandrogenism.[25] This broadening of diagnostic criteria led to many more phenotypes being added to the syndrome, thus increasing the prevalence of PCOS globally.

In 2006 a systematic review by a task force of the Androgen Excess and PCOS Society (AE-PCOS) pooled available evidence on the epidemiologic and phenotypic manifestations of PCOS. The task force concluded that hyperandrogenism (with its various clinical manifestations) remains the central abnormality in patients with PCOS and the diagnosis should not be established without clinical or biochemical evidence of such; and that HA in the presence of either polycystic ovarian morphology and/or ovulatory dysfunction (and its various manifestations, including menstrual irregularity) should be considered as diagnostic. Based on various combinations of these features, the task force identified nine phenotypes that could be considered as PCOS but also recognized that the phenotypic presentation may change even in the same patient based on changes in weight and throughout the life course.[26]

Most recently, in 2012, the NIH conducted an evidence-based methodology workshop on PCOS, where experts discussed not only the benefits and drawbacks of the different diagnostic criteria but also optimal prevention and treatment strategies and made recommendations on future research priorities.[27] The panel recognized that the use of different criteria compromises clinical care and research progress. The task force recommended the continued usage of the Rotterdam criteria but advised to also *add a phenotype classification* to allow clinicians to understand the impact of the syndrome based on the severity of clinical manifestations, associated comorbidities, and reproductive health considerations and the overall effect on the quality of life of a patient.[27]

The Four Phenotypes

The four phenotypes include:

1. Type A (Classic phenotype/frank PCOS), which is characterized by high androgen levels/hyperandrogenism, irregular periods/delayed ovulation, and polycystic ovaries (HA + OD + PCO).
2. Type B (Non-PCO phenotype), which is characterized by high androgen levels/hyperandrogenism, irregular periods/ delayed ovulation, and normal ovaries (HA + OD).
3. Type C (Ovulatory phenotype), which is characterized by high androgen levels/androgenism, regular periods

(35 days or shorter cycles)/ovulation, and polycystic ovaries (HA + PCO).
4. Type D (Nonhyperandrogenic phenotype), which is considered a milder form and is characterized by normal androgens, irregular periods/delayed ovulation, and polycystic ovaries (OD + PCO).

We will discuss the clinical characteristics and the associated abnormalities of the phenotypes.

Phenotypes A and B

In patients with PCOS, phenotypes A and B are more common, with reported prevalence of 50% to 68% and 8% to 11%, respectively.[28,29] Most patients present with classic symptoms of menstrual irregularity, subfertility, and infertility,[29-32] and clinical manifestations of hyperandrogenism, including hirsutism.[33-35] Although females with phenotype A are considered to be at the highest risk of developing adverse cardiometabolic outcomes, hyperandrogenism in the absence of ovulatory disturbances, as seen in phenotype B, can also contribute to an adverse metabolic profile and insulin resistance (IR). Preadipocytes have androgen receptors, and adipose cell function is regulated by androgens at a mechanistic level. Thus hyperandrogenism increases abdominal obesity, which, in turn, increases IR.[36] Increased androgens have also been shown to induce selective IR in cultured adipocytes.[37] Thus both patients with phenotypes A and B are reported to have higher rates of obesity,[38] IR,[34,38,39] dyslipidemia,[34,40] hepatic steatosis,[41,42] and an increased probability for metabolic syndrome.[42,43] These changes put them at a higher risk for adverse metabolic and potentially cardiovascular outcomes.[44,45]

Phenotype C

Females with ovulatory PCOS present with hyperandrogenism and polycystic ovaries but do not have ovulatory dysfunction. They constitute approximately 20% to 30% of PCOS patients.[28,29] Compared with patients with phenotypes A and B, those with ovulatory PCOS not only have intermediate abnormalities in androgen levels but also have lower body mass index (BMI) and associated hyperinsulinism and IR.[28] Nevertheless, research suggests that the reduced IR in ovulatory PCOS is largely a function of reduced abdominal adiposity. Compared with BMI-matched females with type A or B PCOS, females with type C PCOS were found to have higher abdominal fat and higher IR and lower adiponectin levels.[46] Moreover, when matched for BMI and abdominal adiposity, females with phenotype C have the same adverse cardiometabolic risk profile as phenotypes A and B.[47]

Phenotype D

Females with nonhyperandrogenic PCOS constitute approximately 3% to 5% of females with PCOS.[29] They present with irregular menstrual cycles, and the ovulatory dysfunction is associated with polycystic ovaries. They are characterized by increased luteinizing hormone (LH) and LH to follicle-stimulating hormone (FSH) ratio but have minimal increases in testosterone and other androgens.[28] Nevertheless, compared with females without PCOS, females with phenotype D are reported to have higher androgen levels,[33,35] and this can affect their BMI,[47] worsen lipid profiles, and increase IR.[48] Compared with females with phenotypes A and B, however, they have an intermediate or milder metabolic risk profile,[49] lower levels of total and abdominal adiposity, and a lower prevalence of metabolic syndrome.[28,42]

One possibility is that the severity of hyperandrogenism varies in females with PCOS, and although hyperandrogenism drives PCOS in the majority of phenotypes (A, B, and C), in those with a mild abnormality in androgens (phenotype D or nonhyperandrogenic PCOS), a greater contribution of inherent or environmentally induced abdominal-obesity-related IR may be required to induce reproductive and ovarian dysfunction.[36]

Insulin Resistance in PCOS Phenotypes

The role of insulin in ovarian function was first suggested by Burghen et al. who observed that hyperinsulinemia is associated with hyperandrogenaemia.[50] IR is intrinsic to the pathogenesis of PCOS, regardless of the degree of obesity.[51-53] About 50% to 80% of patients with PCOS are reported to have IR.[34] High levels of insulin work synergistically with LH to increase androgen production of theca cells, which lead to lipid abnormalities.[54,55] In addition, elevated insulin level inhibits hepatic synthesis of sex hormone–binding globulin, leading to an increased amount of unbound or free testosterone,[52] thus playing both a direct and indirect role in the pathogenesis of PCOS.

Females with classic phenotypes (A and B) are more insulin resistant than those with either the ovulatory (phenotype C) or normoandrogenic phenotype (phenotype D).[28,56,57] In addition, overweight/obese patients with phenotype A have higher circulating androgens than those with phenotype B. Interestingly, overweight/obese patients with phenotype D also show IR regardless of the absence of hyperandrogenism.[17,42,43,56]

Differences in Risk of Metabolic Complications and Cardiovascular Disease Among Phenotypes

In females with PCOS, androgen excess is directly related to the increased incidence of metabolic syndrome and coronary artery disease.[58] Females with PCOS have an 11-fold higher risk of developing metabolic syndrome compared with their age-matched counterparts.[59-61] Using the phenotypic definitions allows us to distinguish which phenotypes are at a higher cardiometabolic risk and have a higher likelihood of developing diabetes, dyslipidemia, and cardiovascular disease. Studies show that females with phenotypes A, B, and C have a six- to eightfold increased risk of metabolic syndrome compared with females without PCOS.[62] Thus females with these phenotypes should not only be treated for reproductive complaints but must also

be screened and treated for cardiometabolic abnormalities at regular intervals.

High BMI[63] and intensity of menstrual irregularity[64] are other independent predictors of metabolic dysfunction in females with PCOS. Polycystic ovaries alone are not associated with metabolic abnormalities.[65]

Differences in Impact on Fertility

PCOS can affect fertility in several ways. Ovulatory dysfunction because of an increase in testosterone production and immaturity of ovarian follicles are common causes. In ovulatory cycles, hormonal imbalance may prevent the lining of the uterus from developing properly to allow for implantation. Unpredictable menstrual cycles can also make it difficult to plan a pregnancy. Evidence-based guidelines are now available for the assessment and management of infertility in patients with PCOS.[66] Nevertheless, these do not take phenotypic classification into account. There are still few studies that have examined the prevalence of infertility in different PCOS phenotypes and the impact of treatment modalities. Females with phenotype A are reported to have higher resistance to clomiphene compared with other phenotypes.[29]

Therapeutic Approach Based on Phenotypes

Treatment of PCOS and its related clinical manifestations needs to begin after the correct identification of phenotype. Goals for treatment are based on a shared-care approach ensuring that the patient's preference are addressed (e.g., treating infertility; regulating menses for endometrial protection; controlling hyperandrogenic features such as hirsutism and acne). At the same time, a clinician's goal is to screen and monitor and mitigate the risk for development of known cardiometabolic outcomes.

The therapeutic approach can be summarized as follows:
- Lifestyle modifications are helpful for all females with PCOS, especially for those who are overweight or obese. Patients with phenotypes A and B, who are at a higher risk for developing adverse cardiometabolic outcomes, require screening and regular monitoring of blood pressure, lipids, and blood glucose levels. In addition, patients with phenotype D are known to benefit from weight loss with improvement in menstrual irregularity, regardless of a change in androgen levels.
- For menstrual irregularity, seen in phenotypes A, B, and D, use of oral contraceptives and insulin sensitizers such as metformin can help.
- For reproductive concerns, including subfertility and infertility, using insulin sensitizers, clomiphene citrate, letrozole, gonadotropins, and laparoscopic ovarian drilling have been tested.
- Clinical manifestations of hyperandrogenism, such as hirsutism and acne, are noted in phenotypes A, B, and C and are amenable to treatment with oral contraceptives, antiandrogens, cosmetic procedures, eflornithine hydrochloride, and GnRH-agonists.

Clinical phenotypes can overlap or change over the lifespan, starting from adolescence to postmenopause, largely influenced by obesity and metabolic alterations and ethnic background.[67,68] Nevertheless, using the phenotypic approach has several practical implications in patients with PCOS. In clinical practice, females at the highest risk of long-term adverse cardiometabolic outcomes can be identified early (phenotypes A and B) and screening protocols for screening and treatment can be put in place. Similarly, those with phenotype D benefit from weight loss to help with menstrual irregularities.

As our understanding of PCOS continues to evolve, the phenotypic classification will allow research to focus on pathogenesis, treatment, and adverse events related to each subgroup and lead to more personalized care.

References

1. Azziz R, Woods KS, Reyna R, Key TJ, Knochenhauer ES, Yildiz BO. The prevalence and features of the polycystic ovary syndrome in an unselected population. *J Clin Endocrinol Metab.* 2004;89(6):2745-2749.
2. Shen HR, Qiu LH, Zhang ZQ, Qin YY, Cao C, Di W. Genomewide methylated DNA immunoprecipitation analysis of patients with polycystic ovary syndrome. *PLoS One.* 2013;8(5):e64801.
3. Diamanti-Kandarakis E. Polycystic ovarian syndrome: pathophysiology, molecular aspects and clinical implications. *Expert Rev Mol Med.* 2008;10:e3.
4. Ilie IR, Georgescu CE. Polycystic ovary syndrome-epigenetic mechanisms and aberrant microRNA. *Adv Clin Chem.* 2015;71:25-45.
5. Kokosar M, Benrick A, Perfilyev A, et al. Erratum: epigenetic and transcriptional alterations in human adipose tissue of polycystic ovary syndrome. *Sci Rep.* 2016;6:25321.
6. Haffner SM, D'Agostino R, Festa A, et al. Low insulin sensitivity (Si= 0) in diabetic and nondiabetic subjects in the insulin resistance atherosclerosis study: is it associated with components of the metabolic syndrome and nontraditional risk factors? *Diabetes Care.* 2003;26(10):2796-2803.
7. Li L, Yang D, Chen X, Chen Y, Feng S, Wang L. Clinical and metabolic features of polycystic ovary syndrome. *Int J Gynecol Obstet.* 2007;97(2):129-134.
8. Allahbadia GN, Merchant R. Polycystic ovary syndrome in the Indian Subcontinent. *Semin Reprod Med.* 2008;26(1):22-34.
9. Moran C, Tena G, Moran S, Ruiz P, Reyna R, Duque X. Prevalence of polycystic ovary syndrome and related disorders in Mexican women. *Gynecol Obstet Invest.* 2010;69(4):274-280.
10. Diamanti-Kandarakis E, Kouli CR, Bergiele AT, et al. A survey of the polycystic ovary syndrome in the Greek island of Lesbos: hormonal and metabolic profile. *J Clin Endocrinol Metab.* 1999;84(11):4006-4011.
11. Azziz R, Woods KS, Reyna R, Key TJ, Knochenhauer ES, Yildiz BO. The prevalence and features of the polycystic ovary syndrome in an unselected population. *J Clin Endocrinol Metab.* 2004;89(6):2745-2749.
12. Baqai Z, Khanam M, Parveen S. Prevalence of PCOS in infertile patients. *Med Channel.* 2010;16(3):437–440.
13. Goodarzi MO, Quiñones MJ, Azziz R, Rotter JI, Hsueh WA, Yang H. Polycystic ovary syndrome in Mexican-Americans: prevalence and association with the severity of insulin resistance. *Fertil Steril.* 2005;84(3):766-769.
14. Mirza SS, Shafique K, Shaikh AR, Khan NA, Qureshi MA. Association between circulating adiponectin levels and polycystic ovarian syndrome. *J Ovarian Res.* 2014;7(1):1-7.
15. Zhao Y, Qiao J. Ethnic differences in the phenotypic expression of polycystic ovary syndrome. *Steroids.* 2013;78(8):755-760.
16. Wang S, Alvero R, eds. *Racial and Ethnic Differences in Physiology and Clinical Symptoms of Polycystic Ovary Syndrome. Seminars in Reproductive Medicine.* New York, NY. USA: Thieme Medical Publishers; 2013.
17. Amato MC, Verghi M, Galluzzo A, Giordano C. The oligomenorrhoic phenotypes of polycystic ovary syndrome are characterized by a high visceral adiposity index: a likely condition of cardiometabolic risk. *Hum Reprod.* 2011;26(6):1486-1494.
18. Stein E, Leventhal ML. Polycystic ovary syndrome. *Am J Obstet Gynecol.* 1935;29:181.
19. Leventhal ML. Amenorrhea and sterility caused by bilateral polycystic ovaries. *Am J Obstet Gynecol.* 1941;41(3):516-517.
20. Hofmeister FJ, Byce KR. Clinical aspects of the Stein-Leventhal syndrome. *Obstet Gynecol.* 1966;28(2):264-267.
21. Ibrahim MS, Zaki S, Girgis S. The diagnostic problem of the Stein-Leventhal syndrome. A review of the literature and report on 9 cases. *J Egypt Med Assoc.* 1966;49(9):629-638.
22. Raj SG, Thompson I, Berger M, Talert L, Taymor M. Diagnostic value of androgen measurements in polycystic ovary syndrome. *Obstet Gynecol.* 1978;52(2):169-171.
23. Adams J, Polson D, Franks S. Prevalence of polycystic ovaries in women with anovulation and idiopathic hirsutism. *Br Med J (Clin Res Ed).* 1986;293(6543):355-359.
24. Azziz R, Carmina E, Dewailly D, et al. The Androgen Excess and PCOS Society criteria for the polycystic ovary syndrome: the complete task force report. *Fertil Steril.* 2009;91(2):456-488.
25. ESHRE TR, Group A-SPCW. Revised 2003 consensus on diagnostic criteria and long-term health risks related to polycystic ovary syndrome. *Fertil Steril.* 2004;81(1):19-25.
26. Azziz R, Carmina E, Dewailly D, et al. Criteria for defining polycystic ovary syndrome as a predominantly hyperandrogenic syndrome: an androgen excess society guideline. *J Clin Endocrinol Metab.* 2006;91(11):4237-4245.
27. Johnson T, Kaplan L, Ouyang P, Rizza R. Final Report: Evidence-based Methodology Workshop on Polycystic Ovary Syndrome. https://prevention.nih.gov/workshops/2012/pcos/docs/PCOS_Final_Statement.pdf. National Institute of Health. December 3-5, 2012.
28. Guastella E, Longo RA, Carmina E. Clinical and endocrine characteristics of the main polycystic ovary syndrome phenotypes. *Fertil Steril.* 2010;94(6):2197-2201.
29. Sachdeva G, Gainder S, Suri V, Sachdeva N, Chopra S. Comparison of the different PCOS phenotypes based on clinical metabolic, and hormonal profile, and their response to clomiphene. *Indian J Endocrinol Metab.* 2019;23(3):326.
30. Jamil AS, Alalaf SK, Al-Tawil NG, Al-Shawaf T. Comparison of clinical and hormonal characteristics among four phenotypes of polycystic ovary syndrome based on the Rotterdam criteria. *Arch Gynecol Obstet.* 2016;293(2):447-456.
31. Romualdi D, Di Florio C, Tagliaferri V, et al. The role of anti-Müllerian hormone in the characterization of the different polycystic ovary syndrome phenotypes. *Reprod Sci.* 2016;23(5):655-661.
32. Sahmay S, Atakul N, Oncul M, Tuten A, Aydogan B, Seyisoglu H. Serum anti-Mullerian hormone levels in the main phenotypes of polycystic ovary syndrome. *Eur J Obstet Gynecol Reprod Biol.* 2013;170(1):157-161.

33. Hsu MI, Liou TH, Chou SY, Chang CY, Hsu CS. Diagnostic criteria for polycystic ovary syndrome in Taiwanese Chinese women: comparison between Rotterdam 2003 and NIH 1990. *Fertil Steril.* 2007;88(3):727-729.

34. Kim JJ, Hwang KR, Choi YM, et al. Complete phenotypic and metabolic profiles of a large consecutive cohort of untreated Korean women with polycystic ovary syndrome. *Fertil Steril.* 2014;101(5):1424-1430.e3.

35. Welt C, Gudmundsson J, Arason G, et al. Characterizing discrete subsets of polycystic ovary syndrome as defined by the Rotterdam criteria: the impact of weight on phenotype and metabolic features. *J Clin Endocrinol Metab.* 2006;91(12):4842-4848.

36. Escobar-Morreale HF, San Millán JL. Abdominal adiposity and the polycystic ovary syndrome. *Trends Endocrinol Metab.* 2007;18(7):266-272.

37. Corbould A, Dunaif A. The adipose cell lineage is not intrinsically insulin resistant in polycystic ovary syndrome. *Metabolism.* 2007;56(5):716-722.

38. Moran L, Teede H, Moran L, Teede H. Metabolic features of the reproductive phenotypes of polycystic ovary syndrome. *Hum Reprod Update.* 2009;15(4):477-488.

39. Diamanti-Kandarakis E, Panidis D. Unravelling the phenotypic map of polycystic ovary syndrome (PCOS): a prospective study of 634 women with PCOS. *Clin Endocrinol.* 2007;67(5):735-742.

40. Carmina E, Orio F, Palomba S, et al. Endothelial dysfunction in PCOS: role of obesity and adipose hormones. *Am J Med.* 2006;119(4):356.e1-356.e6.

41. Jones H, Sprung VS, Pugh CJ, et al. Polycystic ovary syndrome with hyperandrogenism is characterized by an increased risk of hepatic steatosis compared to nonhyperandrogenic PCOS phenotypes and healthy controls, independent of obesity and insulin resistance. *J Clin Endocrinol Metab.* 2012;97(10):3709-3716.

42. Goverde A, Van Koert A, Eijkemans M, et al. Indicators for metabolic disturbances in anovulatory women with polycystic ovary syndrome diagnosed according to the Rotterdam consensus criteria. *Hum Reprod.* 2009;24(3):710-717.

43. Mehrabian F, Khani B, Kelishadi R, Kermani N. The prevalence of metabolic syndrome and insulin resistance according to the phenotypic subgroups of polycystic ovary syndrome in a representative sample of Iranian females. *J Res Med Sci.* 2011;16(6):763.

44. Pehlivanov B, Orbetzova M. Characteristics of different phenotypes of polycystic ovary syndrome in a Bulgarian population. *Gynecol Endocrinol.* 2007;23(10):604-609.

45. Moran L, Teede H. Metabolic features of the reproductive phenotypes of polycystic ovary syndrome. *Hum Reprod Update.* 2009;15(4):477-488.

46. Carmina E, Bucchieri S, Mansueto P, Rini G, Ferin M, Lobo RA. Circulating levels of adipose products and differences in fat distribution in the ovulatory and anovulatory phenotypes of polycystic ovary syndrome. *Fertil Steril.* 2009;91(4):1332-1335.

47. Dewailly D, Catteau-Jonard S, Reyss AC, Leroy M, Pigny P. Oligoanovulation with polycystic ovaries but not overt hyperandrogenism. *J Clin Endocrinol Metab.* 2006;91(10):3922-3927.

48. Norman RJ, Masters SC, Hague W, Beng C, Pannall P, Wang JX. Metabolic approaches to the subclassification of polycystic ovary syndrome. *Fertil Steril.* 1995;63(2):329-335.

49. Dilbaz B, Özkaya E, Cinar M, Cakir E, Dilbaz S. Cardiovascular disease risk characteristics of the main polycystic ovary syndrome phenotypes. *Endocrine.* 2011;39(3):272-277.

50. Burghen GA, Givens JR, Kitabchi AE. Correlation of hyperandrogenism with hyperinsulinism in polycystic ovarian disease. *J Clin Endocrinol Metab.* 1980;50(1):113-116.

51. Stepto NK, Cassar S, Joham AE, et al. Women with polycystic ovary syndrome have intrinsic insulin resistance on euglycaemic–hyperinsulinaemic clamp. *Hum Reprod.* 2013;28(3):777-784.

52. Diamanti-Kandarakis E, Dunaif A. Insulin resistance and the polycystic ovary syndrome revisited: an update on mechanisms and implications. *Endocr Rev.* 2012;33(6):981-1030.

53. Dunaif A. Drug insight: insulin-sensitizing drugs in the treatment of polycystic ovary syndrome-a reappraisal. *Nat Clin Pract Endocrinol Metab.* 2008;4(5):272-283.

54. Nestler JE, Jakubowicz DJ, Falcon de Vargas A, Brik C, Quintero N, Medina F. Insulin stimulates testosterone biosynthesis by human thecal cells from women with polycystic ovary syndrome by activating its own receptor and using inositolglycan mediators as the signal transduction system. *J Clin Endocrinol Metab.* 1998;83(6):2001-2005.

55. Poretsky L, Smith D, Seibel M, Pazianos A, Moses A, Flier J. Specific insulin binding sites in human ovary. *J Clin Endocrinol Metab.* 1984;59(4):809-811.

56. Yilmaz M, Isaoglu U, Delibas IB, Kadanali S. Anthropometric, clinical and laboratory comparison of four phenotypes of polycystic ovary syndrome based on Rotterdam criteria. *J Obstet Gynaecol Res.* 2011;37(8):1020-1026.

57. Shroff R, Syrop CH, Davis W, Van Voorhis BJ, Dokras A. Risk of metabolic complications in the new PCOS phenotypes based on the Rotterdam criteria. *Fertil Steril.* 2007;88(5):1389-1395.

58. March WA, Moore VM, Willson KJ, Phillips DI, Norman RJ, Davies MJ. The prevalence of polycystic ovary syndrome in a community sample assessed under contrasting diagnostic criteria. *Hum Reprod.* 2010;25(2):544-551.

59. Rizzo M, Longo R, Guastella E, Rini G, Carmina E. Assessing cardiovascular risk in Mediterranean women with polycystic ovary syndrome. *J Endocrinol Invest.* 2011;34(6):422-426.

60. Orio Jr F, Palomba S, Spinelli L, et al. The cardiovascular risk of young women with polycystic ovary syndrome: an observational, analytical, prospective case-control study. *J Clin Endocrinol Metab.* 2004;89(8):3696-3701.

61. Wild RA, Painter P, Coulson PB, Carruth KB, Ranney G. Lipoprotein lipid concentrations and cardiovascular risk in women with polycystic ovary syndrome. *J Clin Endocrinol Metab.* 1985;61(5):946-951.

62. Shroff R, Syrop CH, Davis W, Van Voorhis BJ, Dokras A. Risk of metabolic complications in the new PCOS phenotypes based on the Rotterdam criteria. *Fertil Steril.* 2007;88(5):1389-1395.

63. Ehrmann DA, Liljenquist DR, Kasza K, et al. Prevalence and predictors of the metabolic syndrome in women with polycystic ovary syndrome. *J Clin Endocrinol Metab.* 2006;91(1):48-53.

64. Brower M, Brennan K, Pall M, Azziz R. The severity of menstrual dysfunction as a predictor of insulin resistance in PCOS. *J Clin Endocrinol Metab.* 2013;98(12):E1967-E1971.

65. Legro RS, Chiu P, Kunselman AR, Bentley CM, Dodson WC, Dunaif A. Polycystic ovaries are common in women with hyperandrogenic chronic anovulation but do not predict metabolic or reproductive phenotype. *J Clin Endocrinol Metab.* 2005;90(5):2571-2579.

66. Costello M, Misso M, Balen A, et al. Evidence summaries and recommendations from the international evidence-based guideline for the assessment and management of polycystic ovary syndrome: assessment and treatment of infertility. *Human Reprod Open.* 2019;2019(1):hoy021.

67. Moran C, Arriaga M, Rodriguez G, Moran S. Obesity differentially affects phenotypes of polycystic ovary syndrome. *Int J Endocrinol.* 2012;2012:317241.

68. Papadakis G, Kandaraki EA, Garidou A, et al. Tailoring treatment for PCOS phenotypes. *Expert Rev Endocrinol Metab.* 2021;16(1):9-18.

3
Polycystic Ovary Syndrome in Adolescents

KHADIJA NUZHAT HUMAYUN, MUZNA ARIF, AND FOZIA MEMON

Introduction

Polycystic ovary syndrome (PCOS) is a vastly prevalent disorder in females. It is a heterogeneous condition that characteristically presents with a combination of menstrual irregularity, hyperandrogenism, and polycystic ovarian morphology.[1] Making a diagnosis of PCOS is difficult in adolescents.[2] Although early diagnosis of PCOS can lead to earlier treatment and hence prevention of long-term complications, hasty diagnosis increases the risk of unnecessary treatment and psychological distress.[3]

In adults, five different diagnostic criteria for PCOS have been presented (Table 3.1) by the National Institutes of Health (NIH) in 1990, Rotterdam in 2003, Androgen Excess–PCOS Society (AE-PCOS) in 2006, Amsterdam in 2012, and the Endocrine Society in 2013. The NIH criteria define PCOS as[4-8]:

1. Presence of clinical or biochemical hyperandrogenism
2. Oligomenorrhea/anovulation

Akgül et al.[4] applied all the different PCOS criteria noted in table 3.1 to adolescents with possible PCOS and found that the number of adolescents diagnosed in accordance with the Rotterdam criteria decreased by more than 30% when the evaluation methodology was changed to the Amsterdam and Pediatric Endocrine Society (PES) criteria, thus raising the concern for underdiagnosis or overdiagnosis. It was concerning that there were no specific diagnostic criteria used for adolescents. In 2013 the clinical practice guidelines of the Endocrine Society suggested that the diagnosis of PCOS in an adolescent female can be made if there is persistent oligomenorrhea along with clinical and/or biochemical evidence of hyperandrogenism after exclusion of other pathologies.

Because the anovulatory symptoms and polycystic ovarian (PCO) morphology can be present in early stages of reproductive maturation, the Endocrine Society guidelines advise caution before labeling PCOS in adolescents, particularly within 2 years of menarche.[2] In 2015 the PES consensus endorsed the criteria of the Endocrine Society with some modifications, such as for the persistent hyperandrogenic oligo/anovulatory menstrual abnormality stage, and age-appropriate standards were suggested that are discussed in detail later.[5]

Risk Factors and Pathogenesis of PCOS in Adolescents

PCOS is a multifactorial disease. Literature supports the genesis of PCOS even from intrauterine life. The divergency of clinical manifestations is best explained by the interaction of genetics with the environment, most importantly with lifestyle and diet.[6]

Although the etiology of PCOS is unclear, there is sufficient evidence to suggest it results from a combination of genetic, metabolic, and environmental factors, including insulin resistance (IR), abnormal adrenal and ovarian steroidogenesis and metabolism, modifications in pancreatic beta cell function, neuroendocrine influences, and epigenetic mechanisms acting in a complex pattern.[1,7] It is well established that gonadotrophin secretion patterns in hyperandrogenemic adolescent females with PCOS are similar to those found in adult females with PCOS.[8]

In adolescents with PCOS, there is presence of an imbalance in the hypothalamic-pituitary-GnRH axis through which follicular development occurs because of an exaggerated luteinizing hormone (LH) response. Studies have shown that compared with normal female serum, LH responses after GnRH were distinctly greater in PCOS.[9]

Diagnostic Challenges in Adolescent PCOS

Making a diagnosis of PCOS in adolescence is more challenging compared with the adult population because of a number of factors.

TABLE 3.1 List of Different Diagnostic Criteria for Polycystic Ovary Syndrome

Criteria	Hyperandrogenism	Chronic Anovulation	Polycystic Ovaries
National Institutes of Health 1990	+	+	−
Rotterdam 2003[a]	+/−	+/−	+/−
Androgen Excess Society 2006[b]	+	+/−	+/−
Amsterdam 2012	+	+	+
Endocrine Society 2013	+	+	−
Pediatric Endocrine Society[c]	+	+[d]	−

[a]Two of the 3 criteria must be met.
[b]Hyperandrogenism and at least 1 of the other 2 criteria must be met.
[c]Biochemical hyperandrogenism: Persistent testosterone elevation above adult norms. Clinical hyperandrogenism: Moderate to severe hirsutism or moderate to severe inflammatory acne vulgaris.
[d]Abnormal uterine bleeding pattern for age or gynecologic age; persistent symptoms for 1 to 2 years.
+ indicates definite criterion; +/− indicates might or might not be a criterion.
From Akgül S, Düzçeker Y, Kanbur N, Derman O. Do different diagnostic criteria impact polycystic ovary syndrome diagnosis for adolescents? *J Pediatr Adolesc Gynecol.* 2018;31(3):258–262.

Immaturity of the Hypothalamic-Pituitary-Axis and Menstrual Irregularities

In the early part of normal maturation of the hypothalamic-pituitary-ovarian axis, irregular menses and anovulatory cycles are common.[10] Oligomenorrhea is commonly seen after menarche during normal puberty and is thus not specific to adolescents with PCOS. Anovulatory cycles account for 85%, 59%, and 25 % of the first, third, and sixth year of menstrual cycles, respectively, and were found to be associated with high serum androgen and LH levels.[2] Approximately 75% of adolescents with PCOS present with menstrual issues. It is difficult to differentiate oligomenorrhea caused by PCOS from the normal physiologic oligomenorrhea of adolescence. Nevertheless, absence of menses by 16 years or 2 to 3 years after thelarche has occurred and persistent oligomenorrhea beyond 2 years of menarche may require additional evaluation.[10]

Hyperandrogenism

Hyperandrogenism is the most prevalent characteristic seen in the adolescent age group because normal pubertal changes present very similarly to PCOS. The isolated presence of hirsutism and/or acne should not be taken as clinical evidence of hyperandrogenism of PCOS, but more severe acne and hirsutism could be an indication of this condition.[10,11] Nearly half of hyperandrogenic adolescents will present with cutaneous signs of hyperandrogenism.[12] Adolescents should be evaluated for other causes of hyperandrogenism if clinically or biochemically indicated (Table 3.2). Moreover, there is no standardized grading system for adolescents and the definition of biochemical hyperandrogenism for the age group is also vague because

TABLE 3.2 Differential of Hyperandrogenism in Adolescents

Exaggerated adrenarche	Acromegaly
Late-onset congenital adrenal hyperplasia	Abnormalities of androgen action or of metabolism
Virilizing tumors	Hair–An Syndrome (hyperandrogenism, insulin resistance, acanthosis nigricans)
Cushing syndrome	Ovarian steroidogenic block
Hyperprolactinemia	Androgenic drugs
Disorder of sex development	Epilepsy (Valproic acid therapy)
Glucocorticoid resistance	Idiopathic

Adapted from Oliveira A, Sampaio B, Teixeira A, Castro-Correia C, Fontoura M, Luís Medina J. Síndrome del ovario poliquístico: retos en la adolescencia. *Endocrinol y Nutr.* 2010;57(7):328–336.

of a lack of well-defined cut-offs of androgen levels during physiologic pubertal development.[13]

Physiologic Insulin Resistance and Additive Effects of Obesity in PCOS Adolescents

In healthy adolescents, increased Insulin Resistance (IR) and hyperinsulinemia is more common compared with healthy adults. This normally temporary state of IR in puberty is because of increase in growth hormone.

Moreover, obese adolescent females have raised androgen levels during puberty compared with normal weight females that indicates hyperandrogenemia is exacerbated by obesity.[2]

Differential Diagnosis of PCOS in Adolescents

According to the Endocrine Society, conditions that should first be excluded in females suspected of having PCOS include hypothyroidism, hyperprolactinemia, and nonclassical congenital adrenal hyperplasia.[2,14] Moreover, other diagnoses like Cushing syndrome, pregnancy, primary ovarian insufficiency, hypothalamic amenorrhea, adrenal-secreting tumors, and acromegaly should also be excluded depending on the presentation of PCOS in adolescents.[2,15] It is critical to remember that PCOS is a diagnosis of exclusion. When evaluating an adolescent for suspected PCOS, the provider should be mindful of other possible underlying conditions, such as elevated prolactin levels, thyroid dysfunction, hypercortisolemia, and other reasons for virilization, causing a similar clinical presentation because of androgen excess, such as androgen-secreting tumors, arising from adnexa or adrenal glands, or congenital adrenal hyperplasia.[16] Clinically pituitary and adrenal disease frequently first present during the perimenarchal period and need to be excluded by clinical evaluation.[17] Screening for nonclassic congenital adrenal hyperplasia (NCCAH) is very critical in adolescent girls presenting with symptoms of PCOS. NCCAH may account for 1% to 4% of females with hyperandrogenic anovulation in the reproductive age group.[10] Table 3.3 gives the a summary of conditions to be considered in differential diagnosis of PCOS.

Diagnosis of PCOS in Adolescence

Diagnosing PCOS in adolescents is dependent on the presence of only two criteria according to international consensus based on PES guidelines:
1. Clinical or biochemical signs of hyperandrogenism
2. Oligo/Anovulatory dysfunction

For more information, see Table 3.4.[15] PCOS is diagnosed in adolescent females with otherwise unexplained persistent hyperandrogenic oligo/anovulatory symptoms that are inappropriate for the age and stage of adolescence. As many as 80% of females diagnosed with PCOS will exhibit biochemical and laboratory features of excess androgens.[24] PCOS should be considered in any adolescent female who presents with menstrual irregularity, hirsutism, treatment-resistant acne, alopecia, acanthosis nigricans, and elevated androgens. Evidence of these signs and symptoms should especially be sought in females who are being evaluated for obesity.[11,25]

Clinical Presentation

Oligo/Anovulatory Dysfunction

Menstrual symptoms are present in about two-thirds of adolescents with PCOS, but oligo/anovulatory and irregular menstrual cycles are also seen in the early phase of physiologic maturation of the hypothalamic-pituitary-ovarian

TABLE 3.3 Differential Diagnosis of PCOS in Adolescents

Disorder	Findings Suggestive of PCOS	Reference
Physiologic adolescent anovulation	Physiologic anovulatory cycles	2,12
Nonclassical congenital adrenal hyperplasia	Hyperandrogenic anovulation, hirsutism, clitoromegaly	15
Thyroid dysfunction	Menstrual irregularities; hypothyroidism also causes multicystic changes in ovaries and low SHBG and coarsening of hair can be mistaken for hirsutism	12
Prolactin excess	Disturbances in menstrual function and galactorrhea	18
Cushing syndrome	Striae, obesity, dorsocervical fat, hirsutism in rare occasions, associated with hyperandrogenic anovulation	19
Acromegaly	Oligomenorrhea and hirsutism, IR stat	20
Androgen secreting tumors/exogenous androgen	Virilization, androgenic alopecia, voice change and clitoromegaly	21
Pregnancy	Secondary amenorrhea	22
Ovarian insufficiency or premature ovarian Failure	Primary or secondary oligo/amenorrhea	23

IR, Insulin resistance; *PCOS,* polycystic ovary syndrome; *SHBG,* sex hormone–binding globulin.

TABLE 3.4 Diagnostic Criteria for Diagnosing Polycystic Ovary Syndrome in Adolescents According to International Consensus Guidelines

1. Abnormal uterine bleeding
   a. Abnormal for that specific age or gynecologic age
   b. Persistent symptoms for 1 to 2 years

2. Hyperandrogenism evidence
   a. Raised testosterone level above adult norms
   b. Moderate to severe hirsutism
   c. Moderate to severe acne vulgaris

Witchel S, F, Oberfield S, Rosenfield R, L, et al., The Diagnosis of Polycystic Ovary Syndrome during Adolescence. Horm Res Paediatr 2015;83:376-389. doi: 10.1159/000375530

(HPO) axis. Approximately 85% of menstrual cycles are oligo/anovulatory in the first year after menarche, decreasing to 25% 6 years after menarche.[26] Approximately 75% of adolescent menstrual cycles are 21 to 45 days in duration in the year immediately after menarche (gynecologic year) and 95% of the adolescents are expected to reach an adult cycle duration of 21 to 40 days about 3 to 5 years after menarche.[15,27] Irregular menstrual pattern is the hallmark of oligo/anovulation, and its persistence indicates PCOS. Differentiating oligomenorrhea caused by PCOS from that of normal physiologic immaturity of the HPO axis is difficult; therefore cycles that last more or less than 19 to 90 days, absent menarche until 15 years of age or 2 to 3 years after thelarche, and persistent oligomenorrhea for more than 2 years after menarche require further evaluation.[28]

The various manifestations of abnormal adolescent ovulation, manifested by abnormal uterine bleeding patterns that occur in at least 5% of adolescents, are presented in Table 3.5.

Adolescent females usually seek medical advice when the menstrual irregularity becomes a cause of concern for them and they start developing physical manifestations, like acne or hirsutism, because they are in a period of life when an appearance of normalcy with peers is critically important.[24]

Menstrual dysfunction presenting as amenorrhea, oligomenorrhea, or abnormal uterine bleeding may often be the first clinical symptoms of PCOS. A significant number of oligomenorrheic adolescents are positive for biochemical markers usually seen with PCOS and ultimately develop clinical features of the syndrome as they advance in age.[29]

Clinical Signs of Hyperandrogenism

Physical examination findings include hirsutism, acne, alopecia, obesity, IR, and acanthosis nigricans.

Hirsutism

Hirsutism is the presence of excessive hair growth on androgen-dependent areas of the body (terminal hair proliferation that develops in a male-like pattern) and is seen in nearly 50% to 76% of adolescent females with PCOS. The exact etiology of hirsutism is not known, but it is presumably multifactorial, with the known fact that sexual hair and sebaceous gland development is androgen dependent. PCOS is the most common cause of hirsutism in females and usually develops around the time of puberty.[30] Moderate to severe hirsutism is the most reliable clinical evidence of androgen excess. Hair growth is commonly seen on the face (upper lip and chin), around the areolas, near the umbilicus, and on the lower abdomen; its evaluation can be done using a modified Ferriman–Gallwey score (mFGS; Fig. 3.1),[29,31] which guides toward appropriate management. A score of 6 to 8 corresponds to mild hirsutism, 8 to 15 is serious hirsutism, and greater than 15 corresponds to overt hirsutism. Adolescent females with hirsutism usually have a more severe metabolic disorder.[17]

Acne

Acne is common in peripubertal females but is suggestive of hyperandrogenism when it occurs in combination with an evolving menstrual disorder.[24,32] Hyperandrogenism leads to increased sebum production, resulting in cystic acne and formation of comedones. Sebum production is amplified during adrenarche, and acne in girls with PCOS represents an exaggerated form of adrenarche.[29] Acne vulgaris is seen in 20% to 50% of adolescents with PCOS and often fails to respond to traditional topical treatments.[17] Severity of acne can be categorized as mild, moderate, or severe depending on the lesion type and count. Moderate to severe inflammatory acne vulgaris (Table 3.6) unresponsive to topical treatments is an indication to test for hyperandrogenemia. Comedonal acne is common in adolescent females, but inflammatory acne that is moderate or severe is uncommon during the perimenarchal years.[15]

Alopecia

Alopecia caused by hyperandrogenism resembles male-pattern baldness and is seen at the vertex, crown, and in the frontal and temporal regions.[25] Alopecia is relatively rare and not studied in adolescents very well. Sequestered acne

TABLE 3.5	Types of Abnormal Uterine Bleeding in Adolescent Girls With PCOS	
Type of Abnormal Bleeding	**Definition of Menstrual Irregularity**
Primary amenorrhea	Absence of menarche by 15 yr. of age with normal pubertal development or by 3 yr. after the onset of thelarche
Secondary amenorrhea	Absence of menstrual period for >3 months after initially menstruating
Oligomenorrhea (infrequent abnormal uterine bleeding)	Postmenarchal year 1: average cycle length >90 d (<4 cycles/yr.). Postmenarchal year 2: average cycle length >60 d (<6 cycles/yr.). Postmenarchal years 3–5: average cycle length >45 d (<8 cycles/yr.) Postmenarchal years >6: average cycle length >38–40 d (<9 cycles/yr.)
Excessive anovulatory abnormal uterine bleeding	Menstrual bleeding occurring in less than 21 d, is excessive (lasts >7 d or soaks >1 pad or tampon every 1–2 hours)

d, Days; *PCOS*, polycystic ovary syndrome; *yr.*, year.

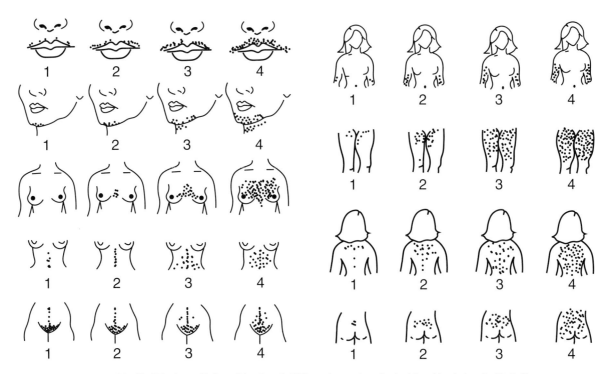

• **Fig.3.1** Modified Ferriman Gallwey hirsutism (mFG) scoring system for facial and body terminal hair. Ferriman, D., and Gallwey, J. D.: Clinical assessment of body hair growth in women, J. Clin. Endocrinol. Metab. 21: 1440. 1961 and Lorenzo, E. M.: Familial study of hirsutism, J. Clin. Endocrinol. Metab. 31:556, 1970.

TABLE 3.6	Acne Scoring System for Adolescents[15]	
Severity	**Comedonal lesions**	**Inflammatory lesions**
Mild	1–10	1–10
Moderate	11–25	11–25
Severe	>25	>25

Data from Rosenfield RL. The diagnosis of polycystic ovary syndrome in adolescents. Pediatrics. 2015;136(6):1154–65.

and alopecia should not be used as diagnostic standards of PCOS in adolescence.

Obesity and Insulin Resistance

The Role of IR and Markers of Metabolic Syndrome in the Diagnosis of PCOS

IR, hyperinsulinemia, and obesity, although relatively frequent in adolescent females with PCOS, cannot be used as diagnostic criteria for PCOS in adolescence. Obesity is a fairly common feature of PCOS and is present in approximately 40% to 60% of females with this condition.[31] Whether obesity is an etiologic factor of PCOS or the prevalence of PCOS is increasing because of the obesity epidemic is still unclear; however, obesity or a history of rapid weight gain in the recent past is usually the initial presentation for 50% of adolescent females presenting with PCOS.[4] Obesity can further aggravate the PCOS-associated menstrual irregularities. Hyperinsulinemia in PCOS appears to be associated with increased central adiposity, which is independent of body mass index (BMI), and this excessive adiposity further increases fat deposition and IR.[28,33] Excessive insulin promotes LH secretion and may add to LH dysregulation. Excessive insulin and LH both, in turn, lead to increased androgen production, oligo/anovulation with menstrual irregularities, obesity, and risk for cardiometabolic abnormalities in the future.[34]

Metabolic syndrome is a combination of abnormal serum glucose levels, central (android) obesity, hypertension, and dyslipidemia, occurring because of IR interacting with obesity and age. Its occurrence is highest in obese individuals and is present in approximately 25% of adolescent females with PCOS. Presence of metabolic syndrome as a comorbidity makes PCOS a risk factor for the early occurrence of type 2 diabetes mellitus (DM), disordered breathing during sleep, and, eventually, the threat of cardiovascular disease.[11,15]

The IR seen in PCOS primarily spins around insulin's effects on glucose metabolism. Other insulin actions are relatively unaffected in PCOS, with resultant compensatory IR hyperinsulinism. Hyperinsulinemia is the root cause of androgen excess because insulin directly promotes the action of LH and raises GnRH indirectly, besides decreasing the sex hormone–binding globulin (SHBG), the main binding protein controlling testosterone levels. As a result of reduced SHBG, free androgen levels are raised, and they, in turn, lead to hyperandrogenic clinical manifestations such as acne, hirsutism, and alopecia. IR can also lead to dyslipidemia, acanthosis, and an elevated risk for cardiovascular disease and diabetes.[35] Clinical features of metabolic syndrome and PCOS are often similar, such as IR, obesity, type 2 DM, hyperlipidemia, and hypertension.[28] These conditions are not a part of the diagnostic criteria of PCOS and must not be considered when making a definitive diagnosis for PCOS. Nevertheless, there is substantial evidence to suggest that PCOS is a risk factor for metabolic syndrome comorbidities.[15]

International, evidence-based guidelines for diagnosis and management of PCOS emphasize recognizing and screening for metabolic abnormalities resulting from PCOS.[36] The presence of obesity and/or signs of IR and acanthosis nigricans should make the health care provider consider the possibility of PCOS along with metabolic syndrome-related comorbidities.[36,37]

Acanthosis Nigricans

Acanthosis nigricans is a dermatologic manifestation of hyperinsulinism and androgen excess that causes poorly defined, thick, dark patches of skin that have a velvety appearance and texture and are typically located on axillae, neck, back, labia, and groins.[38] Hyperpigmentation more frequently occurs in dark-skinned individuals because of epidermal and dermal hyperkeratosis secondary to hyperinsulinemia.

Quality of Life in Adolescents With PCOS

Mental health issues faced by adolescents with PCOS are correlated with impaired health-related quality of life (HRQoL)[17]. There is growing evidence that psychological comorbidities like anxiety, eating disorders, depression, and adverse body image perceptions secondary to dermatologic manifestations such as hirsutism, acne, thinning of hair, and decreased HRQoL, are widely prevalent in adolescent females with PCOS. Hyperinsulinemia, hyperandrogenism, and obesity also contribute to this association.[39] Screening for psychological stress should be included in the comprehensive evaluation of adolescents being diagnosed with PCOS.[39]

Diagnostic Approach to PCOS in Adolescence

Diagnosing PCOS in adolescents is quite challenging because the diagnostic criteria based on evidence-based international guidelines mimic physiologic pubertal development. Adolescent females presenting with menstrual problems, including oligo/amenorrhea, require appropriate screening and awareness teaching, along with appropriate healthcare interventions to improve their reproductive health and HRQoL. An effective diagnostic approach is to identify females with clinical features who would profit from screening, biochemical testing, and imaging studies.[31] Further evaluation is needed in

adolescent females with moderate to severe acne and hirsutism, especially of rapid onset, acanthosis nigricans, associated menstrual irregularities, and central obesity.[31]

A stepwise diagnostic approach is recommended in adolescent females. A detailed history and physical examination are indispensable to identifying any underlying source of androgen excess before a diagnosis of PCOS is made. The history should include onset and duration of hyperandrogenism, detailed menstrual history (menarche, amenorrhea, and oligomenorrhea), history of steroid/androgenic steroid exposure (in utero or exogenous), and medications (antiepileptic or psychiatric) because some medications can cause clinical features like those seen in PCOS. Family history should be reviewed for PCOS, DM, thyroid disorders, or premature cardiovascular disease. Many of these adolescents may have used medication to treat acne, and some of the features of PCOS might have resolved or masked.[16,17]

The physical examination should include an assessment of body hair distribution, alopecia or thinning hair, acne, clitoromegaly, and ovarian enlargement on the pelvic examination. Signs of IR such as acanthosis, central obesity, and hypertension should be sought.[17]

Laboratory Testing for Biochemical Hyperandrogenism

Biochemical testing is done to help in the diagnosis of PCOS and eliminate other causes of hyperandrogenism and menstrual irregularities. Adolescent females with signs and symptoms of androgen excess are candidates for evaluation of hyperandrogenism. The initial endocrine workup for hyperandrogenism includes total and free testosterone, SHBG, dehydroepiandrosterone sulfate (DHEAS), and early morning 17 hydroxyprogesterone (17 OHP) levels. DHEAS will be significantly elevated in blood in the case of adrenal or ovarian secreting tumor but only slightly elevated (20%–30%) in individuals with PCOS. The total testosterone serum concentration will also be significantly raised among those who have a secretory tumor.[15] Commercially available assays that are used for measuring testosterone are not very sensitive at the low levels of testosterone that are found in patients with PCOS. Liquid chromatography-tandem mass spectrometry is the gold standard for measurement of all steroids, but it is quite expensive and also not widely available.[40] Testosterone circulates bound to SHBG; therefore SHBG concentration is the principal factor that regulates the level of free testosterone. Free testosterone assays are less standardized, especially in the pediatric population, and at times are unreliable. Free testosterone or free androgen index can be easily calculated by total testosterone and SHBG concentration. Testosterone levels begin rising as puberty onsets and reach peak levels some years after menarche. There is no absolute value of testosterone beyond which hyperandrogenism can be diagnosed.[7,41] Gonadotropin measurement is not used for diagnosis of PCOS. An elevated LH to follicle-stimulating hormone (FSH) ratio is seen often in PCOS but is not diagnostic.

Antimullerian hormone (AMH) correlates with testosterone levels and is found to be raised in patients with PCOS compared with normally ovulating adolescent females, but again there is no agreement on the use of AMH levels for diagnosing PCOS, mainly because of preanalytic and analytic issues.[42]

As a general rule, following biochemical tests (Table 3.7) should be a part of investigations in an adolescent female presenting with suspicion of PCOS, and a point should be made to exclude other existing pathologies and other causes of hyperandrogenism that can overlap with PCOS.[31,43]

All guidelines endorse screening for nonclassic congenital adrenal hyperplasia (NCCAH), which very closely mimics PCOS, although it accounts for only 5% of hyperandrogenic anovulation.[15] Thyroid screening is recommended because it can cause menstrual irregularity and coarse hair (different from hirsutism). Hyperprolactinemia is reported to be present in up to 14% to 16% of young females presenting with PCOS. Hirsutism and central/truncal adiposity present in PCOS can raise concern over suspicion of Cushing syndrome diagnosis, but other features are different.[15]

17-OHP levels in the early morning require interpretation because a normal random value cannot be used to completely exclude NCCAH because of diurnal variation.[28] Evaluation for type 2 DM and metabolic syndrome should be done in PCOS adolescents, especially those who are obese and have familial risk factors.[11]

Ultrasonography

Classic polycystic ovariany morphology (PCOM) ultrasonographically is defined in adults as an ovary with a thickened capsule, a large volume (>10 cm^3 in volume), and multiple small cysts or 12 or more antral follicles that are 2 to 9 mm in diameter in at least one ovary.[7] Nevertheless, pelvic ultrasound is seldom necessary for diagnosing PCOM in adolescence, especially with a gynecologic age of 8 years (<8 years postmenarche). These criteria are uncertain and problematic in young females because ovaries with multiple follicles are usually seen around the time of menarche and if PCOM is used as criteria for diagnosis of PCOS, approximately 50% of adolescents would meet this criteria, leading to false-positive diagnoses of PCOS in these young females.[10] If clinical findings are indicative of a virilizing tumor and the patient presents with features like rapid progression of hirsutism, pelvic mass, clitoromegaly, a total testosterone level greater than 200 ng/dL, or disorder of sex development, then sonography is indicated. The Endocrine Society guidelines also restraints against the use of PCOM as diagnostic criteria for PCOS in adolescent females.[44]

PCOS is overdiagnosed if pelvic ultrasound is used as a diagnostic modality during adolescence and less than 8 years postmenarche.[35] Normative models have suggested that the gynecologic age of less than 8 years is used as a cut off because maximum ovarian volume is reached at age 20.[46]

Treatment Strategies

To date, there are no specific pharmacologic treatments for PCOS that can completely cure the condition, but medications are available to treat the clinical symptoms associated with PCOS.[35] The treatment strategy in every young female with PCOS varies depending on the clinical presentation and underlying cause. There are two main constituents of therapy. The first is control of symptoms of hyperandrogenism (hirsutism, acne, irregular menstrual cycles, and infertility), and the second is to improve and prevent the long-term comorbidities that are seen in patients with PCOS (metabolic syndrome, cardiovascular abnormalities, type 2 DM, dyslipidemia, and problems with emotional health and self-esteem). Perceived concerns of adolescent females should be taken into consideration and are vital for embarking on the long-term maintenance of cooperation to a treatment plan. The various options available are lifestyle intervention, combined oral contraceptive pills (COCP), antiandrogens, insulin sensitizers, bariatric surgery, and local cosmetic treatments (Table 3.8).[7,31]

TABLE 3.7	Biochemical Evaluation of PCOS in Adolescent Girls[15,44,45]
Diagnostic evaluation	**Rationale**
Estradiol	Ovarian function
17-OHP	If NCCAH is suspected
FSH	Normal to high in PCOS High in primary gonadal failure, a cause of primary amenorrhea
LH	High in PCOS Low in Hypogonadotropic hypogonadism
Prolactin	If Pituitary tumor or mass lesion is suspected
Testosterone	Androgen excess
DHEAS	Androgen producing tumors
Thyroid stimulating hormone	Thyroid dysfunction
Fasting lipid profile	Dyslipidemia
Fating 2-hour OGTT	Insulin resistance and type 2 diabetes
Serum and urine cortisol	Cushing syndrome

17-OHP, 17 Hydroxyprogesterone; *DHEAS,* dehydroepiandrosterone sulfate; *FSH,* follicle-stimulating hormone; *LH,* luteinizing hormone; *NCCAH,* nonclassical congenital adrenal hyperplasia; *OGTT,* oral glucose tolerance test; *PCOS,* polycystic ovary syndrome.

TABLE 3.8	Management Strategies of PCOS in Adolescents	
Hyperandrogenism	First-line medical management is COCP.	
	Cosmetic therapy (laser, waxing, electrolysis); eflornithine topical cream.	
	Combination therapy: Spironolactone and COCPs improve moderate to severe hirsutism.	
Acne	COCPs.	
	Topical antibiotics, retinoic acid and salicylic acid.	
	Generalized body acne is treated with systemic antibiotics and isotretinoin.	
Oligo/amenorrhea	Lifestyle modification: 5%–10% weight reduction, healthy diet. Used for decreasing androgens, IR, and cardiovascular risk factors.	
	COCPs cause reduction in LH and androgen synthesis, which, in turn, reduces testosterone and improves hirsutism score. Cyclical progesterone can also be used.	
	Metformin: Ovulation improves, regularizing the menstrual cycle.	
Metabolic syndrome	Weight reduction is the key to improving IR and hyperandrogenism, along with reducing cardiovascular risk factors and suppressing ovarian androgen production, hence reducing the risk of metabolic syndrome and type 2 diabetes.	
	Metformin for IR-related conditions.	

COCP, Combined oral contraceptive pills; *IR*, insulin resistance; *LH*, luteinizing hormone; *PCOS*, polycystic ovary syndrome.
From Ibáñez L, Oberfield SE, Witchel S, et al. An international consortium update: pathophysiology, diagnosis, and treatment of polycystic ovarian syndrome in adolescence. *Horm Res Paediatr.* 2017;88(6):371–395; Fitzgerald S, Divasta A, Gooding H. An update on PCOS in adolescents. *Curr Opin Pediatr.* 2018;30(4):459–465; and Teede HJ, Misso ML, Costello MF, et al. Recommendations from the international evidence-based guideline for the assessment and management of polycystic ovary syndrome. *Hum Reprod.* 2018;33(9):1602–1618.

Lifestyle Interventions

PCOS is a long-term disease with other comorbidities like type 2 DM associated with it, so lifestyle modification is the first and most important, yet simple, approach to carry out in young females with PCOS. The prevalence and degree of hirsutism and ovulatory dysfunction is found to be higher in obese females with PCOS. Randomized controlled trials in adolescents have shown that lifestyle changes, including a balanced healthy diet and exercise, exert a positive impact on body weight, IR, and testosterone levels, increasing the number of menstrual cycles, decreasing the amount of testosterone (with an increase in SHBG quantity), and reducing the hirsutism score (mFGS).[35] A weight loss of as little as 5% to 10% in obese young females has shown favorable effects within 6 months.[47] Lifestyle modifications are challenging for adolescents over a long period of time, and there is a high grade of relapse and cessation of behavior modification programs.[25] Family support is crucial to ensuring the continuity of these interventions.

Combined Oral Contraceptive Pills

Cyclic administration of COCPs containing estrogen and progesterone is considered a first-line therapy in adolescents with a clear diagnosis of PCOS. This both achieves control of hyperandrogenic symptoms and regularizes menstrual cycles. The estrogen component of COCPs increases SHBG, decreasing free androgens. Progestins in COCPs decrease LH secretion, which, in turn, reduces androgen production by suppressing the pituitary ovarian feedback loop. This androgen-reducing effect of COCPs is valuable also for treating clinical signs of androgen excess like hirsutism and acne. Newer progestins like drospirenone have greater progestogenic and weak antiandrogenic properties and may be used as a treatment modality. The best combination of COCP and duration of treatment is still debated. Major adverse effects associated with these pills are worsening of cardiometabolic profile, increased triglyceride levels, reduced insulin sensitivity, and increased risk of thromboembolic events. Drospirenone has a greater risk of venous thrombosis and may be contraindicated in females with morbid obesity. The lowest effective daily dose of estrogen (20–30 ug of ethinyl estradiol or its equivalent) or natural estrogen-like conjugated equine estrogen is preferred. The use of COCPs should be according to the risk grade of patients and stopped immediately if any contraindication occurs.[35]

Antiandrogens

Androgen receptor blockers, namely spironolactone, flutamide, or third-generation progestin (cyproterone acetate), and 5 alpha reductase inhibitors like finasteride are the antiandrogens used for treating hirsutism. Spironolactone, an aldosterone antagonist, is commonly used; the starting dose is 25 mg/day and can be increased up to a maximum of 200 mg/day. Some side effects of spironolactone are breast tenderness, intermenstrual bleeding, and scalp alopecia.

Flutamide is not widely used because of its hepatotoxic effects at high doses greater than 250 mg/day, but a low dose of 1 mg/kg/day is not hepatotoxic in long-term use and almost similar in efficacy to spironolactone. It is used in combination with metformin to reduce its hepatotoxicity and significantly reduces hirsutism compared with metformin monotherapy.[27] Efficacy of antiandrogens is significantly increased when used in combination with COCPs or metformin. The use of antiandrogen should be avoided in sexually active adolescents to avoid feminizing effects on male fetuses in case of pregnancy.[7,35,48] Cyproterone acetate is an antiandrogen with potent progestogenic activity and is used in combination with Ethinyl estradiol for acne and hirsutism. Finasteride is a 5-alpha reductase inhibitor that decreases the hirsutism score but has limited use because of its teratogenic effects.[35]

Insulin Sensitizers

This class of drugs is used to treat PCOS-associated metabolic comorbidities because they act by decreasing IR and normalizing insulin levels. When IR is decreased, it leads to lowered androgen levels, resulting in regularization of the menstrual cycle.[35]

Metformin

Metformin is the insulin sensitizer used most to reduce IR and hyperinsulinemia, which, in turn, will cause a reduction in androgen levels in PCOS.[31] Metformin used in combination with lifestyle changes has a beneficial effect on metabolic profile, especially improving insulin sensitivity and glucose tolerance by increasing peripheral tissue glucose uptake and utilization, reducing hepatic glucose production, decreasing BMI, subcutaneous and visceral adiposity, and improving anovulatory menstrual irregularities.[47] Metformin improves glucose tolerance and other components of the metabolic syndrome seen in both obese and nonobese adolescents with PCOS.[10] About 18% to 24% of adolescents with PCOS have abnormal glucose metabolism. Menstrual irregularities also show improvement with metformin therapy in adolescents. In females with a contraindication to use of COCPs, metformin is an excellent option. Nevertheless, it does not have any antiandrogen effect and will have very little impact on hirsutism or acne.[29]

No serious side effects have been reported except gastrointestinal disturbance, which is dose dependent. International consensus guidelines recommend the use of metformin along with lifestyle improvements in adolescents with a clear diagnosis of PCOS or with symptoms of PCOS before the diagnosis is made.[40,49]

Metformin has a beneficial role in preventing long-term PCOS-associated comorbidities such as endometrial cancer, type 2 DM, cardiovascular diseases, and hypertension.[35]

Thiazolidinediones

The class of thiazolidinediones (TZDs) is commonly referred to as "glitazones" and includes rosiglitazone and pioglitazone. TZDs decrease the 11-ß-HSD enzyme activity responsible for conversion of cortisol. They are considered a second-line treatment for PCOS patients after metformin to improve IR. TZDs increase SHBG levels and decrease excess androgens. Both metformin and TZDs have comparable efficacy in increasing ovulation, reducing IR, and regularizing the menstrual cycle, but their use in adolescents is less commonly studied and still very limited.[35]

Combination Treatment

Lifestyle changes are the first-line treatment in all adolescents with PCOS, especially those who are overweight or obese. The combination of COCPs and metformin can be considered in adolescents with PCOS and a BMI of over 25kg/m² where COCP and lifestyle changes cannot achieve the desired goals. A combination of antiandrogens with COCP could also be considered in PCOS adolescents with severe hirsutism who have failed to respond to COCP and cosmetic treatment after a duration of 6 months.[44] A low-dose, triple-drug combination of metformin, flutamide, and pioglitazone showed no improvement in decreasing androgens in adolescents compared with COCPs but improved lipid profile, carotid intima media thickness, and body composition parameters.[7]

Antiobesity Treatment (Bariatric Surgery)

Antiobesity medications are not approved for use in children and adolescents. Bariatric surgery for seeking improvement in the problems of PCOS and infertility is also not considered.[7,33]

Contraception

One in 10 females with oligomenorrhoea can ovulate spontaneously, so a sexually active adolescent female should be advised to follow the general principles of contraception. No specific method/agent is recommended for adolescents with PCOS.[7]

Management of Dermatologic Manifestations

Cosmetic problems can be treated with short- and long-term therapies. Hirsutism can be managed with short-term mechanical methods, such as chemical depilation, threading, and waxing, and long-term methods, like electrolysis and laser therapy. In addition, a 13.9% topical solution of Eflornithine hydrochloride can be used to reduce facial hair growth, although it has only a short-term effect and requires daily use.[29]

Summary

PCOS has become a progressively important adolescent reproductive health diagnosis because of its effect of reducing HRQoL in adolescent females. Because of the challenge of diagnosing PCOS in adolescents, experts have suggested devising different criteria for adolescents.[11] Labeling an early adolescent female with the diagnosis of PCOS has long-term implications for metabolic, cardiovascular, mental health, and reproductive health outcomes. Hence, it has been suggested that the diagnosis of PCOS should be deferred at least for 2 years after achieving menarche.[50] Treatment for these patients involves lifestyle changes in all patients regardless of whether they receive diagnosis. In obese and overweight adolescents, weight loss strategies are suggested in the form of calorie-restricted diets and exercise. The medical therapy of PCOS in adolescents is still controversial but should be introduced in at-risk, confirmed, or resistant cases.

References

1. Çelebier M, Kaplan O, Özel Ş, Engin-Üstün Y. Polycystic ovary syndrome in adolescents: Q-TOF LC/MS analysis of human plasma metabolome. *J Pharm Biomed Anal.* 2020;191:113543.

2. Legro RS, Arslanian SA, Ehrmann DA, et al. Diagnosis and treatment of polycystic ovary syndrome: an Endocrine Society clinical practice guideline. *J Clin Endocrinol Metab.* 2013;98(12):4565-4592.

3. Nicandri KF, Hoeger K. Diagnosis and treatment of polycystic ovarian syndrome in adolescents. *Curr Opin Endocrinol Diabetes Obes.* 2012;19(6):497-504.

4. Akgül S, Bonny AE. Metabolic syndrome in adolescents with polycystic ovary syndrome: prevalence on the basis of different diagnostic criteria. *J Pediatr Adolesc Gynecol.* 2019;32(4):383-387.

5. Akgül S, Düzçeker Y, Kanbur N, Derman O. Do different diagnostic criteria impact polycystic ovary syndrome diagnosis for adolescents? *J Pediatr Adolesc Gynecol.* 2018;31(3):258-262.

6. Oliveira A, Sampaio B, Teixeira A, Castro-Correia C, Fontoura M, Luís Medina J. Síndrome del ovario poliquístico: retos en la adolescencia. *Endocrinol y Nutr.* 2010;57(7):328-336.

7. Dabadghao P. Polycystic ovary syndrome in adolescents. *Best Pract Res Clin Endocrinol Metab.* 2019;33(3):101272. Available at: https://doi.org/10.1016/j.beem.2019.04.006.

8. Shayya R, Chang RJ. Reproductive endocrinology of adolescent polycystic ovary syndrome. *BJOG.* 2010;117(2):150-155.

9. Patel K, Coffler MS, Dahan MH, Malcom PJ, Deutsch R, Chang RJ. Relationship of GnRH-stimulated LH release to episodic LH secretion and baseline endocrine-metabolic measures in women with polycystic ovary syndrome. *Clin Endocrinol (Oxf).* 2004;60:67-74.

10. Rothenberg SS, Beverley R, Barnard E, Baradaran-Shoraka M, Sanfilippo JS. Polycystic ovary syndrome in adolescents. *Best Pract Res Clin Obstet Gynaecol.* 2018;48:103-114.

11. Roe AH, Prochaska E, Smith M, Sammel M, Dokras A. Using the androgen excess-PCOS society criteria to diagnose polycystic ovary syndrome and the risk of metabolic syndrome in adolescents. *J Pediatr.* 2013;162(5):937-941. Available at: http://dx.doi.org/10.1016/j.jpeds.2012.11.019.

12. Rosenfield RL. The diagnosis of polycystic ovary syndrome in adolescents. *Pediatrics.* 2015;136(6):1154-1165.

13. Rosner W, Auchus RJ, Azziz R, Sluss PM, Raff H. Position statement: utility, limitations, and pitfalls in measuring testosterone: an Endocrine Society position statement. *J Clin Endocrinol Metab.* 2007;92(2):405-413.

14. Dewailly D, Lujan ME, Carmina E, et al. Definition and significance of polycystic ovarian morphology: a task force report from the Androgen Excess and Polycystic Ovary Syndrome Society. *Hum Reprod Update.* 2014;20(3):334-352.

15. Rosenfield RL. The diagnosis of polycystic ovary syndrome in adolescents. *Pediatrics.* 2015;136(6):1154-1165.

16. Kamboj MK, Bonny AE. Polycystic ovary syndrome in adolescence: diagnostic and therapeutic strategies. *Transl Pediatr.* 2017;6(4):248-255.

17. Hachey LM, Kroger-Jarvis M, Pavlik-Maus T, Leach R. Clinical implications of polycystic ovary syndrome in adolescents. *Nurs Womens Health.* 2020;24(2):115-126. Available at: https://doi.org/10.1016/j.nwh.2020.01.011.

18. Melmed S, Casanueva FF, Hoffman AR, et al. Diagnosis and treatment of hyperprolactinemia: an Endocrine Society clinical practice guideline method of development of evidence-based clinical practice guidelines. *J Clin Endocrinol Metab.* 2011;96:273-288.

19. Kaltsas GA, Korbonits M, Isidori AM, et al. How common are polycystic ovaries and the polycystic ovarian syndrome in women with Cushing's syndrome? *Clin Endocrinol.* 2000;53(4):493-500.

20. Melmed S, Colao A, Barkan A, et al. Guidelines for acromegaly management: an update. *J Clin Endocrinol Metab.* 2009;94(5):1509-1517.

21. Carmina E, Rosato F, Janni, A, Rizzo JM, Longo RA. Extensive clinical experience relative prevalence of different androgen excess disorders in 950 women referred because of clinical hyperandrogenism. *J Clin Endocrinol Metab.* 2006;91(1):2-6.

22. Klein DA, Poth MA. Amenorrhea: an approach to diagnosis and management. *Am Fam Physician.* 2013;87(11):781-788.

23. Peña AS, Witchel SF, Hoeger KM, et al. Adolescent polycystic ovary syndrome according to the international evidence-based guideline. BMC Med. 2020;18(1):1–16.

24. Trent M, Gordon CM. Diagnosis and management of polycystic ovary syndrome in adolescents. *Pediatrics.* 2020;145(suppl 2):S210-S218.

25. Nicolaides NC, Matheou A, Vlachou F, Neocleous V, Skordis N. Polycystic ovarian syndrome in adolescents: from diagnostic criteria to therapeutic management. *Acta Biomed.* 2020;91(3):1-13.

26. Legro RS. Ovulation induction in polycystic ovary syndrome: current options. *Best Pract Res Clin Obstet Gynaecol.* 2016;37:152-159. Available at: http://dx.doi.org/10.1016/j.bpobgyn.2016.08.001.

27. Ibáñez L, Oberfield SE, Witchel S, et al. An international consortium update: pathophysiology, diagnosis, and treatment of polycystic ovarian syndrome in adolescence. *Horm Res Paediatr.* 2017;88(6):371-395.

28. Rosenfield RL, Ehrmann DA. The Pathogenesis of Polycystic Ovary Syndrome (PCOS): the hypothesis of PCOS as functional ovarian hyperandrogenism revisited. *Endocr Rev.* 2016;37(5):467-520.

29. Lizneva D, Gavrilova-Jordan L, Walker W, Azziz R. Androgen excess: investigations and management. *Best Pract Res Clin Obstet Gynaecol.* 2016;37:98-118. Available at: http://dx.doi.org/10.1016/j.bpobgyn.2016.05.003.

30. Mihailidis J, Dermesropian R, Taxel P, Luthra P, Grant-Kels JM. Endocrine evaluation of hirsutism. *Int J Women's Dermatology.* 2017;3(1):S6-S10. Available at: http://dx.doi.org/10.1016/j.ijwd.2017.02.007.

31. Escobar-Morreale HF, Carmina E, Dewailly D, et al. Epidemiology, diagnosis and management of hirsutism: a consensus statement by the androgen excess and polycystic ovary syndrome society. *Hum Reprod Update.* 2012;18(2):146-170.

32. Fitzgerald S, Divasta A, Gooding H. An update on PCOS in adolescents. *Curr Opin Pediatr.* 2018;30(4):459-465.

33. Muscogiuri G, Colao A, Orio F. Insulin-mediated diseases: adrenal mass and polycystic ovary syndrome. *Trends Endocrinol Metab.* 2015;26(10):512-514. Available at: http://dx.doi.org/10.1016/j.tem.2015.07.010.

34. Witchel SF, Burghard AC, Tao RH, Oberfield SE. The diagnosis and treatment of PCOS in adolescents: an update. *Curr Opin Pediatr.* 2019;31(4):562-569.

35. Bulsara J, Patel P, Soni A, Acharya S. A review: brief insight into Polycystic Ovarian syndrome. *Endocr Metab Sci.* 2021;3:100085.

36. Diamanti-Kandarakis E, Dunaif A. Insulin resistance and the polycystic ovary syndrome revisited: an update on mechanisms and implications. *Endocr Rev.* 2012;33(6):981-1030.

37. Eek D, Paty J, Black P, Celeste Elash C, Reaney M. A comprehensive disease model of Polycystic Ovary Syndrome (PCOS). *Value Heal.* 2015;18(7):A722.

38. Jain P, Jain S, Singh A, Goel S. Pattern of dermatologic manifestations in polycystic ovarian disease cases from a tertiary care hospital. *Int J Adv Med.* 2018;5(1):197.

39. Dokras A, Sarwer DB, Allison KC, et al. Weight loss and lowering androgens predict improvements in health-related quality of life in women with PCOS. *J Clin Endocrinol Metab.* 2016;101(8):2966-2974.

40. Teede H, Misso M, Costello M, et al. *International Evidence-Based Guideline for the Assessment and Management of Polycystic Ovary Syndrome 2018.* Monash University, Melbourne Australia: National Health and Medical Research Council (NHMRC; 2018:1–198.

41. Conway G, Dewailly D, Diamanti-Kandarakis E, et al. The polycystic ovary syndrome: a position statement from the European Society of Endocrinology. *Eur J Endocrinol.* 2014;171(4):P1-P29.

42. Rocha AL, Oliveira FR, Azevedo RC, et al. Recent advances in the understanding and management of polycystic ovary syndrome[version 1; peer review: 3 approved]. *F1000Res.* 2019; 8(565):1-11.

43. Guleken Z, Bulut H, Bulut B, Depciuch J. Assessment of the effect of endocrine abnormalities on biomacromolecules and lipids by FT-IR and biochemical assays as biomarker of metabolites in early polycystic ovary syndrome women. *J Pharm Biomed Anal.* 2021;204:114250. Available at: https://doi.org/10.1016/j.jpba.2021.114250.

44. Legro RS, Arslanian SA, Ehrmann DA, et al. Diagnosis and treatment of polycystic ovary syndrome: an Endocrine Society clinical practice guideline. *J Clin Endocrinol Metab.* 2013; 98(12):4565-4592.

45. Teede HJ, Misso ML, Costello MF, et al. Recommendations from the international evidence-based guideline for the assessment and management of polycystic ovary syndrome. *Hum Reprod.* 2018; 33(9):1602-1618.

46. Peña AS, Witchel SF, Hoeger KM, et al. Adolescent polycystic ovary syndrome according to the international evidence-based guideline. *BMC Med.* 2020;18(1):1-16.

47. Hoeger K, Davidson K, Kochman L, Cherry T, Kopin L, Guzick DS. The impact of Metformin, oral contraceptives, and lifestyle modification on polycystic ovary syndrome in obese adolescent women in two randomized, placebo-controlled clinical trials. *J Clin Endocrinol Metab.* 2008;93(11):4299-4306.

48. Kavitha VJ, Devi MG, Puvaneswari N Clinical presentation, risk assessment and management of Polycystic Ovary Syndrome [PCOS]. *International Journal of Biomedical and Advance Research.* 2017;8(3):66–71.

49. Sebastian MR, Wiemann CM, Bacha F, Alston Taylor SJ. Diagnostic evaluation, comorbidity screening, and treatment of polycystic ovary syndrome in adolescents in 3 specialty clinics. *J Pediatr Adolesc Gynecol.* 2018;31(4):367-371. Available at: https://doi.org/10.1016/j.jpag.2018.01.007.

50. Dokras A, Feldman Witchel S. Are young adult women with polycystic ovary syndrome slipping through the healthcare cracks? *J Clin Endocrinol Metab.* 2014;99(5):1583-1585.

4

Pathophysiology of Polycystic Ovary Syndrome

MOHUMMAD HASSAN RAZA RAJA, MUHAMMAD ABDULLAH JAVED, AND REHANA REHMAN

Pathophysiology of Polycystic Ovary Syndrome

Polycystic ovary syndrome (PCOS), an endocrine disorder in reproductive-age females, has a multifactorial etiology, largely defined by the presence of at least two out of the following three conditions: oligo-ovulatory/anovulatory cycles, polycystic ovaries, and hyperandrogenism. Widely considered a diagnosis of exclusion, it continues to be the universal cause of infertility related to anovulation among females of childbearing age and estimates suggest that up to 20% of reproductive-age females may be affected by PCOS. Because of a complex pathophysiologic basis, involving an interwoven interplay of hormonal aberrations and genetic, epigenetic, and environmental factors, PCOS presents as a spectrum of disease with mild to severe presentations.

Hormonal Aberrations

Androgen Excess

Elevated androgen levels are a defining characteristic of PCOS, causing several of the presenting manifestations. Under normal physiologic conditions, ovaries and the adrenal glands each contribute equal amounts of androgens (predominantly androstenedione and testosterone) within reproductive-age females.[1] In PCOS caused by dysfunctional regulation in the process of steroidogenesis, the ovaries (and, in some cases, the adrenal glands) produce excessive androgens (Fig. 4.1).

Functional Ovarian Hyperandrogenism

The main source of ovarian androgens is the theca cells, which produce androstenedione (see Fig. 4.1). Androstenedione is converted to testosterone either directly within the theca cells or may be secreted in the blood to be converted in peripheral tissue. Hyperandrogenism, as seen in PCOS, is driven by both extraovarian and intraovarian factors. In females with PCOS, theca cells have exhibited increased expression of enzymes CYP17A1 and CY11A and decreased expression of CYP19 in granulosa cells.[2]

In theca cells, CYP17A1 is the enzyme that determines the rate of biosynthetic pathway. This enzyme functions as both 17a-hydroxylase and 17,20-lyase, which are capable of converting pregnenolone/progesterone into dehydroandrosterone/androstenedione, respectively. Rosenfield et al. has shown an increased expression of CYP17A1 in theca cells in PCOS subjects, hence leading to increased androgen production.[3] The expression of CYP17A1 remains increased in long-term in-vitro cultures of theca cells, hence demonstrating an intraovarian dysregulatory mechanism.[3] Continuing with the same theme, the upregulation of CYP11A/P450scc causes an increased conversion of cholesterol to pregnenolone, whereas a downregulation of CYP19 in granulosa cells leads to a decreased conversion of testosterone to estrogen, tipping the balance toward hyperandrogenemia (Fig. 4.2).

There is developing evidence suggesting that dysregulation of the steroid biosynthetic pathway, causing functional adrenal hyperandrogenism (FOH), may have fetal origins. High androgen exposure during intrauterine life within rhesus monkeys and ewes has been shown to precipitate an irreversible cascade of events leading to anovulation and ovarian hyperandrogenism during puberty and adulthood.[4,5] During pregnancy, levels of sex hormone–binding globulin (SHBG) and intrinsic aromatase activity in placenta protect the fetus from androgens in the mother.[6] Possible mechanisms leading to increased fetal exposure to androgens may be fetuses born to mothers with congenital adrenal hyperplasia (CAH), variations in gene expression leading to lower levels of SHBG and/or aromatase, or inhibitions of aromatase activity and/or SHBG secretion because of maternal hyperinsulinemia.[7]

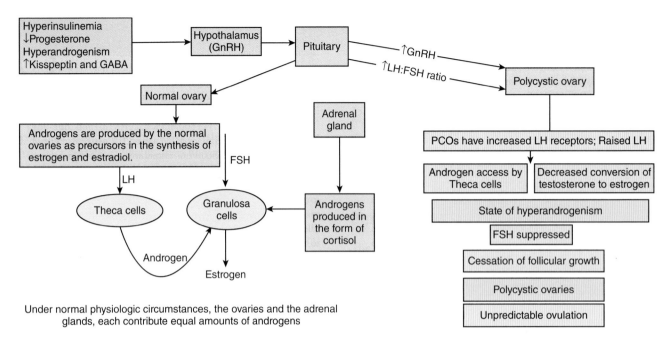

• **Fig. 4.1** Hormonal Aberrations (Androgen Excess) in Polycystic Ovary Syndrome. *FSH*, Follicle-stimulating hormone; *GnRH*, gonadotropin-releasing hormone; *LH*, luteinizing hormone; *PCOs*, polycystic ovaries.

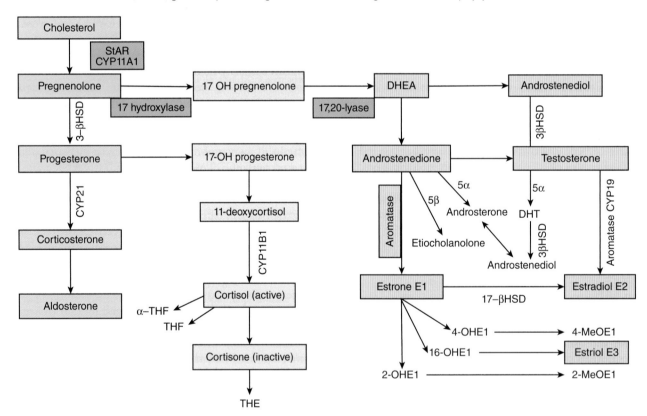

• **Fig. 4.2** Steroidogenic Biosynthetic Pathway.

Hypothalamic-Pituitary-Ovarian Axis Dysregulation

As previously highlighted, although there are intraovarian factors that lead to hyperandrogenism, extraovarian factors, namely dysregulation of the hypothalamic-pituitary-ovarian (HPO) axis, also contribute to the pathogenesis of the disease. Gonadotropin-releasing hormone (GnRH) is normally released by axon terminals in the median eminence of the hypothalamus in a pulsatile fashion resulting in the release of follicle-stimulating hormone (FSH) and luteinizing hormone (LH) from gonadotrophs in the anterior pituitary gland. Both FSH and LH are essential to regulating ovarian function. FSH primarily stimulates folliculogenesis, while also promoting the production of estrogens from androgens in granulosa cells. Furthermore, LH serves as a crucial stimulus for androgen production and ovulation and promotes progesterone production during the luteal phase. Throughout each phase of the menstrual cycle, the levels of FSH and LH remain tightly regulated and controlled by changes in the amplitude and frequency of pulses of GnRH.[8]

In PCOS, there are clear aberrations in the levels of LH and FSH, with markedly elevated LH levels and markedly decreased FSH levels, causing a subsequently increased LH/FSH ratio seen in the majority of females. Increased frequency and amplitude of LH pulses, which are regulated upstream by increased frequency of GnRH pulses, appear to be the cause of this. Although the underlying mechanisms behind this shift in frequency are unclear, several mechanisms have been proposed:

1. Hyperinsulinemia enhances the response of the pituitary gland to GnRH and to intrinsic GnRH neuronal activity.
2. Decreased progesterone, seen in PCOS because of anovulation, disrupts the negative feedback loop of GnRH, leading to increased GnRH secretion.
3. Hyperandrogenism directly disrupts negative feedback loops of progesterone and estrogen on the GnRH/LH production.[9]

The dysfunction of the HPO axis may be explained by alterations in the neuroendocrine physiology at the hypothalamic level. The hypothalamic peptide, kisspeptin, is encoded by the *KISS1* gene.[10] The majority of prior literature has shown females who have PCOS to exhibit higher levels of kisspeptin and appear to influence the HPO axis, through stimulating an increased GnRH pulse rate and amplitude.[11] Additionally, a growing body of evidence also points toward the part played by GABA in the pathophysiology of PCOS. Although GABA tends to be inhibitory elsewhere in the central nervous system (CNS), within the hypothalamus, GABA appears to increase the activity of GnRH neurons via GABAa receptors. Thus increased GABA will lead to increased GnRH and an increased LH/FSH ratio.[12]

Functional Adrenal Hyperandrogenism

Although FOH remains the major mechanism causing androgen excess in PCOS, steroidogenic dysfunction arising from the adrenal glands may also serve a contributory role. Prior literature has shown that the prevalence of functional adrenal hyperandrogenism (FAH) in females with PCOS ranged from 20% to 65%, with less than 3% of cases of PCOS attributable to isolated FAH.[13,14] FAH is marked by increased serum levels of dehydroepiandrosterone sulfate (DHEAS), an androgen secreted only by the adrenal cortex. The underlying mechanism leading to increased adrenal androgen production remains unclear, yet it is hypothesized that similar mechanisms that exist to produce FOH also result in FAH, leading to steroid biosynthetic pathway dysfunction. Additionally, it has also been demonstrated that the adrenal glands are hyperresponsive to ACTH, and hyperinsulinemic conditions seen in PCOS also

play a role in potentiating the activities of 17α-hydroxylase and 17,20-lyase.[15] Differences in androgenic products produced by the adrenal reticularis and ovaries are because of the differential expression of enzymes. The adrenal glands possessing reduced activity of 3β-hydroxysteroid dehydrogenase 2 and increased expression of SULT2A1 sulfotransferase lead to the production of DHEA-S (rather than androstenedione production as seen in the ovaries) from dehydroepiandrosterone (DHEA;).[16]

Insulin Resistance and Hyperinsulinemia

Along with hyperandrogenism, selective insulin resistance (IR) and hyperinsulinemia are key features of the disease in almost two-thirds of patients who show features of reduced insulin sensitivity.[17] The hyperinsulinemic state found in PCOS can be attributed to IR, which develops from abnormal serine phosphorylation of the insulin receptors and insulin receptor substrate-1, leading to defects in postreceptor signaling.[18,19] This hyperphosphorylation is because of increased intracellular serine kinase activity. Furthermore, hyperinsulinemia is strongly associated with the hyperandrogenic state found in PCOS and often both factors work synergistically together. The production of hepatic SHBG is reduced because of hyperinsulinemia, and it elevates free androgens levels.[20,21] Additionally, insulin may directly act as a reproductive hormone, acting to boost GnRH-mediated gonadotropic hormone release from the pituitary gland and later in a synergistic way with LH, inducing androgen production in theca cells.[22,23] There are insulin receptors present in the ovaries, which stimulate steroidogenesis in granulosa cells and theca cells in PCOS.[24] This is surprising considering IR appears to be selective, only affecting glucose metabolism and leading to subsequent metabolic derangement seen in PCOS, whereas insulin's effect on the ovaries remains unchanged, if not enhanced.[25] What continues to remain unclear, however, is whether IR and hyperinsulinemia contributes to the pathologic mechanisms that precipitate PCOS or whether it is simply a metabolic effect of PCOS, with further studies required in this regard.

Vascular Endothelial Growth Factor

Vascular endothelial growth factor (VEGF) is a protein that binds specific receptors on endothelial cells inducing angiogenesis. In ovaries, vascular supply develops on a cyclical basis and VEGF plays a significant role in mediating angiogenesis and permeability of vasculature, which are critical to the process of ovulation and corpus luteum development.[26]

VEGF and its receptors are expressed on multiple ovarian cells, including theca and granulosa cells. The levels of VEGF in the follicular fluid are significantly higher than that in serum.[27] PCOS subjects who underwent in vitro fertilization (IVF) had raised levels of VEGF as reported by a study. Additional studies have found increased VEGF expression in theca, granulosa, and luteal cells.[27] Doppler studies revealed increased blood flow velocity in ovaries to be positively correlated with VEGF levels, and this increase in angiogenesis secondary to high VEGF could be a contributing factor to the increased size of ovaries, a hallmark of the disease.[28] High VEGF can also lead to abnormal growth of theca cells.[29] The role of VEGF gene polymorphisms in the pathologic process contributing to PCOS has been widely studied. Bao et al. found a strong association of the rs1570360 single nucleotide polymorphism with increased risk for PCOS, whereas rs3025020 and rs833061 were marginally associated.[29] The aforementioned findings do suggest that high VEGF levels could contribute to many of the phenotypic features observed in PCOS patients.

Vitamin D

Vitamin D, an important steroid hormone, exists as vitamin D_2 (ergocalciferol) and vitamin D_3 (cholecalciferol) and exerts its actions via vitamin D receptor. The predominant function of vitamin D is calcium and phosphate regulation in the body by way of which it influences bone metabolism.[30]

Apart from its role in bone metabolism, vitamin D also plays a significant role in ovarian function and subsequently PCOS pathogenesis (Fig. 4.3).[30] Deficiency of vitamin D is very common in PCOS patients, with a prevalence of around 67% to 85%.[31] An important association in PCOS lies with anti-Mullerian hormone (AMH) levels. As hypothesized, AMH has the following major functions and leads to inhibition of[32]:

1. Follicular activation and growth
2. FSH stimulated growth
3. Granulosa cell growth
4. Aromatase

High AMH levels in PCOS patients could cause decreased sensitivity of follicle to the effects of FSH, thus impairing ovarian function.[33] Moreover, increased AMH inhibition of aromatase could explain the reduced estrogen levels in PCOS patients. AMH may directly stimulate theca cells to synthesize more androgens.[34] A study revealed vitamin D levels to be negatively regulated with AMH and AMH receptor mRNA levels; thus vitamin D supplementation in PCOS patients may improve folliculogenesis because of lower AMH levels.[35]

Advanced glycation end products (AGEs) are proinflammatory molecules found in PCOS that cause follicular dysfunction. The soluble receptors for AGEs (sRAGE) bind to AGEs to neutralize their harmful effects.[36] An association has been found between vitamin D supplementation and increased circulating levels of sRAGE, and this can potentially reduce the harmful effects of circulatory AGEs.[37]

PCOS patients with IR show a significant association with vitamin D. Vitamin D regulates the expression of numerous genes, including the ones involved in the metabolism of lipids and glucose. Deficiency of vitamin D is thus linked with IR and increased free androgen index.[38] High levels of VEGF as previously mentioned are a risk factor for PCOS and vitamin D supplementation also decreases serum VEGF levels.[39]

Epigenetics

Epigenetic changes are heritable alterations in the expression of genes that are influenced by environment and behavior changes, while the underlying genomic sequences is still preserved.[40] Epigenetic changes modifying gene expression include changes in levels of DNA methylation, histone

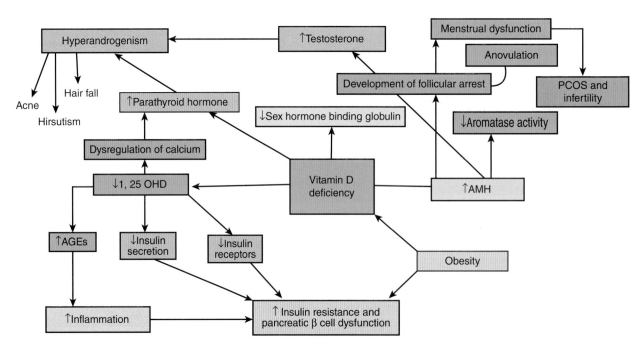

• **Fig. 4.3** Vitamin D Deficiency and Polycystic Ovary Syndrome *(PCOS)*. *AGEs,* Advanced glycation end products; *AMH,* anti-Mullerian hormone.

modification, and microRNAs (miRNAs), and these modifications have been shown to alter the development and clinical severity of PCOS.[41]

MicroRNAs

miRNAs are noncoded small RNAs molecules made of roughly 21 to 22 nucleotides. They regulate gene expression between the transcription and the translation phase via mRNA decay and subsequent cleavage and ultimately repression of translation.[42] MiRNAs interact with sites on mRNAs, most commonly the 3′ untranslated region (UTR), and decrease translation by inducing mRNA degradation. Other sites where they can bind to produce their action include 5′ UTR, gene promoters, and coding sequences. Apart from the cell cytoplasm, miRNAs have been found in a variety of bodily fluids including saliva, plasma, urine, breast milk, seminal plasma, and tears.[43]

Aberrations in miRNA have been identified in the granulosa cells, theca cells, adipose tissue, and serum of females with PCOS, suggesting their role in the pathogenesis of the disease.[42] Multiple miRNAs are implicated in the pathogenesis of PCOS, including miRNA 21, miRNA27b, miRNA-320, and miR-376a.[44,45] Although an explanation of the entirety of biochemical pathways affected by miRNAs would be out of the scope of this chapter, miRNA abnormalities have been shown to induce cellular proliferation, inhibit cell apoptosis, promote insulin resistance, downregulate estrogen production, and alter steroidogenesis in PCOS. Some notable miRNAs known to be dysregulated in PCOS patients are shown in Table 4.1. For example, miR-93 is overexpressed in granulosa cells, leading to cellular proliferation, via inhibition of cdk1a

TABLE 4.1 Notable Dysregulated Intraovarian miRNAs

miRNA	Location	Change in PCOS
miR-93[46]	Granulosa Cells	Upregulation
miR-483-5p[48]		Downregulation
miR-320[55]		
miR-145[56]		
miR-126-5p[47]		
miR-29a-5p[47]		
miR-92b[48]		
miR-92b[48]	Theca Cells	Downregulation
miR-92a[57]		
miR-233[58]	Adipose Tissue	Upregulation
miR-93[46]		Downregulation
miR-30a[59]	Follicular Fluid	Upregulation
miR-320[55]		Downregulation
miR-132[60]		
miR-140[59]		
let-7b[59]		

PCOS, Polycystic ovary syndrome.

gene.[46] Moreover, underexpression of miRs-126-5p, -29a-5p, and -92b in granulosa cells of PCOS subjects can lead to apoptosis of said cells.[47,48] The previous two statements may appear to be contradictory, yet this may have a simple explanation. In PCOS, there is rapid cellular proliferation leading to increased transition of the first follicles into the primary follicle stage, resulting in an increased proportion of follicles.[49] On the other hand, increased granulosa cell apoptosis may follow, leading to atretic follicles, ovarian insufficiency, and subsequently anovulation, as seen in PCOS.[50] Within theca cells, miR-92a and -92b are underexpressed, resulting in increased activity of *GATA6* gene and *IRS-2* gene products, respectively, leading to increased activity of CYP17 and 17a-hydroxylase and hence increased androgen production.[22,51] miR-376a was found to increase primordial follicle expression and inhibit oocyte apoptosis by regulating the expression of proliferating cell nuclear antigen.[45] Another miRNA that works by regulating PCNA is miR-155, which inhibits the release of testosterone by inhibiting PCNA, and its expression is increased in PCOS, and this may serve as a potential biomarker to supervise the effect of therapy.[52] The use of targeted therapy against specific miRNAs implicated in PCOS has been widely studied and has shown very promising results. One such miRNA is mi-R145, which suppresses granulosa cell proliferation by inhibiting IRS1 expression and consequently MAPK/EPK signaling. These findings suggest that mi-R145 can be a potential therapeutic target to improve granulosa cell irregularities.[53] Another potential treatment target for PCOS that works by inducing apoptosis of granulosa cells is miR-30d-5p and accomplishes this by targeting Smad 2.[54]

As mentioned previously, miRNAs are also found in bodily fluids and can serve as potential noninvasive biochemical markers of PCOS.[61] Currently, no single miRNA has been identified to concretely influence the pathogenesis, yet miRNAs could serve as future biomarkers for screening and detection. Results of a case control study showed significantly higher serum levels of miR-222, miR-146a, and miR-30c in cases as opposed to controls validating their use as potential biomarkers.[62] Significantly lower levels of miR-320 were reported in cases of PCOS compared with controls in another study. Because miR-320 negatively regulates serum levels of ET-1 (endothelin), significantly higher levels of ET-1 in PCOS patients show an inverse association between the two.[63] Furthermore, levels of miRNA in follicular fluid have also been studied with variable profiles across different studies. A study analyzed 176 miRNAs and found a significant difference in levels of 29 miRNAs between PCOS patients compared with controls. Out of these 29 miRNAs, 12 were associated with reproductive pathways, 12 with inflammation in disease pathways, and 6 were linked to benign pelvic disease.[64] Another study found significantly lower levels of miR-132 in PCOS subjects. Because miRNAs regulate estradiol concentration in the body, their lower levels explain lower estradiol levels in PCOS subjects.[60]

DNA Methylation

DNA methylation is a process by which the S adenosyl methionine group is added to the DNA molecule by the enzyme DNA methyltransferase. This process can involve different DNA sequences but most notably occurs at the CpG dinucleotide sequence.[41] DNA methylation decreases the transcription of the involved genes because they can no longer be recognized by RNA polymerase.

Research studying the influence of DNA methylation changes in the pathogenesis of PCOS has revealed some interesting results. A study conducted in China concluded that hypomethylation of genes could result in increased expression of genes, leading to increased synthesis of steroid hormones, including androgens, and thus explaining the hyperandrogenism observed in PCOS.[65] Hypermethylation of the promoter region of CYP19A1, which encodes aromatase, could explain the decreased activity of this enzyme in PCOS patients, leading to decreased estrogen production.[66] Similarly, another study found that high leptin levels in PCOS patients could be attributed to a decrease in methylation of the concerned gene.[67] Genome-wide association studies have revealed the thymocyte selection–associated high mobility group box (TOX3) to be hypomethylated or demethylated in PCOS patients, and this was proven by a study that revealed lower levels of TOX3 methylation, TOX3 mRNA, and TOX3 proteins in PCOS patients. It also revealed high levels of LH, thyroid stimulating hormone (TSH), testosterone, and estradiol and lower levels of FSH and prolactin in PCOS patients.[68] An interesting phenomenon was demonstrated in a study whereby the environment of the uterus of females with PCOS could alter methylation levels of certain genes related to metabolic and reproductive pathways and the derangements are carried to both male and female newborns of these mothers.[69]

Genetics

The role of genes in the development of PCOS has long been a topic of interest for decades and has led to many studies trying to establish the association. PCOS has long been considered an autosomal dominant disorder as first identified by Cooper et al. in 1968; however, twin studies conducted in 11 pairs of mono and dizygotic twins point toward an X-linked polygenic inheritance.[70,71] It is thought to occur because of a complex interaction between multiple genes and environmental factors, which can be both intrauterine and extrauterine.[71]

The genetic association is reflected by the high prevalence of PCOS in families, with studies reporting prevalence ranging from 24% to 32% in female relatives (mothers, sisters) of known PCOS patients.[72] Similarly, male relatives have shared characteristics of the syndrome, including IR and endothelial cell dysfunction.[73] Studies have also shown them to be more likely to develop metabolic syndrome, dyslipidemia, and hypertension.[74] Significantly elevated levels of DHEAS in both brothers and sisters of females with PCOS may point toward a shared defect in steroidogenesis.[75]

The complexity of PCOS is evident by the fact that many genes are implicated in its pathogenesis (Fig. 4.4):

1. *CYP11a* encodes for p450, which converts cholesterol to pregnenolone and is the rate-limiting step of steroidogenesis.[76] Gharani et al. show variation in *CYP11a* to be associated with hyperandrogenemia, which is a characteristic

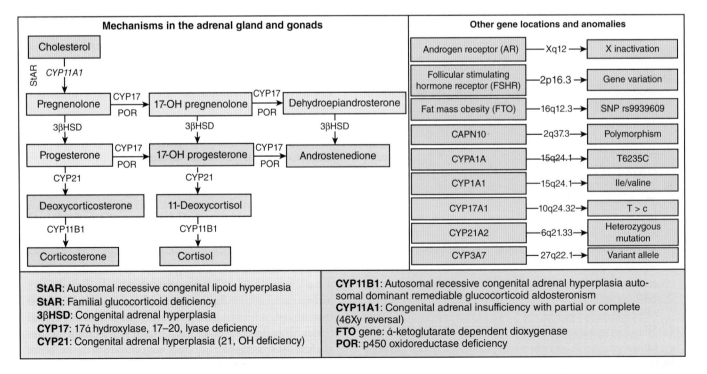

• **Fig. 4.4** The Role of Genes Involved in the Development and Progression of Polycystic Ovary Syndrome (PCOS).

feature of PCOS.[77] Another case-control study conducted in China concluded that polymorphisms in *CYP11A1* are strongly associated with PCOS.[78]

2. *CYP21* encodes for a p450, which converts 17 hydroxy-progesterone to 11 deoxycortisol.[76] A study concluded that in females with hyperandrogenism, heterozygosity for CYP21 was increased.[79]

3. *CYP17* encodes 17 alpha-hydroxylase, which converts pregnenolone and progesterone to 17 shydroxy pregnenolone and 17 hydroxyprogesterone, respectively. These products are then converted to *DHEA* and androstenedione via 17,20 lyase, which is encoded by the same enzyme.[76] Rahimi et al. concluded there is a 2.31 times susceptibility to PCOS in those with *CYP17 TC* genotype compared with control.[80] A2 allele variations of *CYP17* are a significant factor modifying the expression of polycystic ovaries.[81]

4. *CYP19* encodes aromatase, which converts androgens to female sex steroids, in particular estrogen.[76] Multiple studies found single nucleotide polymorphisms (SNP) 2414096 in the *CYP19* gene to be associated with an increased risk of PCOS.[82,83]

5. *StAR* is the short form for "steroidogenic acute regulatory protein." The first step of steroid biosynthesis starts with cholesterol, and StAR is a transport protein responsible for transporting cholesterol through the mitochondrial membrane.[84] Hyperandrogenism in PCOS can be because of increased activity at the very first step involving StAR as demonstrated by Melissa et al.[85]

6. The *AR* (androgen receptor) gene encodes the androgen receptor and is located at Xq11-12 on the X chromosome.[86] Stretches of polyglutamine are encoded by CAG trinucleotide repeats, and the activity of AR is inversely related to the number of CAG repeats.[87] Therefore one possible cause of hyperandrogenism symptoms in patients with normal androgen levels could be fewer CAG repeats, leading to increased AR activity.[88]

7. The *SHBG* gene encodes a serum protein that binds androgens and controls circulating hormone levels in the body.[89] It is located on p12-p13 bands on chromosome 17.[90] A meta-analysis of 62 articles found significantly lower levels of SHBG in PCOS patients compared with controls, highlighting its possible role in the pathogenesis of PCOS.[89]

8. *DENDD1A* is a protein-encoding gene found in theca cells. The gene has previously been associated with metabolic and reproductive abnormalities in PCOS patients. DENDD1A encodes two variants, namely, V1 and V2, and they have been implicated with increased androgen production by way of increasing expression of certain enzymes involved in androgen biosynthetic pathway. A study performed whole genome sequencing on 62 families having at least one case of PCOS and found at least one variant of *DENND1A* in 50% of the studied families[91]

Other genes known to be involved in PCOS pathogenesis include genes encoding for the LH and FSH receptors.[92,93] LH is an important regulator of ovarian androgenesis and plays a role in folliculogenesis, induction of ovulation, and estrogen production.[94] LH mediates its actions by acting on LH receptors located on multiple ovarian cells, including theca, luteal, and granulosa cells.[95] High circulating LH levels are a defining feature of PCOS, and this, in turn, leads to increased androgen production. Polymorphisms in LHβ and LH receptors have been associated with PCOS, and the majority of affected females had elevated levels of LH.[92] Moreover, studies have also found high expression of LH receptor on theca and granulosa cells of PCOS patients.[96] Similarly, polymorphisms in the gene encoding for FSH are associated with alteration in the phenotype of PCOS.[93] Studies have also found genes responsible for insulin production and action like the insulin *VNTR* (variable number tandem repeat) gene, *IGF 2* genes, and Calpain 10 to be implicated in the pathogenesis of the syndrome.[97,98]

References

1. Kirschner MA, Bardin CW. Androgen production and metabolism in normal and virilized women. *Metabolism*. 1972;21(7):667-688. doi:10.1016/0026-0495(72)90090-x.
2. Dadachanji R, Shaikh N, Mukherjee S. Genetic variants associated with hyperandrogenemia in PCOS pathophysiology. *Genet Res Int*. 2018;2018:7624932. doi:10.1155/2018/7624932.
3. Rosenfield RL, Ehrmann DA. The Pathogenesis of Polycystic Ovary Syndrome (PCOS): the hypothesis of PCOS as functional ovarian hyperandrogenism revisited. *Endocr Rev*. 2016;37(5):467-520. doi:10.1210/er.2015-1104.
4. Abbott DH, Dumesic DA, Eisner JR, Colman RJ, Kemnitz JW. Insights into the development of polycystic ovary syndrome (PCOS) from studies of prenatally androgenized female rhesus monkeys. *Trends Endocrinol Metab*. 1998;9(2):62-67. doi:10.1016/s1043-2760(98)00019-8.
5. Padmanabhan V, Veiga-Lopez A. Reproduction symposium: developmental programming of reproductive and metabolic health. *J Anim Sci*. 2014;92(8):3199-3210. doi:10.2527/jas.2014-7637.
6. Morel Y, Roucher F, Plotton I, Goursaud C, Tardy V, Mallet D. Evolution of steroids during pregnancy: maternal, placental and fetal synthesis. *Ann Endocrinol (Paris)*. 2016;77(2):82-89. doi:10.1016/j.ando.2016.04.023.
7. Puttabyatappa M, Cardoso RC, Padmanabhan V. Effect of maternal PCOS and PCOS-like phenotype on the offspring's health. *Mol Cell Endocrinol*. 2016;435:29-39. doi:10.1016/j.mce.2015.11.030.
8. Clarke IJ, Cummins JT. GnRH pulse frequency determines LH pulse amplitude by altering the amount of releasable LH in the pituitary glands of ewes. *J Reprod Fertil*. 1985;73(2):425-431. doi:10.1530/jrf.0.0730425.
9. Liao B, Qiao J, Pang Y. Central regulation of PCOS: abnormal neuronal-reproductive-metabolic circuits in PCOS pathophysiology. *Front Endocrinol (Lausanne)*. 2021;12:667422. doi:10.3389/fendo.2021.667422.
10. Ohtaki T, Shintani Y, Honda S, et al. Metastasis suppressor gene KiSS-1 encodes peptide ligand of a G-protein-coupled receptor. *Nature*. 2001;411(6837):613-617. doi:10.1038/35079135.
11. Tang R, Ding X, Zhu J. Kisspeptin and polycystic ovary syndrome. *Front Endocrinol (Lausanne)*. 2019;10:298. doi:10.3389/fendo.2019.00298.
12. Ruddenklau A, Campbell RE. Neuroendocrine impairments of polycystic ovary syndrome. *Endocrinology*. 2019;160(10):2230-2242. doi:10.1210/en.2019-00428.

13. Carmina E, Koyama T, Chang L, Stanczyk FZ, Lobo RA. Does ethnicity influence the prevalence of adrenal hyperandrogenism and insulin resistance in polycystic ovary syndrome? *Am J Obstet Gynecol.* 1992;167(6):1807-1812. doi:10.1016/0002-9378(92)91779-a.

14. Kumar A, Woods KS, Bartolucci AA, Azziz R. Prevalence of adrenal androgen excess in patients with the polycystic ovary syndrome (PCOS). *Clin Endocrinol (Oxf).* 2005;62(6):644-649. doi:10.1111/j.1365-2265.2005.02256.x.

15. Rosenfield RL. Evidence that idiopathic functional adrenal hyperandrogenism is caused by dysregulation of adrenal steroidogenesis and that hyperinsulinemia may be involved. *J Clin Endocrinol Metab.* 1996;81(3):878-880. doi:10.1210/jcem.81.3.8772543.

16. Rainey WE, Carr BR, Sasano H, Suzuki T, Mason JI. Dissecting human adrenal androgen production. Trends. *Endocrinol Metab.* 2002;13(6):234-239. doi:10.1016/s1043-2760(02)00609-4.

17. Tosi F, Bonora E, Moghetti P. Insulin resistance in a large cohort of women with polycystic ovary syndrome: a comparison between euglycaemic-hyperinsulinaemic clamp and surrogate indexes. *Hum Reprod.* 2017;32(12):2515-2521. doi:10.1093/humrep/dex308.

18. Corbould A, Kim YB, Youngren JF, et al. Insulin resistance in the skeletal muscle of women with PCOS involves intrinsic and acquired defects in insulin signaling. *Am J Physiol Endocrinol Metab.* 2005;288(5):E1047-E1054. doi:10.1152/ajpendo.00361.2004.

19. Dunaif A, Xia J, Book CB, Schenker E, Tang Z. Excessive insulin receptor serine phosphorylation in cultured fibroblasts and in skeletal muscle. A potential mechanism for insulin resistance in the polycystic ovary syndrome. *J Clin Invest.* 1995;96(2):801-810. doi:10.1172/jci118126.

20. Poretsky L, Cataldo NA, Rosenwaks Z, Giudice LC. The insulin-related ovarian regulatory system in health and disease. *Endocr Rev.* 1999;20(4):535-582. doi:10.1210/edrv.20.4.0374.

21. Pugeat M, Crave JC, Elmidani M, et al. Pathophysiology of sex hormone binding globulin (SHBG): relation to insulin. *J Steroid Biochem Mol Biol.* 1991;40(4-6):841-849. doi:10.1016/0960-0760(91)90310-2.

22. Munir I, Yen HW, Geller DH, et al. Insulin augmentation of 17alpha-hydroxylase activity is mediated by phosphatidyl inositol 3-kinase but not extracellular signal-regulated kinase-1/2 in human ovarian theca cells. *Endocrinology.* 2004;145(1):175-183. doi:10.1210/en.2003-0329.

23. Nestler JE, Strauss JF III. Insulin as an effector of human ovarian and adrenal steroid metabolism. *Endocrinol Metab Clin North Am.* 1991;20(4):807-823.

24. Baptiste CG, Battista MC, Trottier A, Baillargeon JP. Insulin and hyperandrogenism in women with polycystic ovary syndrome. *J Steroid Biochem Mol Biol.* 2010;122(1-3):42-52. doi:10.1016/j.jsbmb.2009.12.010.

25. Rice S, Christoforidis N, Gadd C, et al. Impaired insulin-dependent glucose metabolism in granulosa-lutein cells from anovulatory women with polycystic ovaries. *Hum Reprod.* 2005;20(2):373-381. doi:10.1093/humrep/deh609.

26. Geva E, Jaffe RB. Role of vascular endothelial growth factor in ovarian physiology and pathology. *Fertil Steril.* 2000;74(3):429-438. doi:10.1016/s0015-0282(00)00670-1.

27. Li Y, Fang L, Yu Y, et al. Association between vascular endothelial growth factor gene polymorphisms and PCOS risk: a meta-analysis. *Reprod Biomed Online.* 2020;40(2):287-295. doi:10.1016/j.rbmo.2019.10.018.

28. Agrawal R, Conway G, Sladkevicius P, et al. Serum vascular endothelial growth factor and Doppler blood flow velocities in in vitro fertilization: relevance to ovarian hyperstimulation syndrome and polycystic ovaries. *Fertil Steril.* 1998;70(4):651-658. doi:10.1016/s0015-0282(98)00249-0.

29. Bao L, Syed R, Aloahd MS. Analysis of VEGF gene polymorphisms and serum VEGF protein levels contribution in polycystic ovary syndrome of patients. *Mol Biol Rep.* 2019;46(6):5821-5829. doi:10.1007/s11033-019-05015-y.

30. Mu Y, Cheng D, Yin TL, Yang J. Vitamin D and polycystic ovary syndrome: a narrative review. *Reprod Sci.* 2021;28(8):2110-2117. doi:10.1007/s43032-020-00369-2.

31. Lin MW, Wu MH. The role of vitamin D in polycystic ovary syndrome. *Indian J Med Res.* 2015;142(3):238-240. doi:10.4103/0971-5916.166527.

32. Zec I, Tislaric-Medenjak D, Megla ZB, Kucak I. Anti-Müllerian hormone: a unique biochemical marker of gonadal development and fertility in humans. *Biochem Med (Zagreb).* 2011;21(3):219-230. doi:10.11613/bm.2011.031.

33. Pigny P, Jonard S, Robert Y, Dewailly D. Serum anti-Mullerian hormone as a surrogate for antral follicle count for definition of the polycystic ovary syndrome. *J Clin Endocrinol Metab.* 2006;91(3):941-945. doi:10.1210/jc.2005-2076.

34. Diamanti-Kandarakis E. Polycystic ovarian syndrome: pathophysiology, molecular aspects and clinical implications. *Expert Rev Mol Med.* 2008;10:e3. doi:10.1017/s1462399408000598.

35. Kuyucu Y, Çelik LS, Kendirlinan Ö, Tap Ö, Mete U. Investigation of the uterine structural changes in the experimental model with polycystic ovary syndrome and effects of vitamin D treatment: an ultrastructural and immunohistochemical study. *Reprod Biol.* 2018;18(1):53-59. doi:10.1016/j.repbio.2018.01.002.

36. Merhi Z. Advanced glycation end products and their relevance in female reproduction. *Hum Reprod.* 2014;29(1):135-145. doi:10.1093/humrep/det383.

37. Irani M, Minkoff H, Seifer DB, Merhi Z. Vitamin D increases serum levels of the soluble receptor for advanced glycation end products in women with PCOS. *J Clin Endocrinol Metab.* 2014;99(5):E886-E890. doi:10.1210/jc.2013-4374.

38. Irani M, Merhi Z. Role of vitamin D in ovarian physiology and its implication in reproduction: a systematic review. *Fertil Steril.* 2014;102(2):460-468.e3. doi:10.1016/j.fertnstert.2014.04.046.

39. Irani M, Seifer DB, Grazi RV, Irani S, Rosenwaks Z, Tal R. Vitamin D decreases serum VEGF correlating with clinical improvement in vitamin D-deficient women with PCOS: a randomized placebo-controlled trial. *Nutrients.* 2017;9(4):334. doi:10.3390/nu9040334.

40. Xu N, Azziz R, Goodarzi MO. Epigenetics in polycystic ovary syndrome: a pilot study of global DNA methylation. *Fertil Steril.* 2010;94(2):781-783.e1. doi:10.1016/j.fertnstert.2009.10.020.

41. Jin Z, Liu Y. DNA methylation in human diseases. *Genes Dis.* 2018;5(1):1-8. doi:10.1016/j.gendis.2018.01.002.

42. Chen B, Xu P, Wang J, Zhang C. The role of MiRNA in polycystic ovary syndrome (PCOS). *Gene.* 2019;706:91-96. Available at: https://doi.org/10.1016/j.gene.2019.04.082.

43. O'Brien J, Hayder H, Zayed Y, Peng C. Overview of MicroRNA biogenesis, mechanisms of actions, and circulation. *Front Endocrinol (Lausanne).* 2018;9:402. doi:10.3389/fendo.2018.00402.

44. Butler AE, Ramachandran V, Sathyapalan T, et al. microRNA Expression in women with and without polycystic ovarian syndrome matched for body mass index. *Front Endocrinol (Lausanne).* 2020;11:206. doi:10.3389/fendo.2020.00206.

45. Zhang H, Jiang X, Zhang Y, et al. microRNA 376a regulates follicle assembly by targeting PCNA in fetal and neonatal mouse ovaries. *Reproduction (Cambridge, England)*. 2014;148(1):43-54. doi:10.1530/rep-13-0508.

46. Jiang L, Huang J, Li L, et al. MicroRNA-93 promotes ovarian granulosa cells proliferation through targeting CDKN1A in polycystic ovarian syndrome. *J Clin Endocrinol Metab*. 2015;100(5):E729-E738. doi:10.1210/jc.2014-3827.

47. Mao Z, Fan L, Yu Q, et al. Abnormality of klotho signaling is involved in polycystic ovary syndrome. *Reprod Sci*. 2018;25(3):372-383. doi:10.1177/1933719117715129.

48. Xu B, Zhang YW, Tong XH, Liu YS. Characterization of microRNA profile in human cumulus granulosa cells: identification of microRNAs that regulate Notch signaling and are associated with PCOS. *Mol Cell Endocrinol*. 2015;404:26-36. doi:10.1016/j.mce.2015.01.030.

49. Das M, Djahanbakhch O, Hacihanefioglu B, et al. Granulosa cell survival and proliferation are altered in polycystic ovary syndrome. *J Clin Endocrinol Metab*. 2008;93(3):881-887. doi:10.1210/jc.2007-1650.

50. Worku T, Rehman ZU, Talpur HS, et al. MicroRNAs: new insight in modulating follicular atresia: a review. *Int J Mol Sci*. 2017;18(2):333. doi:10.3390/ijms18020333.

51. Ho CKM, Wood JR, Stewart DR, et al. Increased transcription and increased messenger ribonucleic acid (mRNA) stability contribute to increased GATA6 mRNA abundance in polycystic ovary syndrome theca cells. *J Clin Endocrinol Metab*. 2005;90(12):6596-6602. doi:10.1210/jc.2005-0890.

52. Arancio W, Calogero Amato M, et al. Serum miRNAs in women affected by hyperandrogenic polycystic ovary syndrome: the potential role of miR-155 as a biomarker for monitoring the estro-progestinic treatment. *Gynecol Endocrinol*. 2018;34(8):704-708. doi:10.1080/09513590.2018.1428299.

53. Cai G, Ma X, Chen B, et al. MicroRNA-145 Negatively regulates cell proliferation through targeting IRS1 in isolated ovarian granulosa cells from patients with polycystic ovary syndrome. *Reprod Sci*. 2017;24(6):902-910. doi:10.1177/1933719116673197.

54. Yu M, Liu J. MicroRNA-30d-5p promotes ovarian granulosa cell apoptosis by targeting Smad2. *Exp Ther Med*. 2020;19(1):53-60. doi:10.3892/etm.2019.8184.

55. Yin M, Wang X, Yao G, et al. Transactivation of micrornA-320 by microRNA-383 regulates granulosa cell functions by targeting E2F1 and SF-1 proteins. *J Biol Chem*. 2014;289(26):18239-18257. doi:10.1074/jbc.M113.546044.

56. Zhang CL, Wang H, Yan CY, Gao XF, Ling XJ. Deregulation of RUNX2 by miR-320a deficiency impairs steroidogenesis in cumulus granulosa cells from polycystic ovary syndrome (PCOS) patients. *Biochem Biophys Res Commun*. 2017;482(4):1469-1476. doi:10.1016/j.bbrc.2016.12.059.

57. Lin L, Du T, Huang J, Huang LL, Yang DZ. Identification of differentially expressed microRNAs in the ovary of polycystic ovary syndrome with hyperandrogenism and insulin resistance. *Chin Med J (Engl)*. 2015;128(2):169-174. doi:10.4103/0366-6999.149189.

58. Chuang TY, Wu HL, Chen CC, et al. MicroRNA-223 expression is upregulated in insulin resistant human adipose tissue. *J Diabetes Res*. 2015;2015:943659. doi:10.1155/2015/943659.

59. Scalici E, Traver S, Mullet T, et al. Circulating microRNAs in follicular fluid, powerful tools to explore in vitro fertilization process. *Sci Rep*. 2016;6(1):24976. doi:10.1038/srep24976.

60. Sang Q, Yao Z, Wang H, et al. Identification of microRNAs in human follicular fluid: characterization of microRNAs that govern steroidogenesis in vitro and are associated with polycystic ovary syndrome in vivo. *J Clin Endocrinol Metab*. 2013;98(7):3068-3079. doi:10.1210/jc.2013-1715.

61. Abdalla M, Deshmukh H, Atkin SL, Sathyapalan T. miRNAs as a novel clinical biomarker and therapeutic targets in polycystic ovary syndrome (PCOS): a review. *Life Sci*. 2020;259:118174. doi:10.1016/j.lfs.2020.118174.

62. Long W, Zhao C, Ji C, et al. Characterization of serum microRNAs profile of PCOS and identification of novel non-invasive biomarkers. *Cell Physiol Biochem*. 2014;33(5):1304-1315. doi:10.1159/000358698.

63. Rashad NM, Ateya MA, Saraya YS, et al. Association of miRNA-320 expression level and its target gene endothelin-1 with the susceptibility and clinical features of polycystic ovary syndrome. *J Ovarian Res*. 2019;12(1):39. doi:10.1186/s13048-019-0513-5.

64. Butler AE, Ramachandran V, Hayat S, et al. Expression of microRNA in follicular fluid in women with and without PCOS. *Sci Rep*. 2019;9(1):16306. doi:10.1038/s41598-019-52856-5.

65. Pan JX, Tan YJ, Wang FF, et al. Aberrant expression and DNA methylation of lipid metabolism genes in PCOS: a new insight into its pathogenesis. *Clin Epigenetics*. 2018;10(1):6. doi:10.1186/s13148-018-0442-y.

66. Yu YY, Sun CX, Liu YK, Li Y, Wang L, Zhang W. Promoter methylation of CYP19A1 gene in Chinese polycystic ovary syndrome patients. *Gynecol Obstet Invest*. 2013;76(4):209-213. doi:10.1159/000355314.

67. Liu L, He D, Wang Y, Sheng M. Integrated analysis of DNA methylation and transcriptome profiling of polycystic ovary syndrome. *Mol Med Rep*. 2020;21(5):2138-2150. doi:10.3892/mmr.2020.11005.

68. Ning Z, Jiayi L, Jian R, Wanli X. Relationship between abnormal TOX3 gene methylation and polycystic ovarian syndrome. *Eur Rev Med Pharmacol Sci*. 2017;21(9):2034-2038.

69. Echiburú B, Milagro F, Crisosto N, et al. DNA methylation in promoter regions of genes involved in the reproductive and metabolic function of children born to women with PCOS. *Epigenetics*. 2020;15(11):1178-1194. doi:10.1080/15592294.2020.1754674.

70. Cooper HE, Spellacy W, Prem K, Cohen WD. Hereditary factors in the Stein-Leventhal syndrome. *Am J Obstet Gynecol*. 1968;100(3):371-387.

71. Jahanfar S, Eden JA, Warren P, Seppälä M, Nguyen TV. A twin study of polycystic ovary syndrome. *Fertil Steril*. 1995;63(3):478-486.

72. Kahsar-Miller MD, Nixon C, Boots LR, Go RC, Azziz R. Prevalence of polycystic ovary syndrome (PCOS) in first-degree relatives of patients with PCOS. *Fertil Steril*. 2001;75(1):53-58. doi:10.1016/s0015-0282(00)01662-9.

73. Kaushal R, Parchure N, Bano G, Kaski JC, Nussey SS. Insulin resistance and endothelial dysfunction in the brothers of Indian subcontinent Asian women with polycystic ovaries. *Clin Endocrinol (Oxf)*. 2004;60(3):322-328. doi:10.1111/j.1365-2265.2004.01981.x.

74. Coviello AD, Sam S, Legro RS, Dunaif A. High prevalence of metabolic syndrome in first-degree male relatives of women with polycystic ovary syndrome is related to high rates of obesity. *J Clin Endocrinol Metab*. 2009;94(11):4361-4366. doi:10.1210/jc.2009-1333.

75. Legro RS, Kunselman AR, Demers L, Wang SC, Bentley-Lewis R, Dunaif A. Elevated dehydroepiandrosterone sulfate levels as the reproductive phenotype in the brothers of women with polycystic ovary syndrome. *J Clin Endocrinol Metab*. 2002;87(5):2134-2138. doi:10.1210/jcem.87.5.8387.

76. Payne AH, Hales DB. Overview of steroidogenic enzymes in the pathway from cholesterol to active steroid hormones. *Endocr Rev.* 2004;25(6):947-970. doi:10.1210/er.2003-0030.

77. Gharani N, Waterworth DM, Batty S, et al. Association of the steroid synthesis gene CYP11a with polycystic ovary syndrome and hyperandrogenism. *Hum Mol Genet.* 1997;6(3):397-402. doi:10.1093/hmg/6.3.397.

78. Zhang CW, Zhang XL, Xia YJ, et al. Association between polymorphisms of the CYP11A1 gene and polycystic ovary syndrome in Chinese women. *Mol Biol Rep.* 2012;39(8):8379-8385. doi:10.1007/s11033-012-1688-7.

79. Witchel SF, Aston CE. The role of heterozygosity for CYP21 in the polycystic ovary syndrome. *J Pediatr Endocrinol Metab.* 2000;13(suppl 5):1315-1317.

80. Rahimi Z, Mohammadi MSE. The CYP17 MSP AI (T-34C) and CYP19A1 (Trp39Arg) variants in polycystic ovary syndrome: a case-control study. *Int J Reprod Biomed.* 2019;17(3):201-208. doi:10.18502/ijrm.v17i3.4519.

81. Carey AH, Waterworth D, Patel K, et al. Polycystic ovaries and premature male pattern baldness are associated with one allele of the steroid metabolism gene CYP17. *Hum Mol Genet.* 1994;3(10):1873-1876. doi:10.1093/hmg/3.10.1873.

82. Ashraf S, Rasool SUA, Nabi M, Ganie MA, Masoodi SR, Amin S. Impact of rs2414096 polymorphism of CYP19 gene on susceptibility of polycystic ovary syndrome and hyperandrogenism in Kashmiri women. *Sci Rep.* 2021;11(1):12942. doi:10.1038/s41598-021-92265-1.

83. Mehdizadeh A, Kalantar SM, Sheikhha MH, Aali BS, Ghanei A. Association of SNP rs.2414096 CYP19 gene with polycystic ovarian syndrome in Iranian women. *Int J Reprod Biomed.* 2017;15(8):491-496.

84. Miller WL. Steroidogenic acute regulatory protein (StAR), a novel mitochondrial cholesterol transporter. *Biochim Biophys Acta.* 2007;1771(6):663-676. doi:10.1016/j.bbalip.2007.02.012.

85. Kahsar-Miller MD, Conway-Myers BA, Boots LR, Azziz R. Steroidogenic acute regulatory protein (StAR) in the ovaries of healthy women and those with polycystic ovary syndrome. *Am J Obstet Gynecol.* 2001;185(6):1381-1387. doi:10.1067/mob.2001.118656.

86. Trapman J, Klaassen P, Kuiper GG, et al. Cloning, structure and expression of a cDNA encoding the human androgen receptor. *Biochem Biophys Res Commun.* 1988;153(1):241-248. doi:10.1016/s0006-291x(88)81214-2.

87. Chamberlain NL, Driver ED, Miesfeld RL. The length and location of CAG trinucleotide repeats in the androgen receptor N-terminal domain affect transactivation function. *Nucleic Acids Res.* 1994;22(15):3181-3186. doi:10.1093/nar/22.15.3181.

88. Mifsud A, Ramirez S, Yong EL. Androgen receptor gene CAG trinucleotide repeats in anovulatory infertility and polycystic ovaries. *J Clin Endocrinol Metab.* 2000;85(9):3484-3488. doi:10.1210/jcem.85.9.6832.

89. Deswal R, Yadav A, Dang AS. Sex hormone binding globulin - an important biomarker for predicting PCOS risk: a systematic review and meta-analysis. *Syst Biol Reprod Med.* 2018;64(1):12-24. doi:10.1080/19396368.2017.1410591.

90. Bérubé D, Séralini GE, Gagné R, Hammond GL. Localization of the human sex hormone-binding globulin gene (SHBG) to the short arm of chromosome 17 (17p12–p13). *Cytogenet Cell Genet.* 1990;54(1-2):65-67. doi:10.1159/000132958.

91. Dapas M, Sisk R, Legro RS, Urbanek M, Dunaif A, Hayes MG. Family-based quantitative trait meta-analysis implicates rare noncoding variants in DENND1A in polycystic ovary syndrome. *J Clin Endocrinol Metab.* 2019;104(9):3835-3850. doi:10.1210/jc.2018-02496.

92. Deswal R, Nanda S, Dang AS. Association of Luteinizing hormone and LH receptor gene polymorphism with susceptibility of polycystic ovary syndrome. *Syst Biol Reprod Med.* 2019;65(5):400-408. doi:10.1080/19396368.2019.1595217.

93. Laven JSE. Follicle stimulating hormone receptor (FSHR) polymorphisms and polycystic ovary syndrome (PCOS). *Front Endocrinol (Lausanne).* 2019;10:23. doi:10.3389/fendo.2019.00023.

94. Howles CM. Role of LH and FSH in ovarian function. *Mol Cell Endocrinol.* 2000;161(1-2):25-30. doi:10.1016/s0303-7207(99)00219-1.

95. Choi J, Smitz J. Luteinizing hormone and human chorionic gonadotropin: origins of difference. *Mol Cell Endocrinol.* 2014;383(1-2):203-213. doi:10.1016/j.mce.2013.12.009.

96. Jakimiuk AJ, Weitsman SR, Navab A, Magoffin DA. Luteinizing hormone receptor, steroidogenesis acute regulatory protein, and steroidogenic enzyme messenger ribonucleic acids are overexpressed in thecal and granulosa cells from polycystic ovaries. *J Clin Endocrinol Metab.* 2001;86(3):1318-1323. doi:10.1210/jcem.86.3.7318.

97. Ajmal N, Khan SZ, Shaikh R. Polycystic ovary syndrome (PCOS) and genetic predisposition: a review article. *Eur J Obstet Gynecol Reprod Biol X.* 2019;3:100060. doi:10.1016/j.eurox.2019.100060.

98. Ferk P, Perme MP, Gersak K. Insulin gene polymorphism in women with polycystic ovary syndrome. *J Int Med Res.* 2008;36(6):1180-1187. doi:10.1177/147323000803600603.

5

Interplay of Adipocytokines With Polycystic Ovary Syndrome

MUKHTIAR BAIG, TAUSEEF AHMAD, AND SABA TARIQ

Introduction

Adipose tissues essentially maintain body homeostasis. The released bioactive substances of adipose tissue regulate glucose and lipid metabolism, as well as energy and immune system activity. Adipose tissue inflammation activates signaling pathways that have been shown to disrupt metabolic homeostasis.[1] Moreover, the dysregulation routes of bioactive substances cause metabolic abnormalities and chronic consequences, particularly in obese people.[2,3]

Adipokines are bioactive substances generated solely by adipose tissue, whereas adipocytokines are produced by various cells, including fat cells.[4] Other organs that produce adipocytokines include the ovaries, placenta, liver, kidney, muscles, heart, bone marrow, and peripheral mononuclear cells.[5] Nonetheless, to avoid confusion, the name "adipokine" refers to these bioactive molecules throughout this review.

Adipokines can be pro- or anti-inflammatory. Obesity was found to increase proinflammatory adipokines and decrease anti-inflammatory adipokines[6] that uphold a low-grade inflammatory response for an extended period.[7] A substantial number of studies worldwide have shown that adipokines play a role in the pathogenesis of diseases that affect nearly all body systems.[8] Additionally, research has established that adipokines are critical in the etiology of obesity and obesity-related disorders.[9] Various characteristics of adipokines are shown in Table 5.1 and Fig. 5.1.

Polycystic ovary syndrome (PCOS) is the most frequent endocrine-metabolic illness in reproductive-aged females. Patients with PCOS are more likely to develop metabolic problems such as type 2 diabetes mellitus (T2DM), insulin resistance (IR), and adipose tissue malfunction.[28,29] PCOS patients have 10 times the rate of T2DM as the general population, and glucose intolerance is 30% to 50% greater in obese PCOS patients.[30] IR affects between 10% to 25% of the general population, whereas PCOS individuals are at a two to three times higher risk of IR.[31] Furthermore, patients with PCOS have a higher rate of obesity than those without the condition.[32] PCOS symptoms are significantly worsened in those who have both PCOS and obesity, but the mechanisms of PCOS are unknown. Many studies have established that obese PCOS patients have frequent adipose tissue malfunctioning and consequently altered adipokine levels, showing that adipokines have a role in PCOS patients.[33,34]

One theory states that variations in adipokine levels in PCOS patients are driven by obesity rather than PCOS.[15] This is demonstrated in that adipokine levels are proportional to body mass index (BMI), and PCOS patients have a higher BMI.[35] Furthermore, a meta-analysis (MA) discovered that females with PCOS have a higher prevalence of overweight obesity and central obesity.[32] An MA included data on nonobese PCOS patients to testify to this notion of the influence of obesity on adipokine levels and to assess the connections between PCOS and adipokine levels.[15] Nevertheless, MA findings demonstrated a change in adipokine levels in nonobese PCOS individuals; thus the results invalidate the theory that obesity rather than PCOS causes modifications in adipokine levels in PCOS patients. It implies that adipokines may have a role in PCOS patients regardless of their weight; however, the precise mechanism through which adipokines contribute to the development of PCOS is unknown.

Determining variations in circulating adipokine levels in PCOS patients has recently grown in popularity. It has also been postulated that these adipokines may play a role in the etiology of PCOS. Vaspin, chemerin, resistin,[36,37] leptin,[38,39] chemerin,[40,41] omentin,[23] adiponectin,[42] and visfatin[18] have all been associated with PCOS in previous investigations using a systematic review and MA technique (Table 5.2).

Nevertheless, the literature is scanty and incomplete with discordant results. Researchers are still trying to figure out what role each adipokine plays in PCOS. Presently, therefore, the role of adipokines in PCOS is a hot topic of discussion. Findings that interplay between adipokines and PCOS may help clinicians better diagnose and manage PCOS and its problems. The current review would include existing evidence on the interaction between adipokines and PCOS.

TABLE 5.1	Adipokines Production Site and Relation to Inflammation, Reproductive Function, and Metabolic Function			
Adipokine	Production site	Relation to Inflammation	Relation to Reproductive function	Relation to Metabolic function
Adiponectin[5,10,11]	Adipocytes placenta, osteoblasts, cardiomyocytes	Anti-inflammatory	Pubertal onset and regulation	Fatty acid oxidation, insulin sensitivity, glucose metabolism
Leptin[12-14]	Adipose tissue placenta	Regulation of immune response	Regulation of gonadotropin secretion	Regulation of food intake, lipid and glucose metabolism
Resistin[11,15,16]	Peripheral-blood mononuclear cells, placenta	Regulation of inflammatory response	Ovarian function and PCOS	Insulin resistance
Visfatin[17,18]	Adipose tissue, liver, muscle, kidney, heart, bone marrow, placenta	Regulation of inflammatory response	Ovarian function and PCOS	Insulin resistance, glucose metabolism
Apelin[19-21]	Brain, uterus, ovary, lungs, small arteries of endothelium	Regulation of inflammatory response	Ovarian function and PCOS	Augment secretion of estradiol and progesterone
Omentin[22-24]	Visceral depots of adipose tissues	Upregulated by proinflammatory conditions	Ovarian function and PCOS	Insulin resistance, glucose metabolism
Chemerin[25-27]	Adipose tissues G-protein coupled receptor	Negative regulator of ovarian steroidogenesis	Ovarian function and PCOS	Suppress FSH-induced expression of p450 enzymes

FSH, Follicle-stimulating hormone; *PCOS*, polycystic ovary syndrome.

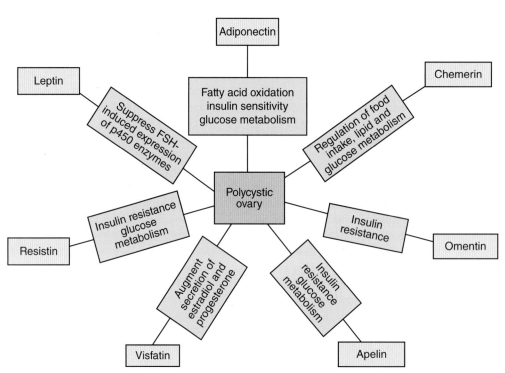

• **Fig. 5.1** Graphical Representation of the Effect of Various Adipocytokines in Polycystic Ovary Syndrome (PCOS). *FSH*, Follicle-stimulating hormone.

TABLE 5.2   Several Meta-Analysis Findings Regarding the Role of Adipokines in PCOS

Study	No. of Studies	No. of Subjects (Case/Control)	Findings in PCOS	Conclusion
Lin et al., 2021[15]	71	5015(2495/2520)	Serum adiponectin = Lower Serum chemerin and resistin = Higher Apelin and omentin = No change	Regardless of the degree of obesity, dys-regulated adipokine levels may play critical roles in the onset and progression of PCOS.
Mehrabani et al., 2021[36]	77	8239	Serum vaspin, chemerin, and resistin = Higher Serum apelin levels = No change	The levels of serum vaspin, chemerin, and resistin can be used to predict the onset of PCOS.
Mansoori et al. 2022[41]	22	2256 (1191/1065)	Serum and FF chemerin and mRNA expression = Higher	Chemerin may be linked to both PCOS and BMI independently.
Wang et al., 2022[40]	8	897(524/373)	Serum chemerin = Higher	Chemerin could play a role in the etiology of PCOS.
Raeisi et al., 2021[37]	38	4328(2424/1904)	Serum resistin = Higher	Serum resistin may play a role in PCOS pathogenesis.
Seth et al., 2021[38]	35	3782(2015/1767)	Serum leptin = No change (in high methodologic quality studies) Serum leptin = Higher (in low methodologic quality studies)	In high-methodologic-quality research, serum leptin is not linked to the risk of PCOS. More research is required.
Zheng et al., 2017[39]	19	1889(991/898)	Serum leptin = Higher	Higher leptin levels were associated with IR, metabolic disorder, infertility, and even cardiovascular disease risk in PCOS, suggesting that they may play a role in the etiology and progression of the condition.
Tang et al., 2017[23]	10	1264(733/531)	Serum omentin-1 = Lower	Serum Omentin-1 could be involved in PCOS pathogenesis.
Li et al., 2014[42]	38	3598(1944/1654)	Serum adiponectin = Lower	Adiponectin levels in the blood could play a role in PCOS development.
Sun et al., 2015[18]		1341(695/646)	Serum visfatin = Higher	Serum visfatin may serve as a biomarker for PCOS.

BMI, Body mass index; *IR*, insulin resistance; *PCOS*, polycystic ovary syndrome.

Adiponectin

Adiponectin is a 30 kDa protein secreted mainly through adipocytes, but to some extent, it is also produced by osteoblasts, placenta, and cardiomyocytes. It has anti-inflammatory, anti-atherogenic, and insulin-sensitizing properties. Obesity is a characteristic of PCOS that can affect adiponectin sensitivity by altering the expression of adiponectin receptors. It causes IR, which exacerbates hyperinsulinemia in PCOS females.[44] Also, several adiponectin gene polymorphisms are more prevalent in PCOS.[45]

Low adiponectin levels are mostly related to the presence or interplay of PCOS and obesity in obese females with PCOS.[46] Indicators of IR are associated with adiponectin levels,[11] which were further supported by an MA.[47] In contrast, several studies reported no link between serum adiponectin levels and IR.[10,42] These contradictory findings are most likely because of genetic variances in obesity and IR susceptibility in different populations.[10]

Serum adiponectin levels were significantly lower in overweight/obese PCOS patients.[46] Similarly, Croatian patients with PCOS had significantly lower serum levels of adiponectin than healthy females.[10] A recent MA exhibited that nonobese PCOS females had lower adiponectin levels.[36]

Genetic and functional research done on adiponectin have reported a role of reduced levels of adiponectin in the causal development of metabolic syndrome (MetS), T2DM, IR, PCOS, and even atherosclerosis.[48] Because adiponectin is found to have anti-inflammatory effects, it can be decreased in conditions of low-grade chronic inflammation such as obesity and PCOS. Adiponectin stimulates the secretion of interleukin (IL)-10 and IL-1 receptor antagonists, both of which are reported to have anti-inflammatory effects while inhibiting cytokine (proinflammatory) production. Furthermore, adiponectin augments the secretion of insulin by inhibiting hepatic gluconeogenesis. Therefore in conditions of inflammation like obesity and PCOS, low levels of adiponectin might be a possible explanation for inflammation.[49] Nevertheless, the mechanism of action of adiponectin in females with PCOS requires additional exploration.

Leptin

Leptin is a product of 167-amino acids secreted primarily by white adipose tissues; however, it is also secreted by other organs. Various functions of leptin have been demonstrated, including food intake mediation, secretion of hepatic glucose and gonadotropins, immune response modulation, and lipogenesis suppression within adipose tissue. Depending on the mass of adipose tissues, circulating leptin levels are determined. Levels of leptin are correlated to the secretion of luteinizing hormone (LH) and gonadotropin hormone-releasing hormone (GnRH).[12]

According to a recent MA, the circulating levels of leptin in nonobese PCOS patients were considerably higher.[15] Several studies found that PCOS patients had higher leptin concentrations than the control group.[10,46,50] A study reported no difference in serum leptin level between PCOS and the control group.[51]

A study observed significantly higher blood leptin levels in PCOS patients compared with control subjects, irrespective of BMI stratification, implying that the elevated serum leptin level in PCOS patients is because of causes other than increased body mass.[10] As an antiobesity hormone, leptin plays a central and peripheral regulatory role in reducing food intake and promoting fat oxidation, raising insulin sensitivity. The increased leptin levels in obese females with PCOS may be connected to the hyperinsulinemic state associated with obesity and PCOS. It promotes hyperandrogenism by promoting steroidogenesis and blocking neuropeptide Y, which inhibits GnRH and results in elevated GnRH and LH levels.[52]

Several types of research have demonstrated that in obese individuals, leptin's mode of action is disrupted; despite an elevated level of this hormone in the bloodstream, appetite is not controlled, and therefore leptin resistance develops.[13,14] IR or hyperinsulinemia might be a precipitating factor that might influence serum levels of leptin. It is observed that insulin directly causes induction of leptin mRNA in adipose tissue in vitro; this suggests insulin might be a stimulating factor for leptin's secretion in PCOS.[39] Hyperinsulinemia and IR are frequently linked with leptin resistance, leading to energy homeostasis problems and the development of various metabolic disorders.[14]

Nevertheless, there is currently no definitive evidence as to what role leptin plays in PCOS development. Escobar-Morreale et al. (1997)[53] found that hyperandrogenemia can raise the leptin level, whereas leptin can influence the gonadal axis in PCOS. Furthermore, elevated leptin concentrations

suppress the expression of proinsulin mRNA by reducing insulin gene promoter transcription activity and insulin receptor phosphorylation in peripheral organs.[54]

Resistin

Resistin is an adipocytokine predominantly produced in macrophages and adipocytes in humans.[11] Resistin was initially reported to contribute to IR leading to DM; however, its role is not completely understood regarding its effects on obesity, insulin sensitivity, and T2DM. Studies have found that circulating levels of resistin are raised in obesity and metabolic conditions like PCOS. Much published data have reported a linkage between resistin and IR. Some studies suggest that resistin causes direct endothelial dysfunction. It stimulates the secretion of proinflammatory cytokines like IL-6 and TNX-alpha.[16]

In their recent MA, Lin et al. (2021)[15] reported significantly higher resistin levels among nonobese PCOS patients. A study reported a significant reduction in serum resistin levels after metformin treatment in PCOS patients.[55] Similarly, another MA demonstrated that the PCOS group's serum resistin levels were significantly greater than controls.[36]

A Croatian study reported significantly higher resistin levels in females with PCOS than healthy females.[10] The same study found no correlation between resistin levels and HOMA-IR or androgen hormone levels in patients with PCOS.

The resistin gene is close to the PCOS-linked D19S884 polymorphism marker, and both are possible PCOS vulnerability loci.[56] An Indian study indicated that the 420 C G (promoter region) and 299 G A polymorphisms in the resistin gene are linked to PCOS occurrence.[57] Both polymorphisms are significantly related to cerebrovascular disease and the development of IR in T2DM patients, explaining the emergence of IR in PCOS patients.[58] Research on adipokine gene polymorphisms and their function in PCOS is currently scarce and inconsistent, and additional research is needed to establish their significance.

Considering obesity in PCOS, it is found that the expression of resistin mRNA by adipocytes substantially increases. It is also observed that in human theca cells (cultured), resistin showed enhancement in 17 alpha-hydroxylase activities, which is a marker of ovarian hyperandrogenism among PCOS patients; therefore it might be possible resistin may impart a local role in PCOS pathogenesis.[59] Nevertheless, more research is needed to determine its role in PCOS.

Visfatin

Visfatin is regarded as a proinflammatory adipokine linked to IL-6 and tumor necrosis factor (TNF),[17,60] which may contribute to the development of obesity-related IR.[61] Visfatin is thought to work similarly to insulin in physiologic settings, reducing blood glucose levels[27,62]; excess visfatin expression, on the other hand, does not have a significant enough effect of preventing high glucose levels and increased IR in obese, T2DM, and PCOS patients. Visfatin can also boost proinflammatory activity by increasing TNF-a and IL-6 release, which raises IR even further.[61] A Turkish study reported that in patients with PCOS, serum visfatin levels were considerably greater than in controls. Visfatin levels significantly decreased with metformin treatment compared with baseline. Serum visfatin levels correlated positively with BMI, waist circumference, triglyceride, HOMA-IR, and insulin levels.[55] A Polish study reported no significant difference in serum visfatin levels between PCOS and the control group.[50] A MA observed significantly increased serum visfatin levels in nonobese PCOS patients.[15] Similarly, another MA revealed that PCOS patients had considerably greater visfatin levels than controls. The stratified and univariate analyses indicated that elevated visfatin levels were not associated with BMI, IR, or total testosterone ratio.[18]

Behboudi-Gandevani et al. (2017)[46] demonstrated significantly higher visfatin levels in the overweight/obese females than normal-weight females with PCOS. It implies that visfatin levels are linked to obesity in PCOS females. This rise could compensate for reduced visfatin signaling, enhancing insulin sensitivity in target tissues.[63] Furthermore, it has been proposed that visfatin is linked to inflammation in PCOS females.[64] Ozkaya et al. (2010)[65] discovered that metformin treatment lowered circulating visfatin levels in PCOS patients after 3 months of therapy. The key mechanism is metformin's increase of insulin sensitivity in PCOS patients.[66] As a result, increased visfatin secretion in PCOS may represent a compensatory mechanism avoiding a rise in IR. Furthermore, circulating visfatin levels were lower with greater insulin sensitivity.[66] A study found increased visfatin secretion in both lean and obese PCOS patients, suggesting that visfatin is an inherent feature of PCOS. In this way, visfatin could be used as a possible biomarker for PCOS treatment and could aid in identifying high-risk PCOS individuals.[18]

Molecular pathway involvement of visfatin in PCOS is proposed to be insulin and glucose metabolism that affects the secretion of visfatin via phosphatidylinositol 3-kinase and protein kinase B pathway. Furthermore, visfatin and increased androgens together form a vicious cycle, which raises the risk of PCOS and other endocrine-related disorders.[18] More research is needed to understand better the regulation of visfatin and its probable repercussions in the pathophysiology of obesity and PCOS.

Apelin

Apelin is a 36 amino acids peptide (the most frequent isoform of apelin) that originated in the stomach (bovine) extract as endogenous ligands of G protein-coupled receptor, known as APJ. Along with the stomach, however, apelin's expression has also been reported in various organs such as brain, uterus, ovary, lungs, and even in the endothelium of small arteries.[19] This indicates that APJ/apelin system might

impart an important part in various physiologic processes. Apelin has been linked to the progression of metabolic illnesses, the regulation of appetite center activity, adipose tissue growth, and the pathogenesis of obesity.[27,43,67] Apelin lowers blood glucose levels by enhancing uptake and absorption by muscle and adipose tissue. It also boosts cell insulin sensitivity.[68]

The expression of adipose apelin and circulation apelin levels are shown to be higher with IR and obesity.[69] Previous research has established that insulin stimulates apelin secretion, whereas apelin inhibits insulin secretion.[70] Furthermore, inflammation can play an active role in apelin synthesis and receptor regulation.[71] An MA found no statistically significant difference in apelin levels between PCOS and control groups.[36]

The presence of an association in between serum levels of apelin and IR in PCOS is still under debate, yet the scarce published data show that apelin is a characteristic of PCOS in ovarian dysfunction rather than a marker for insulin sensitivity. Expression of APJ and apelin has been observed in human ovarian follicles, theca cells (TCs), granulosa cells (GCs), and oocytes, and even in vitro research has demonstrated apelin's potential role in controlling the various function of the ovary.[20] Apelin also has been shown to regulate the process of luteolysis of corpus luteum and maturation of oocytes.[21] It has been observed that apelin mRNA levels in GCs correlate negatively to levels of plasma FSH. Although positively associated with the duration of the menstrual cycle, apelin can also take part in disturbing hormone levels, being the originating cause for the pathogenesis of PCOS.[21]

Apelin and its receptors are found to be expressed in ovaries in follicles and GCs. They play a vital role in the angiogenesis and metabolism of ovarian hormones. This shows that apelin and its receptors might have an essential role in follicular development. These are found to be raised in PCOS, causing disturbances in the menstrual cycle, leading to disorders of menstruation and even anovulation. Furthermore, apelin is also reported to increase in metabolic disorders, such as T2DM and obesity, both of which are risk factors for PCOS.[72]

Kolan et al. (2021)[50] reported apelin's significantly lower levels in the PCOS group than in the healthy group. The apelin level in the PCOS group was unaffected by BMI or carbohydrate metabolism factors. Nevertheless, apelin investigations have yielded contradictory and equivocal results.[21,73,74] Research findings suggest apelin's predictive usefulness in the context of metabolic abnormalities associated with PCOS, such as glucose metabolism.[50]

More research on apelin is needed to confirm the idea that adipokine, which is found in significantly lower amounts in PCOS patients, may be helpful in predicting metabolic abnormalities that arise as a result of PCOS.

Omentin

Omentin is also called intelectin-1, regarded as novel adipokine secreted predominantly by visceral depots of fats. It has been reported that omentin's expression is substantially higher in both the GCs and follicular fluid (FF) of PCOS females compared with the controlled group.[75] The majority of the investigations have reported low levels of plasma omentin among PCOS females in addition to lowered omentin mRNA levels. Published data have observed an inverse relation of serum omentin to HOMA-IR/fasting insulin. In vitro research has supported hyperinsulinemia's role in decreasing the expression of omentin in adipose tissues. Disturbance in hormonal levels, mostly hyperandrogenism, has been declared a key component contributing to the lower synthesis of omentin in PCOS females.[76]

Regulation of omentin is also postulated by inflammation because its expression tends to show altered levels in inflammation, and PCOS is regarded as a proinflammatory disorder. The increased omentin expression in GCs and FF proposes that omentin production at the ovarian level is independently linked to the action of insulin and, therefore, regulated by some other mechanism.[24] It was reported that higher levels of serum omentin were observed among PCOS females having irregular cycles compared with those females having regular cycles. This suggests that a positive correlation persists in between adipokine expression in ovulatory dysfunction, which is marked in PCOS.[23]

In human adipocytes, omentin operates as an insulin sensitizer hormone. It also acts as an anti-inflammatory agent by reducing the release of TNF-induced superoxide.[77] In females with PCOS, hyperandrogenemia and hyperinsulinemia may also lead to lower omentin concentrations.[22]

Omentin levels were considerably lower in overweight/obese females with PCOS compared with normal weight PCOS. Its levels, however, remained consistent across BMI groups in healthy females.[46] Nevertheless, the interactive effect of obesity and PCOS was not statistically significant in their study, so they have hypothesized that multifactorial processes could modulate circulating omentin-1 levels in addition to PCOS and obesity. As a result, more research is needed to elucidate this ambiguous link.

With the change in omentin levels in obese PCOS patients, it is possible that reduced omentin levels are involved in the metabolic abnormalities observed in PCOS patients. Omentin and PCOS have been linked in certain studies, but additional work is needed to fully understand the connection.

Chemerin

Chemerin is a multifaced adipocytokine present in the ligand of G protein-coupled receptor CMKLRI and is predominantly regarded as a proinflammatory cytokine involved in innate and adaptive immunity.[25] Studies have reported that chemerin plus CMKLR1 levels in both FF and mRNA levels in GCs are predominantly higher among females with PCOS.[78] Chemerin's role in inflammation and MetS connects its pathophysiologic mechanism to IR and body fat storage.[79] Yet another adipokine, chemerin, modulates insulin sensitivity and secretion, whereas insulin, in

turn, increases chemerin release from adipose tissue.[80] Chemerin levels were shown to be higher in obese PCOS patients, and there was a considerable increase in chemerin mRNA expression in subcutaneous and omental adipose tissue depots among PCOS patients.[81] Several other studies also found higher chemerin levels in obese PCOS individuals who also had IR.[82,83] According to a recent MA, serum chemerin levels in the PCOS group were considerably higher than in the controls.[36]

Furthermore, chemerin levels have been linked to insulin regulation function.[81] Fat mass is the most important determinant of high chemerin levels.[82] Tan et al. (2009)[81] showed that 6 months of metformin treatment resulted in a significant decrease in serum chemerin levels and concurrent reduction in IR in PCOS patients.

A study found no statistically significant difference in serum chemerin levels between overweight and normal-weight PCOS patients and the control group.[46] In comparison, a study reported substantially greater chemerin levels in overweight PCOS patients than in normal-weight PCOS individuals. It was found to positively correlate with BMI, triglycerides, insulin, and HOMA-IR in the PCOS group. These findings imply that BMI alone is not a reliable predictor of circulating chemerin levels.[76]

These disagreements could be attributed to differences in adiposity and chemo-inflammatory responses of adipose tissue in different PCOS groups and differences in assay settings and PCOS phenotypes with larger ovarian capacity.[84] Furthermore, it has been proposed that chemerin serum levels may not necessarily represent changes caused by the varied type and amount of adipose tissue. Because of the wide range of results from different studies, it is proposed that the relationship between chemerin, obesity, and PCOS be investigated further in more detail.

Even though there are discordant results in PCOS models, most studies have reported increased chemerin levels both in adipose tissue and plasma in PCOS females. Published literature has suggested that chemerin might be involved in arresting the growth of antral follicles linked to hyperandrogenic proinflammatory states that are characteristic features of PCOS.[26]

Molecular mechanisms involving chemerin in PCOS that have been proposed include transcription and translation of chemerin and its receptor known as chemR23, which is significantly raised in the ovaries of PCOS patients. Chemerin's complicated connection with PCOS parameters and other processes warrants further investigation.

Asprosin

Asprosin is comparatively a newly discovered peptide produced by white adipose tissue. It activates the G protein-cAMP-PKA pathway, which promotes glucose production from the liver, and its levels are abnormally high with IR or obesity.[85] In participants with T2DM, asprosin levels were significantly higher than in controls, and IR was also linked to asprosin levels in T2DM patients.[86,87]

A Turkish study found that patients with PCOS had considerably higher levels of asprosin than controls.[88] In contrast, one study found no statistically significant difference in serum asprosin levels between PCOS and control groups. It was, however, significantly lower in the PCOS patient groups with hyperandrogenism and IR compared with the equivalent PCOS nonhyperandrogenism and non-IR groups.[89] Two more investigations found considerably higher levels of asprosin in PCOS women than in controls.[90,91] According to Chang et al. (2019),[73] asprosin levels in females with PCOS were comparable to those in matching controls.

Alan et al. (2019)[90] hypothesized that asprosin contributes significantly to PCOS development by interfering with pathophysiological pathways like IR and inflammation.

The discovery of asprosin was one of the most important topics for future research into treating numerous metabolic illnesses related to IR. Nevertheless, at present, the research is still in its infancy in terms of concluding if asprosin is associated with PCOS, IR, and metabolic parameters. As a result, additional investigation is recommended.

Conclusion

The role of adipokines in PCOS is still not explicitly understood. There is a lot to learn about their roles in the pathophysiology of the disease. Interestingly, few studies found increased, decreased, or no change in the same adipokine levels in PCOS, such as asprosin and leptin. Several findings have been drawn regarding their functions in PCOS.

- Some adipokines have receptors on the ovaries and hence perform a direct role.
- Several adipokines exert their effects indirectly via interacting with androgens and insulin.
- Many adipokine levels vary because the majority of PCOS patients are obese.
- TCs and GCs are involved in the action of some adipokines.
- An imbalance of pro- and anti-inflammatory adipokines may exacerbate PCOS symptoms.
- Adipokine polymorphisms may affect their levels in PCOS.
- It is also possible that adipokines are not the cause of PCOS, but metabolic alterations such as IR and hyperandrogenism may cause adipose tissue dysregulation, leading to changes in adipokine levels.
- Optimal adipokine levels are likely required to recover from PCOS; thus a greater understanding of abnormal adipokine levels and their connection with PCOS is required.
- Metformin is reported to cure PCOS and its symptoms by balancing aberrant levels of adipokines such as chemerin, resistin, irisin, and visfatin. Metformin may improve testosterone levels and insulin sensitivity, and because these biochemical alterations are normalized, adipokine levels return to normal. Nevertheless, metformin has no direct influence on these adipokines. More research is needed to see if metformin can help with PCOS by regulating adipokine levels that are out of whack.
- As the exact mechanism of PCOS is unknown, adipokines are likely to play a role in the onset and progression of the condition.

Adipokines appear to play a crucial role in health and disease in general, and especially in PCOS. The link between adipokines and IR, obesity, steroid hormones, lipid profile, tumor pathogenesis, endothelial dysfunction, bone pathology, and infertility emphasizes these bioactive substances' active role in the pathophysiology of the extensive range of diseases. As a result, more research is needed to identify the interplay between adipokines and PCOS and draw a conclusion concerning the participation of adipokines in PCOS.

References

1. Xu X, Grijalva A, Skowronski A, van Eijk M, Serlie MJ, Ferrante Jr AW. Obesity activates a program of lysosomal-dependent lipid metabolism in adipose tissue macrophages independently of classic activation. *Cell Metab.* 2013;18(6):816-830.
2. Ezeh U, Chen IY, Chen YH, Azziz R. Adipocyte insulin resistance in PCOS: relationship with GLUT-4 expression and whole-body glucose disposal and β-cell function. *J Clin Endocrinol Metab.* 2020;105(7):e2408-e2420.
3. Reilly SM, Saltiel AR. Adapting to obesity with adipose tissue inflammation. *Nat Rev Endocrinol.* 2017;13(11):633-643.
4. Azamar-Llamas D, Hernandez-Molina G, Ramos-Avalos B, Furuzawa-Carballeda J. Adipokine contribution to the pathogenesis of osteoarthritis. *Mediators Inflamm.* 2017;2017:5468023.
5. Achari AE, Jain SK. Adiponectin, a therapeutic target for obesity, diabetes, and endothelial dysfunction. *Int J Mol Sci.* 2017;18(6):1321.
6. Shibata R, Ouchi N, Ohashi K, Murohara T. The role of adipokines in cardiovascular disease. *J Cardiol.* 2017;70(4):329-334.
7. Ouchi N, Parker JL, Lugus JJ, Walsh K. Adipokines in inflammation and metabolic disease. *Nat Rev Immunol.* 2011;11(2):85-97.
8. Maximus PS, Al Achkar Z, Hamid PF, Hasnain SS, Peralta CA. Adipocytokines: are they the theory of everything? *Cytokine.* 2020;133:155144.
9. Chen T, Wang F, Chu Z, et al. Serum CTRP3 levels in obese children: a potential protective adipokine of obesity, insulin sensitivity and pancreatic β cell function. *Diabetes Metab Syndr Obes.* 2019;12:1923.
10. Baldani DP, Skrgatic L, Kasum M, Zlopasa G, Kralik Oguic S, Herman M. Altered leptin, adiponectin, resistin and ghrelin secretion may represent an intrinsic polycystic ovary syndrome abnormality. *Gynecol Endocrinol.* 2019;35(5):401-405.
11. Arikan Ş, Bahceci M, Tuzcu A, Kale E, Gökalp D. Serum resistin and adiponectin levels in young non-obese women with polycystic ovary syndrome. *Gynecol Endocrinol.* 2010;26(3):161-166.
12. Jahromi BN, Dabaghmanesh MH, Parsanezhad ME, Fatehpoor F. Association of leptin and insulin resistance in PCOS: a case-controlled study. *Int J Reprod Biomed.* 2017;15(7):423.
13. Borsuk A, Biernat W, Zieba D. Multidirectional action of resistin in the organism. *Postepy Hig Med Dosw.* 2018;72:327-338.
14. Góralska M, Majewska-Szczepanik M, Szczepanik M. Immunological mechanisms involved in obesity and their role in metabolic syndrome. *Postepy Hig Med Dosw.* 2015;69:1384-1404.

15. Lin K, Sun X, Wang X, Wang H, Chen X. Circulating adipokine levels in nonobese women with polycystic ovary syndrome and in nonobese control women: a systematic review and meta-analysis. *Front Endocrinol.* 2021;11:537809.

16. Sarray S, Madan S, Saleh LR, Mahmoud N, Almawi WY. Validity of adiponectin-to-leptin and adiponectin-to-resistin ratios as predictors of polycystic ovary syndrome. *Fertil Steril.* 2015;104(2):460-466.

17. Kralisch S, Klein J, Lossner U, et al. Interleukin-6 is a negative regulator of visfatin gene expression in 3T3-L1 adipocytes. *Am J Physiol Heart Circ Physiol.* 2005;289(4):E586-E590.

18. Sun Y, Wu Z, Wei L, Liu C, Zhu S, Tang S. High-visfatin levels in women with polycystic ovary syndrome: evidence from a meta-analysis. *Gynecol Endocrinol.* 2015;31(10):808-814.

19. Rak A, Drwal E, Rame C, et al. Expression of apelin and apelin receptor (APJ) in porcine ovarian follicles and in vitro effect of apelin on steroidogenesis and proliferation through APJ activation and different signaling pathways. *Theriogenology.* 2017;96:126-135.

20. Roche J, Ramé C, Reverchon M, et al. Apelin (APLN) regulates progesterone secretion and oocyte maturation in bovine ovarian cells. *Reproduction.* 2017;153(5):589-603.

21. Altinkaya SÖ, Nergiz S, Küçük M, Yüksel H. Apelin levels in relation with hormonal and metabolic profile in patients with polycystic ovary syndrome. *Eur J Obstet Gynecol Reprod Biol.* 2014;176:168-172.

22. Yang HY, Ma Y, Lu XH, et al. The correlation of plasma omentin-1 with insulin resistance in non-obese polycystic ovary syndrome. *Ann Endocrinol (Paris).* 2015;76(5):620-627.

23. Tang YL, Yu J, Zeng ZG, Liu Y, Liu JY, Xu JX. Circulating omentin-1 levels in women with polycystic ovary syndrome: a meta-analysis. *Gynecol Endocrinol.* 2017;33(3):244-249.

24. Özgen İT, Oruçlu Ş, Selek S, Kutlu E, Guzel G, Cesur Y. Omentin-1 level in adolescents with polycystic ovarian syndrome. *Pediatr Int.* 2019;61(2):147-151.

25. Fatima SS, Rehman R, Baig M, Khan TA. New roles of the multidimensional adipokine: chemerin. *Peptides.* 2014;62:15-20.

26. Wang Q, Leader A, Tsang BK. Inhibitory roles of prohibitin and chemerin in FSH-induced rat granulosa cell steroidogenesis. *Endocrinology.* 2013;154(2):956-967.

27. Bongrani A, Mellouk N, Rame C, et al. Ovarian expression of adipokines in polycystic ovary syndrome: a role for chemerin, omentin, and apelin in follicular growth arrest and ovulatory dysfunction? *Int J Mol Sci.* 2019;20(15):3778.

28. Spritzer PM, Lecke SB, Satler F, Morsch DM. Adipose tissue dysfunction, adipokines, and low-grade chronic inflammation in polycystic ovary syndrome. *Reproduction.* 2015;149(5):R219-R227.

29. Legro RS, Kunselman AR, Dodson WC, Dunaif A. Prevalence and predictors of risk for type 2 diabetes mellitus and impaired glucose tolerance in polycystic ovary syndrome: a prospective, controlled study in 254 affected women. *J Clin Endocrinol Metab.* 1999;84(1):165-169.

30. Jakubowicz D, Wainstein J, Homburg R. The link between polycystic ovarian syndrome and type 2 diabetes: preventive and therapeutic approach in Israel. *Isr Med Assoc J.* 2012;14(7):442-447.

31. Sirmans SM, Pate KA. Epidemiology, diagnosis, and management of polycystic ovary syndrome. *Clin Epidemiol.* 2014;6:1-13.

32. Lim SS, Davies MJ, Norman RJ, Moran LJ. Overweight, obesity and central obesity in women with polycystic ovary syndrome: a systematic review and meta-analysis. *Hum Reprod Update.* 2012;18(6):618-637.

33. Itoh H, Kawano Y, Furukawa Y, Matsumoto H, Yuge A, Narahara H. The role of serum adiponectin levels in women with polycystic ovarian syndrome. *Clin Exp Obstet Gynecol.* 2021;40(4):531-535.

34. Kumawat M, Ram M, Agarwal S, Singh V. Role of serum Leptin, insulin and other hormones in women with Polycystic ovarian syndrome. *Indian J Clin Biochem.* 2018;33:S88-S89.

35. Barrea L, Arnone A, Annunziata G, et al. Adherence to the Mediterranean diet, dietary patterns and body composition in women with polycystic ovary syndrome (PCOS). *Nutrients.* 2019;11(10):2278.

36. Mehrabani S, Arab A, Karimi E, Nouri M, Mansourian M. Blood circulating levels of adipokines in polycystic ovary syndrome patients: a systematic review and meta-analysis. *Reprod Sci.* 2021;28:3032-3050.

37. Raeisi T, Rezaie H, Darand M, et al. Circulating resistin and follistatin levels in obese and non-obese women with polycystic ovary syndrome: a systematic review and meta-analysis. *PLoS One.* 2021;16(3):e0246200.

38. Seth MK, Gulati S, Gulati S, et al. Association of leptin with polycystic ovary syndrome: a systematic review and meta-analysis. *J Obstet Gynaecol India.* 2021;71:567-576.

39. Zheng SH, Du DF, Li XL. Leptin levels in women with polycystic ovary syndrome: a systematic review and a meta-analysis. *Reprod Sci.* 2017;24(5):656-670.

40. Wang X, Zhang Q, Zhang L, et al. Circulating chemerin levels in women with polycystic ovary syndrome: a meta-analysis. *Gynecol Endocrinol.* 2022;38:22-27.

41. Mansoori A, Amoochi-Foroushani G, Zilaee M, Hosseini SA, Azhdari M. Serum and follicular fluid chemerin and chemerin mRNA expression in women with polycystic ovary syndrome: systematic review and meta-analysis. *Endocrinol Diabetes Metab.* 2022;5:e00307.

42. Li S, Huang X, Zhong H, et al. Low circulating adiponectin levels in women with polycystic ovary syndrome: an updated meta-analysis. *Tumour Biol.* 2014;35(5):3961-3973.

43. Sun X, Wu X, Zhou Y, Yu X, Zhang W. Evaluation of apelin and insulin resistance in patients with PCOS and therapeutic effect of drospirenone-ethinylestradiol plus metformin. *Med Sci Monit.* 2015;21:2547.

44. Drolet R, Bélanger C, Fortier M, et al. Fat depot-specific impact of visceral obesity on adipocyte adiponectin release in women. *Obesity.* 2009;17(3):424-430.

45. Xita N, Georgiou I, Chatzikyriakidou A, et al. Effect of adiponectin gene polymorphisms on circulating adiponectin and insulin resistance indexes in women with polycystic ovary syndrome. *Clin Chem.* 2005;51(2):416-423.

46. Behboudi-Gandevani S, Tehrani FR, Yarandi RB, Noroozzadeh M, Hedayati M, Azizi F. The association between polycystic ovary syndrome, obesity, and the serum concentration of adipokines. *J Endocrinol Invest.* 2017;40(8):859-866.

47. Toulis KA, Goulis DG, Farmakiotis D, et al. Adiponectin levels in women with polycystic ovary syndrome: a systematic review and a meta-analysis. *Hum Reprod Update.* 2009;15:297-307.

48. Oliveira BS, Costa JA, Gomes ET, et al. Expression of adiponectin and its receptors (AdipoR1 and AdipoR2) in goat ovary and its effect on oocyte nuclear maturation in vitro. *Theriogenology.* 2017;104:127-133.

49. Febriza A, Ridwan R, As'ad Suryani, Kasim VN, Idrus HH. Adiponectin and its role in inflammatory process of obesity. *Mol Cell Biomed Sci.* 2019;3(2):60-66.

50. Kolan E, Boinska J, Socha MW. Adipokine levels and carbohydrate metabolism in patients diagnosed de novo with polycystic ovary syndrome. *Qatar Med J.* 2021;2021(2):34.

51. Baig M, Rehman R, Tariq S, Fatima SS. Serum leptin levels in polycystic ovary syndrome and its relationship with metabolic and hormonal profile in Pakistani females. *Int J Endocrinol.* 2014;2014:132908.

52. Veldhuis JD, Pincus SM, Garcia-Rudaz MC, Ropelato MG, Escobar ME, Barontini M. Disruption of the synchronous secretion of leptin, LH, and ovarian androgens in nonobese adolescents with the polycystic ovarian syndrome. *J Clin Endocrinol Metab.* 2001;86(8):3772-3778.

53. Escobar-Morreale HF, Serrano-Gotarredona J, Varela C, Garcia-Robles R, Sancho J. Circulating leptin concentrations in women with hirsutism. *Fertil Steril.* 1997;68(5):898-906.

54. Tan BK, Adya R, Farhatullah S, et al. Omentin-1, a novel adipokine, is decreased in overweight insulin-resistant women with polycystic ovary syndrome: ex vivo and in vivo regulation of omentin-1 by insulin and glucose. *Diabetes.* 2008;57(4):801-808.

55. Tarkun İ, Dikmen E, Çetinarslan B, Cantürk Z. Impact of treatment with metformin on adipokines in patients with polycystic ovary syndrome. *Eur Cytokine Netw.* 2010;21(4):272-277.

56. Urbanek M, Du Y, Silander K, et al. Variation in resistin gene promoter not associated with polycystic ovary syndrome. *Diabetes.* 2003;52(1):214-217.

57. Nambiar V, Vijesh VV, Lakshmanan P, Sukumaran S, Suganthi R. Association of adiponectin and resistin gene polymorphisms in South Indian women with polycystic ovary syndrome. *Eur J Obstet Gynecol Reprod Biol.* 2016;200:82-88.

58. Kunnari A, Ukkola O, Kesäniemi YA. Resistin polymorphisms are associated with cerebrovascular disease in Finnish Type 2 diabetic patients. *Diabet Med.* 2005;22(5):583-589.

59. Pine GM, Batugedara HM, Nair MG. Here, there and everywhere: resistin-like molecules in infection, inflammation, and metabolic disorders. *Cytokine.* 2018;110:442-451.

60. Kralisch S, Klein J, Lossner U, et al. Hormonal regulation of the novel adipocytokine visfatin in 3T3-L1 adipocytes. *J Endocrinol.* 2005;185(3):R1-R8.

61. Kern PA, Ranganathan S, Li C, Wood L, Ranganathan G. Adipose tissue tumor necrosis factor and interleukin-6 expression in human obesity and insulin resistance. *Am J Physiol Endocrinol Metab.* 2001;280(5):E745-E751.

62. Farshchian F, Tehrani FR, Amirrasouli H, et al. Visfatin and resistin serum levels in normal-weight and obese women with polycystic ovary syndrome. *Int J Endocrinol Metab.* 2014;12(3):e15503.

63. Tan BK, Chen J, Digby JE, Keay SD, Kennedy CR, Randeva HS. Increased visfatin mRNA and protein levels in adipose tissue and adipocytes in women with polycystic ovary syndrome (PCOS): parallel increase in plasma visfatin. *J Clin Endocrinol Metab.* 2006;91:5022-5028.

64. Lajunen TK, Purhonen AK, Haapea M, et al. Full-length visfatin levels are associated with inflammation in women with polycystic ovary syndrome. *Eur J Clin Invest.* 2012;42(3):321-328.

65. Ozkaya M, Cakal E, Ustun Y, Engin-Ustun Y. Effect of metformin on serum visfatin levels in patients with polycystic ovary syndrome. *Fertil Steril.* 2010;93(3):880-884.

66. Nawrocka J, Starczewski A. Effects of metformin treatment in women with polycystic ovary syndrome depends on insulin resistance. *Gynecol Endocrinol.* 2007;23(4):231-237.

67. Jiang T, Pan J, Ying SU, Zhou H, Qiu M, Xiaoyi LI. The relationship between polycystic ovary syndrome and vaspin, apelin and leptin. *J Kunming Med Univ.* 2016;37(10):41-46.

68. Zhu S, Sun F, Li W, et al. Apelin stimulates glucose uptake through the PI3K/Akt pathway and improves insulin resistance in 3T3-L1 adipocytes. *Mol Cell Biochem.* 2011;353(1):305-313.

69. Ma WY, Yu TY, Wei JN, et al. Plasma apelin: a novel biomarker for predicting diabetes. *Clin Chim Acta.* 2014;435:18-23.

70. Xu S, Tsao PS, Yue P. Apelin and insulin resistance: another arrow for the quiver? *J Diabetes.* 2011;3(3):225-231.

71. Karimi E, Moini A, Yaseri M, et al. Effects of synbiotic supplementation on metabolic parameters and apelin in women with polycystic ovary syndrome: a randomised double-blind placebo-controlled trial. *Br J Nutr.* 2018;119(4):398-406.

72. Kanwal S, Allahwasaya A, Anjum N, Fatima SS. Serum apelin levels in polycystic ovary syndrome and its relationship with adiposity profile in females. *Prof Med J.* 2021;28(6):902-906.

73. Chang CL, Huang SY, Hsu YC, Chin TH, Soong YK. The serum level of irisin, but not asprosin, is abnormal in polycystic ovary syndrome patients. *Sci Rep.* 2019;9(1):1-11.

74. Kurowska P, Barbe A, Różycka M, Chmielińska J, Dupont J, Rak A. Apelin in reproductive physiology and pathology of different species: a critical review. *Int J Endocrinol.* 2018;2018:9170480.

75. Zabetian-Targhi F, Mirzaei K, Keshavarz SA, Hossein-Nezhad A. Modulatory role of omentin-1 in inflammation: cytokines and dietary intake. *J Am Coll Nutr.* 2016;35(8):670-678.

76. Guvenc Y, Var A, Goker A, Kuscu NK. Assessment of serum chemerin, vaspin and omentin-1 levels in patients with polycystic ovary syndrome. *J Int Med Res.* 2016;44(4):796-805.

77. Kazama K, Usui T, Okada M, Hara Y, Yamawaki H. Omentin plays an anti-inflammatory role through inhibition of TNF-α-induced superoxide production in vascular smooth muscle cells. *Eur J Pharmacol.* 2012;686(1-3):116-123.

78. Yang X, Yao J, Wei Q, et al. Role of chemerin/CMKLR1 in the maintenance of early pregnancy. *Front Med.* 2018;12(5):525-532.

79. Fatima SS, Bozaoglu K, Rehman R, Alam F, Memon AS. Elevated chemerin levels in Pakistani men: an interrelation with metabolic syndrome phenotypes. *PLoS One.* 2013;8(2):e57113.

80. Bauer S, Bala M, Kopp A, et al. Adipocyte chemerin release is induced by insulin without being translated to higher levels in vivo. *Eur J Clin Invest.* 2012;42(11):1213-1220.

81. Tan BK, Chen J, Farhatullah S, et al. Insulin and metformin regulate circulating and adipose tissue chemerin. *Diabetes.* 2009;58(9):1971-1977.

82. Guzel EC, Celik C, Abali R, et al. Omentin and chemerin and their association with obesity in women with polycystic ovary syndrome. *Gynecol Endocrinol.* 2014;30(6):419-422.

83. Martínez-García MÁ, Montes-Nieto R, Fernández-Durán E, Insenser M, Luque-Ramírez M, Escobar-Morreale HF. Evidence for masculinization of adipokine gene expression in visceral and subcutaneous adipose tissue of obese women with polycystic ovary syndrome (PCOS). *J Clin Endocrinol Metab.* 2013;98(2):E388-E396.

84. Kort DH, Kostolias A, Sullivan C, Lobo RA. Chemerin as a marker of body fat and insulin resistance in women with polycystic ovary syndrome. *Gynecol Endocrinol.* 2015;31(2):152-155.

85. Romere C, Duerrschmid C, Bournat J, et al. Asprosin, a fasting-induced glucogenic protein hormone. *Cell.* 2016;165(3):566-579.

86. Zhang L, Chen C, Zhou N, Fu Y, Cheng X. Circulating asprosin concentrations are increased in type 2 diabetes mellitus and independently associated with fasting glucose and triglyceride. *Clin Chim Acta.* 2019;489:183-188.

87. Wang Y, Qu H, Xiong X, et al. Plasma asprosin concentrations are increased in individuals with glucose dysregulation and

correlated with insulin resistance and first-phase insulin secretion. *Mediators Inflamm.* 2018;2018:9471583.

88. Deniz R, Yavuzkir S, Ugur K, et al. Subfatin and asprosin, two new metabolic players of polycystic ovary syndrome. *J Obstet Gynaecol.* 2021;41(2):279-284.

89. Jiang Y, Liu Y, Yu Z, Yang P, Zhao S. Serum asprosin level in different subtypes of polycystic ovary syndrome: a cross-sectional study. *Rev Assoc Med Bras.* 2021;67:590-596.

90. Alan M, Gurlek B, Yilmaz A, et al. Asprosin: a novel peptide hormone related to insulin resistance in women with polycystic ovary syndrome. *Gynecol Endocrinol.* 2019;35(3):220-223.

91. Li X, Liao M, Shen R, et al. Plasma asprosin levels are associated with glucose metabolism, lipid, and sex hormone profiles in females with metabolic-related diseases. *Mediators Inflamm.* 2018;2018:7375294.

6

Crosstalk between Oxidative Stress and Chronic Inflammation in Pathogenesis of Polycystic Ovary Syndrome

FAIZA ALAM

Introduction: The Role of Oxidative Stress and Chronic Inflammation in the Pathogenesis of Polycystic Ovary Syndrome

Reproductive processes require ovarian follicles to develop continuously. To achieve this development, a number of structural changes occur during each estrous cycle, including endometrial, ovarian, and uterine changes. In addition to these changes, the basal body temperature also fluctuates, corresponding to the alteration endometrium thickness. Furthermore, with the entrance of the sperm into the female reproductive system, there is a three-step process that occurs if an egg is present within 24 hours of entry, known as "fertilization" of the egg or pregnancy. A very important process, implantation follows fertilization to progress with a successful pregnancy. This whole course from maturation of granulosa cells to the implantation of the fertilized ovum demands a certain environment to attain reproductive capability. Reactive oxidant species (ROS) within their range are essential for the signaling transduction pathways during folliculogenesis, oocyte maturation, and embryologic development.

The Oxidant and Antioxidant System

A moderately generated ROS is favorably required by the oocyte for maturity; nonetheless, unopposed levels of oxidants deteriorate the oocyte quality, negatively affecting the reproductive outcomes.[1-4]

During the process of energy production by the mitochondria, free radicals are produced that do not produce harmful effects if opposed by the antioxidants. Otherwise, free radical oxidation may cause follicular atresia and aging of oocytes.[1] Thus a balance and restoration of the oxidative milieu is crucial for the natural progressive growth of oocytes, cell integrity, and the hormonal balance required for positive reproductive activity.[5]

Aging of oocytes with the increased age of a female and persistent psychological stress are two main risk factors that influence their fertilization capacity. Near menopause, the graph of the ovarian reserve declines, decreasing the hormonal stability and functional capability of the oocytes essential for fertility.[6] It is accepted that with increasing age of the oocyte, the oxidative stress (OS) is also increased and causes the quality of oocyte to deteriorate. A large number of studies indicate the presence of OS in polycystic ovary syndrome (PCOS) patients with increased expression and activity of prolidase in serum along with raised total oxidants. PCOS has frequently been associated with inflammation, OS, insulin resistance (IR) regardless of obesity, and weak follicular maturity.

Oxidative Stress and Chronic Inflammation

Chronic inflammation is defined as unresolved inflammation because of tissue damage with unregulated and persistent cytokine production and secretion.[7] Chronic inflammation is capable of inducing OS by overproduction of ROS that overpowers the cells' antioxidant power.[8,9] During persistent inflammation, expression of NADPH oxidases (NOX) is promoted by the increased NFκB-p65 phosphorylation, which, in turn, produces large amounts of oxygen radicals.[10,11] These radicals convert to $H2O2$ via the enzymatic action of superoxide dismutase (SOD). This H_2O_2 then freely moves into the cytoplasm of the cell, activating NFκB-p65 phosphorylation and leading to overproduction of proinflammatory cytokines (tumor necrosis factor alpha [TNF-α] and interleukin-6 [IL-6]).[12,13]

Certain cytokines have been proven to cause defective oocyte maturation. Metabolic syndrome, including obesity, hyperinsulinemia, and IR, is accompanied by a chronic inflammatory state and raised levels of cytokines. Increased body mass index (BMI) has been shown to negatively affect reproductive outcomes in PCOS patients.[14] Obesity serves as a low-grade chronic inflammation leading to OS and contributing to metabolic and neural noncommunicative diseases.[15] OS is well known for inducing local inflammation, leading to elevated production of cytokines. With the perspective of obesity, increased circulating triglycerides deposited in adipocytes cause adipocyte hypertrophy. This induces necrosis of the adipocytes because of hypoxia. As a result, secretion of monocyte-chemoattractant1 (MCP-1/CCL2) and nicotinamide phosphoribosyltransferase (NAMPT) instigate penetration of circulating phagocytes like macrophages and T helper cells from the circulation into the adipocytes. The macrophages successively produce proinflammatory cytokines and proinflammatory interleukins (TNF-α and IL-6, respectively). The NFκB signal transduction pathway is activated by these cytokines, and a vicious cycle starts for the production of cytokines. Other adipokines, such as leptin and lipocalin, are also secreted to promote supplementary release of TNF-α and IL-6. Presence of the cytokines and adipokines in the circulation prompts inflammatory cascades in other body tissues, including the ovary[16-18]

Insulin signaling recruits protein tyrosine kinase receptors for its functionality, maintaining the insulin sensitivity. In PCOS patients, undue serine phosphorylation activity has been noted to inhibit tyrosine kinase receptor function, resulting in insulin-resistant PCOS patients. Furthermore, it results in hyperandrogenism in PCOS females by affecting P450c17 enzyme activity. Hyperinsulinemia also augments the effects of luteinizing hormone (LH) on theca interstitial cells, resulting in increased androgen production. IR rates are quite significant among PCOS patients, ranging from 50% to 70%. IR also facilitates OS existence because hyperglycemia and elevated free fatty acid instigate ROS production.[19]

Oxidative Stress and Polycystic Ovary Syndrome

ROS are frequently considered a "double-edged sword." Their function as second messenger is critical for the intracellular signaling cascades to occur, but overabundance of an ROS exerts indispensable consequences on the cellular processes. The frequently involved ROS are superoxide anion ($O_2 \cdot$), hydrogen peroxide (H_2O_2), and hydroxyl ($\cdot$OH). By default, the main ROS-producing organelle is mitochondria because it is involved in the energy production pathway of

electron transport chain reactions. Hydrogen peroxide itself is not harmful, but it easily crosses the biologic cell membranes to break down into the highly reactive $\cdot$OH radicals.

The body does offer defense against the ROS produced in the body in the form of antioxidants (i.e. superoxide dismutase [SOD], catalase [CAT], glutathione peroxidase [GPx], and glutathione reductase [GSR]). They all, except GPx, act as the primary defense proteins. GPx has a peroxidase activity and, along with oxidoreductases, nuclear enzymes, and vitamin E (VE), protects the body as a secondary defense protein.

An ROS is an eminent element in the smooth run of the cellular functions but is also capable of inducing cellular oxidative damage by interacting with various proteins in the cell. The macromolecules in the cell membrane, organelles, and specifically DNA are vulnerable for ROS target. This profuse production of OS frequently affects the maturation of oocytes by various pathways.

In PCOS patients, IR may develop because of OS. A high oxidative environment activates protein kinases, inducing phosphorylation of the serine/threonine component of the insulin receptor substrate (IRS) and inhibiting their typical tyrosine phosphorylation. This induces degradation of the IRS.[20,21]

DNA oxidation may be another attribute of PCOS. Guanine residues have higher oxidation potential compared with cytosine, thymine, and adenine. ROS outbreak secondary to O_2- generation from the energy-generating electron transport chain, absence of histone defense, and nonexistence or insignificant repair mechanisms that exist are great threats to the mitochondrial DNA.[22] A significant increase in hydrogen peroxide instigates breakage of the DNA strands, promoting maturation failure of cells in PCOS females.[23]

Another school of thought presents an inverse relationship between OS and PCOS. The factors expressed in PCOS lead to OS, which will, in turn, cause IR and hyperinsulinemia. This theory is not well established yet; however, the etiology of PCOS is accepted to be multifactorial, whereas the pathogenesis of PCOS is led by genetic variations, resulting in an inability to preserve the physiologic cellular functions. In such clinical cases, an imbalance between oxidants and ROS is generated with pronounced implications such as impaired glucose tolerance, diabetes mellitus (DM) type II, and increased risk of hypertension, dyslipidemia, and endothelial dysfunction (Fig. 6.1).

Effects of Reactive Oxygen Species on Cellular Functions in Polycystic Ovary Syndrome Patients

Transcription Factor Activation

Expression of proinflammatory cytokines and adipokines, cell differentiation, and apoptosis are all regulated by the transcription factors (AP-1, p53, and NF-κB). As discussed earlier, PCOS is a state where low-grade inflammation and raised

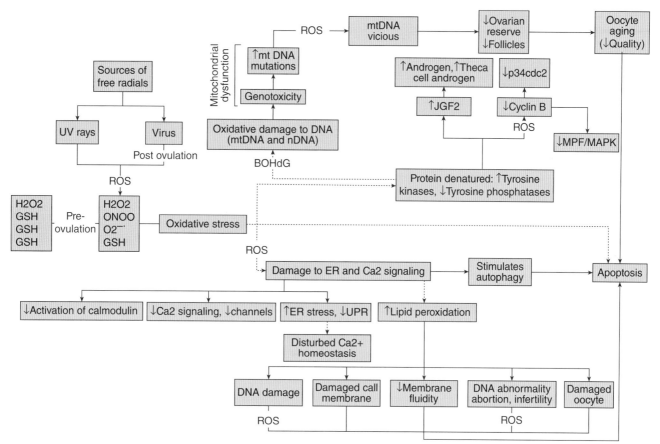

• **Fig. 6.1** Effect of Oxidative Stress on Oocyte Development. *8OHdG*, 8-Hydroxydeoxyguanosine; *CaM*, calmodulin (an abbreviation for the calcium-modulated protein); *ER*, endoplasmic reticulum; *IGF2*, growth factor; *MPF*, M-phase promoting factor; *MAPK*, mitogen-activated protein kinase; *ROS*, reactive oxygen species; *UPR*, unfolded protein response; *UV*, ultraviolet.

inflammatory cytokines exist simultaneously, usually measured by C-reactive protein (CRP), TNF-α, IL-6, and IL-18.[24,25]

Protein Kinase Activation

Cells respond to various extracellular signals and stress by activating protein kinases, which may cause cell damage or death (necrosis or apoptosis).[26]

The triggering of the mitogen-activated protein kinase signaling pathways by increased ROS serves as a major regulator of gene transcription by enhancing the activities of tyrosine kinase receptors, protein tyrosine kinases, cytokines receptors, and growth factors.[27,28] An ROS has the ability to activate other pathways as well, like c-Jun *N*-terminal kinases (JNK) and p38 pathways, which regulate the expression of various cytokines, growth factors, inflammatory enzymes, matrix metalloproteinase, and immunoglobulins by affecting their transcription genes.

In PCOS patients, OS activates protein kinases, which, in turn, degrades the IRS by inducing serine/threonine phosphorylation and inhibiting tyrosine phosphorylation of IRS[20,29] (Fig. 6.2).

Ion Channel Opening

With an increase in ROS, Ca^{+2} ions are released from the endoplasmic reticulum, leading to disturbed intracellular Ca^{+2} homeostasis. This overload of cytosolic Ca^{+2} ion adversely affects the stability of the mitochondrial membrane and results in a decrease in adenosine triphosphate (ATP) synthesis, pushing the cell into necrosis. This may be a reason for ineffective maturation of the oocytes in PCOS patients.

Protein Oxidation

OS easily targets amino acids for damaging them by directly oxidizing their side chains, transforming them into carbonyl products. Carbonyl products are unable to function as proteins; thus protein dysfunction occurs, which is also an attribute of OS and disease-derived protein dysfunction. PCOS patients exhibit significantly raised levels of serum plasma advanced oxidation protein products (AOPPs), which are accepted as novel biomarkers of ROS-mediated protein damage[30]

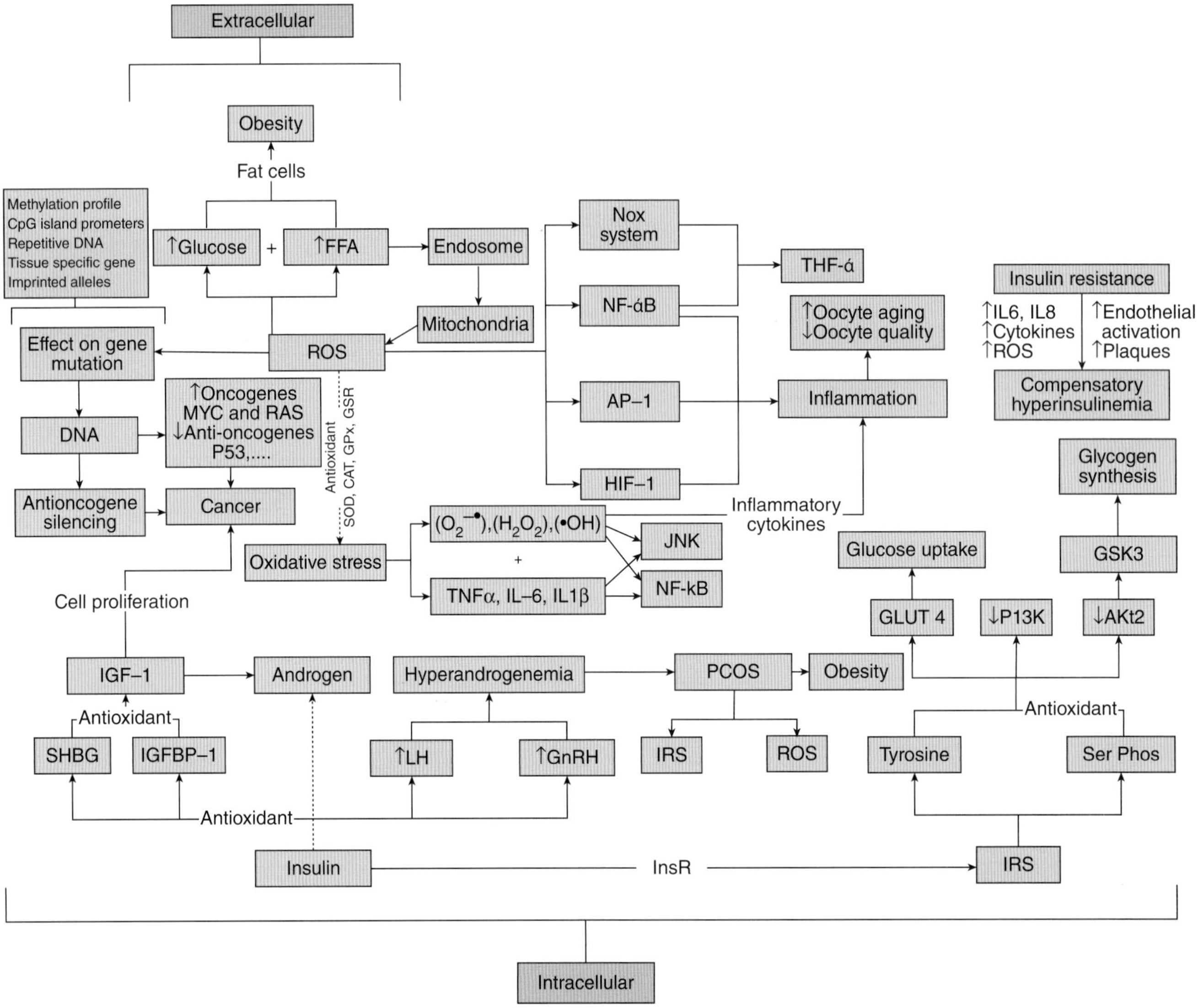

• **Fig. 6.2** Interplay of Oxidative Stress, Inflammation, Insulin Resistance, and Hyperandrogenemia in Polycystic Ovary Syndrome (PCOS). *Akt*, Protein kinase B; *AP-1*, activator protein-1; *FFA*, free fatty acid; *GLUT4*, glucose transporter-4; *GnRH*, gonadotropin-releasing hormone; *HIF-1,* hypoxia-induced factor-1; *IGFBP-1*, insulin growth factor binding protein; *IGF-1*, insulin growth factor-1; *IL*, interleukin; *InsR*, insulin receptor; *IRS*, insulin receptor substrate; *JNK*, c-Jun N-terminal kinase; *LH*, luteinizing hormone; *NF-κB*, nuclear factor kappa B; *Nox*, nicotinamide adenine dinucleotide phosphate oxidase system; *PI3K*, phosphatidyl inositol 3-kinase; *ROS*, reactive oxygen species; *Ser Phos*, serine phosphorylation; *SHBG*, sex hormone–binding globulin; *TNF-α*, tumor necrosis factor-α; *Tyr Phos*, tyrosine phosphorylation.

Lipid Peroxidation

ROS causes lipid peroxidation of the polyunsaturated fatty acid side chains present in the cell membranes and organelles that contain lipid (mitochondria). This damage leads to cell death.

Levels of biomarkers, like oxidized low-density lipoprotein and malondialdehyde (MDA), are found to be raised in the PCOS patients with high levels of serum lipid peroxide concentrations[31]

Oxidative Stress Biomarkers Detected in Polycystic Ovary Syndrome

The biomarkers recognized to be involved in the pathogenesis of PCOS are malondialdehyde and nitric oxide (oxidants); however, the antioxidants also examined are total antioxidant capacity (TAC), superoxide dismutase (SOD), glutathione peroxidase (GPx), VE, vitamin C, and glutathione reductase (GSH).

Malondialdehyde

Lipid peroxidation of polyunsaturated fatty acids is a commonly found mechanism in OS and PCOs. MDA is the resultant of this lipid peroxidation and thus act as a biomarker of OS not only in serum but also in the follicular fluid of PCOS patients. Serum MDA concentration can be found raised in obese and nonobese PCOS patients. Independent of obesity, body mass index (BMI), and age, it becomes a biomarker of choice. Follicular MDA in PCOS patients is perhaps because of the low progesterone secretion and high levels of the follicle-stimulating hormone to luteinizing hormone ratio.[32]

Nitric Oxide

NO is an essential free radical and a cellular signaling molecule required to an appropriate extent for all physiologic and pathologic processes. Enzyme nitric oxide synthase (NOS) coverts L-arginine using oxygen and nicotinamide adenine dinucleotide phosphate (NADPH) as cofactors to synthesize NO. It is also released during the immune operations through phagocytic activities of monocytes, macrophages, and neutrophils. NO has a short half-life, which makes it really difficult to be detected in vivo. Nevertheless, it acts as a neuronal transmitter in the vessels and plays an important role in regulating vessel tone, blood pressure, vascular repair, and inflammation. With toxic levels, NO may affect cellular structural elements in combination with the other inflammatory factors.[33]

Young and metabolically fit PCOS patients have demonstrated high levels of NO (low levels of nitrites) and fibrinogen as biomarkers of vascular disease associated with IR. The nitrite to nitrate concentration ratio serves as an index of endothelium-derived NO. These mechanisms are independent of age and obesity; however, high BMI and IR are the confounding factors for easy manifestation of PCOS when existing simultaneously.

Furthermore, NO has been found to coexist with OS. Increased consumption of dietary nitrate can affect the plasma nitrite and nitrate levels, reflecting as increased endogenous NO production. Thus it can be concluded that low levels of nitrites may be a causative factor of the OS, leading to endothelial injury in PCOS patients.[34,35]

Advanced Glycation End Products

Advanced glycation end products (AGEs), also known as "glycotoxins," arc produced in the Maillard reaction, where the carbonyl groups of carbohydrates nonenzymatically react with the lipid or protein amino groups, inducing OS and resulting in inflammation and the promulgation of tissue damage. This further enhances the Maillard reaction and becomes a vicious cycle. With these effects, AGEs may alter enzyme functions, induce inflammatory modifications, and cause IR by the steroidal biosynthesis in the polycystic ovaries of PCOS patients. This atypical steroidogenesis occurring in PCOS women has led to eminent androgen synthesis and dysfunctional folliculogenesis. Serum concentrations of AGEs and expression of its receptor (RAGE) in monocytes have been found to be raised in PCOS patients, with an increase in serum AGEs and testosterone as a positive association.[36]

Xanthine Oxidase

Xanthine oxidase (XO) enzymatically helps in the oxidation of hypoxanthine to xanthine and furthermore catalyzes the xanthine to uric acid via the oxidation process.[37] This renders XO as a potential source of superoxide anion radical production, leading to OS. This role of XO of catabolizing purines in humans and generating ROS has been observed in cardiovascular disease, diabetes, metabolic syndrome, and PCOS patients. It has been found to be high along with the OS biomarkers with a simultaneous decrease in antioxidants.[38,39]

Total Antioxidant Capacity

Total antioxidant capacity (TAC) is the ability of scavenger present in the blood to encounter the free radical production. The association of TAC with PCOS has not yet been established. TAC has been found to be adequate in some studies, whereas others demonstrate low levels of TAC in PCOS patients. Nevertheless, one proposed theory of its high levels in PCOS is as a compensatory or reactionary increase to increased OS.[40]

Superoxide Dismutase

Mixed associations have been reported for SOD and PCOS. Females with PCOS exhibited increased SOD levels compared with controls, suggesting that the byproduct of oxidative damage is expected to be increased in women with PCOS.[41] SOD is an essential antioxidant that recognizes and eliminates superoxide anions (O_2-), by its enzymatic action, converting them to H_2O_2 and then by GPx to water.

SOD has been examined in the serum and in the follicular fluid (FF) of PCOS patients. Serum levels of SOD may decrease in PCOS patients but be increased in the follicular fluid. Decreased serum concentration with increase of SOD activity has been explained by the increased consumption of SOD against the provoked production of ROS occurring from the confounding factors like IR and obesity, coexisting in PCOS patients. In the FF, SOD attempts to counteract the ROS-mediated apoptosis. Furthermore, the decreased levels may also influence the second messenger system functioning for the oocytes. Because PCOS is characterized by a large number of large follicles in the ovary, a lot of cells need to undergo apoptosis as well. A decrease in FF SOD concentration and decreased expression of mRNA in the GC cells of PCOS patients indicate the high turnover of degenerating or dead granulosa cells, demonstrating the

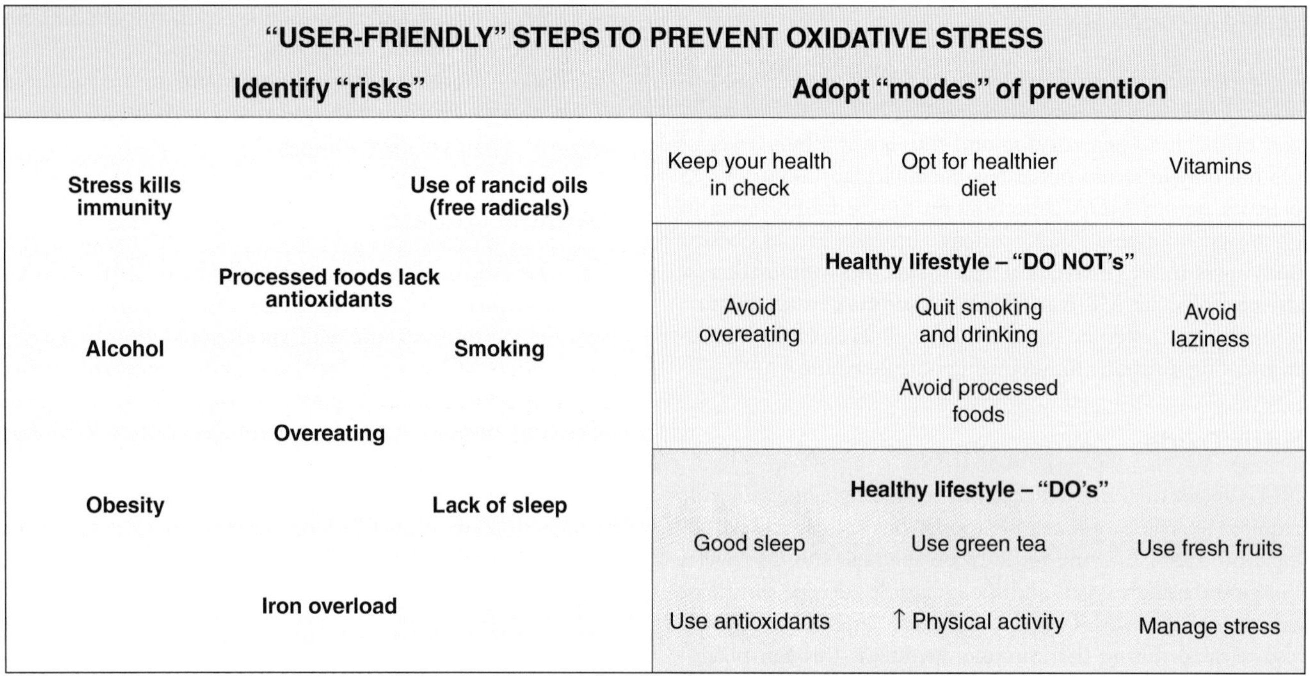

"USER-FRIENDLY" STEPS TO PREVENT OXIDATIVE STRESS

Identify "risks"	Adopt "modes" of prevention

Stress kills immunity	Use of rancid oils (free radicals)	Keep your health in check	Opt for healthier diet	Vitamins

Processed foods lack antioxidants

Alcohol	Smoking	**Healthy lifestyle – "DO NOT's"**	

		Avoid overeating	Quit smoking and drinking	Avoid laziness

Overeating

Avoid processed foods

Obesity	Lack of sleep	**Healthy lifestyle – "DO's"**

		Good sleep	Use green tea	Use fresh fruits

Iron overload

Use antioxidants	↑ Physical activity	Manage stress

• **Fig. 6.3** "Nip the Evil in the Bud." Oxidative Stress: Risks and Prevention.

---

significance of SOD in the process and maintenance of oocyte maturation.[42]

Glutathione Peroxidase

GPx belongs to the family of enzymes that provides protection from oxidative damage. It does this by reducing lipid hydroperoxides into their respective alcohols and then converting H_2O_2 to water. Nevertheless, researchers have been unable to report decreased levels of GPx in PCOS patients. This might be because of the compensatory increase against ROS. Further studies are warranted to find the causal relationship.[43]

Vitamin E

VE is a lipid-soluble molecule known as tocopherol. It acts vitally in female fertility because of its antioxidant and anti-inflammatory properties on female pregnancy, childbirth, and overall reproductive outcomes.[44] VE possess an antioxidant property because it is a peroxyl free radical scavenger. It prevents the free radicals from proliferating in membranes and plasma lipoproteins, thus acting as a "chain breaking antioxidant." Furthermore, because of its lipid solubility, it guards polyunsaturated fatty acids (PUFAs) from peroxidation (LPO).[45] Tolerable levels of VE in follicular fluid augments the probability of oocyte maturation, resulting in improved intracytoplasmic sperm injection (ICSI) outcomes.[46] VE improves OS and helps in decreasing human chorionic gonadotropin (HMG) dosage

(with no effect on the follicular development), endometrium thickness, and estradiol level in PCOS patients. It increases the serum TAC content and decreases the levels of MDA.

Identification and Prevention of OS Enhancing Factors

PCOS is recognized as a compound condition that can exist because of several precursors of OS and chronic inflammation. Identification of factors in daily lifestyle and understanding their effect on the aggravation of PCOs can play a vital role in preventing the advancement of the disease. Obesity and IR stand as prominent outcomes of OS and chronic inflammation. Unhealthy diet, lack of exercise and sleep, emotional stress, and smoking are some of the aspects that demand lifestyle modifications to aid better reproductive outcomes in potential PCOS patients (Fig. 6.3).

Conclusion

PCOS is frequently characterized by the existence of hormonal dysfunction, oocyte maturation, IR, DM, endothelial dysfunction, increased risk of hypertension, and dyslipidemia. Regardless of the apparent associated disease, the underlying cause rests on the crosstalk between OS and chronic inflammation. Evaluation of OS and cytokines/adipokines for the grade of inflammation would play an important role in treating PCOS patients.

References

1. Agarwal A, Gupta S, Sharma RK. Role of oxidative stress in female reproduction. *Reprod Biol Endocrinol.* 2005;3:28.

2. Pandey AN, Tripathi A, Premkumar KV, Shrivastav TG, Chaube SK. Reactive oxygen and nitrogen species during meiotic resumption from diplotene arrest in mammalian oocytes. *J Cell Biochem.* 2010;111(3):521-528. doi:10.1002/jcb.22736.

3. Tatemoto H, Sakurai N, Muto N. Protection of porcine oocytes against apoptotic cell death caused by oxidative stress during In vitro maturation: role of cumulus cells. *Biol Reprod.* 2000;63(3): 805-810.

4. Ishii T, Miyazawa M, Takanashi Y, et al. Genetically induced oxidative stress in mice causes thrombocytosis, splenomegaly and placental angiodysplasia that leads to recurrent abortion. *Redox Biol.* 2014;2:679-685.

5. Shkolnik K, Tadmor A, Ben-Dor S, Nevo N, Galiani D, Dekel N. Reactive oxygen species are indispensable in ovulation. *Proc Natl Acad Sci U S A.* 2011;108(4):1462-1467. doi:10.1073/pnas.1017213108.

6. Eichenlaub-Ritter U. Oocyte ageing and its cellular basis. *Int J Dev Biol.* 2012;56(10-12):841-852.

7. Landskron G, De la Fuente M, Thuwajit P, Thuwajit C, Hermoso MA. Chronic inflammation and cytokines in the tumor microenvironment. *J Immunol Res.* 2014;2014:149185.

8. Biswas SK. Does the interdependence between oxidative stress and inflammation explain the antioxidant paradox? *Oxid Med Cell Longev.* 2016;2016:5698931.

9. Hussain T, Tan B, Yin Y, Blachier F, Tossou MC, Rahu N. Oxidative stress and inflammation: what polyphenols can do for us? *Oxid Med Cell Longev.* 2016;2016:7432797.

10. Bedard K, Krause KH. The NOX family of ROS-generating NADPH oxidases: physiology and pathophysiology. *Physiol Rev.* 2007;87(1):245-313.

11. Lu X, Murphy TC, Nanes MS, Hart CM. PPARγ regulates hypoxia-induced Nox4 expression in human pulmonary artery smooth muscle cells through NF-κB. *Am J Physiol Lung Cell Mol Physiol.* 2010;299(4):L559-L566.

12. Oliveira-Marques V, Marinho HS, Cyrne L, Antunes F. Role of hydrogen peroxide in NF-κB activation: from inducer to modulator. *Antioxid Redox Signal.* 2009;11(9):2223-2243.

13. Yin J, Duan J, Cui Z, Ren W, Li T, Yin Y. Hydrogen peroxide-induced oxidative stress activates NF-κB and Nrf2/Keap1 signals and triggers autophagy in piglets. *RSC Adv.* 2015;5(20):15479-15486.

14. Rehman R, Mehmood M, Ali R, Shaharyar S, Alam F. Influence of body mass index and polycystic ovarian syndrome on ICSI/IVF treatment outcomes: a study conducted in Pakistani women. *Int J Reprod Biomed.* 2018;16(8):529.

15. Piya MK, McTernan PG, Kumar S. Adipokine inflammation and insulin resistance: the role of glucose, lipids and endotoxin. *J Endocrinol.* 2013;216(1):T1-T15.

16. Ouchi N, Parker JL, Lugus JJ, Walsh K. Adipokines in inflammation and metabolic disease. *Nat Rev Immunol.* 2011;11(2): 85-97.

17. Wang Y, Huang F. N-3 polyunsaturated fatty acids and inflammation in obesity: local effect and systemic benefit. *Biomed Res Int.* 2015;2015:581469.

18. Xie F, Anderson CL, Timme KR, Kurz SG, Fernando SC, Wood JR. Obesity-dependent increases in oocyte mRNAs are associated with increases in proinflammatory signaling and gut microbial abundance of Lachnospiraceae in female mice. *Endocrinology.* 2016;157(4):1630-1643.

19. Yeon Lee J, Baw CK, Gupta S, Aziz N, Agarwal A. Role of oxidative stress in polycystic ovary syndrome. *Curr Womens Health Rev.* 2010;6(2):96-107.

20. Pollak M. The insulin and insulin-like growth factor receptor family in neoplasia: an update. *Nat Rev Cancer.* 2012;12(3): 159-169.

21. Zhang D, Luo WY, Liao H, Wang CF, Sun Y. The effects of oxidative stress to PCOS. *Sichuan Da Xue Xue Bao Yi Xue Ban.* 2008;39(3): 421-423.

22. Cooke MS, Evans MD, Dizdaroglu M, Lunec JJ. Oxidative DNA damage: mechanisms, mutation, and disease. *FASEB J.* 2003;17(10):1195-1214.

23. Dinger Y, Akcay T, Erdem T, Ilker Saygili E, Gundogdu S. DNA damage, DNA susceptibility to oxidation and glutathione level in women with polycystic ovary syndrome. *Scand J Clin Lab Invest.* 2005;65(8):721-728.

24. Amato G, Conte M, Mazziotti G, et al. Serum and follicular fluid cytokines in polycystic ovary syndrome during stimulated cycles. *Obstet Gynecol.* 2003;101(6):1177-1182.

25. Kelly CC, Lyall H, Petrie JR, Gould GW, Connell JM, Sattar N. Low grade chronic inflammation in women with polycystic ovarian syndrome. *J Clin Endocrinol Metab.* 2001;86(6): 2453-2455.

26. Wang X, Martindale JL, Liu Y, Holbrook N. The cellular response to oxidative stress: influences of mitogen-activated protein kinase signalling pathways on cell survival. *Biochem J.* 1998;333(2):291-300.

27. Boutros T, Chevet E, Metrakos PJ. Mitogen-activated protein (MAP) kinase/MAP kinase phosphatase regulation: roles in cell growth, death, and cancer. *Pharmacol Rev.* 2008;60(3):261-310.

28. Brown MD, Sacks DB. Protein scaffolds in MAP kinase signalling. *Cell Signal.* 2009;21(4):462-469.

29. Diamanti-Kandarakis E, Dunaif A. Insulin resistance and the polycystic ovary syndrome revisited: an update on mechanisms and implications. *Endocr Rev.* 2012;33(6):981-1030.

30. Kaya C, Erkan AF, Cengiz SD, et al. Advanced oxidation protein products are increased in women with polycystic ovary syndrome: relationship with traditional and nontraditional cardiovascular risk factors in patients with polycystic ovary syndrome. *Fertil Steril.* 2009;92(4):1372-1377.

31. Nur Torun A, Vural M, Cece H, Camuzcuoglu H, Toy H, Aksoy N. Paraoxonase-1 is not affected in polycystic ovary syndrome without metabolic syndrome and insulin resistance, but oxidative stress is altered. *Gynecol Endocrinol.* 2011;27(12):988-992.

32. Yildirim B, Demir S, Temur I, Erdemir R, Kaleli B. Lipid peroxidation in follicular fluid of women with polycystic ovary syndrome during assisted reproduction cycles. *J Reprod Med.* 2007;52(8):722-726.

33. Stichtenoth D, Frölich JC. Nitric oxide and inflammatory joint diseases. *Br J Rheumatol.* 1998;37(3):246-257.

34. Meng C. Nitric oxide (NO) levels in patients with polycystic ovary syndrome (PCOS): a meta-analysis. *J Int Med Res.* 2019;47(9):4083-4094.

35. Sprung VS, Atkinson G, Cuthbertson DJ, et al. Endothelial function measured using flow-mediated dilation in polycystic ovary syndrome: a meta-analysis of the observational studies. *Clin Endocrinol (Oxf).* 2013;78(3):438-446.

36. Garg D, Merhi Z. Relationship between advanced glycation end products and steroidogenesis in PCOS. *Reprod Biol Endocrinol.* 2016;14(1):1-13.

37. Puddu P, Puddu GM, Cravero E, Vizioli L, Muscari A. The relationships among hyperuricemia, endothelial dysfunction,

and cardiovascular diseases: molecular mechanisms and clinical implications. *J Cardiol.* 2012;59(3):235-242.

38. Galassetti P. Inflammation and oxidative stress in obesity, metabolic syndrome, and diabetes. *Exp Diabetes Res.* 2012;2012:943706.

39. Miric DJ, Kisic BB, Zoric LD, Mitic RV, Miric BM, Dragojevic IM. Xanthine oxidase and lens oxidative stress markers in diabetic and senile cataract patients. *J Diabetes Complications.* 2013;27(2):171-176.

40. Verit FF, Erel O. Oxidative stress in nonobese women with polycystic ovary syndrome: correlations with endocrine and screening parameters. *Gynecol Obstet Invest.* 2008;65(4):233-239.

41. Talat A, Satyanarayana P, Anand P. Association of superoxide dismutase level in women with polycystic ovary syndrome. *J Obstet Gynaecol India.* 2022;72:6-12.

42. Seleem AK, El Refaeey AA, Shaalan D, Sherbiny Y, Badawy A. Superoxide dismutase in polycystic ovary syndrome patients undergoing intracytoplasmic sperm injection. *J Assist Reprod Genet.* 2014;31(4):499-504.

43. Savic-Radojevic A, Antic IB, Coric V, et al. Effect of hyperglycemia and hyperinsulinemia on glutathione peroxidase activity in non-obese women with polycystic ovary syndrome. *Hormones (Athens).* 2015;14(1):101-108.

44. Shamim AA, Schulze K, Merrill RD, et al. First-trimester plasma tocopherols are associated with risk of miscarriage in rural Bangladesh. *Am J Clin Nutr.* 2015;101(2):294-301.

45. Lebold KM, Traber MG. Interactions between α-tocopherol, polyunsaturated fatty acids, and lipoxygenases during embryogenesis. *Free Radic Biol Med.* 2014;66:13-19.

46. Ashraf M, Mustansir F, Baqir SM, Alam F, Rehman R. Changes in vitamin E levels as a marker of female infertility. *J Pak Med Assoc.* 2020;70(10):1762-1766.

7

Polycystic Ovary Syndrome and Subfertility: Ovulation Dysregulation and Fertility Problems (Clinical Features and Pathophysiology)

NADEEM F. ZUBERI AND SUMERA BATOOL

Introduction

Polycystic ovary syndrome (PCOS) affects mainly reproductive-age females. The prevalence can vary between 8% to 13% based on ethnicity, and the variability is because of different criteria used for the diagnosis.[1] The most common concerning problem related to PCOS is the physical appearance in adolescence females, but metabolic abnormalities, cardiovascular risk factors, and psychosocial problems are also part of a broader disease spectrum. Another very important and distressing aspect for middle-aged females is subfertility/infertility. Although family size has not been found to be different in females with and without PCOS in different studies, those with PCOS are more likely to require treatment or some assistance to conceive. Multiple factors have been studied to understand the pathophysiologic processes involved in infertility among females with PCOS. Chronic anovulation is considered to be the main reason among these. Oligo/anovulation is also considered one of the major diagnostic criteria of PCOS.[2]

Subfertility is having reduced fertility in couples trying to conceive and is considered after unprotected intercourse of 12 months' duration. About 8% to 12% of couples are affected by this, and the main reason is found to be male factor infertility in 50% of cases.[3] In females seeking treatment for ovulation dysregulation–related infertility, however, PCOS is the most common diagnosis in 70% of cases.[4] The American Society for Reproductive Medicine recommends that a female with PCOS undergo infertility evaluation if she is unable to conceive after 6 months of unprotected intercourse, provided the intercourse is regular (2 to 3 times/week).[5]

Normal Ovulation Physiology

Ovulation is characterized by the development and subsequent release of one dominant follicle from the ovary in each menstrual cycle. The follicle then enters the fallopian tube where fertilization can occur. The whole process of ovulation requires an active hypothalamic-pituitary axis.[6]

During embryogenesis, primordial follicles are formed, which are mainly oocytes arrested at the prophase I during meiosis. There are around 1 to 2 million primordial follicles in each ovary. In prepubertal females, the follicles develop to the antral stage; after that, maturation is mainly dependent on gonadotropins. During puberty, the rise in gonadotropins stimulates the completion of meiosis I in primordial follicles, resulting in formation of secondary follicles. These secondary follicles enter meiosis II and continue to develop until the preovulatory stage. One of the follicles is selected as a dominant follicle, which sustains its development, and it undergoes ovulation. The rest of the follicles undergo atresia. In this way, a significant number of follicles are lost in a single ovulatory cycle, and there is a linear correlation between the number of follicles lost and age[7]. Each month, both the ovaries release follicles alternately. With the onset of menopause, the ovulatory function ceases[8] (Fig. 7.1).

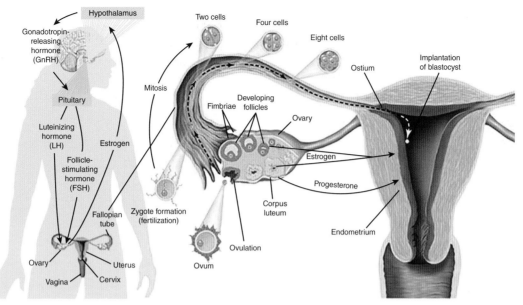

• **Fig. 7.1** The Hypothalamus-Pituitary-Ovarian Axis, from Ovulation to Implantation.

Hormones Involved in Ovulation

Gonadotropin-releasing hormone (GnRH) is secreted by the arcuate nucleus within the hypothalamus. It is secreted in pulses and regulates the secretion of follicle-stimulating hormone (FSH) and luteinizing hormone (LH) from the anterior pituitary. Low frequency pulses of GnRH stimulate the FSH secretion, whereas high frequency ones cause LH secretion.[9]

Gonadotropins are glycoprotein molecules, and they have two subunits (i.e., alpha and beta). All glycoproteins, like thyroid stimulating hormone and human chorionic gonadotropin hormone, have common alpha subunits, just like FSH and LH. The beta subunit is specific to each hormone.

In females, FSH is responsible for the secretion of estrogen, and it controls the maturation of the dominant follicle. LH, on the other hand, causes androgen production from the ovarian theca cells. Low levels of estrogen give a negative feedback to the gonadotropins.[10]

FSH acts on the G-protein coupled receptors on the surface of granulosa cells, initiating estrogen production. This estrogen is required for the development and maturation of follicles during the follicular phase of menstrual cycle. It also causes granulosa cells to increase their own production of estrogen autonomously. When estrogen reaches a critical level, it starts giving positive feedback for LH and results in an LH surge.[11]

This LH surge causes rupture of dominant follicle, inducing ovulation and luteinization of granulosa cells forming corpus luteum. This corpus luteum then secretes progesterone, marking the start of luteal phase. If fertilization does not occur, then corpus luteum degrades spontaneously and progesterone levels drop. This marks the start of shedding of the uterine endometrium and menstrual bleeding.[12]

The complex interaction between GnRH, FSH, and LH is essential for follicular development and maturation, ovulation, and uterine endometrium reception or shedding[13] (Fig. 7.2).

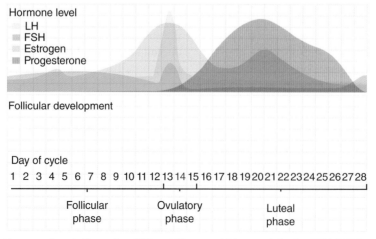

• **Fig. 7.2** Hormone Levels Regarding Different Phases of Menstrual Cycle. *FSH*, Follicle stimulating hormone; *LH*, luteinizing hormone. (Reproduced with permission from Nevada Center for Reproductive Medicine, https://nevadafertility.com/phasesofthemenstrualcycle/)

Pathology in Polycystic Ovary Syndrome

The pathology involved in PCOS is complex and multifactorial involving hyperandrogenism, ovulation and menstrual abnormalities, and polycystic morphology of ovaries on ultrasonography. Excessive androgen production either in ovaries or adrenals, is because of defects in steroidogenesis and an increase in insulin levels. The majority of females with PCOS (60%–80%) also have metabolic abnormalities, such as overweight/obesity and insulin resistance (IR).

The abnormalities involved at different levels of hypothalamus, pituitary and ovaries are discussed as follow:

Hypothalamic: Pituitary Axis

In PCOS, there is excess secretion of GnRH from the hypothalamus. The pulse frequency of GnRH increases up to 40% from normal, and some evidence even suggests that the anterior pituitary becomes more sensitive toward the action of GnRH.[14] LH secretion is enhanced by the higher pulse frequency, whereas the FSH levels are stimulated by lower GnRH pulses. Thus the high pulse frequency of GnRH results in relatively high levels of LH. So, in PCOS, the LH to FSH ratio is typically two or three times higher than normal, although it is not included in the diagnostic criteria.[15] Because of low FSH and estradiol levels and the absence of an LH surge, ovulation does not occur and corpus luteum does not form. Normally progesterone is secreted by corpus luteum and gives a negative feedback to GnRH at hypothalamus; therefore this negative feedback is lost. Moreover, because of high androgen levels, the hypothalamus also becomes less sensitive to this negative feedback from the estradiol and progesterone; thus a vicious cycle develops.[14]

At the Level of Ovaries

LH acts on LH receptors on ovarian theca cells, which undergo hyperplasia and start producing excessive androgens. Normally the androgens produced by theca cells are converted into estrogen by an enzyme called aromatase. This enzyme is produced by granulosa cells and is a rate-limiting enzyme for estrogen production. Aromatase activity is sometimes assessed by the ratio of estradiol to testosterone. In PCOS, however, either the aromatase activity is reduced or dysregulated; the exact reason why is still under investigation.[16]

Similarly, the effects of IR and obesity on aromatase activity are still controversial. The high androgen levels can manifest clinically as acne, hirsutism, or temporal baldness. The clinical or biochemical evidence of hyperandrogenism is one of the major criteria of PCOS adopted by almost all of the guidelines.

The relatively low estradiol and FSH levels and high androgens disrupt the process of follicle maturation. Multiple follicles start growing at the same time, but their growth arrests prematurely. There is inhibition of ovulation. This anovulation is the principal cause of subfertility in PCOS females and is why ovulation induction is the first-line treatment option for such patients.

Another important problem is menstrual irregularities which is also one of the major diagnostic criteria for PCOS. This is a common presentation of PCOS and results in unpredicted ovulation causing a difficulty in planning a pregnancy. About 75% to 80% of PCOS females have some menstrual abnormalities.[17] Moreover, in PCOS, sometimes even when the cycles are regular, ovulation does not occur regularly, resulting in decreased chances to conceive.

The majority of androgens in PCOS are produced in the ovaries, but some are also produced in the adrenal glands as well.

Obesity and Insulin Resistance

Different cutoffs are used for overweight and obese patients, but the majority (35%–80%) of PCOS females fall under these categories. Obesity, specifically central obesity, potentiates the clinical and biochemical features of PCOS and increases IR.

The hyperinsulinemia decreases the sex hormone–binding globulin (SHBG), resulting in high free testosterone levels, thus further contributing to hyperandrogenism.

Another important pathology is IR, which is a hallmark of PCOS, affecting 65% to 70% of patients. Acanthosis nigricans is a clinical sign of IR and is commonly found in PCOS patients. IR is even found independent or disproportionate to the grade of obesity in PCOS, which forms the basis for lean PCOS. It acts synergistically with LH and potentiates ovarian hyperandrogenism. It upregulates LH receptors at the surface of theca cells and induces enzymes involved in steroidogenesis. This is considered a functional hyperandrogenism because it does not involve any enzyme deficiency. These biochemical abnormalities (hyperandrogenism and IR) also induce the microcyst formation in ovaries arranged at the periphery, the characteristic polycystic morphology on ultrasonography.

At the Level of Endometrium

Because of continuous estrogen exposure without adequate progesterone, endometrial hyperplasia can occur in PCOS females, and they are considered to be at high risk for developing endometrial cancer compared with the normal population. Nevertheless, routine screening for endometrial cancer for PCOS females is still not recommended. Moreover, these endometrial changes render the uterus less receptive for pregnancy, with increased incidence of failed implantation or early pregnancy loss. About 50% of PCOS females experience first trimester miscarriages[18] (Fig. 7.3).

Intrauterine Exposure of Androgens

Multiple environmental and genetic factors have been hypothesized to be responsible for such a broad range of disease

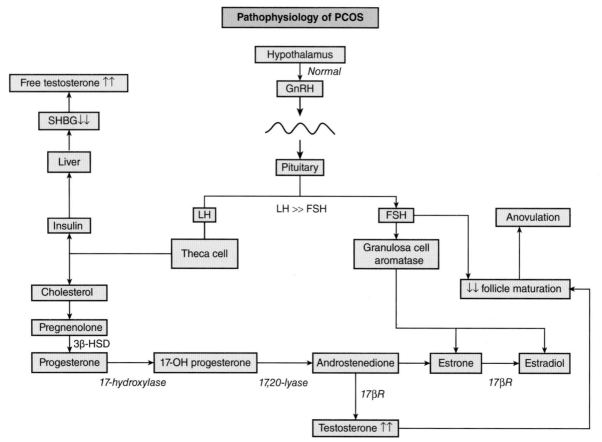

• **Fig. 7.3** Multifactorial Pathology of Polycystic Ovary Syndrome *(PCOS)*. *FSH,* Follicle stimulating hormone; *GnRH,* gonadotropin-releasing hormone; *LH,* luteinizing hormone; *SHBG,* sex hormone binding globulin.

symptoms. Genetic factors have been taken into consideration because of cases clustering in families. Nevertheless, so far only a few genes have been linked to PCOS. Some of the important environmental factors include sedentary lifestyle, overweight/obesity, and exposure to androgens in prenatal life.[19]

The female child of a mother with congenital adrenal hyperplasia when get exposed to high androgen levels during intrauterine life; their ovaries develop PCOS morphology in adolescence. The same has been observed with other virilizing diseases and tumors, which supports the link of PCOS and prenatal androgen exposure.

Other Factors

Depression and mood disorders are common in females with PCOS (23%–64% of patients).[8] Sexual dysfunction has also been reported to be as high as 57.7% in PCOS females.[20] This can be because of psychological issues like anxiety, low self-esteem, or altered body image because of obesity, hirsutism, or acne. These factors have also been considered important in couples with infertility/subfertility–related issues. Another reason is high androgen levels, which directly reduce sexual drive in females.

Conclusion

In conclusion, the data gathered through epidemiologic and observational studies points toward the multifactorial pathogenesis in PCOS and subfertility. Hyperandrogenism is the key biochemical abnormality, but obesity and IR are commonly found in PCOS females and further exacerbate the hyperandrogenism and negatively affect their fertility potential.

References

1. Sanchez-Garrido MA, Tena-Sempere M. Metabolic dysfunction in polycystic ovary syndrome: pathogenic role of androgen excess and potential therapeutic strategies. *Mol Metab.* 2020;35:100937. Available at: https://www.ncbi.nlm.nih.gov/pmc/articles/PMC7115104/. doi:10.1016/j.molmet.2020.01.001.

2. Mohammad MB, Seghinsara AM. Polycystic ovary syndrome (PCOS), diagnostic criteria, and AMH. *Asian Pac J Cancer Prev.* 2017;18(1):17-21. doi:10.22034/APJCP.2017.18.1.17.

3. Vander Borght M, Wyns C. Fertility and infertility: definition and epidemiology. *Clin Biochem.* 2018;62:2-10. doi:10.1016/j.clinbiochem.2018.03.012.

4. Cunha A, Póvoa AM. Infertility management in women with polycystic ovary syndrome: a review. *Porto Biomed J.* 2021;6(1):e116. doi:10.1097/j.pbj.0000000000000116.

5. Melo AS, Ferriani RA, Navarro PA. Treatment of infertility in women with polycystic ovary syndrome: approach to clinical practice. *Clinics (Sao Paulo)*. 2015;70(11):765-769. doi:10.6061/clinics/2015(11)09.

6. Holesh JE, Bass AN, Lord M. Physiology, ovulation. In: *StatPearls* [Internet]. Treasure Island (FL): StatPearls Publishing; 2021. Available at: http://www.ncbi.nlm.nih.gov/books/NBK441996/.

7. Cox E, Takov V. Embryology, Ovarian Follicle Development. In: StatPearls [Internet]. Treasure Island (FL): StatPearls Publishing; 2022 [cited 2022 Aug 24]. Available from: http://www.ncbi.nlm.nih.gov/books/NBK532300/

8. Richards JS, Russell DL, Robker RL, Dajee M, Alliston TN. Molecular mechanisms of ovulation and luteinization. *Mol Cell Endocrinol*. 1998;145(1-2):47-54. doi:10.1016/s0303-7207(98)00168-3.

9. Laven JSE. Follicle stimulating hormone receptor (FSHR) polymorphisms and polycystic ovary syndrome (PCOS). *Front Endocrinol*. 2019;10:23. doi:10.3389/fendo.2019.00023.

10. Gardner DG, Shoback D, eds. *Greenspan's Basic & Clinical Endocrinology*. 10th ed. McGraw Hill; 2017. Available at: https://accessmedicine.mhmedical.com/content.aspx?bookid=2178&sectionid=166246461.

11. Mikhael S, Punjala-Patel A, Gavrilova-Jordan L. Hypothalamic-pituitary-ovarian axis disorders impacting female fertility. *Biomedicines*. 2019;7(1):5. doi: 10.3390/biomedicines7010005.

12. Reed BG, Carr BR. The normal menstrual cycle and the control of ovulation. In: Feingold KR, Anawalt B, Boyce A, et al., eds. *Endotext* [Internet]. South Dartmouth (MA): MDText.com, Inc.; 2000. Available at: https://www.ncbi.nlm.nih.gov/books/NBK279054/.

13. Richards JS, Pangas SA. The ovary: basic biology and clinical implications. *J Clin Invest*. 2010;120(4)963-972. doi: 10.1172/JCI41350.

14. Abbara A, Dhillo WS. Targeting elevated GnRH pulsatility to treat polycystic ovary syndrome. *J Clin Endocrinol Metab*. 2021;106(10): e4275-e4277. doi:10.1210/clinem/dgab422.

15. Saadia Z. Follicle stimulating hormone (LH: FSH) ratio in polycystic ovary syndrome (PCOS) - obese vs. non- obese women. *Med Arch*. 2020;74(4):289-293. doi:10.5455/mearh.2020.74.289-293.

16. Chen J, Shen S, Tan Y, et al. The correlation of aromatase activity and obesity in women with or without polycystic ovary syndrome. *J Ovarian Res*. 2015;8:11. doi:10.1186/s13048-015-0139-1.

17. Harris HR, Titus LJ, Cramer DW, Terry KL. Long and irregular menstrual cycles, polycystic ovary syndrome, and ovarian cancer risk in a population-based case-control study. *Int J Cancer*. 2017;140(2):285-291. doi:10.1002/ijc.30441.

18. Li X, Feng Y, Lin JF, Billig H, Shao R. Endometrial progesterone resistance and PCOS. *J Biomed Sci*. 2014;21(1):2. doi:10.1186/1423-0127-21-2.

19. Ruddenklau A, Campbell RE. Neuroendocrine impairments of polycystic ovary syndrome. *Endocrinology*. 2019;160(10): 2230-2242. doi:10.1210/en.2019-00428.

20. Eftekhar T, Sohrabvand F, Zabandan N, Shariat M, Haghollahi F, Ghahghaei-Nezamabadi A. Sexual dysfunction in patients with polycystic ovary syndrome and its affected domains. *Iran J Reprod Med*. 2014;12(8):539-546.

8

Clinical Features and Presentation of Polycystic Ovary Syndrome

SOBIA SABIR ALI AND SUMERAH JABEEN

Introduction

Polycystic ovarian syndrome (PCOS) is a complex disorder with systemic metabolic manifestations affecting 4% to 20% of reproductive-aged females worldwide.[1] It is characterized by signs and symptoms of androgen excess, anovulatory cycles, and/or presence of cysts in one or both ovaries. PCOS has a variable phenotypic presentation, and its underlying pathophysiology is still not completely understood.[2] Multiple genetic and environmental factors play an important role in the occurrence of this heterogenous disorder. PCOS dates back to 1935, when it was then known as Stein Leventhal syndrome after two prominent gynecologists who were the first to present a case series of seven females with menstrual irregularities, sterility, and hyperandrogenemia.[3] The year 1990 heralded the first international definition of PCOS, which has since evolved and been classified by various professional bodies. PCOS, although currently defined by three different definitions, is still considered a diagnosis of exclusion.

Clinical Features of Polycystic Ovary Syndrome: A Brief Overview

There are three main diagnostic criteria proposed for PCOS. The classical features of clinical or biochemical evidence of hyperandrogenemia and chronic anovulation with oligomenorrhea or amenorrhea are the common components of all three criteria, but the Rotterdam criteria incorporates the morphologic appearance of polycystic ovaries on ultrasound examination as an additional feature.

In 2012 the Evidence-Based Methodology PCOS Workshop sponsored by the National Institutes of Health characterized PCOS into four main phenotypes as follows:[4]
- Hyperandrogenism, ovulatory dysfunction, and polycystic ovary morphology

- Hyperandrogenism with ovulatory dysfunction
- Hyperandrogenism and polycystic ovary morphology
- Ovulatory dysfunction with polycystic ovary morphology

The hyperandrogenemia in PCOS usually presents with hirsutism, acne, androgenic alopecia, and thinning of scalp hair. Virilization, including male pattern balding, deepening of voice, and increased muscle mass, are not features of PCOS but suggestive of an underlying adrenal or ovarian neoplasm or severe insulin resistance (IR). Females with PCOS are prone to develop weight gain, which could lead to IR causing hyperandrogenemia and worsening the symptoms of PCOS.

Irregular or absent menstrual cycles are among the most common manifestations of PCOS symptoms. Irregular cycles are defined as cycles that are either less than 21 days or more than 35 days in duration or fewer than 8 cycles per year, but adolescent females presenting with primary amenorrhea at 15 or 16 years merits the exclusion of other causes as well.[5] Similarly, secondary amenorrhea lasting for more than 90 days is uncommon and requires further investigation. Because of anovulatory cycles, PCOS females are at an increased risk for infertility with spontaneous miscarriages seen more frequently in obese PCOS than the general population.

Clinical Features

The detailed narrative of clinical features of PCOS can be elaborated as:
1. Cutaneous or cosmetic manifestations
   i. Hirsutism
   ii. Acne
   iii. Androgenic alopecia
   iv. Acanthosis nigricans
   v. Seborrhea

2. Ovulatory dysfunction
    i. Oligomenorrhoea
    ii. Infertility
3. Metabolic dysfunction
    i. Obesity
    ii. IR
    iii. Dysglycemia
4. Psychological vulnerability
5. Other associations of PCOS
    i. Thyroid dysfunction
    ii. Endometrial carcinoma
    iii. Lipid disorders
    iv. Obstructive sleep apnea (OSA)
    v. Nonalcoholic fatty liver disease (NAFLD)/Nonalcoholic steatohepatitis (NASH)
    vi. Adverse pregnancy outcomes

Cutaneous Manifestations

Hyperinsulinemia and IR are commonly identified in females with PCOS. Hyperinsulinemia, in concert with LH, can result in hyperandrogenemia by enhancing the theca cell ovarian androgen production at one end and lowering the hepatic production of sex hormone–binding globulin (SHBG) at the other end, thus resulting in raised free testosterone levels with the clinical manifestations of hirsutism, acne, seborrhea, and scalp hair loss. Acanthosis nigricans and skin tags are the other cutaneous manifestations of PCOS suggesting underlying IR in such patients.

Androgens play an important role in the cutaneous manifestations of PCOS, but they have also been observed in patients in the absence of biochemical hyperandrogenemia, which has led to the inclusion of either clinical or biochemical hyperandrogenism as one of the components of PCOS criteria.[6]

Although obesity tends to precipitate hyperinsulinemia, females with PCOS are shown to have significant IR independent of the extent of obesity and androgenic concentration.[7] Thus the cutaneous manifestations in PCOS are a complex interplay between various hormonal and metabolic factors.

Hirsutism

Hirsutism is defined as male-pattern terminal hair growth in an androgen-dependent area of a female. Hirsutism remains the most common clinical feature of hyperandrogenism. It is present in approximately 65% to 75% of patients with PCOS. It should be differentiated from hypertrichosis, which is the presence of abnormal excessive villus hair all over the body. The development of hirsutism is subject to genetic and geographic variations with lower incidence seen in Asian population.[8]

The extent of clinical presentation of hyperandrogenism is dependent on both the circulating and local androgen concentrations and the sensitivity of the pilosebaceous unit to the androgens. In metabolically obese patients, hirsutism tends to be more severe. Hirsutism may be the hallmark of

the metabolic sequelae of PCOS and also may herald an adverse prognosis for conception and pregnancy during infertility treatment.[9,10]

The modified Ferriman-Gallwey scoring system is a widely used tool by most clinicians to define hirsutism. It includes scoring the nine body areas most sensitive to androgen from 0 (no hair) to 4 (frankly virile), and these separate scores are summed to provide a hormonal hirsutism score. A score of 8 or greater is considered as significant, 8 to 15 is taken as mild hirsutism, and a score of 16 to 36 is moderate to severe hirsutism. Nevertheless, this scoring system has its own limitations because it depends on patient subjectivity and does not include hair growth on side burns, the nape of the neck, and the phalangeal and perianal region. A woman with a thick upper lip can have a score of less than 8, thus not reflecting the cosmetic concern of the patient.

Acne

Acne is considered one of the common dermatologic conditions of PCOS; the prevalence is reported in the range of 9.8% to 34%.[11] It results from the formation of comedones along with sebum accumulation and desquamated follicular epithelial cells, which provide a substrate for colonization by the bacterium *Propionibacterium acnes*. Acne in females with PCOS can present with lesions on the face, neck, upper chest, upper back, and upper arms. Although androgens play an important role in the pathophysiology of acne by increasing the sebum production within the pilosebaceous unit, in adolescent and postpubertal PCOS, the acne could also be a result of normal puberty because of an adrenal androgen surge with adrenarche. Thus androgen-dependent and androgen-independent acne can both occur in females with PCOS.

Androgenic Alopecia

Androgenic alopecia, described as the preservation of the frontal hairline with progressive thinning of the crown by Ludwig, is a recognized symptom of PCOS. Androgenic alopecia has a late presentation during the disease course but is a significant cause of psychological distress in women.

It can present in several patterns including diffuse reduction in volume and thinning of hair. The reported prevalence of alopecia in PCOS ranges between 67% to 77.8%, confirming an association between PCOS and androgenic alopecia.[11,12] With studies showing both a positive and negative correlation of alopecia with circulating androgens levels, it is hypothesized that for the development of androgenic alopecia the local androgens may be important mediators compared with the level of circulating androgens. The Ludwig score is a well-known subjective method for grading androgenic alopecia.

Acanthosis Nigricans

Acanthosis nigricans is defined as hyperpigmented, thickened, soft velvety plaques present primarily over the axillae, neck, and the angular extensor surfaces on the elbows and knuckle. It is an important feature in females with PCOS and considered a clinical indicator of IR with an increased risk for type 2 diabetes mellitus (DM). Females with obesity are more prone to develop acanthosis nigricans. An Indian study showed a prevalence of 56% acanthosis nigricans among females with PCOS, which was significantly higher than the general population, reiterating the importance of lifestyle modifications in patients presenting with this readily apparent and identifiable physical examination to prevent the impending metabolic sequalae of the syndrome.[13]

Seborrhea

Seborrhea, a common skin problem that can cause red, itchy rash and white scales over the scalp and parts of the face, has also been defined as a cutaneous feature in PCOS with a prevalence of 34.7% in one study.[9] The clinical presentation of seborrhea is associated with higher levels of free testosterone, fasting glucose, and insulin levels. Besides hyperandrogenemia, the genetic predisposition, climate, and emotional factors are other important elements affecting seborrhea occurrence; therefore in females with PCOS, a clinical, serologic, and radiologic examination is important for the diagnosis of this entity in relation to PCOS.[9]

Ovulatory Dysfunction

Ovulatory dysfunction is one of the most common features of PCOS. Because PCOS is considered an IR state, the raised insulin levels serve as a stimulator to ovarian steroidogenesis, leading to ovarian dysfunction in such females.

Oligomenorrhea

The spectrum of ovulatory dysfunction includes both oligomenorrhea, defined as either a cycle duration of more than 35 days or fewer than 8 cycles per year or polyamenorrhea, defined as cycles of less than 21 days in duration. There is also a small subset of females with PCOS who may appear eumenorrheic until evaluated more closely by measuring a midluteal phase (day 21–23) progesterone level.

Because PCOS is characterized by eu-estrogenic chronic anovulation, leading to a well estrogenized endometrium, a withdrawal bleeding can be induced in such females after a 5 to 10 day course of progesterone. The occurrence of a withdrawal bleed in a patient with secondary amenorrhea can further support the anovulation being secondary to PCOS and exclude ovarian insufficiency or hypogonadotropic hypogonadism, which are hypoestrogenic states.

Infertility

PCOS remains one of the leading causes of anovulatory infertility, accounting for 25% to 40% of cases in population-based studies of infertility.[2] Although oligo/anovulation remains the most common cause behind PCOS infertility, there are other potential factors that could contribute to PCOS infertility, including reduced oocyte competency and diminished endometrial receptivity because of increased androgen receptors in the endometrium of females with PCOS.[14,15]

The accompanying obesity in such females also serves to potentiate delayed conception and subfertility. Once the aforementioned factors have been excluded, male factor infertility should also be considered during the workup of infertility.

Metabolic Dysfunction

PCOS is a common endocrinopathy affecting both the reproductive and metabolic functions. The IR, along with other metabolic abnormalities of PCOS, translates into an increased risk of developing obesity, type 2 DM, dyslipidemia, hypertension, and cardiovascular diseases.

Obesity

Obesity continues to remain a common feature of PCOS. The relationship between obesity and PCOS is complex. Although there is evidence suggesting an increased prevalence of obesity in females with PCOS, it is debatable if the incidence of PCOS may parallel the growing epidemic of obesity.

There is a higher rate of upper-body obesity in women with PCOS, independent of body mass index (BMI), as demonstrated by increased waist circumference and waist-hip ratio compared with BMI-matched control females.[16]

Obesity and, in particular, abdominal obesity cause relative hyperandrogenemia by initiating a reduction in SHBG levels and increasing the delivery of bioavailable androgens to the target tissues. There is also an increased production rate of non-SHBG–bound dehydroepiandrosterone and androstenedione, which explains the basis for more frequent menstrual abnormalities and chronic anovulation in adult overweight and obese compared with normal weight females.[17,18]

In comparison to normal weight PCOS females, the obese PCOS patients are found to have more severe clinical features, increased central fat distribution, worsened metabolic parameters, hyperandrogenemia, and metabolic abnormalities. Thus obesity tends to exacerbate the reproductive and metabolic abnormalities, including the relative risk of anovulatory infertility, in such females. Obesity has also been shown to hamper the stimulation in ovulation induction cycles, requiring higher doses with longer periods of stimulation.[10]

Insulin Resistance

IR and hyperinsulinemia is a common finding in females with PCOS, particularly seen in females with polycystic ovary morphology and chronic anovulation.[19] Insulin-mediated glucose uptake by skeletal muscles is reduced by 35% to 40% in females with PCOS compared with weight comparable non-PCOS females, suggesting that IR is independent of obesity. Obesity, on the other hand, exacerbates the IR by causing resistance to insulin-mediated suppression of endogenous hepatic glucose production. Therefore there is a combined deleterious effect of obesity and PCOS on endogenous glucose production, forming a basis for the pathogenesis of glucose intolerance.[19]

Dysglycemia in Polycystic Ovary Syndrome

PCOS patients present with a fivefold to 10-fold higher risk for abnormal glucose metabolism (ABG), occurring a little earlier (approximately in the third or fourth decade of life) compared with the general population.[20] The IR with hyperinsulinemia and some PCOS showing alteration in beta cell function leads to metabolic abnormalities, including impaired glucose tolerance, type 2 DM, and lipid abnormalities, important risk factors for cardiovascular diseases. Obesity, positive family history of type 2 DM, and hyperandrogenemia are additional factors contributing to this metabolic milieu of PCOS.

Psychological Vulnerability

The various cosmetic, gynecologic, and metabolic features associated with PCOS may have serious implications on the psychological wellbeing of an individual. The physical appearance of a PCOS female can interfere with the norms of femininity, leading to life-long emotional distress and depression. These patients are prone to develop anxiety, poor self-esteem, body image dissatisfaction, and eating and sexual disorders. Therefore addressing the psychological problems from the very start of management is as important as treating their physical symptoms.[21]

Other Associations of Polycystic Ovary Syndrome

Thyroid Dysfunction

PCOS and autoimmune thyroid diseases are two of the most common endocrinopathies. Studies have shown a significantly higher prevalence of goiter and subclinical hypothyroidism in PCOS patients compared with controls. Although the connection between these two entities has not been clearly defined, increased BMI and IR are conditions common to both. PCOS females are also shown to have higher thyroid antibody levels, larger thyroid volumes, and thyroid echogenicity compared with controls. PCOS has also been shown to have increased autoimmunity for organs other than thyroid as well.[22,23]

Endometrial Carcinoma

There are also studies suggesting an association between PCOS and endometrial cancer. PCOS is considered a risk factor for developing endometrial cancer, with one study suggesting a threefold increased risk of endometrial carcinoma in females with PCOS.[24,25]

Lipid Disorders

The metabolic abnormalities are a common feature of females with PCOS. PCOS patients have certain metabolic characteristics, predominantly defective insulin action and beta cell function, that confer a substantially increased risk for glucose intolerance and type 2 DM. Studies have also shown PCOS females to have alterations in lipid metabolism including high triglycerides, low-density lipoproteins (LDL) cholesterol, and lower high-density lipoproteins (HDL), accompanied with elevated C reactive protein (CRP) levels, and chronic low-grade inflammation makes them more susceptible to cardiovascular diseases, such as atherosclerosis.[26]

Obstructive Sleep Apnea

OSA is a complication seen in females with PCOS predominantly because of hyperandrogenemia and obesity, although these two factors cannot fully account for the pathogenesis because, even after controlling BMI, PCOS females were still seen to have multiple-fold increased sleep disordered breathing and daytime somnolence compared with controls.[27]

NAFLD/NASH

NAFLD/NASH has also been confirmed as an impending complication of PCOS because of the underlying metabolic dysfunction, with increasing age, ethnicity, obesity, IR, dyslipidemia, and glucose intolerance contributing as compounding factors in the underlying pathogenesis.[28]

Adverse Pregnancy Outcomes

PCOS is also considered one of the most common causes of anovulatory infertility. These females are shown to have difficult ovulation induction with higher doses and longer periods required for stimulation of ovulation induction. There is also evidence suggesting adverse pregnancy outcomes in females with PCOS with preterm delivery, gestational diabetes, and pre-eclampsia. A meta-analysis has suggested an independent association between PCOS, gestational DM, and hypertension.[29]

References

1. Deswal R, Narwal V, Dang A, Pundir CS. The prevalence of polycystic ovary syndrome: a brief systematic review. *J Hum Reprod Sci.* 2020;13(4):261.
2. Legro RS, Arslanian SA, Ehrmann DA, et al. Diagnosis and treatment of polycystic ovary syndrome: an Endocrine Society clinical practice guideline. *J Clin Endocrinol Metab.* 2013;98:4565-4592.
3. Stein IF. Amenorrhea associated with bilateral polycystic ovaries. *Am J Obstet Gynecol.* 1935;29:181-191.
4. Johnson T, Kaplan L, Ouyang P, Rizza P. *National Institutes of Health Evidence-Based Methodology Workshop on Polycystic Ovary Syndrome. NIH EbMW Reports.* Bethesda, MD: National Institutes of Health. 2012;1:1-14. Available at: https://prevention.nih.gov/sites/default/files/2018-06/FinalReport.pdf.
5. Witchel SF, Oberfield SE, Peña AS. Polycystic ovary syndrome: pathophysiology, presentation, and treatment with emphasis on adolescent girls. *J Endocr Soc.* 2019;3(8):1545-1573.
6. Li L, Yang D, Chen X, Chen Y, Feng S, Wang L. Clinical and metabolic features of polycystic ovary syndrome. *Int J Gynecol Obstet.* 2007;97(2):129-134.
7. Dunaif A, Segal KR, Futterweit W, Dobrjansky A. Profound peripheral insulin resistance, independent of obesity, in polycystic ovary syndrome. *Diabetes.* 1989;38(9):1165-1174.

8. Bozdag G, Mumusoglu S, Zengin D, Karabulut E, Yildiz BO. The prevalence and phenotypic features of polycystic ovary syndrome: a systematic review and meta-analysis. *Hum Reprod.* 2016;31(12): 2841-2855.

9. Özdemir S, Özdemir M, Görkemli H, Kiyici A, Bodur S. Specific dermatologic features of the polycystic ovary syndrome and its association with biochemical markers of the metabolic syndrome and hyperandrogenism. *Acta Obstet Gynecol Scand.* 2010;89(2):199-204.

10. Rausch ME, Legro RS, Barnhart HX, et al. Predictors of pregnancy in women with polycystic ovary syndrome. *J Clin Endocrinol Metab.* 2009;94(9):3458-3466.

11. Azziz R, Sanchez LA, Knochenhauer ES, et al. Androgen excess in women: experience with over 1000 consecutive patients. *J Clin Endocrinol Metab.* 2004;89(2):453-462.

12. Cela E, Robertson C, Rush K, et al. Clinical study prevalence of polycystic ovaries in women with androgenic alopecia. *Eur J Endocrinol.* 2003;149(5):439-442.

13. Rathnakar U, Gopalakrishna H, Jagadish RP. Acanthosis nigricans in PCOS patients and its relation with type 2 diabetes mellitus and body mass at a tertiary care hospital in southern India. *J Clin Diagn Res.* 2013;7(2):317-319.

14. Trounson A, Wood C, Kausche A. In vitro maturation and the fertilization and developmental competence of oocytes recovered from untreated polycystic ovarian patients. *Fertil Steril.* 1994;62(2): 353-362.

15. Apparao KB, Lovely LP, Gui Y, Lininger RA, Lessey BA. Elevated endometrial androgen receptor expression in women with polycystic ovarian syndrome. *Biol Reprod.* 2002;66(2):297-304.

16. Sam S. Obesity and polycystic ovary syndrome. *Obes Manag.* 2007;3(2):69-73.

17. Pasquali R. Obesity and androgens: facts and perspectives. *Fertil Steril.* 2006;85(5):1319-1340.

18. Pasquali R, Gambineri A, Pagotto U. The impact of obesity on reproduction in women with polycystic ovary syndrome. *BJOG.* 2006;113(10):1148-1159.

19. Dunaif A. Insulin action in the polycystic ovary syndrome. *Endocrinol Metab Clin North Am.* 1999;28(2):341-359.

20. Pelusi B, Gambineri A, Pasquali R. Type 2 diabetes and the polycystic ovary syndrome. *Minerva Ginecol.* 2004;56(1):41-51.

21. Farkas J, Rigó A, Demetrovics Z. Psychological aspects of the polycystic ovary syndrome. *Gynecol Endocrinol.* 2014;30(2): 95-99.

22. Singla R, Gupta Y, Khemani M, Aggarwal S. Thyroid disorders and polycystic ovary syndrome: an emerging relationship. *Indian J Endocrinol Metab.* 2015;19(1):25.

23. Fénichel P, Gobert B, Carré Y, Barbarino-Monnier P, Hiéronimus S. Polycystic ovary syndrome in autoimmune disease. *Lancet.* 1999;353(9171):2210.

24. Chittenden BG, Fullerton G, Maheshwari A, Bhattacharya S. Polycystic ovary syndrome and the risk of gynaecological cancer: a systematic review. *Reprod Biomed Online.* 2009;19(3):398-405.

25. Haoula Z, Salman M, Atiomo W. Evaluating the association between endometrial cancer and polycystic ovary syndrome. *Hum Reprod.* 2012;27(5):1327-1331.

26. Alves AC, Valcarcel B, Mäkinen VP, et al. Metabolic profiling of polycystic ovary syndrome reveals interactions with abdominal obesity. *Int J Obes.* 2017;41(9):1331-1340.

27. Vgontzas AN. Legro RS, Bixler EO, Grayev A, Kales A, Chrousos GP. Polycystic ovary syndrome is associated with obstructive sleep apnea and daytime sleepiness: role of insulin resistance. *J Clin Endocrinol Metab.* 2001;86:517-520.

28. Setji TL, Holland ND, Sanders LL, Pereira KC, Diehl AM, Brown AJ. Nonalcoholic steatohepatitis and nonalcoholic fatty liver disease in young women with polycystic ovary syndrome. *J Clin Endocrinol Metab.* 2006;91(5):1741-1747.

29. Boomsma CM, Eijkemans MJ, Hughes EG, Visser GH, Fauser BC, Macklon NS. A meta-analysis of pregnancy outcomes in women with polycystic ovary syndrome. *Hum Reprod Update.* 2006;12(6):673-683.

9

Diagnostic Criteria for Polycystic Ovary Syndrome

ZAREEN KIRAN

Introduction

One of the most common endocrine diseases in females worldwide is polycystic ovary syndrome (PCOS).[1] In females of reproductive age, it is characterized by hyperandrogenic anovulation. Stein and Leventhal, who discovered a link between amenorrhea and hyperandrogenism and infertility in 1935, were the first to describe PCOS.[2] It covers a wide range of symptoms, including hirsutism and virilization, oligomenorrhea, amenorrhea, hypomenorrhea, or even polymenorrhea, and subfertility to infertility. In almost all cases, there is a concomitant or delayed association of several features of metabolic syndrome risking diabetes mellitus (DM) and cardiovascular disease (CVD) because of hormonal interplay in this syndrome.[3,4]

The heterogeneous and complex clinical presentation of PCOS have made the definition and terminology of the condition difficult over time. Although we now use the term PCOS to refer to a variety of "multisystem reproductive-metabolic disorders," the evolution of different phenotypes explains the need for more defined diagnostic criteria and, most likely, a better term for this disorder.[5]

Diagnosis of Polycystic Ovary Syndrome in Adults

PCOS can be suspected in any female of reproductive age who has irregular menstruation and hyperandrogenism symptoms (acne, hirsutism, male-pattern hair loss). Females who have experienced a sudden or gradual weight gain and meet frank overweight or obesity criteria should be evaluated for the presence of PCOS. Patients who have polycystic ovaries on ultrasound but no other clinical features of PCOS (hyperandrogenism or menstrual dysfunction) are not considered to have PCOS and should avoid extensive testing.[6] Simultaneously, having a high index of suspicion for PCOS is important because these patients may have associated risk factors for CVD, such as glucose intolerance, dyslipidemia, fatty liver, and obstructive sleep apnea, which require evaluation and treatment.

Clinical Features

PCOS is recognized as a clinical syndrome with multiple potential etiologies and variable clinical manifestations. It is characterized by ovulatory dysfunction, androgen excess, and polycystic ovarian morphology. Infertility or subfertility is a common complaint among patients. Many patients can be diagnosed based on their medical history and physical examination, as well as the Rotterdam criteria (detailed later).[7,8] Therefore for a better understanding of the diagnostic approach, these distinguishing features will be described in greater detail.

Menstrual Dysfunction

Menstrual Irregularities

Patients with PCOS may experience frequent bleeding at less than 21-day intervals or infrequent bleeding at intervals greater than 35 days.[8,9] Occasionally, despite falling at a normal interval, bleeding may be anovulatory (25–35 days). Menstrual dysfunction in PCOS can thus be characterized by polymenorrhea, oligomenorrhea, or even amenorrhea, with the latter two being closely associated with infrequent or absent ovulation. In such cases, midluteal progesterone may be used to detect anovulation.[10] Affected females typically have a slightly delayed or normal menarche followed by irregular cycles. As a result, menstrual irregularities may begin around the peripubertal period. Other patients may present in their late twenties or thirties, initially reporting normal cycles, and then develop menstrual irregularity in association with weight gain.[11]

Gonadotropin Effects

Patients with PCOS have higher mean luteinizing hormone (LH) levels and higher LH pulse frequency and amplitude.[12] Nevertheless, many factors must be considered before

• BOX 9.1 **Factors Affecting Luteinizing Hormone Levels in Females With Polycystic Ovary Syndrome**

1. Timing of the sample relative to the last menstrual period
2. Ovarian activity
3. Use of oral contraceptive pills
4. Body mass index
5. Frequency of luteinizing hormone sampling

interpreting the true rise in serum LH levels (Box 9.1). As a result, the absence of an elevated serum LH level does not rule out PCOS. Serum follicle-stimulating hormone (FSH) levels, on the other hand, may be normal or low in PCOS; however, neither an elevated serum LH concentration nor an elevated LH/FSH ratio is required to diagnose PCOS.

Endometrial Dysplasia and Cancer

Aside from the more typical symptoms of oligomenorrhea or amenorrhea in patients with PCOS, chronic unopposed stimulation of the endometrium by the estrogens associated with anovulation may increase the risk of endometrial hyperplasia and endometrial carcinoma. A link between PCOS and endometrial carcinoma was first proposed in 1949,[13] but scientific evidence in the literature has been debated for decades.[14,15] The reason for this is the lack of an independent association of anovulation with cancer risk,[16] despite the fact that several endocrine and metabolic factors have been linked to an increased risk for endometrial cancer.[17] Although there is a lack of consensus with a background of varying diagnostic criteria, a recent meta-analysis of five studies found that females with PCOS had an increased risk of endometrial cancer (odds ratio [OR] 2.79, 95% confidence interval [CI] 1.31–5.95).[18]

Ovarian Dysfunction

Ovarian Morphology and Role of Ultrasound

Patients with PCOS have enlarged ovaries with numerous peripheral small antral follicles and increased central stroma on histology. An important diagnostic criterion for PCOS is the presence of 12 or more follicles 2 to 9 mm in diameter and/or an increased ovarian volume greater than 10 mL (without a cyst or dominant follicle) in either ovary.[19] Newer guidelines have proposed a minimum of 20 follicles per ovary, with no corpora lutea, dominant follicles, or cysts in the ovaries.[8] Nevertheless, because of age-related variations and diagnostic discrepancies based on ultrasound criteria, ovarian morphology alone is no longer sufficient to make the diagnosis.[8] As a result, if the patient has both oligomenorrhea and evidence of hyperandrogenism, and all causes other than PCOS have been ruled out, they meet the criteria for PCOS, and an ultrasound is not required. An ultrasound examination, on the other hand, contributes to a better understanding of the various phenotypes of PCOS.[20,21] Ultrasound is also frequently used in patients

with hyperandrogenic symptoms and normal menstrual cycles to look for polycystic ovarian morphology (PCOM). When possible, the transvaginal approach should be used rather than the transabdominal approach in this context.

Swanson described the ultrasound findings for polycystic ovaries, or PCOM, for the first time in 1981.[22] It is important to note that the number and size of follicles, rather than cysts, are important in ultrasound diagnosis. The Rotterdam criteria, which are thought to have sufficient specificity and sensitivity to define PCOM, include the presence of 12 or more follicles measuring 2 to 9 mm in diameter in either ovary and/or increased ovarian volume (>10 mL; calculated using the formula 0.5 × length × width × thickness). PCOM is defined by any one of the ovaries that meets this definition ("Revised 2003 consensus on diagnostic criteria and long-term health risks related to polycystic ovary syndrome (PCOS)," 2004).[23] According to some reports, however, more than half of normal-cycling females met the criteria of 12 or more small follicles in each ovary,[24] prompting experts to reconsider the 2003 Rotterdam ultrasound criteria.

Ultrasound Criteria for Polycystic Ovary Syndrome

A number of alternative criteria have been proposed since 2003, but there is currently no consensus on the optimal ultrasound criteria.

1. A higher threshold (25 follicles per ovary) has been proposed based on a 2014 systematic review, but only if the clinician uses a transducer frequency that provides maximum resolution (e.g., 8 MHz).[25] Most clinicians do not have easy access to this technology.
2. In 2018, an international evidence-based medicine group recommended a follicle count of 20 in each ovary.[8]
3. In females with or without PCOS, ovarian volume and follicle number decrease with age. As a result, age-based criteria for defining polycystic ovaries have been proposed.[26,27]

Patients who are referred for PCOS because of an incidental finding of cystic ovaries on pelvic ultrasound or other abdominal imaging do not need to be evaluated further if no other clinical features of PCOS are found. Polycystic ovaries detected sonographically or radiographically are thus a nonspecific finding.[20]

Ovarian Follicular Defects

In PCOS ovaries, both follicular development and function are disordered, with an abnormal hormonal milieu in follicular fluid.[28] There is clear evidence of a defect in ovarian folliculogenesis. Anovulatory females with polycystic ovaries have a higher density of small preantral follicles than normal controls.[29,30] The percentage of primary, secondary, and tertiary follicles is significantly higher overall,[31,32] whereas the percentage of primordial (resting) follicles is lower, and there is a trend toward an increase in the number of atretic follicles.[33]

Anovulatory Infertility

Patients with PCOS have infrequent ovulation, making it more difficult to conceive. Many, if not most, patients with

PCOS and oligo-ovulation who desire conception eventually undergo ovulation induction therapy. Patients with PCOS may have additional reasons for infertility because they have a lower rate of conception relative to the rate of ovulation after clomiphene citrate therapy than those with hypothalamic amenorrhea. The original definition of PCOS also included infertility.[2] Many studies have also reported an increased rate of early pregnancy loss in PCOS patients, the mechanism of which is unknown[34] but may be related to obesity.

Hyperandrogenism (Clinical Evaluation)

The second symptom of PCOS is hyperandrogenism. Both clinical and biochemical features should be carefully assessed and interpreted for diagnosis. Clinical manifestations of hyperandrogenism include hirsutism, acne, and male-pattern hair loss. Extreme forms may manifest as masculinization, hoarseness of the voice, or clitoromegaly. In most cases, these findings point to other causes of virilization, such as hyperthecosis or androgen-producing ovarian or adrenal tumors.[35,36]

Hirsutism

The most common clinical manifestation of hyperandrogenemia is hirsutism. It is defined as excess terminal (thick, pigmented) body hair in a male distribution,[37] and it is commonly diagnosed using the modified Ferriman-Gallwey scoring system, which includes nine androgen-sensitive body areas (Refer Figure 3.1).[38,39] This approach, however, has a number of limitations in clinical practice. Most importantly, hair growth expression varies across racial groups.[40] Even though serum androgen concentrations are similar in all groups, most East Asian and Native American females have little body hair, White and Black females have an intermediate amount, and most Mediterranean, South Asian, and Middle Eastern females have significantly more body hair.[40,41] Therefore even minor acne or facial hair in an East Asian female should raise the possibility of a hyperandrogenic disorder, most commonly PCOS.[42,43]

A common cosmetic complaint is localized areas of excessive sexual hair growth ("focal hirsutism") with a normal score ("even a single hair casts a shadow"). As a result, not all "patient-significant hirsutism" is abnormal. Adult hirsutism guidelines have also defined "idiopathic hirsutism" as hirsutism that occurs without elevated circulating levels of androgen or menstrual abnormality.[44]

Acne

Acne vulgaris in females can be an indication of PCOS. There is evidence that acne vulgaris has a hormonal and metabolic influence in patients with PCOS. Acne severity in PCOS patients with higher androstenedione concentrations was associated with higher levels of total testosterone, free testosterone, dehydroepiandrosterone sulfate (DHEAS), and cortisol. Similarly, increased glucose concentration correlates with the severity of acne.[45]

Virilization

Virilization is a rare symptom of hyperandrogenism. Androgenic alopecia, clitoromegaly, voice deepening, increased muscle mass, and decreased breast size are all symptoms of virilization. Females who have virilization are almost always amenorrheic. In virilization, alopecia usually manifests as male-pattern baldness with bitemporal recession.[46] Clitoromegaly is defined as a clitoral index (the product of the sagittal and transverse diameters of the clitoris glans) greater than 35 mm.[47] The presence of an androgen-secreting neoplasm should always be suspected in any female who develops virilization symptoms, especially if the onset is sudden and progresses quickly. Nevertheless, virilization does not always indicate severe hyperandrogenism because any pattern or degree of androgen excess features can be seen in females with hyperandrogenism caused by nonneoplastic causes, such as PCOS and idiopathic hirsutism.[48]

Baldness is an unusual symptom of adolescent hyperandrogenemia. When it occurs, it can be male pattern (affecting the fronto-temporo-occipital scalp) or female pattern (affecting the crown, typically manifesting early as a widened midline part).[49] Seborrhea, hyperhidrosis, and hidradenitis suppurativa are some of the alternate cutaneous manifestations of hyperandrogenemia.[50] Hidradenitis suppurativa is distinguished by painful inflammatory nodules in intertriginous areas, most notably the axillae.

Biochemical Testing in Polycystic Ovary Syndrome

Between 50% and 90% of PCOS females have elevated serum androgen levels, depending on the androgen measured and the technique used.[51] Serum total testosterone concentration is thought to provide the best overall estimate of androgen production in clinically hyperandrogenic females for biochemical diagnosis. Other androgens are also elevated, but the mechanism of excess androgens in PCOS is gonadotropin dependent, with theca cells increasing androgen production in response to chronically elevated LH and insulin levels.[52,53] Although PCOS is the most common cause of hirsutism in females, it is critical to distinguish those who have other disorders, such as nonclassic congenital adrenal hyperplasia (NCCAH), or a more serious cause (androgen-secreting tumors and ovarian hyperthecosis).

Tests in Females With Normal Menstrual Cycles

Females who have hyperandrogenic symptoms (most commonly hirsutism) and normal menstrual cycles are more likely to have PCOS or idiopathic hirsutism and are unlikely to have a more serious cause for their hirsutism. Only measuring serum total testosterone is an appropriate first step for these patients.[44]

Tests in Females With Oligomenorrhea

PCOS is a diagnosis of exclusion in terms of biochemistry. Other causes of irregular menstruation should be investigated in any female who has oligomenorrhea/oligo-ovulation.

Human chorionic gonadotropin (hCG) should be tested to rule out pregnancy; prolactin and thyroid-stimulating hormone (TSH) should be tested to rule out hyperprolactinemia and thyroid disorders; and FSH should be tested to rule out ovarian insufficiency. Once these causes have been excluded, determining androgen excess and an early morning 17-hydroxyprogesterone (17-OHP) level in females with hyperandrogenic symptoms and oligomenorrhea is warranted.

1. **Serum total testosterone:** The most accurate and specific method for determining serum total testosterone is liquid chromatography-tandem mass spectroscopy (LC-MS/MS). Serum total testosterone concentration is thought to provide the most accurate overall estimate of androgen production in clinically hyperandrogenic females. The upper limit of normal for serum testosterone in females using LC-MS/MS is 45 to 60 ng/dL (1.6–2.1 nmol/L); those with serum testosterone levels greater than 150 ng/dL require evaluation for the most serious causes of hyperandrogenism (ovarian and adrenal androgen-secreting tumors). The immunoassays that are available in most hospital laboratories are not suitable to accurately measure testosterone in females.[54,55]

2. **Serum–free testosterone:** Serum-free testosterone may be a more sensitive test for the presence of hyperandrogenic disorders[56] because current direct assays are inconclusive. If free testosterone is requested, equilibrium dialysis should be used.[57] Elevated total or free testosterone levels are thus a key diagnostic feature of biochemical hyperandrogenism in PCOS.

3. **Sex hormone–binding globulin (SHBG):** SHBG measurements are another option for determining free testosterone levels indirectly. Although less accurate, a laboratory that calculates free testosterone levels from total testosterone and SHBG levels can provide a close estimate by using a formula with results that agree with equilibrium dialysis results.[58,59] In addition, direct measurement of SHBG is beneficial in other ways. An abnormally low SHBG in a patient with PCOS is a risk factor for increased biologically active testosterone and, as a result, a more severe phenotype.[60]

4. **DHEAS:** DHEAS levels are elevated in approximately 25% of PCOS patients, despite the fact that the diagnosis requires the use of age-related cut-off values because DHEAS levels decrease with age. Furthermore, only 10% of PCOS patients have isolated DHEAS elevation.[61] Therefore routine DHEAS measurement is not recommended by international consensus.[8] It can, however, be measured as part of the overall workup for hyperandrogenism when the cause is unlikely to be PCOS.[53]

5. **Serum androstenedione**: Serum androstenedione is sometimes elevated in patients with PCOS; however, its role in evaluating PCOS and/or hirsutism is unknown.[62] It is found to be elevated in 18% of PCOS patients; however, isolated elevations are observed in only 9% of cases.[63]

6. **17-OHP:** Serum 17-OHP measurement in the morning sample is recommended to rule out NCCAH because of 21-hydroxylase deficiency.[44] This should be done in the early follicular phase for females who have some spontaneous menstrual cycles and on a random day for those who do not.[64] NCCAH's clinical presentation can be similar, if not identical, to that of PCOS (hyperandrogenism, oligomenorrhea, and polycystic ovaries). NCCAH is less common than PCOS, but it should be ruled out because there is a risk that offspring will have the more severe classic 21-hydroxylase deficiency. It is especially important to screen females who live in high-risk areas, such as Ashkenazi Jews, and certain Caucasians, and Eastern European females.[65]

7. **Role of the LH and FSH ratio:** An elevated LH-to-FSH ratio is not a criterion for PCOS diagnosis.[66] Many clinicians used to measure LH and FSH and use an elevated LH-to-FSH ratio ($\geq$2) as evidence for PCOS diagnosis.[67] Nevertheless, the LH-to-FSH ratio can be deceptive. For example, if there has been a recent ovulation, LH will be suppressed and the ratio will be less than or equal to 2.[67] In fact, increased pituitary LH secretion cannot always be determined by serum concentration because approximately one-third of patients have circulating levels of LH in the normal range.[68,69]

8. **Serum prolactin levels:** Prolactin levels in some hyperandrogenic females may be mildly elevated, but the significance is unknown.[70] Prolactin levels greater than 40 mg/dL should prompt further investigation for other causes.

9. **Function of anti-Müllerian hormone (AMH):** Because serum AMH is produced by small preantral and early antral follicles, serum concentrations reflect the size of the primordial follicle pool (ovarian reserve). AMH levels in adult females gradually decline with age (as the primordial follicle pool shrinks) and become undetectable at menopause.[71] Compared with age-matched controls, mean AMH concentrations in patients with PCOS are found to be high.[72-74] A serum AMH concentration of greater than 4.7 ng/mL had a specificity and sensitivity of 79% and 83%, respectively, for diagnosing PCOS in a meta-analysis of 10 observational studies of patients with PCOS.[75] Despite emerging evidence of AMH's role as a surrogate marker for PCOS diagnosis, an elevated AMH is not currently considered a criterion for PCOS diagnosis.[76] Several limitations include significant heterogeneity in the study population, with variations in the cut-offs used for adolescents and adults, and inconsistency in defining polycystic morphology in imaging, assays, and sample handling.[76]

Tests in Females on Pharmacotherapy

Some patients may already be receiving pharmacologic therapy, typically estrogen-progestin oral contraceptives (OC). In this case, measuring serum androgens is worthless because OC suppresses serum gonadotropins and ovarian androgens, particularly testosterone. Similarly, androgen measurements should be avoided in females who are taking metformin or spironolactone because the interpretation of the results is complicated by the effects of these medications on androgen levels.[77] According to recommendations, patients should discontinue their medications at least 4 to 6 weeks before measuring serum androgens.[8,44,78]

Tests in Females With Features of Other Endocrine Disorders

Females with other endocrine disorders, such as Cushing syndrome, can occasionally present with symptoms similar to PCOS (oligomenorrhea, hirsutism, and obesity). They do, however, have symptoms and signs of cortisol excess, such as centripetal obesity, hypertension, purple striae, and proximal muscle weakness.[79,80] Similarly, females with acromegaly may present with oligomenorrhea and hirsutism, which may necessitate the measurement of serum insulin-like growth factor-1 (IGF-1).[44,79]

Diagnostic Criteria

Rotterdam Criteria

Most expert groups use Rotterdam criteria to make the diagnosis of PCOS,[8,44,57] although there are certain limitations when using these criteria, as detailed in Table 9.1. Any two out of three of the following criteria are required to make the diagnosis ("Revised 2003 consensus on diagnostic criteria and long-term health risks related to polycystic ovary syndrome (PCOS)," 2004)[23]:

1. Oligo- and/or anovulation
2. Clinical and/or biochemical signs of hyperandrogenism
3. Polycystic ovaries (by ultrasound)

Many females with irregular menstruation and hyperandrogenic symptoms can be diagnosed based solely on their medical history and physical exam. Nevertheless, PCOS is only confirmed when all other conditions that cause oligo/anovulation and/or hyperandrogenism, such as thyroid disease, NCCAH, hyperprolactinemia, and androgen-secreting neoplasms, are ruled out.

National Institutes of Health Criteria

The 1990 National Institutes of Health (NIH) criteria allow for a clinical diagnosis without the use of an imaging study. In addition, the NIH criteria require the presence of irregular menses, whereas the other criteria do not.[81]

Androgen Excess and Polycystic Ovary Syndrome Society Criteria

The Androgen Excess (AE) and PCOS Society proposed the AE-PCOS Criteria in 2006.[56] In contrast to the Rotterdam criteria, the majority of the AE-PCOS task force agreed that there were insufficient data to diagnose PCOS in females who had ovulatory dysfunction and polycystic ovaries but no evidence of hyperandrogenism.[56]

The use of multiple classification systems confuses clinicians and patients. According to a summary report from the NIH Evidence-Based Methodology Workshop on PCOS in December of 2012, the Rotterdam criteria should be used for the time being because they are the most inclusive (Table 9.2).[82] They also proposed changing the name "PCOS" because it focuses on polycystic ovarian morphology (PCOM), which is neither sufficient nor necessary for diagnosis, and fluid-filled structures in the ovary are not "cysts." One proposed name is the "metabolic reproductive syndrome," which reflects the multifaceted nature of the syndrome, but the workshop participants acknowledge the difficulty changing the name.

Diagnosis of Polycystic Ovary Syndrome in Postmenopausal Females

Postmenopausal Androgens

In both premenopausal and postmenopausal females, the adrenal glands and the ovaries produce endogenous androgens.[83] From their peak in early adulthood, adrenal androgens, particularly dehydroepiandrosterone (DHEA) and its sulfate (DHEAS), decrease dramatically with age.[84] Changes in ovarian androgen secretion as a function of age and menopause are far less dramatic, with longitudinal studies focusing on the last menstrual period revealing that total testosterone levels decrease only slightly, with a slightly greater decrease in SHBG.[83,85]

Clinical Presentation

The most common symptoms of hyperandrogenism in postmenopausal females are hirsutism and alopecia, whereas

TABLE 9.1	Limitations of the Rotterdam Criteria
Androgen Excess	• Diurnal variations in concentrations • Age-related difference in concentrations • Assays are not standardized across laboratories • Ethnic variations in clinical hyperandrogenism • Subjective variations in quantifying hyperandrogenism
Ovulatory Dysfunction	• Poorly defined ovulation standards • Variable ovulation over a female's lifetime • Objective measurement of ovulatory dysfunction is poorly understood • Normally interpreted anovulatory cycles
PCO Morphology	• Observer and technique dependent • Lack of normative standards across the menstrual phase and reproductive age • Intrinsically nonspecific and can mimic other disorders

PCO, Polycystic ovary.

TABLE 9.2   Proposed Diagnostic Criteria for Polycystic Ovary Syndrome

NIH Consensus Criteria 1990 (all required)	Rotterdam Criteria 2003 (two out of three required)	AES Definition 2008 (all required)
Menstrual irregularity because of oligo- or anovulation	Oligo- or anovulation	Clinical and/or biochemical signs of hyperandrogenism
Clinical and/or biochemical signs of hyperandrogenism	Clinical and/or biochemical signs of hyperandrogenism	Ovarian dysfunction – oligo/anovulation and/or polycystic ovaries on ultrasound
Exclusion of other disorders: NCCAH, androgen-secreting tumors	Polycystic ovaries (by ultrasound)	Exclusion of other androgen excess or ovulatory disorders

AES, Androgen Excess Society; *NCCAH*, nonclassic congenital adrenal hyperplasia; *NIH*, National Institutes of Health.

clitoromegaly, lowering of the voice, increased muscle strength, and an anabolic appearance are associated with higher androgen levels.[86-88] Some postmenopausal patients with tumor-induced hyperandrogenism experience uterine bleeding as a result of peripheral aromatization of androgens to estrogens.[86] Some patients may also develop endometrial hyperplasia or endometrial carcinoma.

In postmenopausal females, new-onset hyperandrogenism is extremely uncommon. PCOS is the most common cause of androgen excess in premenopausal females. A history of irregular menstrual cycles combined with clinical hyperandrogenism before menopause may indicate premenopausal PCOS.[89] Androgen levels typically fall after menopause in both PCOS and healthy females; however, postmenopausal females with a history of PCOS continue to have higher androgen levels than healthy postmenopausal females.[90] When hyperandrogenism develops or worsens in postmenopausal females, it is usually because of another cause, such as ovarian hyperthecosis or an androgen-secreting neoplasms.[86]

Diagnostic Criteria

According to the 2013 Endocrine Society Clinical Practice Guidelines for the Diagnosis and Treatment of PCOS, the Rotterdam criteria should be used to diagnose PCOS in adult premenopausal females.[7] They acknowledge that establishing the diagnosis in postmenopausal patients is difficult, but they suggest that a "well-documented long-term history of oligomenorrhea and hyperandrogenism during the reproductive years" can be used to make a presumptive diagnosis. In such cases, the discovery of PCOS morphology on pelvic ultrasound would provide additional evidence.

Nevertheless, ovarian volume and follicle number decrease with age in both PCOS and non-PCOS females. Although age-based PCOS criteria for females over the age of 40 have been proposed,[27] there are currently no well-established criteria in postmenopausal females. Transvaginal ultrasound (TVUS) should always be performed to rule

out disorders such as ovarian hyperthecosis and androgen-secreting tumors in postmenopausal females who present with new-onset or worsening hirsutism or other symptoms of severe hyperandrogenism.

Diagnosis in Adolescents

Clinical Presentation

Adolescent hyperandrogenemia may be a precursor to adult PCOS, and clinical manifestations of PCOS frequently begin in adolescence. Obesity appears to contribute to hyperandrogenemia in two studies of peripubertal females because increasing body mass index (BMI) was associated with increases in serum total testosterone, free testosterone, and (DHEAS) concentrations.[91,92] It is unclear whether a PCOS phenotype exists in which obesity is accompanied by intrinsic ovarian hyperandrogenism in the absence of hirsutism, acne, and anovulatory symptoms.[93]

Hirsutism

According to sparse normative data, sexual hair growth matures throughout puberty and reaches maturity 2 years after menarche, at around 15 years of age (see Fig. 9.1).[38,94] Because idiopathic hirsutism accounts for half of all cases of mild hirsutism, adolescent PCOS guidelines[95] consider only moderate to severe hirsutism to be clinical evidence of hyperandrogenism, and even this is considered less reliable evidence of hyperandrogenism than persistent testosterone elevation determined by a reliable reference assay.

Acne

Excessive acne vulgaris is a common but variable cutaneous manifestation of adolescent hyperandrogenemia.[96] The severity of acne can be determined by the number of lesions present.[97] Although comedonal acne is common in adolescent females, the presence of moderate (>10 facial lesions) or severe inflammatory acne during the perimenarchal years indicates hyperandrogenemia.[95,98]

Challenges in the Diagnosis of Polycystic Ovary Syndrome in Adolescents

For a variety of reasons, applying adult PCOS diagnostic criteria to adolescents has proven difficult. First, normal adolescent females have anovulatory cycles and menstrual irregularities. Second, because hirsutism is in a developmental phase and acne vulgaris is common in adolescents, the common signs of hyperandrogenism in adults are less reliable when applied to adolescents. Third, measuring testosterone levels in adolescents is difficult because serum concentrations rise during anovulatory cycles, there are few reliable norms for androgen levels in adolescent females, and the extent to which adolescent hyperandrogenism predicts adult hyperandrogenism is unknown. Fourth, by adult standards, PCOM is common in normal adolescents.[99]

Diagnostic Criteria in Adolescents

Three international expert conferences have published recommendations for the diagnosis of adolescent PCOS.[8,95,100] These documents agree on the following essential criteria: otherwise unexplained persistent evidence of ovulatory dysfunction (as indicated by a menstrual abnormality based on chronologic and gynecologic age-appropriate standards) and clinical and/or biochemical evidence of androgen excess (hyperandrogenism; Table 9.3).[101]

These recommendations, however, differ in some clinical details regarding appropriate evidence to satisfy these criteria.[101] They disagree on whether a menstrual abnormality should last 1 or 2 years to distinguish PCOS from normal menstrual cycle immaturity ("physiologic adolescent anovulation"). They also differ in how far hirsutism or acne can be considered evidence of hyperandrogenism on equal level with accurate biochemical evidence of hyperandrogenism. They do agree, however, that adolescent females who show

TABLE 9.3 International Diagnostic Criteria for Polycystic Ovary Syndrome in Adolescents

Otherwise unexplained combination of:

1. Abnormal menstrual pattern as evidence of ovulatory dysfunction
   a. Abnormal for age or gynecologic age, and
   b. Persistent symptoms for 1–2 years

2. Clinical and/or biochemical evidence of hyperandrogenism
   a. Hirsutism, especially if moderate-severe, is clinical evidence of hyperandrogenism.
   b. Elevation of serum total or free testosterone by a specialty reference assay is biochemical evidence of hyperandrogenism.

(From Rosenfield RL. Perspectives on the international recommendations for the diagnosis and treatment of polycystic ovary syndrome in adolescence. *J Pediatr Adolesc Gynecol.* 2020;S1083.)

signs of PCOS 1 to 2 years after menarche should be given a provisional diagnosis of "at risk for PCOS" and treated symptomatically.

Differential Diagnosis

PCOS is an exclusionary diagnosis. Once other conditions with features similar to PCOS, such as NCCAH, thyroid disease, and hyperprolactinemia, have been ruled out, a diagnosis of PCOS can be made using the Rotterdam diagnostic criteria. Females with severe hyperandrogenism and virilization necessitate a more thorough examination to rule out the most serious causes of androgen excess (androgen-secreting ovarian and adrenal neoplasms and ovarian hyperthecosis). Table 9.4 lists important conditions to rule out when making a PCOS diagnosis.

Nonclassic Congenital Adrenal Hyperplasia

NCCAH has a clinical presentation similar to or identical to PCOS (hyperandrogenism, oligomenorrhea, and polycystic ovaries). NCCAH is less common than PCOS, but it should be ruled out because there is a risk that offspring will have the more severe classic 21-hydroxylase deficiency. This test is especially important in high-risk females, such as those of Mediterranean, Hispanic, and Ashkenazi Jewish descent.[65] This diagnosis is unlikely if the value in the early

TABLE 9.4 Conditions to Exclude Before Diagnosing Polycystic Ovary Syndrome

Disorder	Test
Thyroid disease	Serum thyrotropin stimulating hormone
Prolactin excess	Serum prolactin
Nonclassical congenital adrenal hyperplasia	Early morning (before 8 am) serum 17-hydroxyprogesterone
Pregnancy	Serum or urine human chorionic gonadotropin (HCG)
Hypothalamic amenorrhea	Serum follicle-stimulating hormone (FSH) and luteinizing hormone (LH)
Primary ovarian insufficiency	Serum FSH and serum estradiol
Androgen secreting tumor	Serum testosterone, dehydroepiandrosterone sulfate level, transvaginal ultrasound of ovaries, MRI of adrenal glands
Cushing syndrome	24-hour urinary cortisol, overnight dexamethasone suppression test
Acromegaly	Serum-free insulin-like growth factor-1 level, MRI of pituitary

MRI, Magnetic resonance imaging.

follicular phase is less than 200 ng/dL (6 nmol/L). A morning value of 17-OHP greater than 200 ng/dL in the early follicular phase strongly suggests the diagnosis, which can be confirmed by a corticotropin (ACTH) 1 to 24 (cosyntropin) stimulation test at a high dose (250 mcg). Cosyntropin response is exaggerated, with most patients having values greater than 1500 ng/dL (43 nmol/L).[64,65]

Androgen-Secreting Tumors/Ovarian Hyperthecosis

Females with androgen-secreting ovarian or adrenal tumors or ovarian hyperthecosis typically present with new-onset severe hirsutism, sudden progressive worsening of hirsutism, and symptoms or signs of virilization, such as frontal baldness, severe acne, clitoromegaly, increased muscle mass, or voice deepening. Serum testosterone concentrations are almost always greater than 150 ng/dL (5.2 nmol/L),[88] and serum DHEAS concentrations are typically greater than 800 mcg/dL (21.6 micromol/L). Although all of these disorders are more common in postmenopausal females, they are also seen in premenopausal females on occasion.

Other Causes

Oligomenorrhea can occur in the presence of hypothyroidism, hyperthyroidism, or hyperprolactinemia. Hyperandrogenic symptoms, on the other hand, are not common in these disorders. Clinical features and biochemical testing (high TSH, low TSH, high prolactin) distinguish these disorders.[79]

Differentials to Consider in Adolescents

Physiologic Adolescent Anovulation

The most common cause of adolescent menstrual irregularity is physiologic adolescent anovulation.[102] It may appear in approximately half of cases of hyperandrogenemia without clinical evidence of androgen excess, but the hyperandrogenemia and anovulation do not persist.[103-105]

Virilizing/Classic Congenital Adrenal Hyperplasia

Classic congenital adrenal hyperplasia (CAH) because of 21-hydroxylase deficiency is the most well-known form of CAH. It is almost always diagnosed during infancy, with genital ambiguity because of congenital virilization of affected females, and may be associated with a salt-losing crisis. Affected individuals may develop PCOS-like signs and symptoms during adolescence, particularly if their disorder is poorly controlled by glucocorticoid therapy. Menstrual irregularities, hirsutism, and clitoromegaly are all possible symptoms. Polycystic ovaries can be caused by virilizing extraovarian androgen excess and adrenal rests of the ovaries (ectopic adrenal tissue in the ovaries).[106] In the absence of androgen excess, adrenal progesterone excess may be sufficient to cause ovarian dysfunction by inhibiting LH pulsatility.[107]

Congenital Disorders of Adrenal Steroid Metabolism or Action

Defects in glucocorticoid receptor signaling cause glucocorticoid resistance. It is a rare congenital form of

ACTH-dependent adrenal hyperandrogenism caused by insufficient negative feedback from cortisol, resulting in excessive ACTH release.[108] Premature pubarche is followed by hyperandrogenic anovulation and a skeletal growth defect in affected adolescent females.

Insulin-Resistance Disorders

PCOS is associated with all extreme states of insulin-resistant (IR) hyperinsulinemia, such as congenital DM caused by insulin-receptor mutations (e.g., Donohue syndrome or leprechaunism) or lipodystrophy.[109] IR is also associated with PCOS in the setting of pseudo-Cushing syndrome and pseudoacromegalic gigantism, disorders that clinically mimic glucocorticoid excess and childhood growth hormone excess without excess production of these hormones. IR symptoms frequently precede PCOS in these disorders.[110] Furthermore, mild forms of IR, in type 1[111] and type 2 DM, are linked to PCOS.[112] Elevated insulin levels seem to promote PCOS by increasing the activity of steroidogenic enzymes in the ovaries and adrenal glands, similarly to IGF-1.

Idiopathic Hyperandrogenism

Approximately 3.9% of hyperandrogenic patients have no identifiable ovarian or adrenal source of androgen after thorough clinical evaluation.[113] Those who present with hirsutism and normal menstruation but do not have a polycystic ovary are traditionally diagnosed with this condition.[114,115] Obesity may be responsible for the majority of cases of idiopathic hyperandrogenism. Obesity, on the other hand, can occasionally cause hyperandrogenic anovulation ("the atypical PCOS of obesity"),[116] and symptoms should improve with weight loss.[117]

Referral to Specialist

The most important aspect of managing PCOS is a multidisciplinary approach. Females with PCOS may first consult a gynecologist, infertility specialist, dermatologist, or endocrinologist. In all cases, the specialist must decide whether or not to refer the patient to another relevant specialty by using a holistic approach to the investigation or management step.[118] When it comes to diagnostic testing for suspected PCOS, there is significant practice heterogeneity even within a single domain (e.g., gynecology).[119] Therefore the use of a multidisciplinary clinic model that includes dermatology and endocrinology, gynecology, psychology, and lifestyle experts provides care for the majority of PCOS symptoms (Table 9.5).[120]

Follow-Up

PCOS has two major consequences: metabolic risk and decreased fecundity. There is very little information available about both of these effects. Most studies have a small sample size and lack uniform criteria for developing common recommendations.[121,122] Nevertheless, several long-term effects can be predicted from these data, necessitating

TABLE 9.5	Role of Providers in the Evaluation Of Polycystic Ovary Syndrome, By Specialty
Specialty	**Role**
Dermatology	• Hirsutism: Measure modified Ferriman-Gallwey (mFG score) • Presence or absence of acne by physical examination with score of severity • Presence or absence of acanthosis nigricans, androgenic alopecia, hidradenitis suppurativa by physical examination
Gynecology/adolescent medicine	• Chronic anovulation: menstrual irregularities and diary • Clinical and/or biochemical signs of hyperandrogenism: total/free testosterone, dehydroepiandrosterone sulfate • Polycystic ovarian morphology: pelvic ultrasound • Endometrial hyperplasia: endometrial biopsy • Discussion regarding future infertility issues
Endocrinology	• Obesity: body mass index measurement. • Hormonal disturbances: total/free testosterone, Dehydroepiandrosterone sulfate (prolactin,17-hydroxyprogesterone, androstenedione, thyroid-stimulating hormone) • Glucose intolerance/diabetes mellitus: glucose tolerance test, hemoglobin A1c • Dyslipidemia: lipid panel (ideally fasting) • Fatty liver: liver function test • Hypertension: measured blood pressure • Screen overweight/obese adolescents with PCOS for symptoms of obstructive sleep • Apnea
Psychology	• Mental health symptoms (e.g., anxiety, depression) • Appetite self-regulation • Emotional eating • Goal setting for lifestyle modification • Optimizing sleep health
Exercise	• Describe goals of exercise • Set activity and exercise goals at every appointment
Nutrition	• Weight trend from baseline and follow up visits • Provide education regarding healthy eating habits

PCOS, Polycystic ovary syndrome.
(From Torres-Zegarra C, Sundararajan D Benson J, et al. Care for adolescents with polycystic ovary syndrome: development and prescribing patterns of a multidisciplinary clinic. *J Ped Adolesc Gynecol.* 2021;34[5]:617–625).

careful monitoring and follow-up strategies in each domain of this "metabolic reproductive syndrome."

Follow-up will be determined by the individual constellation of symptoms and signs,[48] and can be divided into two categories: cardiometabolic review and review of reproductive outcomes.

Cardiometabolic Review

In patients without PCOS, the risk of CVD, cerebrovascular disease, DM, hypertension, dyslipidemia, obesity, and nonalcoholic fatty liver disease should be routinely evaluated in accordance with individual guidelines and recommendations.[3,4,122] Females with high-risk characteristics, on the other hand, should be followed up at minimum with the following parameters:

1. Check weight, BMI, waist circumference
2. Blood pressure
3. Fasting blood sugar and, if required, standard oral glucose tolerance test (OGTT) and fasting lipids
4. Evaluation of bone mineral density

Review of Reproductive Outcomes

Many females with PCOS experience infertility, subfertility, or miscarriages as their first symptom.[48] These can be easily evaluated to determine the cause (absence or presence of PCOS) and then managed to achieve their conception goals through multidisciplinary management involving lifestyle changes and artificial reproductive techniques.[123] Furthermore, the risk of endometrial carcinoma necessitates a thorough assessment and timely review (see previous text) for both prevention and management.[17] Finally, pregnancy-related complications such as gestational diabetes (GDM), gestational hypertension, pre-eclampsia, and preterm birth, as well as several neonatal complications, are more common in females with PCOS and should be kept in mind when providing obstetric care to such patients.[124] The following objectives should be kept in mind when monitoring and following up on the reproductive aspects of PCOS:

1. Endometrial hyperplasia and carcinoma prevention, which may occur as a result of chronic anovulation. Anovulatory

dysfunctional uterine bleeding (especially with endometrial hyperplasia) requires oral or intrauterine progestogen therapy (at first every 3–6 months).

2. Contraception for those who do not wish to become pregnant, because females with oligomenorrhea ovulate intermittently and an unwanted pregnancy may occur.

3. Ovulation induction for those wishing to become pregnant and follow-up for pregnancy-related complications, as previously described.

4. Antiandrogen therapy monitoring (at first every 3–6 months).

5. Routine breast examination, cervical smear, and mammograms for all females.

Conclusion

PCOS is a complicated metabolic reproductive syndrome. A thorough understanding of its signs and symptoms is required for clinical evaluation. Each clinical feature has its own set of criteria and definitions, which are determined by a variety of clinical and biochemical scoring systems. The Rotterdam criteria is universally accepted for adult females with PCOS and is best used after excluding important differential diagnosis. Diagnosis is more difficult for adolescent age groups and, in some cases, postmenopausal females who may have androgenic malignancies to rule out. Most diagnoses are delayed or incomplete as a result of presentation to multiple clinical specialties. Adequate referral to a relevant expert, on the other hand, results in multidisciplinary management protocols and benefits the long-term follow-up and monitoring required.

References

1. Wolf WM, Wattick RA, Kinkade ON, Olfert MD. Geographical prevalence of polycystic ovary syndrome as determined by region and race/ethnicity. *Int J Environ Res Public Health*. 2018;15(11):2589.

2. Stein I, Leventhal M. Amenorrhea associated with bilateral polycystic ovaries. *Am J Obstet Gynecol*. 1935;29:181-191.

3. Bahadur A, Mundhra R, Kashibhatla J, Rajput R, Verma N, Kumawat M. Prevalence of metabolic syndrome among women with different PCOS phenotypes - a prospective study. *Gynecol Endocrinol*. 2021;37(1):21-25. doi:10.1080/09513590.2020.1775193.

4. Zaeemzadeh N, Sadatmahalleh SJ, Ziaei S, et al. Prevalence of metabolic syndrome in four phenotypes of PCOS and its relationship with androgenic components among Iranian women: a cross-sectional study. *Int J Reprod Biomed*. 2020;18(4):253-264. doi:10.18502/ijrm.v13i4.6888.

5. Johnson T, Kaplan L, Ouyang P, Rizza PJ. *National Institutes of Health Evidence-Based Methodology Workshop on Polycystic Ovary Syndrome. NIH EbMW Reports*. Bethesda, MD: National Institutes of Health; 2019:1-14.

6. Witchel SF, Burghard AC, Tao RH, Oberfield SE. The diagnosis and treatment of PCOS in adolescents: an update. *Curr Opin Pediatr*. 2019;31(4):562-569. doi:10.1097/MOP.0000000000000778.

7. Legro RS, Arslanian SA, Ehrmann DA, et al. Diagnosis and treatment of polycystic ovary syndrome: an Endocrine Society clinical practice guideline. *J Clin Endocrinol Metab*. 2013;98(12):4565-4592. doi:10.1210/jc.2013-2350.

8. Teede HJ, Misso ML, Costello MF, et al. Recommendations from the international evidence-based guideline for the assessment and management of polycystic ovary syndrome. *Fertil Steril*. 2018;110(3):364-379. doi:10.1016/j.fertnstert.2018.05.004.

9. Strowitzki T, Capp E, von Eye Corleta H. The degree of cycle irregularity correlates with the grade of endocrine and metabolic disorders in PCOS patients. *Eur J Obstet Gynecol Reprod Biol*. 2010;149(2):178-181.

10. Hull MG, Savage PE, Bromham DR, Ismail AA, Morris AF. The value of a single serum progesterone measurement in the midluteal phase as a criterion of a potentially fertile cycle ("ovulation") derived from treated and untreated conception cycles. *Fertil Steril*. 1982;37(3):355-360.

11. Sheehan MT. Polycystic ovarian syndrome: diagnosis and management. *Clin Med Res*. 2004;2(1):13-27.

12. Taylor AE, McCourt B, Martin KA, et al. Determinants of abnormal gonadotropin secretion in clinically defined women with polycystic ovary syndrome. *J Clin Endocrinol Metab*. 1997;82(7):2248-2256. doi:10.1210/jcem.82.7.4105.

13. Speert H. Carcinoma of the endometrium in young women. *Surg Gynecol Obstet*. 1949;88(3):332-336.

14. Haoula Z, Salman M, Atiomo W. Evaluating the association between endometrial cancer and polycystic ovary syndrome. *Hum Reprod*. 2012;27(5):1327-1331. doi:10.1093/humrep/des042.

15. Hardiman P, Pillay OS, Atiomo W. Polycystic ovary syndrome and endometrial carcinoma. *Lancet*. 2003;361(9371):1810-1812.

16. Furberg A, Thune I. Metabolic abnormalities, lifestyle and endometrial cancer risk in a Norwegian cohort. *Int J Cancer*. 2003;104:669-676.

17. Ignatov A, Ortmann O. Endocrine risk factors of endometrial cancer: polycystic ovary syndrome, oral contraceptives, infertility, tamoxifen. *Cancers (Basel)*. 2020;12(7):1766.

18. Barry JA, Azizia MM, Hardiman PJ. Risk of endometrial, ovarian and breast cancer in women with polycystic ovary syndrome: a systematic review and meta-analysis. *Hum Reprod Update*. 2014;20(5):748-758. doi:10.1093/humupd/dmu012.

19. Broekmans FJ, Knauff EA, Valkenburg O, Laven JS, Eijkemans MJ, Fauser BC. PCOS according to the Rotterdam consensus criteria: change in prevalence among WHO-II anovulation and association with metabolic factors. *BJOG*. 2006;113(10):1210-1217. doi:10.1111/j.1471-0528.2006.01008.x.

20. Adams JM, Taylor AE, Crowley Jr WF, Hall JE. Polycystic ovarian morphology with regular ovulatory cycles: insights into the pathophysiology of polycystic ovarian syndrome. *J Clin Endocrinol Metab*. 2004;89(9):4343-4350. doi:10.1210/jc.2003-031600.

21. Welt CK, Arason G, Gudmundsson JA, et al. Defining constant versus variable phenotypic features of women with polycystic ovary syndrome using different ethnic groups and populations. *J Clin Endocrinol Metab*. 2006;91(11):4361-4368. doi:10.1210/jc.2006-1191.

22. Swanson M, Sauerbrei EE, Cooperberg PL. Medical implications of ultrasonically detected polycystic ovaries. *J Clin Ultrasound*. 1981;9(5):219-222. doi:10.1002/jcu.1870090504.

23. Rotterdam ESHRE/ASRM-Sponsored PCOS Consensus Workshop Group. Revised 2003 consensus on diagnostic criteria and long-term health risks related to polycystic ovary syndrome (PCOS). *Hum Reprod*. 2004;19(1):41-47. doi:10.1093/humrep/deh098.

24. Johnstone EB, Rosen MP, Neril R, et al. The polycystic ovary post-Rotterdam: a common, age-dependent finding in ovulatory

women without metabolic significance. *J Clin Endocrinol Metab.* 2010;95(11):4965-4972. doi:10.1210/jc.2010-0202.

25. Dewailly D, Lujan ME, Carmina E, et al. Definition and significance of polycystic ovarian morphology: a task force report from the Androgen Excess and Polycystic Ovary Syndrome Society. *Hum Reprod Update.* 2014;20(3):334-352. doi:10.1093/humupd/dmt061.

26. Ahmad AK, Quinn M, Kao CN, Greenwood E, Cedars MI, Huddleston HG. Improved diagnostic performance for the diagnosis of polycystic ovary syndrome using age-stratified criteria. *Fertil Steril.* 2019;111(4):787-793.e2. doi:10.1016/j.fertnstert.2018.11.044.

27. Alsamarai S, Adams JM, Murphy MK, et al. Criteria for polycystic ovarian morphology in polycystic ovary syndrome as a function of age. *J Clin Endocrinol Metab.* 2009;94(12):4961-4970. doi:10.1210/jc.2009-0839.

28. Mason HD, Willis DS, Beard RW, Winston RM, Margara R, Franks S. Estradiol production by granulosa cells of normal and polycystic ovaries: relationship to menstrual cycle history and concentrations of gonadotropins and sex steroids in follicular fluid. *J Clin Endocrinol Metab.* 1994;79(5):1355-1360. doi:10.1210/jcem.79.5.7962330.

29. Hughesdon P. Morphology and morphogenesis of the Stein-Leventhal ovary and of so-called "hyperthecosis." *Obstet Gynecol Surv.* 1982;37(2):59-77.

30. Webber LJ, Stubbs S, Stark J, et al. Formation and early development of follicles in the polycystic ovary. *Lancet.* 2003;362(9389):1017-1021. doi:10.1016/s0140-6736(03)14410-8.

31. Abbott DH, Dumesic DA, Franks S. Developmental origin of polycystic ovary syndrome - a hypothesis. *J Endocrinol.* 2002;174(1):1-5. doi:10.1677/joe.0.1740001.

32. Maciel GA, Baracat EC, Benda JA, et al. Stockpiling of transitional and classic primary follicles in ovaries of women with polycystic ovary syndrome. *J Clin Endocrinol Metab.* 2004;89(11):5321-5327. doi:10.1210/jc.2004-0643.

33. Franks S, McCarthy MI, Hardy K. Development of polycystic ovary syndrome: involvement of genetic and environmental factors. *Int J Androl.* 2006;29(1):278-285.

34. Balen AH, Tan SL, MacDougall J, Jacobs HS. Miscarriage rates following in-vitro fertilization are increased in women with polycystic ovaries and reduced by pituitary desensitization with buserelin. *Hum Reprod.* 1993;8(6):959-964. doi:10.1093/oxfordjournals.humrep.a138174.

35. Makrantonaki E, Zouboulis CC. [Hyperandrogenism, adrenal dysfunction, and hirsutism]. *Hautarzt.* 2020;71(10):752-761. doi:10.1007/s00105-020-04677-1.

36. Meczekalski B, Szeliga A, Maciejewska-Jeske M, et al. Hyperthecosis: an underestimated nontumorous cause of hyperandrogenism. *Gynecol Endocrinol.* 2021;37(8):677-682. doi:10.1080/09513590.2021.1903419.

37. Fanta M. [Hirsutism]. *Ceska Gynekol.* 2017;82(3):237-242.

38. Ferriman D, Gallwey JD. Clinical assessment of body hair growth in women. *J Clin Endocrinol Metab.* 1961;21(11):1440-1447.

39. Hatch R, Rosenfield RL, Kim MH, Tredway D. Hirsutism: implications, etiology, and management. *Am J Obstet Gynecol.* 1981;140(7):815-830.

40. Wijeyaratne CN, Balen AH, Barth JH, Belchetz PE. Clinical manifestations and insulin resistance (IR) in polycystic ovary syndrome (PCOS) among South Asians and Caucasians: is there a difference? *Clin Endocrinol (Oxf).* 2002;57(3):343-350. doi:10.1046/j.1365-2265.2002.01603.x.

41. Mangelsdorf S, Otberg N, Maibach HI, Sinkgraven R, Sterry W, Lademann J. Ethnic variation in vellus hair follicle size and distribution. *Skin Pharmacol Physiol.* 2006;19(3):159-167. doi:10.1159/000093050.

42. Cheewadhanaraks S, Peeyananjarassri K, Choksuchat C. Clinical diagnosis of hirsutism in Thai women. *J Med Assoc Thai.* 2004;87(5):459-463.

43. Zhao X, Ni R, Li L, et al. Defining hirsutism in Chinese women: a cross-sectional study. *Fertil Steril.* 2011;96(3):792-796. doi:10.1016/j.fertnstert.2011.06.040.

44. Martin KA, Anderson RR, Chang RJ, et al. Evaluation and treatment of hirsutism in premenopausal women: an endocrine society clinical practice guideline. *J Clin Endocrinol Metab.* 2018;103(4):1233-1257. doi:10.1210/jc.2018-00241.

45. Franik G, Bizoń A, Włoch S, Kowalczyk K, Biernacka-Bartnik A, Madej P. Hormonal and metabolic aspects of acne vulgaris in women with polycystic ovary syndrome. *Eur Rev Med Pharmacol Sci.* 2018;22(14):4411-4418. doi:10.26355/eurrev_201807_15491.

46. Ludwig E. Classification of the types of androgenetic alopecia (common baldness) occurring in the female sex. *Br J Dermatol.* 1977;97(3):247-254. doi:10.1111/j.1365-2133.1977.tb15179.x.

47. Tagatz GE, Kopher RA, Nagel TC, Okagaki T. The clitoral index: a bioassay of androgenic stimulation. *Obstet Gynecol.* 1979;54(5):562-564.

48. Fraser IS, Kovacs G. Current recommendations for the diagnostic evaluation and follow-up of patients presenting with symptomatic polycystic ovary syndrome. *Best Pract Res Clin Obstet Gynaecol.* 2004;18(5):813-823.

49. Carmina E, Azziz R, Bergfeld W, et al. Female pattern hair loss and androgen excess: a report from the multidisciplinary androgen excess and PCOS committee. *J Clin Endocrinol Metab.* 2019;104(7):2875-2891. doi:10.1210/jc.2018-02548.

50. Karagiannidis I, Nikolakis G, Sabat R, Zouboulis CC. Hidradenitis suppurativa/Acne inversa: an endocrine skin disorder? *Rev Endocr Metab Disord.* 2016;17(3):335-341. doi:10.1007/s11154-016-9366-z.

51. DeVane GW, Czekala NM, Judd HL, Yen SS. Circulating gonadotropins, estrogens, and androgens in polycystic ovarian disease. *Am J Obstet Gynecol.* 1975;121(4):496-500. doi:10.1016/0002-9378(75)90081-2.

52. Ehrmann DA, Barnes RB, Rosenfield RL. Polycystic ovary syndrome as a form of functional ovarian hyperandrogenism due to dysregulation of androgen secretion. *Endocr Rev.* 1995;16(3):322-353. doi:10.1210/edrv-16-3-322.

53. Lizneva D, Gavrilova-Jordan L, Walker W, Azziz R. Androgen excess: investigations and management. *Best Pract Res Clin Obstet Gynaecol.* 2016;37:98-118. doi:10.1016/j.bpobgyn.2016.05.003.

54. Rosner W, Auchus RJ, Azziz R, Sluss PM, Raff H. Position statement: utility, limitations, and pitfalls in measuring testosterone: an Endocrine Society position statement. *J Clin Endocrinol Metab.* 2007;92(2):405-413. doi:10.1210/jc.2006-1864.

55. Rosner W, Vesper H. Toward excellence in testosterone testing: a consensus statement. *J Clin Endocrinol Metab.* 2010;95(10):4542-4548. doi:10.1210/jc.2010-1314.

56. Azziz R, Carmina E, Dewailly D, et al. The Androgen Excess and PCOS Society criteria for the polycystic ovary syndrome: the complete task force report. *Fertil Steril.* 2009;91(2):456-488. doi:10.1016/j.fertnstert.2008.06.035.

57. Goodman NF, Cobin RH, Futterweit W, et al. American Association of Clinical Endocrinologists, American College of Endocrinology, and androgen excess and PCOS society disease state clinical review: guide to the best practices in the evaluation and treatment of polycystic ovary syndrome-part 1. *Endocr Pract.* 2015;21(11):1291-1300.

58. Ly LP, Handelsman DJ. Empirical estimation of free testosterone from testosterone and sex hormone-binding globulin immunoassays. *Eur J Endocrinol*. 2005;152(3):471-478. doi:10.1530/eje.1.01844.

59. Sartorius G, Ly LP, Sikaris K, McLachlan R, Handelsman DJ. Predictive accuracy and sources of variability in calculated free testosterone estimates. *Ann Clin Biochem*. 2009;46(Pt 2):137-143. doi:10.1258/acb.2008.008171.

60. Lim SS, Norman RJ, Davies MJ, Moran LJ. The effect of obesity on polycystic ovary syndrome: a systematic review and meta-analysis. *Obes Rev*. 2013;14(2):95-109. doi:10.1111/j.1467-789X.2012.01053.x.

61. Huang A, Landay M, Azziz R. O-26: The association of androgen levels with the severity of hirsutism in the polycystic ovary syndrome (PCOS). *Fertil Steril*. 2006;86(3):S12.

62. Pinola P, Piltonen TT, Puurunen J, et al. Androgen profile through life in women with polycystic ovary syndrome: a Nordic multicenter collaboration study. *J Clin Endocrinol Metab*. 2015;100(9):3400-3407. doi:10.1210/jc.2015-2123.

63. Azziz R, Sanchez LA, Knochenhauer ES, et al. Androgen excess in women: experience with over 1000 consecutive patients. *J Clin Endocrinol Metab*. 2004;89(2):453-462. doi:10.1210/jc.2003-031122.

64. Nordenström A, Falhammar H. Management of endocrine disease: diagnosis and management of the patient with non-classic CAH due to 21-hydroxylase deficiency. *Eur J Endocrinol*. 2019;180(3):R127-R145. doi:10.1530/eje-18-0712.

65. Carmina E, Dewailly D, Escobar-Morreale HF, et al. Non-classic congenital adrenal hyperplasia due to 21-hydroxylase deficiency revisited: an update with a special focus on adolescent and adult women. *Hum Reprod Update*. 2017;23(5):580-599. doi:10.1093/humupd/dmx014.

66. Saucedo de la Llata E, Moraga-Sánchez MR, Romeu-Sarrió A, Carmona-Ruiz IO. [LH-FSH ratio and polycystic ovary syndrome: a forgotten test?]. *Ginecol Obstet Mex*. 2016;84(2):84-94.

67. Cho LW, Jayagopal V, Kilpatrick ES, Holding S, Atkin SL. The LH/FSH ratio has little use in diagnosing polycystic ovarian syndrome. *Ann Clin Biochem*. 2006;43(Pt 3):217-219. doi:10.1258/000456306776865188.

68. Banaszewska B, Spaczyński RZ, Pelesz M, Pawelczyk L. Incidence of elevated LH/FSH ratio in polycystic ovary syndrome women with normo- and hyperinsulinemia. *Rocz Akad Med Bialymst*. 2003;48:131-134.

69. Baskind NE, Balen AH. Hypothalamic-pituitary, ovarian and adrenal contributions to polycystic ovary syndrome. *Best Pract Res Clin Obstet Gynaecol*. 2016;37:80-97. doi:10.1016/j.bpobgyn.2016.03.005.

70. Delcour C, Robin G, Young J, Dewailly D. PCOS and hyperprolactinemia: what do we know in 2019? *Clin Med Insights Reprod Health*. 2019;13:1179558119871921. doi:10.1177/1179558119871921.

71. Seifer DB, Baker VL, Leader B. Age-specific serum anti-Müllerian hormone values for 17,120 women presenting to fertility centers within the United States. *Fertil Steril*. 2011;95(2):747-750. doi:10.1016/j.fertnstert.2010.10.011.

72. Casadei L, Madrigale A, Puca F, et al. The role of serum anti-Müllerian hormone (AMH) in the hormonal diagnosis of polycystic ovary syndrome. *Gynecol Endocrinol*. 2013;29(6):545-550.

73. Saxena U, Ramani M, Singh P. Role of AMH as diagnostic tool for polycystic ovarian syndrome. *J Obstet Gynaecol India*. 2018;68(2):117-122.

74. Wiweko B, Maidarti M, Priangga MD, et al. Anti-mullerian hormone as a diagnostic and prognostic tool for PCOS patients. *J Assist Reprod Genet*. 2014;31(10):1311-1316.

75. Iliodromiti S, Kelsey TW, Anderson RA, Nelson SM. Can anti-Mullerian hormone predict the diagnosis of polycystic ovary syndrome? A systematic review and meta-analysis of extracted data. *J Clin Endocrinol Metab*. 2013;98(8):3332-3340. doi:10.1210/jc.2013-1393.

76. Teede H, Misso M, Tassone EC, et al. Anti-Müllerian hormone in PCOS: a review informing international guidelines. *Trends Endocrinol Metab*. 2019;30(7):467-478.

77. Hahn S, Quadbeck B, Elsenbruch S, et al. [Metformin, an efficacious drug in the treatment of polycystic ovary syndrome]. *Dtsch Med Wochenschr*. 2004;129(19):1059-1064. doi:10.1055/s-2004-824847.

78. Sánchez LA, Pérez M, Centeno I, David M, Kahi D, Gutierrez E. Determining the time androgens and sex hormone-binding globulin take to return to baseline after discontinuation of oral contraceptives in women with polycystic ovary syndrome: a prospective study. *Fertil Steril*. 2007;87(3):712-714. doi:10.1016/j.fertnstert.2006.07.1507.

79. Kyritsi EM, Dimitriadis GK, Kyrou I, Kaltsas G, Randeva HS. PCOS remains a diagnosis of exclusion: a concise review of key endocrinopathies to exclude. *Clin Endocrinol (Oxf)*. 2017;86(1):1-6. doi:10.1111/cen.13245.

80. Rachoń D. Differential diagnosis of hyperandrogenism in women with polycystic ovary syndrome. *Exp Clin Endocrinol Diabetes*. 2012;120(4):205-209. doi:10.1055/s-0031-1299765.

81. Zawadski JK, Dunaif A Diagnostic Criteria for Polycystic Ovary Syndrome: Towards a Rational Approach. In: Dunaif A, Givens JR, Haseltine F, eds. *Polycystic Ovary Syndrome*. Boston: Blackwell Scientific; 1992:377–384.

82. National Institute of Health. *Evidence-Based Methodology Workshop on Polycystic Ovary Syndrome*. 2013. Available at: https://prevention.nih.gov/sites/default/files/2018-06/FinalReport.pdf.

83. Burger HG. Androgen production in women. *Fertil Steril*. 2002;77(suppl 4):S3-S5. doi:10.1016/s0015-0282(02)02985-0.

84. Burger HG, Dudley EC, Cui J, Dennerstein L, Hopper JL. A prospective longitudinal study of serum testosterone, dehydroepiandrosterone sulfate, and sex hormone-binding globulin levels through the menopause transition. *J Clin Endocrinol Metab*. 2000;85(8):2832-2838. doi:10.1210/jcem.85.8.6740.

85. Rannevik G, Jeppsson S, Johnell O, Bjerre B, Laurell-Borulf Y, Svanberg L. A longitudinal study of the perimenopausal transition: altered profiles of steroid and pituitary hormones, SHBG and bone mineral density. *Maturitas*. 1995;21(2):103-113. doi:10.1016/0378-5122(94)00869-9.

86. Kaltsas GA, Isidori AM, Kola BP, et al. The value of the low-dose dexamethasone suppression test in the differential diagnosis of hyperandrogenism in women. *J Clin Endocrinol Metab*. 2003;88(6):2634-2643. doi:10.1210/jc.2002-020922.

87. Kaltsas GA, Mukherjee JJ, Kola B, et al. Is ovarian and adrenal venous catheterization and sampling helpful in the investigation of hyperandrogenic women? *Clin Endocrinol (Oxf)*. 2003;59(1):34-43. doi:10.1046/j.1365-2265.2003.01792.x.

88. Outwater EK, Marchetto B, Wagner BJ. Virilizing tumors of the ovary: imaging features. *Ultrasound Obstet Gynecol*. 2000;15(5):365-371. doi:10.1046/j.1469-0705.2000.00123.x.

89. Daniilidis A, Dinas K. Long term health consequences of polycystic ovarian syndrome: a review analysis. *Hippokratia*. 2009;13(2):90-92.

90. Markopoulos MC, Rizos D, Valsamakis G, et al. Hyperandrogenism in women with polycystic ovary syndrome persists

after menopause. *J Clin Endocrinol Metab.* 2011;96(3):623-631. doi:10.1210/jc.2010-0130.

91. McCartney CR, Prendergast KA, Chhabra S, et al. The association of obesity and hyperandrogenemia during the pubertal transition in girls: obesity as a potential factor in the genesis of postpubertal hyperandrogenism. *J Clin Endocrinol Metab.* 2006;91(5):1714-1722. doi:10.1210/jc.2005-1852.

92. Reinehr T, de Sousa G, Roth CL, Andler W. Androgens before and after weight loss in obese children. *J Clin Endocrinol Metab.* 2005;90(10):5588-5595. doi:10.1210/jc.2005-0438.

93. Zore T, Lizneva D, Brakta S, Walker W, Suturina L, Azziz R. Minimal difference in phenotype between adolescents and young adults with polycystic ovary syndrome. *Fertil Steril.* 2019;111(2):389-396. doi:10.1016/j.fertnstert.2018.10.020.

94. Lucky AW, Biro FM, Daniels SR, Cedars MI, Khoury PR, Morrison JA. The prevalence of upper lip hair in black and white girls during puberty: a new standard. *J Pediatr.* 2001;138(1):134-136. doi:10.1067/mpd.2001.109790.

95. Ibáñez L, Oberfield SE, Witchel S, et al. An international consortium update: pathophysiology, diagnosis, and treatment of polycystic ovarian syndrome in adolescence. *Horm Res Paediatr.* 2017;88(6):371-395. doi:10.1159/000479371.

96. Deplewski D, Rosenfield RL. Role of hormones in pilosebaceous unit development. *Endocr Rev.* 2000;21(4):363-392. doi:10.1210/edrv.21.4.0404.

97. Rosenfield RL. The diagnosis of polycystic ovary syndrome in adolescents. *Pediatrics.* 2015;136(6):1154-1165. doi:10.1542/peds.2015-1430.

98. Lucky AW, Biro FM, Simbartl LA, Morrison JA, Sorg NW. Predictors of severity of acne vulgaris in young adolescent girls: results of a five-year longitudinal study. *J Pediatr.* 1997;130(1):30-39. doi:10.1016/s0022-3476(97)70307-x.

99. Rothenberg SS, Beverley R, Barnard E, Baradaran-Shoraka M, Sanfilippo JS. Polycystic ovary syndrome in adolescents. *Best Pract Res Clin Obstet Gynaecol.* 2018;48:103-114. doi:10.1016/j.bpobgyn.2017.08.008.

100. Witchel SF, Oberfield S, Rosenfield RL, et al. The diagnosis of polycystic ovary syndrome during adolescence. *Horm Res Paediatr.* 2015. doi:10.1159/000375530.

101. Rosenfield RL. Perspectives on the international recommendations for the diagnosis and treatment of polycystic ovary syndrome in adolescence. *J Pediatr Adolesc Gynecol.* 2020;33(5):445-447. doi:10.1016/j.jpag.2020.06.017.

102. Rosenfield RL. Clinical review: adolescent anovulation: maturational mechanisms and implications. *J Clin Endocrinol Metab.* 2013;98(9):3572-3583. doi:10.1210/jc.2013-1770.

103. van Hooff MH, Voorhorst FJ, Kaptein MB, Hirasing RA, Koppenaal C, Schoemaker J. Predictive value of menstrual cycle pattern, body mass index, hormone levels and polycystic ovaries at age 15 years for oligo-amenorrhoea at age 18 years. *Hum Reprod.* 2004;19(2):383-392. doi:10.1093/humrep/deh079.

104. Venturoli S, Porcu E, Fabbri R, et al. Menstrual irregularities in adolescents: hormonal pattern and ovarian morphology. *Horm Res.* 1986;24(4):269-279. doi:10.1159/000180567.

105. Wiksten-Almströmer M, Hirschberg AL, Hagenfeldt K. Prospective follow-up of menstrual disorders in adolescence and prognostic factors. *Acta Obstet Gynecol Scand.* 2008;87(11):1162-1168. doi:10.1080/00016340802478166.

106. Barnes RB, Rosenfield RL, Ehrmann DA, et al. Ovarian hyperandrogynism as a result of congenital adrenal virilizing disorders: evidence for perinatal masculinization of neuroendocrine

function in women. *J Clin Endocrinol Metab.* 1994;79(5):1328-1333. doi:10.1210/jcem.79.5.7962325.

107. Bachelot A, Chakhtoura Z, Plu-Bureau G, et al. Influence of hormonal control on LH pulsatility and secretion in women with classical congenital adrenal hyperplasia. *Eur J Endocrinol.* 2012;167(4):499-505. doi:10.1530/eje-12-0454.

108. Charmandari E, Kino T, Ichijo T, Chrousos GP. Generalized glucocorticoid resistance: clinical aspects, molecular mechanisms, and implications of a rare genetic disorder. *J Clin Endocrinol Metab.* 2008;93(5):1563-1572. doi:10.1210/jc.2008-0040.

109. Lungu AO, Zadeh ES, Goodling A, Cochran E, Gorden P. Insulin resistance is a sufficient basis for hyperandrogenism in lipodystrophic women with polycystic ovarian syndrome. *J Clin Endocrinol Metab.* 2012;97(2):563-567. doi:10.1210/jc.2011-1896.

110. Littlejohn EE, Weiss RE, Deplewski D, Edidin DV, Rosenfield R. Intractable early childhood obesity as the initial sign of insulin resistant hyperinsulinism and precursor of polycystic ovary syndrome. *J Pediatr Endocrinol Metab.* 2007;20(1):41-51. doi:10.1515/jpem.2007.20.1.41.

111. Codner E, Escobar-Morreale HF. Clinical review: hyperandrogenism and polycystic ovary syndrome in women with type 1 diabetes mellitus. *J Clin Endocrinol Metab.* 2007;92(4):1209-1216. doi:10.1210/jc.2006-2641.

112. Peppard HR, Marfori J, Iuorno MJ, Nestler JE. Prevalence of polycystic ovary syndrome among premenopausal women with type 2 diabetes. *Diabetes Care.* 2001;24(6):1050-1052. doi:10.2337/diacare.24.6.1050.

113. Sanchón R, Gambineri A, Alpañés M, Martínez-García M, Pasquali R, Escobar-Morreale HF. Prevalence of functional disorders of androgen excess in unselected premenopausal women: a study in blood donors. *Hum Reprod.* 2012;27(4):1209-1216. doi:10.1093/humrep/des028.

114. Carmina E. Mild androgen phenotypes. *Best Pract Res Clin Endocrinol Metab.* 2006;20(2):207-220. doi:10.1016/j.beem.2006.02.001.

115. Rosenfield RL. Evidence that idiopathic functional adrenal hyperandrogenism is caused by dysregulation of adrenal steroidogenesis and that hyperinsulinemia may be involved. *J Clin Endocrinol Metab.* 1996;81(3):878-880. doi:10.1210/jcem.81.3.8772543.

116. Rosenfield RL, Mortensen M, Wroblewski K, Littlejohn E, Ehrmann DA. Determination of the source of androgen excess in functionally atypical polycystic ovary syndrome by a short dexamethasone androgen-suppression test and a low-dose ACTH test. *Hum Reprod.* 2011;26(11):3138-3146. doi:10.1093/humrep/der291.

117. Escobar-Morreale HF, Santacruz E, Luque-Ramírez M, Botella Carretero JI. Prevalence of 'obesity-associated gonadal dysfunction' in severely obese men and women and its resolution after bariatric surgery: a systematic review and meta-analysis. *Hum Reprod Update.* 2017;23(4):390-408. doi:10.1093/humupd/dmx012.

118. Sivayoganathan D, Maruthini D, Glanville JM, Balen AH. Full investigation of patients with polycystic ovary syndrome (PCOS) presenting to four different clinical specialties reveals significant differences and undiagnosed morbidity. *Hum Fertil (Camb).* 2011;14(4):261-265. doi:10.3109/14647273.2011.632058.

119. Bonny AE, Appelbaum H, Connor EL, et al. Clinical variability in approaches to polycystic ovary syndrome. *J Pediatr Adolesc Gynecol.* 2012;25(4):259-261. doi:10.1016/j.jpag.2012.03.004.

120. Torres-Zegarra C, Sundararajan D, Benson J, et al. Care for adolescents with polycystic ovary syndrome: development and

prescribing patterns of a multidisciplinary clinic. *J Pediate Adolesc Gynecol.* 2021;34(5):617-625.

121. Hudecova M, Holte J, Olovsson M, Sundström Poromaa I. Long-term follow-up of patients with polycystic ovary syndrome: reproductive outcome and ovarian reserve. *Hum Reprod.* 2009;24(5):1176-1183.

122. Wekker V, van Dammen L, Koning A, et al. Long-term cardiometabolic disease risk in women with PCOS: a systematic review and meta-analysis. *Hum Reprod Update.* 2020;26(6): 942-960. doi:10.1093/humupd/dmaa029.

123. Sha T, Wang X, Cheng W, Yan Y. A meta-analysis of pregnancy-related outcomes and complications in women with polycystic ovary syndrome undergoing IVF. *Reprod Biomed Online.* 2019;39(2):281-293. doi:10.1016/j.rbmo.2019.03.203.

124. Qin JZ, Pang LH, Li MJ, Fan XJ, Huang RD, Chen HY. Obstetric complications in women with polycystic ovary syndrome: a systematic review and meta-analysis. *Reprod Biol Endocrinol.* 2013;11:56. doi:10.1186/1477-7827-11-56.

10

Polycystic Ovary Syndrome and Metabolic Syndrome: Risks in Later Life

AISHA SHEIKH

Introduction

Polycystic ovary syndrome (PCOS) is the most frequent endocrine-metabolic-reproductive condition affecting females in their reproductive life. PCOS is closely linked to metabolic disorders such as obesity and insulin resistance (IR), which plays a central role in its pathogenesis. A large proportion of females with PCOS are obese or overweight and demonstrate IR with associated compensatory hyperinsulinemia, which plays an important role in the development of some phenotypic features of PCOS and, together with beta-cell dysfunction, increases the risk of developing other metabolic abnormalities such as type 2 diabetes mellitus (T2DM), hypertension, dyslipidemia, and cardiovascular diseases (CVD). On the other hand, a subset of lean females with PCOS also exhibit IR.[1,2]

Metabolic syndrome (MetS) is a group of impairments in the metabolism of glucose and lipids and consists of central obesity, glucose intolerance, dyslipidemia, and hypertension.[3] It is a well-documented risk factor for T2DM and CVD. IR and central obesity are proven to play important roles in the etiopathogenesis of both MetS and PCOS. Globally, several definitions of MetS are in use based on the presence of multiple CVD risk factors in an individual (Table 10.1). Studies investigating MetS in PCOS have used one or several of these criteria to find the prevalence of MetS in their study subjects.

Polycystic Ovary Syndrome and Obesity

PCOS is a condition that is associated with obesity, IR, and cardiometabolic risk, although these features do not form part of the diagnostic criteria for PCOS. Females with PCOS are at a higher risk for being overweight or obese and have higher prevalence of central obesity (risk ratio 1.73)

compared with healthy females.[7] There is ambiguity as to whether PCOS causes weight gain and obesity or if obesity is linked to the development of PCOS.[8] Weight gain and obesity contribute to the development of PCOS through worsening of IR as one of the pathophysiologic mechanisms, which leads to impaired glucose tolerance (IGT) and risk of T2DM. In fact, genetically predisposed females who gain weight over the course of their lives have a much higher risk of developing manifestations of PCOS. The association between PCOS and obesity is evident from epidemiologic studies that reveal that the majority of patients (38%–88%) with PCOS are either overweight or obese.[9] Primarily, central or visceral (abdominal) obesity is often observed in patients with PCOS regardless of their body mass index (BMI). Obesity aggravates the hormonal irregularities and metabolic consequences, not only worsening the clinical features of PCOS but also leading to compromised fertility outcomes and increasing the risks for MetS, T2DM, and CVD.[10,11] On the other hand, even modest weight loss of just 5% body weight with improvement in insulin sensitivity often results in clinically significant benefits in hyperandrogenic, reproductive, and metabolic features. Nevertheless, it is also clear that, independent of obesity and fat mass, PCOS is inherently associated with metabolic aberrations that include IR, dyslipidemia, and nonalcoholic fatty liver disease (NAFLD).

Polycystic Ovary Syndrome and Insulin Resistance

Besides the genetic and environmental factors, the pathogenic role of IR in PCOS was first recognized in 1980s. Thereafter the compensatory hyperinsulinemia in response to IR was established that leads to increased androgen production from ovaries through a range of mechanisms, including stimulation

TABLE 10.1	Commonly Used Definitions of Metabolic Syndrome Based on Various Criteria

	NCEP-ATP III[4]	International Diabetes Federation (IDF)[5]	Joint criteria[6]
Required	—	WC (≥80 cm in females (South Asian, Chinese ≥80 cm in females, Japanese ≥90 cm in females)	—
No. of abnormalities	≥3 of:	≥2 of:	≥3 of:
Obesity	WC ≥ 88 cm in females		WC: Population- and country-specific definitions
Triglycerides	≥150 mg/dL	≥150 mg/dL	≥150 mg/dL
HDL cholesterol	<50 mg/dL in females	<50 mg/dL in females	<50 mg/dL in females
Hypertension	≥130/85 mm Hg	≥130/85 mm Hg	≥130/85 mm Hg
Glucose	≥110 mg/dL	≥100 mg/dL	≥100 mg/dL

HDL, High density lipoprotein; *NCEP-ATP III*, National Cholesterol Education Program Adult Treatment Panel III (ATP III); *WC*, waist circumference

of gonadotropin hormone-releasing hormone (GnRH) gene transcription in the hypothalamus and a subsequent rising frequency of luteinizing hormone (LH) pulse at the pituitary. Insulin thus acts to interrupt all levels of the hypothalamic-pituitary-ovarian axis, and IR in ovarian tissue causes a series of metabolic signaling derangements, which favor hyperandrogenemia (HA) in the presence of an unaffected mitogenic and steroidogenic activity. Increased androgens further aggravate IR by enhancing free fatty acids and modifying muscle tissue structure and performance, thus continuing the IR-hyperinsulinemia-HA cycle.[2] HA further worsens the IR and

thus a vicious cycle of IR-hyperinsulinemia-HA continues. Furthermore, obesity augments all events in this cycle by increasing androgen production not only in ovaries but also in subcutaneous adipose tissue and adrenal glands. Leptin plays its role by disrupting ovarian physiology and inducing a chronic systemic inflammatory state.[2] Eventually, both IR and chronic inflammation flourish on all endocrine-metabolic disturbances related to PCOS, putting the affected females at risk for T2DM and CVD (Fig. 10.1).

IR is a common pathology in patients with PCOS. Nevertheless, it is not present in all subjects. Data on 526

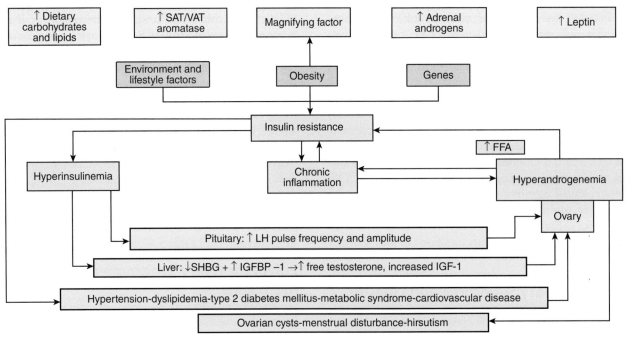

• **Fig. 10.1** A representation of the Pathogenesis and Progression of Polycystic Ovary Syndrome and Related Comorbidities. *FFA*, Free fatty acids; *IGF-1*, insulin-like growth factor 1; *IGFBP-1*, insulin-like growth factor binding protein-1; *LH*, luteinizing hormone; *SAT*, subcutaneous adipose tissue; *SHBG*, sex hormone–binding globulin; *VAT*, visceral adipose tissue.

reproductive-aged females reported IR in 112 (42.6%) of the PCOS females and 45 (17.1%) of the control ($P <$ .001).[12] A study from Iran showed 36.5% prevalence of IR among the PCOS patients. The prevalence of MetS in the IR versus insulin sensitive (IS) PCOS patients was significantly higher (43.5% vs. 20%; $p =$ .034).[13]

Another interesting study compared markers of IR and circulating androgens between females with PCOS and females with MetS; 1223 White females with PCOS and 277 females without PCOS, matched for BMI, were included in the study. The results showed a statistically significant difference in terms of higher IR in PCOS females with MetS versus those with PCOS without MetS. Interestingly, the authors found that control females with MetS were more IR than PCOS females without MetS ($P <$ .001 for the comparisons in all markers of IR). Only females with PCOS irrespective of the MetS status had higher circulating androgen levels.[14]

Assessment of Insulin Resistance

Hyperinsulinemic Euglycemic Clamp Technique

The gold standard to measure IS is through the hyperinsulinemic euglycemic clamp (M-clamp) technique. The procedure relies on a constant insulin infusion, which results in a new steady-state insulin level above the fasting level, which eventually augments glucose uptake in skeletal muscle and adipose tissue on one hand and slows hepatic gluconeogenesis; 20% dextrose is given to "clamp" blood glucose levels in the euglycemic range. This technique directly measures all body glucose disposal under steady-state insulin conditions, but it is tedious, laborious, costly, and professionally challenging.[15]

Surrogate Markers of Insulin Resistance

Because of the difficulties with clinical use of M-Clamp, researchers have developed various surrogate markers to assess IS/IR based on mathematical formulations using fasting glucose and insulin levels either in basal conditions or after glucose load (Table 10.2). These surrogate indexes have been compared with M-clamp and have been used extensively in clinical research. The correlation of surrogate indexes of IR with M-Clamp has been reasonable. Moghetti et al. studied 375 patients with PCOS, out of whom 74.9% of the patients were identified as IR through an M-Clamp. IR was more frequent in obese PCOS (93.9% in obese vs. 77.5% in overweight vs. 59.3% in normal-weight PCOS patients). The researchers further compared the surrogate indexes with the M-clamp values, which highly correlated. Nevertheless, the authors noted that these markers have low sensitivity to identify IR, particularly in normal-weight PCOS, which led to inaccurate labeling of normal-weight PCOS patients as IS. Based on this, the authors proposed that these indexes can be used to rule in, but not rule out,

TABLE 10.2	Surrogate Indexes of Insulin Resistance
Index (reference)	Calculation
HOMA (homeostasis model assessment)[17]	Fasting glucose, mmol/L × fasting insulin, mU/L/22.5
G/I (glucose/insulin) ratio[18]	Fasting glucose, mg/dL/fasting insulin, mU/L
QUICKI (quantitative insulin sensitivity check index)[19]	1/Log (fasting insulin, mU/L) + log (fasting glucose, mg/dL)
Gutt index[20]	$\{[75\,000 + (\text{fasting glucose, mg/dL} - \text{glucose}_{120}') \times 0.19 \times \text{body weight, kg}/120]/ [(\text{fasting glucose} + \text{glucose}_{120}')/2]\}/\log [(\text{fasting insulin, mU/L}, + \text{insulin}_{120}')/2]$
Stumvoll[21]	$0.156 - 0.0000459 \times \text{insulin}_{120}', \text{pmol/L} - 0.000321 \times \text{fasting insulin} - 0.00541 \times \text{glucose}_{120}', \text{mmol/L}$
Matsuda[22]	$10000/ [(\text{Fasting glucose, mg/dL} \times \text{fasting insulin, mU/L}) \times (\text{glucose}_{30}' + \text{glucose}_{60}' + \text{glucose}_{90}' + \text{glucose}_{120}')/4 \times (\text{insulin}_{30}' + \text{insulin}_{60}' + \text{insulin}_{90}' + \text{insulin}_{120}')/4]^{0.5}$

IR in PCOS.[16] Many researchers have tried to use these surrogate indexes to estimate IR and antedate the diagnosis of MetS and cardiovascular outcomes in PCOS. Thus those studies have demonstrated an improvement in use of medical resources, cost savings, and reduction of side effects.

Novel Biomarkers

In recent years, quite a few proteins are emerging as possible biomarkers of IR in PCOS. A strong association has been found between adipocytokines (i.e., adiponectin, visfatin, vaspin, and apelin), copeptin, irisin, plasminogen activator inhibitor-1 (PAI-1), and zonulin with IR and PCOS physiopathology.[23]

Polycystic Ovary Syndrome and Metabolic Syndrome

Patients with PCOS are at risk for MetS. Numerous studies have reported higher frequencies of MetS in females with PCOS compared with females without PCOS and a higher risk in obese PCOS females compared with nonobese PCOS. Table 10.3 shows a few published studies.

A meta-analysis of 35 studies reported that females with PCOS had a greater prevalence of the metabolic syndrome than females without PCOS (odds ratio [OR] 2.88). The authors gave the frequencies of different components of the

TABLE 10.3   A Few Recent Publications on the Prevalence of Metabolic Syndrome in Females With Polycystic Ovary Syndrome

Study	n	Control Group	Criteria of MetS Used	IR Marker	Percentage of MetS	Other CVD Risks Reported	Comments
(Jamil et al., 2015)[12]	526	Yes	NCEP-ATPIII	Fasting glucose to insulin ratio, HOMA-IR, HOMA-B, QUICKI, Metsuda index	53.6% vs. 32.7% (p <0.001)	TG/HDL, 3.17 ± 3.03 vs 2.28 ± 1.61 (p < .001)	Females undergoing fertility treatment. Higher BMI and WC reported in PCOS group
(Abdelazim & Elsawah, 2015)[24]	220	No	NCEP-ATPIII	Not reported	30.5%	Not reported	Infertile females with PCOS MetS prevalence 100% in females >35
(Montazerifar, Ghasemi, Arabpour, Karajibani, & Keikhah, 2020)[25]	240	Yes	NCEP-ATPIII		29.2% vs. 7.5% (p <0.0001)	Low HDL, high TG, high TG/HDL ratio, increased WC	Infertile females
(N. Anjum, Zohra, Arif, Azhar, & Qureshi, 2013)[26]	425	Yes	NCEP-ATP III	FBS/Insulin ratio	35.6% vs. 9.5% (p < .0001)	BMI, WC, systolic BP, diastolic BP, TG increased, HDL low, high TG/HDL ratio	
(Panidis et al., 2013)[27]	1500	yes	All criteria of MetS	G/I ratio HOMA-IR QUICKI	Age group 31–39: Joint criteria: 39.1% vs. 28.5 % (p .045) NCEP-ATPIII criteria 27.1% vs. 12.1% (p .001)	WC, WHR, BP, lipids NS among PCOS vs. control when adjusted for BMI	No difference in MetS in age groups below 31 and in any age group if adjusted for BMI. Females with PCOS were more IR than controls across all BMI groups
(Moghetti et al., 2013)[28]	137	No	IDF/NCEP-ATPIII	M-clamp	32.8% (IDF) 31.3% (NCEP-ATPIII)	Increased WC (73.7%) and low HDL cholesterol (54.1%)	71.4% were IR
(Meyer et al., 2020)[29]	1427	Yes	Joint	Not reported	19.3% (Joint)	Abdominal obesity (>66%) and low HDL-C (cholesterol) (>42%), elevated BP (20.6%)	No significant associations between MetS and OC use to regulate periods or acne The interaction with BMI greater than or equal to 30 kg/m² was not statistically significant (p > .26)

TABLE 10.3   A Few Recent Publications on the Prevalence of Metabolic Syndrome in Females With Polycystic Ovary Syndrome—cont'd

Study	n	Control Group	Criteria of MetS Used	IR Marker	Percentage of MetS	Other CVD Risks Reported	Comments
(Liang et al., 2012)[30]	290	yes	NCEP-ATP III	HOMA-IR	30% vs. 18% (p .008)	High BMI, WC, WHR, and TG in PCOS females vs controls	Obesity was the only significant variable that increased the risk of MetS (OR 54)
(Le et al., 2018)[31]	441	No	NCEP-ATP III	Modified ACE criteria[32]	10.4%	High BMI, abdominal obesity (84.8%), SBP (18.2%), TG (78.8%) and low HDL (93.9%) in PCOS females with MetS	Infertile females IRS 27%
(Kyrkou et al., 2016)[33]	385	yes	IDF	-	12.6% vs 1.9%	High BMI, BP, TG	
(Karee, Gundabattula, Sashi, Boorugu, & Chowdhury, 2020)[34]	382	No	NCEP ATPIII	-	38.5%	Low HDL, increased WC	Significant association of BMI and age
(Hosseinpanah, Barzin, Tehrani, & Azizi, 2011)[35]	559	Yes	Joint interim statement	HOMA-IR	18.5% vs 18.3% (p = NS)	Abdominal obesity, dyslipidemia, BP nonsignificant	IR 27.2% vs 24.2% (p<0.01)
(S. Anjum, Askari, Riaz, & Basit, 2020)[36]	153	No	AHA/NHLB1	HOMA-IR	46.4%	Obesity 82.4% Dyslipidemia 56.2%	No difference in IR among PCOS females with and without MetS

ACE, Amercian College of Endocrinology; AHA/NHLB1, American Heart Association/National Heart, Lung, and Blood Institute; BMI, Body mass index; BP, blood pressure; CVD, cardiovascular disease; HDL, high density lipoprotein; HOMA, homeostatic model assessment; IR, insulin resistance; MetS, metabolic syndrome; NCEP-ATP III, National Cholesterol Education Program Adult Treatment Panel III (ATP III); NS, not significant; OC, oral contraceptives; OR, odds ratio; PCOS, polycystic ovary syndrome; TG, triglycerides; WC, waist circumference; WHR, waist-hip ratio.

metabolic syndrome in females with PCOS: waist circumference (WC) or BMI (11%–98%), decreased high density lipoprotein (HDL)-cholesterol (C) (28.6%–95%), increased triglycerides (5.5%–56%), elevated blood pressure (BP; 7.3%–70%), and elevated fasting glucose (0%–43.5%).[37] Another systematic review and meta-analysis reported the pooled prevalence of MetS among PCOS females as 26.30% but varied from 7.1% to 37.5%, depending on the diagnostic criteria used. Reduced HDL and increased WC were the most common components of MetS reported in 61.87% and 52.23% of PCOS females with MetS, respectively. Compared with healthy controls, the overall pooled OR of MetS in PCOS patients was 2.09, but this ranged from 0.31 to 4.69 depending on the diagnostic criteria used.[38]

Ethnic Differences in Risk of Metabolic Syndrome

Various studies have investigated the risk of MetS in different ethnicities, either living in the same geographic location or in different geographic locations. Increased risk of MetS is reported in both Black adolescents (risk ratio [RR] 2.65) and adult females (RR 1.44) with PCOS compared with White subjects with PCOS.[39] Another study reported that Hispanic females with PCOS have marked HA and risk for MetS compared with non-Hispanic Black and White females.[40] Both Hispanic White and Black females with PCOS have higher basal state IR and accelerated β-cell response and postchallenge hyperinsulinemia in contrast to non-Hispanic White and Asian American subjects. Asian American females, however, showed a reduced insulin response.[41] The prevalence of MetS components varies in females with PCOS, such that compared with White females (28.3%) from the United States, Black U.S. females had the highest prevalence (52%), whereas females from India (38.2%) and Norway (41.1%) had a higher prevalence of MetS independent of obesity (OR 6.53 and 2.16, respectively).[42] White, South Asian, and East Asian females with PCOS living in the same geographic location have similar metabolic profiles to one another, whereas Asian females have higher 2-hour insulin levels and East Asian females, specifically, have higher 2-hour glucose levels.[43]

These findings suggest that race and ethnicity should be taken into consideration when screening females with PCOS for metabolic dysfunction. There is a need for longitudinal studies to examine the independent effect of PCOS and race on CVD risk in these patients.

Metabolic Disturbances in Nonobese Females With Polycystic Ovary Syndrome

Several authors have reported higher frequencies of metabolic disturbances even in nonobese patients with PCOS using the adult treatment panel III definition. These metabolic disturbances involve IR, IGT, high triglycerides (TG), low HDL, and MetS in nonobese patients with PCOS.

One hundred lean patients with PCOS were studied for the effect of IR as detected by the homeostatic model assessment for IR (HOMA-IR; 2.5 cut-off) on metabolic parameters. The results showed 47% of patients with IR that was positively correlated with waist-hip ratio (WHR), systolic BP, diastolic BP, estradiol levels, Ferriman–Gallwey score (FGS), and total testosterone levels.[44] A meta-analyses of 22 studies that compared prevalence of MetS in nonobese PCOS compared with nonobese controls (BMI <30 kg/m² in White patients, and <25 kg/m² in Asian patients) showed a higher prevalence of hyperinsulinemia (OR, 36.27, IR [OR, 5.70], IGT [OR, 3.42], T2DM [OR, 1.47], hypertriglyceridemia [OR, 10.46], low-HDL [OR, 4.03], and MetS [OR, 2.57]).[45] No significant difference was observed for impaired fasting glucose (IFG), pre-DM, dyslipidemia, hypercholesterolemia, and hypertension in this meta-analysis. In subgroup analysis, White patients exhibited increased risks of IR, IGT, IFG, T2DM, hypertension, and MetS, whereas no significant metabolic change was found in Asian patients. No study reported specifically an incidence of myocardial infarction, stroke, cerebrovascular accident, arterial occlusive disease, or coronary heart disease in nonobese patients with PCOS.[45]

Combined Oral Contraceptive COC Use and Risk of MetS in PCOS

Combined oral contraceptives (COCs) are frequently used in patients with PCOS to achieve menstrual cycle regularity and improve manifestations of HA because they can increase sex hormone–binding globulin (SHBG) and reduce androgen levels significantly. Small observational studies on the use of COCs in patients with PCOS have raised concerns about worsening of metabolic profile, inciting an inflammatory response and coagulation parameters, thus posing a higher risk for T2DM, CVD, and venous thromboembolism.[46] Nevertheless, a recent meta-analysis concluded that there are inconsistent data on the impact of COCs on glucose tolerance status. With regards to lipids, COCs led to increased HDL, total cholesterol and triglycerides consistently but to assess the clinical impact of such dyslipidemia, more longitudinal studies are needed.[47] Another recent study suggested that COC use to regulate periods or acne had similar MetS prevalence compared with those with no oral contraceptive use (20.1% vs. 21.0%, respectively).[29] Based on the existing evidence, it is important to individualize COC use for patients with PCOS considering the singular cardiovascular risk and risk-benefit ratio of using these agents.

Association of Vitamin D Deficiency With Metabolic Markers in PCOS

Vitamin D deficiency is common globally, but patients with PCOS are more likely to have severe vitamin D deficiency compared with controls (44.0% vs. 11.2%), and this was associated with multiple MetS risk factors.[48] Vitamin D deficiency is more marked in obese PCOS patients with IR.[49,50] A statistically significant negative correlation between 25(OH)D levels and BMI, WHR, fasting insulin, HOMA-IR, total cholesterol, low-density lipoprotein cholesterol [LDL-C]), and high-sensitivity C-reactive protein (hs-CRP) was found ($P < .05$). In contrast, there was a positive correlation between serum 25(OH)D concentration HDL-C ($P < .05$), thus deliberating a possible protective effect.[50]

Hyperandrogenism and Risk of Metabolic Syndrome

PCOS patients with androgen excess are at high risk for metabolic consequences like liver diseases and IR. HA was found to be an independent contributor to the high prevalence of MetS in PCOS patients.[51]

A study evaluated the testosterone to dihydrotestosterone ratio (TT/DHT) as a biomarker for an adverse metabolic profile in 275 females with PCOS compared with 35 BMI-matched, healthy controls. In PCOS patients, the TT/DHT ratio was significantly higher ($P < .001$) in obese females and those with MetS, IGT, or IR. The TT/DHT ratio correlated significantly with adverse anthropometric, hormonal, and various parameters of liver, lipid, and glucose metabolism.[52] Still others have reported that SHBG, rather than testosterone, is independently associated with MetS in overweight females with PCOS and is associated with IR and PCOS diagnostic criteria. Thus SHBG may be representing an independent marker of MetS irrespective of the androgen status.[53] In patients with PCOS, a positive correlation between

SHBG and HDL levels is reported in literature. On the other hand, there is significant negative correlation of SHBG with BMI, systolic BP, diastolic BP, TG, fasting insulin, HOMA-IR, and 2-h (postglucose load) plasma glucose level. The SHBG cut-off value of 21.3 nmol/L (sensitivity of 100% and specificity of 85%) is described for predicting MetS in PCOS.[54]

For various PCOS phenotypes, insulin action was significantly impaired in patients with either the classic or the ovulatory phenotype but not in those with the normo-androgenic phenotype.[28] Others have found an inverse association of SHBG with WC, systolic BP, TG, LDL, APOB (apolipoprotein B), alanine transaminase (ALT), aspartate transaminase (AST), and blood urea nitrogen (BUN) but positively associated with HDL and APOA1 (apolipoprotein A1). SHBG was found to be a protective predictor for MetS on logistic regression with an OR of 0.96.[55]

Metabolic Syndrome and Polycystic Ovary Syndrome Phenotype

The Rotterdam classification divided PCOS into four distinct phenotypes based on oligo/anovulation (OA), clinical and/or biochemical HA, and polycystic ovary morphology (PCO) phenotype A (HA+OA+PCO), phenotype B (HA+OA), phenotype C (HA+PCO), and phenotype D (OA+PCO).[56] Investigators have estimated the risk of MetS among different PCOS phenotypes (Table 10.4). As previously discussed, the frequency of MetS is significantly higher in all phenotypes of PCOS compared with the control group but the nonhyperandrogenic phenotype of PCOS (phenotype OA + PCO) has the lowest frequency of MetS in all PCOS phenotypes.[57] Besides the increased risk of MetS in phenotype A, anti-Müllerian hormone (AMH) levels were reported to be the highest in this phenotype as well.[12]

Thus it is clear that PCOS patients with HA phenotypes are at a higher metabolic risk than the normoandrogenic phenotype. Likewise, the frequency of IR in the classic, ovulatory, and normoandrogenic phenotype subgroups was reported as 80.4%, 65.0%, and 38.1%, respectively ($P < .001$).[28] The emergent normoandrogenic phenotypes from Rotterdam criteria have lesser risk of MetS compared with more severe phenotypes based on the National Institutes of Health (NIH) consensus criteria. A recent meta-analysis reported the least favorable metabolic profile with the classic phenotype A. Generally, the normoandrogenic PCOS phenotype has the most favorable metabolic profile, which is akin to the metabolic profile of healthy control females. Nevertheless, in the studies conducted in East Asian populations, even the normoandrogenic phenotype was associated with an increased metabolic risk.[63]

Abnormalities of Glucose Tolerance and Diabetes in Polycystic Ovary Syndrome

IR and MetS predispose patients with PCOS to higher risk of abnormalities of glucose tolerance. A meta-analyses of 35 studies reported that females with PCOS had increased prevalence of IGT (OR 2.48), T2DM (OR 4.43), and MetS (OR 2.88) compared with females without PCOS for BMI-matched groups.[37] Even lean females with PCOS had a greater prevalence of IGT (OR 3.22). Females reporting PCOS also had a higher prevalence of IFG (32.5%) compared with females not reporting PCOS (17.4%).[29] Most often, females with PCOS have IGT reflecting primarily IR at the level of skeletal muscles. IGT was present in 59.3% and 10.3% of the females with and without IR, respectively.[31] The likelihood of having T2DM was higher in females with PCOS compared with controls (4.6% vs. 2.3%, respectively).[12] Patients with PCOS develop abnormalities of glucose tolerance in their fourth or fifth decade of life, which is earlier than the general population.[8]

TABLE 10.4   Prevalence of Metabolic Syndrome for Different Phenotypes Across Various Ethnicities

Author	Ethnicity	PCO+OA+HA	OA+HA	PCO+HA	OA+PCO	Control
(Wiweko et al., 2020)[58]	South Asian	36.1%	8.3%	6.2%	17.8%	-
(Moghetti et al., 2013)[28]	Caucasian	39.1%	28.6%	Not reported	9.5%	-
(Krentowska et al., 2021)[59]	Caucasian	19.05%	20%	0	4.35%	-
Bahadur 2020	South Asian	9.9%	8%	0	14.9%	-
(Zaeemzadeh et al., 2020)[57]	Middle Eastern	17.1%	13.5%	3.0%	2.5%	0.0%
(Zhang et al., 2018)[60]	East Asian	30.6%	36.4%	21.1%	15.0%	-
(Jamil et al., 2015)[12]	Middle Eastern	58.3%	80.0%	47.2%	44.9%	32.7%
(Borzan et al., 2021)[61]	Australian	14.5%	14.7%	9.6%	5.3%	4.3%
(Yildirim et al., 2017)[62]	Turkish	19.5%	20.0%	16.0%	7.4%	3.8%

HA, Hyperandrogenism; *OA*, oligo-anovulation; *PCO*, polycystic ovarian morphology.

Association of Body Mass Index With Glucose Abnormalities

The risk of glucose abnormalities (fasting glucose ≥100 mg/dL, and/or 2-hour post 75-g [glucose load] glucose ≥ 140 mg/dL), which were mainly evident in postglucose load levels, increased with weight, being highest in those with BMI greater than 30 kg/m². Nevertheless, even lean females with PCOS had increased rates of IGT and T2DM.[1] The study by Liang et al. on 220 females with PCOS versus 70 control females showed that obesity was the only factor that predicted IGT and MetS (OR 8). IGT frequencies were 43% for obese PCOS versus 25% for obese non-PCOS, whereas 10% of nonobese PCOS had IGT, and there were no cases in nonobese, non-PCOS females.[30] Thus obesity should be treated as the major factor determining long-term health consequences associated with PCOS.

Risk of Incident Glucose Abnormalities on Longitudinal Studies

Long-term longitudinal studies on progression of metabolic abnormalities and incident IGT/T2DM are lacking. An Italian cohort study on patients with PCOS confirmed an increased risk of T2DM during the follow-up of over 10 years. More specifically, the age-standardized prevalence of T2DM at the end of the follow-up was 39.3% compared with 5.8% in the general female population of similar age.[64] An Australian study on a small cohort of patients with PCOS who were normoglycemic at baseline showed that 9% developed IGT and a further 8% developed T2DM on less than 10-year follow-up. Moreover, 54% of patients with PCOS who had IGT at baseline developed T2DM during the follow-up. BMI at baseline was found to be an independent predictor of this adverse glycemic profile in later life.[65]

Determining Glucose Abnormalities

Patients with PCOS are more at risk for IGT compared with other glucose abnormalities; consequently, the OGTT (2 h-post glucose challenge glucose) is the ideal test to determine glucose abnormalities (i.e. IGT and T2DM). Compared with OGTT, glycosylated hemoglobin (Hb A_{1c}) has low sensitivity in detecting glucose abnormalities in PCOS.[1] Recent position statements and guidelines from the Androgen Excess Society and Royal College of Obstetrics and Gynaecology recommends that all patients with PCOS be screened with OGTT. If the OGTT is normal, a rescreening is required at least every 2 years or even earlier if there are additional risk factors present (e.g., advancing age, overweight or obesity, history of gestational diabetes in past or family history of T2DM). Patients who have IGT should be rescreened annually.[66-69]

Risks in Later Life

Patients with PCOS are exposed to multiple cardiovascular risk factors from an earlier age as evident by clustering of components of MetS. The presence of central or visceral obesity, IR, T2DM, hypertension, and dyslipidemia puts these patients at increased risk for future cardiovascular events compared with non-PCOS females. In general, females are at increased risk for CVD because of a tendency toward weight gain in the perimenopausal period; however, it is still uncertain whether this risk aggravates further in females with PCOS during the perimenopausal stage of life.[70] Biochemical HA tends to improve with aging in PCOS females, whereas glucose abnormalities and dyslipidemia worsen over time in both PCOS and non-PCOS females.[71] Contrary to this finding, others have reported a lower than expected prevalence of CVD with advancing age in females with PCOS.

Livadas et al. studied the impact of age on IR and MetS in 1345 females with PCOS with control group of 302 non-PCOS females. The authors reported an increase in IR and aging but only in obese PCOS.[72] In a subset of PCOS and control subjects older than 30 years of age, it was shown that HOMA-IR was significantly higher in females with PCOS, in both lean and obese subjects. A positive association of IR with BMI and androgens level was reported.[72] With the well-known fact that androgens decline with aging, nonobese PCOS may present a better metabolic profile with time and PCOS may even remain a silent disorder. This observation strongly confirms the need for implementing lifestyle modifications against weight gain, which may ameliorate adverse cardiometabolic profile in PCOS females.

In a longitudinal study, 117 females with PCOS (mean age 45.8 years) had higher prevalence of IGT compared with control females (25% vs. 9.2%; P < .001). Those with both HA and OA had the highest prevalence of worse metabolic and hormonal parameters.[73]

Several studies have observed a higher prevalence of MetS in older patients with presumed PCOS diagnosis compared with controls. Some of these studies also showed a higher prevalence of MetS in the HA PCOS phenotype compared with the normoandrogenic phenotype. A follow-up study at 12 years reported higher rates of MetS in patients with PCOS who did not have MetS at baseline (incidence rates: PCOS 3.57 vs. control 2.26). Nevertheless, after adjustment for BMI, the difference became insignificant that might suggest that PCOS patients without MetS in their reproductive years may represent a lower risk group to develop MetS in the long term.[74] A Swedish study on long-term follow-up of patients with PCOS (mean age 43) documented 23.8% prevalence of MetS in patients with PCOS compared with 8% in controls. This study failed to show any association of PCOS phenotype with prevalence on MetS either at baseline or on long-term follow-up. In addition, higher WC, hypertriglyceridemia, and use of antidiabetic agents was more frequent, whereas hypertension or use of antihypertensives was less frequent in the PCOS group compared with controls.[75]

Still others have assessed the cardiometabolic phenotype and prevalence of CVD in middle-aged females older than 45 years (n = 200) with PCOS, compared with age-matched controls (n = 200), and assessed the cardiovascular health and 10-year CVD risk. Patients with PCOS were more likely to have increased WC, BMI, hypertension and glucose intolerance, but the prevalence of T2DM, MetS and dyslipidemia was not higher in patients with PCOS. Carotid intima-media thickness (cIMT) was lower in those with PCOS (P < .001). Calculated cardiovascular health and 10-year CVD risk were similar in females with PCOS and controls. The median 10-year CVD risk was 5.79% in those with PCOS and 7.38% in controls (P = .214).[76]

Although conflicting, the data suggest that despite an unfavorable profile at a younger age, long-term cardiovascular health in patients with PCOS seems to be similar to that of the general population. Whether this is because of the healthier lifestyles and proper preventive treatment that most patients with PCOS get at an early age that results in better DNA repair and maintenance genes is yet to be determined.

Screening for Metabolic Syndrome

History

It is important to take a detailed history of patients with PCOS, which must include information on age, ethnicity, personal history of smoking, gestational diabetes or prediabetes, weight changes, response/adherence to lifestyle modification or antiobesity medication, use of insulin sensitizing agents and their response in past, and assessment for obstructive sleep apnea. The pertinent features should be reevaluated on clinical follow-up. In addition, details of family history of metabolic syndrome, prediabetes, T2DM, hypertension, or atherosclerotic cardiovascular disease (ASCVD) should be recorded and reviewed on follow-up visits.

Physical Assessment and Laboratory Assessment

Patients with PCOS need to undergo evaluation for abnormalities of glucose tolerance, lipids, and liver function (see algorithm). Thus an OGTT, complete lipid profile, and liver function tests (LFTs) should be offered at baseline to every patient with PCOS. If those tests are normal at baseline, then monitoring of those tests should be done at periodic intervals, which can take place every 2 years or earlier if there is weight gain or identification of other risk factors (Fig. 10.2;).[66-69,77]

Clinical Implications

Patients with PCOS have a higher risk of underlying IR and a substantial number of these patients have MetS, which can predispose them to future CVD risk.

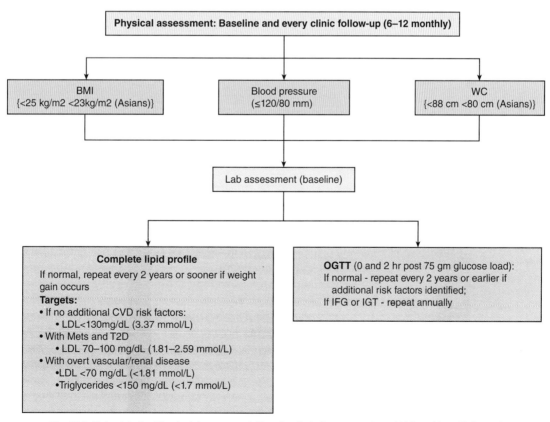

• **Fig. 10.2** Schedule for Physical Assessment, Baseline Lab Assessment, and Follow-Up at Polycystic Ovary Syndrome (PCOS) Clinics. *BMI*, Body mass index; *CVD*, cardiovascular disease; *IFG*, impaired fasting glucose; *IGT*, impaired glucose tolerance; *LDL*, low density lipoprotein; *OGTT*, oral glucose tolerance test; *WC*, waist circumference.

The observed differences in the prevalence of MetS among four distinct phenotypes highlight the need for individualized screening and intervention for patients with PCOS.

Patients with PCOS need assessment for MetS including markers of central adiposity, weight, BP screening with OGTT, lipid profile at baseline, and then on periodic intervals.

Lifestyle intervention, including medical nutrition therapy and exercise along with metformin as an insulin sensitizer, stay as the cornerstone of PCOS management with a focus on reducing the risk of T2DM and ASCVD.

Future Research Needs

Future research needs to focus on clarifying the mechanisms of IR and MetS in patients with PCOS and its phenotypes. There is a need to elucidate the reasons of observed differences in prevalence of MetS among different ethnicities.

There is a lack of longitudinal studies in patients with PCOS, and there is a need for well-controlled and appropriately designed long-term longitudinal studies on cohorts of females with PCOS to find out the ideal time point for screening of MetS and associated cardiovascular risks and the optimal time of interventions for their prevention. On the other hand, these longitudinal studies can answer the definite risk of development of T2DM, hypertension, MetS, and CVD in patients with PCOS.

PCOS registries for different regions of the world and various ethnicities can help researchers find out many of the yet unanswered questions for this condition that has a significant impact on a person's life.

References

1. Diamanti-Kandarakis E, Dunaif A. Insulin resistance and the polycystic ovary syndrome revisited: an update on mechanisms and implications. *Endocr Rev.* 2012;33(6):981-1030. doi:10.1210/er.2011-1034.
2. Rojas J, Chavez M, Olivar L, et al. Polycystic ovary syndrome, insulin resistance, and obesity: navigating the pathophysiologic labyrinth. *Int J Reprod Med.* 2014;2014:719050. doi:10.1155/2014/719050.
3. Samson SL, Garber AJ. Metabolic syndrome. *Endocrinol Metab Clin North Am.* 2014;43(1):1-23. doi:10.1016/j.ecl.2013.09.009.
4. National Institute of Health. *National Institutes of Health Third Report of the National Cholesterol Education Program Expert Panel on Detection, Evaluation, and Treatment of High Blood Cholesterol in Adults (Adult Treatment Panel III). Executive Summary.* Bethesda, MD: National Institutes of Health, National Heart, Lung, and Blood; 2001.
5. Alberti KGM, Zimmet P, Shaw J. The metabolic syndrome—a new worldwide definition. *Lancet.* 2005;366(9491):1059-1062.
6. Alberti KG, Eckel RH, Grundy SM, et al. Harmonizing the metabolic syndrome: a joint interim statement of the International Diabetes Federation Task Force on Epidemiology and Prevention; National Heart, Lung, and Blood Institute; American Heart Association; World Heart Federation; International Atherosclerosis Society; and International Association for the Study of Obesity. *Circulation.* 2009;120(16):1640-1645.
7. Lim SS, Kakoly NS, Tan JWJ, et al. Metabolic syndrome in polycystic ovary syndrome: a systematic review, meta-analysis and meta-regression. *Obes Rev.* 2019;20(2):339-352. doi:10.1111/obr.12762.
8. Jeanes YM, Reeves S. Metabolic consequences of obesity and insulin resistance in polycystic ovary syndrome: diagnostic and methodological challenges. *Nutr Res Rev.* 2017;30(1):97-105. doi:10.1017/S0954422416000287.
9. Dadachanji R, Patil A, Joshi B, Mukherjee S. Elucidating the impact of obesity on hormonal and metabolic perturbations in polycystic ovary syndrome phenotypes in Indian women. *PLoS One.* 2021;16(2):e0246862. doi:10.1371/journal.pone.0246862.
10. Legro RS. *Obesity and PCOS: implications for diagnosis and treatment.* Paper presented at the Seminars in reproductive medicine; 2012.
11. Alves AC, Valcarcel B, Mäkinen VP, et al. Metabolic profiling of polycystic ovary syndrome reveals interactions with abdominal obesity. *Int J Obes (Lond).* 2017;41(9):1331-1340.
12. Jamil AS, Alalaf SK, Al-Tawil NG, Al-Shawaf T. A case–control observational study of insulin resistance and metabolic syndrome among the four phenotypes of polycystic ovary syndrome based on Rotterdam criteria. *Reprod Health.* 2015;12:7.
13. Ebrahimi-Mamaghani M, Saghafi-Asl M, Pirouzpanah S, et al. Association of insulin resistance with lipid profile, metabolic syndrome, and hormonal aberrations in overweight or obese women with polycystic ovary syndrome. *J Health Popul Nutr.* 2015;33(1):157-167.
14. Tziomalos K, Katsikis I, Papadakis E, Kandaraki EA, Macut D, Panidis D. Comparison of markers of insulin resistance and circulating androgens between women with polycystic ovary syndrome and women with metabolic syndrome. *Hum Reprod.* 2013;28(3):785-793. doi:10.1093/humrep/des456.
15. DeFronzo RA, Tobin JD, Andres RJ. Glucose clamp technique: a method for quantifying insulin secretion and resistance. *Am J Physiol.* 1979;237(3):E214-E223.
16. Tosi F, Bonora E, Moghetti P. Insulin resistance in a large cohort of women with polycystic ovary syndrome: a comparison between euglycaemic-hyperinsulinaemic clamp and surrogate indexes. *Hum Reprod.* 2017;32(12):2515-2521. doi:10.1093/humrep/dex308.
17. Matthews DR, Hosker J, Rudenski A, Naylor B, Treacher D, Turner RC. Homeostasis model assessment: insulin resistance and β-cell function from fasting plasma glucose and insulin concentrations in man. *Diabetologia.* 1985;28(7):412-419.
18. Legro RS, Finegood D, Dunaif A. A fasting glucose to insulin ratio is a useful measure of insulin sensitivity in women with polycystic ovary syndrome. *J Clin Endocrinol Metab.* 1998;83(8):2694-2698.
19. Katz A, Nambi SS, Mather K, et al. Quantitative insulin sensitivity check index: a simple, accurate method for assessing insulin sensitivity in humans. *J Clin Endocrinol Metab.* 2000;85(7):2402-2410.
20. Gutt M, Davis CL, Spitzer SB, et al. Validation of the insulin sensitivity index (ISI0, 120): comparison with other measures. *Diabetes Res Clin Pract.* 2000;47(3):177-184.
21. Stumvoll M, Van Haeften T, Fritsche A, Gerich J. Oral glucose tolerance test indexes for insulin sensitivity and secretion based on various availabilities of sampling times. *Diabetes Care.* 2001;24(4):796-797.
22. Matsuda M, DeFronzo RA. Insulin sensitivity indices obtained from oral glucose tolerance testing: comparison with the euglycemic insulin clamp. *Diabetes Care.* 1999;22(9):1462-1470.

23. Polak K, Czyzyk A, Simoncini T, Meczekalski B. New markers of insulin resistance in polycystic ovary syndrome. *J Endocrinol Invest.* 2017;40(1):1-8. doi:10.1007/s40618-016-0523-8.

24. Abdelazim IA, Elsawah WF. Metabolic syndrome among infertile women with polycystic ovary syndrome. *Asian Pac J Reprod.* 2015;4(1):44-48. doi:10.1016/s2305-0500(14)60057-9.

25. Montazerifar F, Ghasemi M, Arabpour N, Karajibani M, Keikhah NJ Metabolic syndrome in women with and without polycystic syndrome, a case control study in Iran. Caspian J Reprod Med. 2020;6(1):9–15.

26. Anjum N, Zohra S, Arif A, Azhar A, Qureshi M. Prevalence of metabolic syndrome in Pakistani women with polycystic ovarian syndrome. *Pak J Biochem Mol Biol.* 2013;46(3):97-100.

27. Panidis D, Tziomalos K, Macut D, et al. Age- and body mass index-related differences in the prevalence of metabolic syndrome in women with polycystic ovary syndrome. *Gynecol Endocrinol.* 2013;29(10):926-930. doi:10.3109/09513590.2013.819079.

28. Moghetti P, Tosi F, Bonin C, et al. Divergences in insulin resistance between the different phenotypes of the polycystic ovary syndrome. *J Clin Endocrinol Metab.* 2013;98(4):E628-E637. doi:10.1210/jc.2012-3908.

29. Meyer ML, Sotres-Alvarez D, Steiner AZ, et al. Polycystic ovary syndrome signs and metabolic syndrome in premenopausal hispanic/latina women: the HCHS/SOL study. *J Clin Endocrinol Metab.* 2020;105(3):e447-e456. doi:10.1210/clinem/dgaa012.

30. Liang SJ, Liou TH, Lin HW, Hsu CS, Tzeng CR, Hsu MI. Obesity is the predominant predictor of impaired glucose tolerance and metabolic disturbance in polycystic ovary syndrome. *Acta Obstet Gynecol Scand.* 2012;91(10):1167-1172. doi:10.1111/j.1600-0412.2012.01417.x.

31. Le MT, Nguyen VQH, Truong QV, Le DD, Le VNS, Cao NT. Metabolic syndrome and insulin resistance syndrome among infertile women with polycystic ovary syndrome: a cross-sectional study from central Vietnam. *Endocrinol Metab (Seoul).* 2018;33(4):447-458. doi:10.3803/EnM.2018.33.4.447.

32. Einhorn DJ, Reaven GM, Cobin RH, et al. American College of Endocrinology position statement on the insulin resistance syndrome. *Endocr Pract.* 2003;9:237-252.

33. Kyrkou G, Trakakis E, Attilakos A, et al. Metabolic syndrome in Greek women with polycystic ovary syndrome: prevalence, characteristics and associations with body mass index. A prospective controlled study. *Arch Gynecol Obstet.* 2016;293(4):915-923. doi:10.1007/s00404-015-3964-y.

34. Karee M, Gundabattula SR, Sashi L, Boorugu H, Chowdhury A. Prevalence of metabolic syndrome in women with polycystic ovary syndrome and the factors associated: a cross sectional study at a tertiary care center in Hyderabad, south-eastern India. *Diabetes Metab Syndr.* 2020;14(4):583-587. doi:10.1016/j.dsx.2020.05.006.

35. Hosseinpanah F, Barzin M, Tehrani FR, Azizi F. The lack of association between polycystic ovary syndrome and metabolic syndrome: Iranian PCOS prevalence study. *Clin Endocrinol (Oxf).* 2011;75(5):692-697. doi:10.1111/j.1365-2265.2011.04113.x.

36. Anjum S, Askari S, Riaz M, Basit A. Clinical presentation and frequency of metabolic syndrome in women with polycystic ovary syndrome: an experience from a tertiary care hospital in Pakistan. *Cureus.* 2020;12(12):e11860. doi:10.7759/cureus.11860.

37. Moran LJ, Misso ML, Wild RA, Norman RJ. Impaired glucose tolerance, type 2 diabetes and metabolic syndrome in polycystic ovary syndrome: a systematic review and meta-analysis. *Hum Reprod Update.* 2010;16(4):347-363. doi:10.1093/humupd/dmq001.

38. Hallajzadeh J, Khoramdad M, Karamzad N, et al. Metabolic syndrome and its components among women with polycystic ovary syndrome: a systematic review and meta-analysis. *J Cardiovasc Thorac Res.* 2018;10(2):56-69. doi:10.15171/jcvtr.2018.10.

39. Hillman JK, Johnson LN, Limaye M, Feldman RA, Sammel M, Dokras A. Black women with polycystic ovary syndrome (PCOS) have increased risk for metabolic syndrome and cardiovascular disease compared with white women with PCOS. *Fertil Steril.* 2014;101(2):530-535. doi:10.1016/j.fertnstert.2013.10.055.

40. Engmann L, Jin S, Sun F, et al. Racial and ethnic differences in the polycystic ovary syndrome metabolic phenotype. *Am J Obstet Gynecol.* 2017;216(5):493.e1-493.e13. doi:10.1016/j.ajog.2017.01.003.

41. Ezeh U, Ida Chen YD, Azziz R. Racial and ethnic differences in the metabolic response of polycystic ovary syndrome. *Clin Endocrinol (Oxf).* 2020;93(2):163-172. doi:10.1111/cen.14193.

42. Chan JL, Kar S, Vanky E, et al. Racial and ethnic differences in the prevalence of metabolic syndrome and its components of metabolic syndrome in women with polycystic ovary syndrome: a regional cross-sectional study. *Am J Obstet Gynecol.* 2017;217(2):189.e1-e189.e8. doi:10.1016/j.ajog.2017.04.007.

43. Chahal N, Quinn M, Jaswa EA, Kao CN, Cedars MI, Huddleston HG. Comparison of metabolic syndrome elements in White and Asian women with polycystic ovary syndrome: results of a regional, American cross-sectional study. *F S Rep.* 2020;1(3):305-313. doi:10.1016/j.xfre.2020.09.008.

44. Yildizhan B, Anik Ilhan G, Pekin T. The impact of insulin resistance on clinical, hormonal and metabolic parameters in lean women with polycystic ovary syndrome. *J Obstet Gynaecol.* 2016;36(7):893-896. doi:10.3109/01443615.2016.1168376.

45. Zhu S, Zhang B, Jiang X, et al. Metabolic disturbances in non-obese women with polycystic ovary syndrome: a systematic review and meta-analysis. *Fertil Steril.* 2019;111(1):168-177. doi:10.1016/j.fertnstert.2018.09.013.

46. Manzoor S, Ganie MA, Amin S, et al. Oral contraceptive use increases risk of inflammatory and coagulatory disorders in women with polycystic ovarian syndrome: an observational study. *Sci Rep.* 2019;9(1):10182.

47. de Medeiros SF. Risks, benefits size and clinical implications of combined oral contraceptive use in women with polycystic ovary syndrome. *Reprod Biol Endocrinol.* 2017;15(1):93.

48. Li HW, Brereton RE, Anderson RA, Wallace AM, Ho CK. Vitamin D deficiency is common and associated with metabolic risk factors in patients with polycystic ovary syndrome. *Metabolism.* 2011;60(10):1475-1481. doi:10.1016/j.metabol.2011.03.002.

49. Joham AE, Teede HJ, Cassar S, et al. Vitamin D in polycystic ovary syndrome: relationship to obesity and insulin resistance. *Mol Nutr Food Res.* 2016;60(1):110-118. doi:10.1002/mnfr.201500259.

50. Wang L, Lv S, Li F, Yu X, Bai E, Yang X. Vitamin D deficiency is associated with metabolic risk factors in women with polycystic ovary syndrome: a cross-sectional study in Shaanxi China. *Front Endocrinol (Lausanne).* 2020;11:171. doi:10.3389/fendo.2020.00171.

51. Albu A, Radian S, Fica S, Barbu CG. Biochemical hyperandrogenism is associated with metabolic syndrome independently of adiposity and insulin resistance in Romanian polycystic ovary syndrome patients. *Endocrine.* 2015;48(2):696-704. doi:10.1007/s12020-014-0340-9.

52. Munzker J, Hofer D, Trummer C, et al. Testosterone to dihydrotestosterone ratio as a new biomarker for an adverse metabolic phenotype in the polycystic ovary syndrome. *J Clin Endocrinol Metab.* 2015;100(2):653-660. doi:10.1210/jc.2014-2523.

53. Moran LJ, Teede HJ, Noakes M, Clifton PM, Norman RJ, Wittert GA. Sex hormone binding globulin, but not testosterone, is associated with the metabolic syndrome in overweight

and obese women with polycystic ovary syndrome. *J Endocrinol Invest.* 2013;36(11):1004-1010. doi:10.3275/9023.

54. Fu C, Minjie C, Weichun Z, et al. Efficacy of sex hormone-binding globulin on predicting metabolic syndrome in newly diagnosed and untreated patients with polycystic ovary syndrome. *Hormones (Athens).* 2020;19(3):439-445. doi:10.1007/s42000-020-00219-5.

55. Luo X, Yang XM, Cai WY, et al. Decreased sex hormone-binding globulin indicated worse biometric, lipid, liver, and renal function parameters in women with polycystic ovary syndrome. *Int J Endocrinol.* 2020;2020:7580218. doi:10.1155/2020/7580218.

56. Lizneva D, Suturina L, Walker W, Brakta S, Gavrilova-Jordan L, Azziz R. Criteria, prevalence, and phenotypes of polycystic ovary syndrome. *Fertil Steril.* 2016;106(1):6-15.

57. Zaeemzadeh N, Sadatmahalleh SJ, Ziaei S, et al. Prevalence of metabolic syndrome in four phenotypes of PCOS and its relationship with androgenic components among Iranian women: a cross-sectional study. *Int J Reprod Biomed.* 2020;18(4):253-264. doi:10.18502/ijrm.v13i4.6888.

58. Wiweko B, Handayani LK, Harzif AK, et al. Correlation of anti-Mullerian hormone levels with metabolic syndrome events in polycystic ovary syndrome: a cross-sectional study. *Int J Reprod Biomed.* 2020;18(3):187-192. doi:10.18502/ijrm.v18i3.6716.

59. Krentowska A, Lebkowska A, Jacewicz-Swiecka M, et al. Metabolic syndrome and the risk of cardiovascular complications in young patients with different phenotypes of polycystic ovary syndrome. *Endocrine.* 2021;72(2):400-410. doi:10.1007/s12020-020-02596-8.

60. Zhang L, Fang X, Li L, et al. The association between circulating irisin levels and different phenotypes of polycystic ovary syndrome. *J Endocrinol Invest.* 2018;41(12):1401-1407. doi:10.1007/s40618-018-0902-4.

61. Borzan V, Lerchbaum E, Missbrenner C, et al. Risk of insulin resistance and metabolic syndrome in women with hyperandrogenemia: a comparison between PCOS phenotypes and beyond. *J Clin Med.* 2021;10(4):829. doi:10.3390/jcm10040829.

62. Yildirim E, Karabulut O, Yuksel UC, et al. Echocardiographic evaluation of diastolic functions in patients with polycystic ovary syndrome: a comperative study of diastolic functions in subphenotypes of polycystic ovary syndrome. *Cardiol J.* 2017;24(4):364-373. doi:10.5603/CJ.a2017.0032.

63. Krentowska A, Kowalska I. Metabolic syndrome and its components in different phenotypes of polycystic ovary syndrome. *Diabetes Metab Res Rev.* 2021;38:e3464. doi:10.1002/dmrr.3464.

64. Gambineri A, Patton L, Altieri P, et al. Polycystic ovary syndrome is a risk factor for type 2 diabetes: results from a long-term prospective study. *Diabetes.* 2012;61(9):2369-2374. doi:10.2337/db11-1360.

65. Norman RJ, Masters L, Milner CR, Wang JX, Davies MJ. Relative risk of conversion from normoglycaemia to impaired glucose tolerance or non-insulin dependent diabetes mellitus in polycystic ovarian syndrome. *Hum Reprod.* 2001;16(9):1995-1998.

66. Goodman NF, Cobin RH, Futterweit W, et al. American Association of Clinical Endocrinologists, American College of Endocrinology,

and Androgen Excess and PCOS Society disease state clinical review: guide to the best practices in the evaluation and treatment of polycystic ovary syndrome-part 1. *Endocr Pract.* 2015;21(11):1291-1300.

67. Goodman NF, Cobin RH, Futterweit W, et al. American Association of Clinical Endocrinologists, American College of Endocrinology, and Androgen Excess and PCOS Society disease state clinical review: guide to the best practices in the evaluation and treatment of polycystic ovary syndrome-part 2. *Endocr Pract.* 2015;21(12):1415-1426.

68. American College of Obstetricians and Gynecologists' Committee on Practice Bulletins—Gynecology. ACOG Practice Bulletin No. 194: Polycystic Ovary Syndrome [published correction appears in Obstet Gynecol. 2020 Sep;136(3):638]. *Obstet Gynecol.* 2018;131(6):e157-e171. doi:10.1097/AOG.0000000000002656.

69. Wild RA, Carmina E, Diamanti-Kandarakis E, et al. Assessment of cardiovascular risk and prevention of cardiovascular disease in women with the polycystic ovary syndrome: a consensus statement by the Androgen Excess and Polycystic Ovary Syndrome (AE-PCOS) Society. *J Clin Endocrinol Metab.* 2010;95(5):2038-2049.

70. Lobo RA. Metabolic syndrome after menopause and the role of hormones. *Maturitas.* 2008;60(1):10-18. doi:10.1016/j.maturitas.2008.02.008.

71. de Medeiros SF, Yamamoto MMW, Souto de Medeiros MA, Barbosa BB, Soares JM, Baracat EC. Changes in clinical and biochemical characteristics of polycystic ovary syndrome with advancing age. *Endocr Connect.* 2020;9(2):74-89. doi:10.1530/EC-19-0496.

72. Livadas S, Kollias A, Panidis D, Diamanti-Kandarakis E. Diverse impacts of aging on insulin resistance in lean and obese women with polycystic ovary syndrome: evidence from 1345 women with the syndrome. *Eur J Endocrinol.* 2014;171(3):301-309. doi:10.1530/EJE-13-1007.

73. Polotsky AJ, Allshouse A, Crawford SL, et al. Relative contributions of oligomenorrhea and hyperandrogenemia to the risk of metabolic syndrome in midlife women. *J Clin Endocrinol Metab.* 2012;97(6):E868-E877. doi:10.1210/jc.2011-3357.

74. Louwers YV, Laven JSE. Characteristics of polycystic ovary syndrome throughout life. *Ther Adv Reprod Health.* 2020;14:2633494120911038. doi:10.1177/2633494120911038.

75. Hudecova M, Holte J, Olovsson M, Larsson A, Berne C, Sundstrom-Poromaa I. Prevalence of the metabolic syndrome in women with a previous diagnosis of polycystic ovary syndrome: long-term follow-up. *Fertil Steril.* 2011;96(5):1271-1274. doi:10.1016/j.fertnstert.2011.08.006.

76. Meun C, Gunning MN, Louwers YV, et al. The cardiovascular risk profile of middle-aged women with polycystic ovary syndrome. *Clin Endocrinol (Oxf).* 2020;92(2):150-158. doi:10.1111/cen.14117.

77. Al Wattar BH, Fisher M, Bevington L, et al. Clinical practice guidelines on the diagnosis and management of polycystic ovary syndrome: a systematic review and quality assessment study. *J Clin Endocrinol Metab.* 2021;106(8):2436-2446. doi:10.1210/clinem/dgab232.

11

Polycystic Ovary Syndrome and Mental Health

NARGIS ASAD, TANIA NADEEM, AND AISHA NOORULLAH

Introduction

Polycystic ovary syndrome (PCOS) is one of the most common endocrine disorders affecting females of reproductive age, with varying prevalence reported by different studies using contrasting diagnostic criteria.[1]

The clinical symptomatology that characterizes PCOS, such as menstrual irregularities, hirsutism, acne, obesity, and infertility, not only has adverse physical consequences but also has an immense long-term effect on the psychological wellbeing of the patient.[2]

Depressive and Anxiety Disorder

An extensive plethora of research provides the data that females diagnosed with PCOS have varying levels of anxiety and depression.[3] The depression and anxiety disorders in females have a biopsychosocial cause. Dysregulation of the hypothalamic-pituitary-adrenal axis has been implicated in the pathophysiology of both disorders in patients with PCOS.[4] Neuroimaging studies also support greater activity in the prefrontal cortex in PCOS that may be linked to anxiety disorders.[5] The findings of one study revealed that patients with high body mass index (BMI), more children, and less education are predisposed for depression.[6]

Anxiety disorders are common among patients with PCOS, manifesting symptoms ranging from mild, moderate and severe.[7] Anxiety may emerge from various factors, such as the potential inability to have children and apprehensions pertinent to building their family, which may be threatening and predispose them to future fears. A high level of social anxiety can be explained by the negative attitudes from society because of gross changes in physical appearance.[8]

Body Image and Polycystic Ovary Syndrome

Body image is a complex and multidimensional phenomenon. It is how a person imagines, thinks, and feels about their own body. It is an amalgam of various components, such as body weight, shape, and overall physical appearance. A healthy body image means feeling satisfied with the way one looks. Negative body image is found among patients with PCOS.[9] The body dissatisfaction and altered body image may contribute to decreased self-confidence and significantly impair social interactions.[10]

The Complex Trio of Culture, Stigma, and Polycystic Ovary Syndrome

Cultures have an innate tendency to judge people by their general physical appearance. Meeting these standards of beauty has become a responsibility for women and an inability to fulfill this has a deeper impact.[11] The revelation of femininity embodies diverse patterns. One of the spectrums includes having regular menses, which represent fertility, and the general physical appearance involving a glabrous face and hairless body. Once these features are lost as part of PCOS, females are subjected to public stigma and the discriminatory attitude of others around them. Later, these negative attitudes and beliefs are internalized by the patients themselves as self-stigma. Stigma has been a thoroughly reviewed area in the context of ethnicity,[12] mental illnesses,[13] and human immunodeficiency virus (HIV)/acquired immunodeficiency syndrome (AIDS).[14] Nevertheless, the problem of stigma and PCOS is underresearched. Interesting qualitative research revealed that a third of the female patients surveyed used the term "freak," particularly to share their subjective experience of being different from other non-PCOS females.[15] A stigmatizing attitude from society may lead to a decrease in self-esteem followed by impaired social interpersonal relationships.

Quality of life (QOL), which is also significantly impaired in PCOS, is defined by the World Health Organization (WHO) in relation to the culture in which a person operates.[16] It encompasses various domains such as physical health, emotional status, and social relations. A female with

PCOS, a deteriorating physical illness, suffers from emotional distress. This distress will ultimately cause impairment in the social and interpersonal functioning of life. Moreover, in the context of traditional local culture, physical appearance and weight are considered significant features for matchmaking by the groom's family who often looks for perfection in the physical attributes of their daughter-in-law. Another milestone expected of females is to give birth; if a female is unable to achieve this, it will impact their QOL overall. Societal stigma, cultural expectations, social pressure, and the compulsion to fulfill the socially expected role of a woman puts PCOS patients at risk for a spectrum of psychological problems.

Sexuality and Marital Life

Sexuality has an overall impact on the emotional wellbeing of a person. PCOS manifests at reproductive age when finding a sexual partner, developing intimacy, building romantic relationships, and desiring to give birth to children are cardinal milestones. The inability to have children may have a significant long-lasting effect on marital relationships and sexual functioning. Sexual impairment lies on a spectrum and involve decreased sexual thoughts, desire, and arousal.[17] Females with PCOS report less satisfaction with their sex life and find themselves less attractive.[18] There is a possibility that the partners may feel less attracted to their spouse, or it may be their cognitive distortion emerging from low self-esteem and body dissatisfaction. Depression, which is very common in patients with PCOS, is associated with decreased libido. Insufficiency in sexual encounters is also correlated with hirsutism.[19]

Quality of Life

The physical and psychological constellation of symptoms of PCOS contributes to a significant deterioration in QOL. QOL may be impaired by various factors. The most crucial factors reported are obesity and infertility.[20] Acne in an otherwise non-PCOS patient also affects QOL.[21] Robust evidence also considers hirsutism as a symptom that impairs QOL[22] because not only its presence but also the cosmetic steps to hide it as much as possible can add to emotional distress.

Coping Strategies

Coping strategies can be predominantly classified as problem solving or emotion reducing. Problem-solving strategies include practical ways of tackling a stressful situation, whereas emotion-reducing strategies regulates the emotional response to the stressors. Literature suggests that patients with PCOS are more likely to use emotional coping strategies,[23] which are subsumed under passive coping and may be maladaptive in various circumstances.[24] These steps suppress the emotional response in the short term but lead to greater difficulties in the long term. Avoidance may not be adaptive in the early stages of any physical illness because it can lead to a delay in seeking early treatment, which worsens the prognosis.

Eating Disorders

Many patients with PCOS have clinical and subclinical eating disorders.[25] It may be associated with an attempt to lose weight, which may lead to binge eating and purging. Eating disorders can have a negative impact on the outcome of the PCOS itself.

Bipolar Affective Disorder

The mood stabilizer valproic acid, which is used in the acute management of episodes and for maintenance in bipolar affective disorder, may induce menstrual irregularities, metabolic syndrome, and features of hyperandrogenism, but no evidence exists to prove that it causes PCOS directly.[26]

The Complex Relationship Between Obesity, Polycystic Ovary Syndrome, and Psychological Issues

The relationship between PCOS and obesity is complex. Obesity is a risk factor for PCOS[27] and also occurs as part of the symptomatology of the illness itself through complex pathophysiology. Any psychological disorder or emotional issues can interfere significantly with lifestyle modifications, which can further worsen the prognosis of PCOS. Obesity is also a risk factor for obstructive sleep apnea, which is common in patients with PCOS.[28]

See Table 11.1 for common psychological disorders and how frequently they are associated with PCOS.

TABLE 11.1	Psychological Disorders in Patients With Polycystic Ovary Syndrome	
S. No	Psychiatric Disorder[a]	Estimated Prevalence/ Frequency
1.	Depressive disorder[28]	23.1%
2.	Anxiety disorder[28]	11.5%
3.	Bipolar disorder[28]	3.2%
4.	Sexual dysfunction[b,15]	57.7%
5.	Eating disorder[29] Bulimia nervosa Binge-eating disorder Night eating disorder	6.1% 17.6% 12.9%
6.	Obstructive sleep apnea syndrome[30]	0.22%

[a]The estimates may vary from one study to another depending on the diverse methodology used.
[b]It is the frequency, not the prevalence per se.
S, Serial number.

Management of Polycystic Ovary Syndrome

Keeping in mind the high burden of psychiatric comorbidity in patients with PCOS, it is important to screen for psychiatric disorders in females suffering from PCOS followed by appropriate interventions.[31] An individualized treatment plan tailored according to the need of the individual is required for specific psychiatric disorders.

Psychoeducation

Psychoeducation regarding the illness is an essential step based on evidence-based literature.[32]

Treatment of the Primary Condition Is Cardinal to the Outcome of the Illness

It is essential to understand the etiology behind the increased risk of mood and other psychiatric disorders in PCOS. It is not only dependent on the psychosocial stressors created by this diagnosis but also on the hormonal imbalance that is part of PCOS. Therefore when considering treatment strategies, the first must be better control of the primary disease. Helping with infertility, obesity, and hirsutism will improve an individual's overall mental health.

Screen for Psychiatric Disorders

All females getting treatment for PCOS should be screened for depression and anxiety disorders at regular intervals.[4] A basic screening for eating disorders and sexual dysfunctions is also desirable. Depending on the severity of the illness, a patient can be referred to psychiatry outpatient clinics for interventions.[33]

Lifestyle Modifications

A healthy routine with proper sleep, regular exercise, and scheduled mindful activities or relaxation techniques can help with both mood disorders and PCOS.[34]

Psychotherapy

An optimistic, humble, and empathic attitude on the part of healthcare professionals will help them understand the distress many patients feel when diagnosed with PCOS.[35] Among nonpharmacologic interventions, psychotherapy is an important treatment option.

Cognitive Behavioral Therapy

Cognitive behavioral therapy (CBT) has been shown to help.[36] Therapy can be focused on accepting the disease, recognizing how it affects a person's thoughts and feelings, and learning how to limit negative thoughts and cope with overwhelming feelings. CBT emphasizes motivation and building a positive body image, which helps improve self-esteem. Because many females with PCOS use maladaptive coping strategies, teaching adaptive coping strategies is helpful.[22] Group counseling has also been shown to be effective.[37]

Specific Management for Anxiety and Depressive Disorders

Whether PCOS is comorbid with anxiety or depression, treatment of the underlying physical illness (PCOS) as previously mentioned is necessary. The stepped-care model for generalized anxiety disorder described by the National Institute for Health and Clinical Excellence[38] provides guidance for the most effective intervention that needs to be tailored according to the severity of the illness. The treatment modalities lie on a spectrum, starting with psychoeducation about the illness and treatment along with active monitoring in the initial phases to self-help (non-guided/guided) and psychoeducational groups. CBT or/and pharmacologic interventions are recommended for more severe symptoms or for those who do not respond to low-intensity treatments. Among pharmacologic interventions, selective serotonin reuptake inhibitors (SSRIs) have shown efficacy in the management of anxiety spectrum disorder.[39,40] For the management of mild depression, antidepressants are not recommended; instead, self-help, regular exercise, and the maintenance of adequate sleep are recommended. Moderate to severe depression, however, can be treated with a combination of pharmacotherapy and/or psychological interventions. Most authorities recommend an SSRI, or mirtazapine if sedation is desirable.[41]

See Fig. 11.1 for The complex psychological sequelae of polycystic ovary syndrome (PCOS) among females.

Specific Biologic Interventions for Mood Disorder in Polycystic Ovary Syndrome

Ultimately, if mood disorder symptoms are very severe or are not improving after 3 months of PCOS treatment, then medication should be considered.[8] The antiandrogenic effects of medicine like spironolactone can also decrease depressive symptoms.[42]

Referral to Specialized Psychiatric Services

Referral will depend immensely on the expertise of the treating physician and the availability of mental health services. Uncomplicated cases of anxiety and depressive disorders can be managed in primary care; however, complicated cases that require more in-depth assessment and intervention need a specialist referral.[43]

Conclusion

To sum up, females who have PCOS experience a vicious cycle of traumatic life events from the time of diagnosis followed by long-term treatment with varying outcomes.

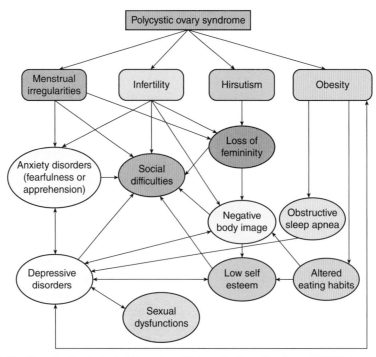

• **Fig. 11.1** The Complex Psychological Sequelae of Polycystic Ovary Syndrome (PCOS) Among Females.

There is no single factor that predisposes them to emotional distress, but throughout the course of the illness itself, they are fortified with unbearable symptoms grossly affecting their femininity, which can make them vulnerable to psychological disorders. A holistic biopsychosocial multidisciplinary approach in the management of patients with PCOS would improve the overall outcome of PCOS-affected females.

See Fig. 11.2 for The stepped-care approach for generalized anxiety disorder. *CBT,* Cognitive behavioral therapy.

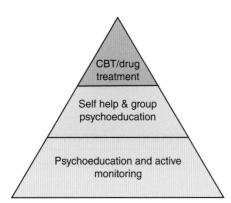

• **Fig. 11.2** The Stepped-Care Approach for Generalized Anxiety Disorder. *CBT,* Cognitive behavioral therapy.

References

1. March WA, Moore VM, Willson KJ, Phillips DI, Norman RJ, Davies MJ. The prevalence of polycystic ovary syndrome in a community sample assessed under contrasting diagnostic criteria. *Hum Reprod.* 2010;25(2):544-551.
2. Jones GL, Hall JM, Lashen HL, Balen AH, Ledger WL. Health-related quality of life among adolescents with polycystic ovary syndrome. *J Obstet Gynecol Neonatal Nurs.* 2011;40(5):577-588.
3. Sayyah-Melli M, Alizadeh M, Pourafkary N, et al. Psychosocial factors associated with polycystic ovary syndrome: a case control study. *J Caring Sci.* 2015;4(3):225.
4. Mueller SC, Ng P, Sinaii N, et al. Psychiatric characterization of children with genetic causes of hyperandrogenism. *Eur J Endocrinol.* 2010;163(5):801.
5. Marsh CA, Berent-Spillson A, Love T, et al. Functional neuroimaging of emotional processing in women with polycystic ovary syndrome: a case-control pilot study. *Fertil Steril.* 2013;100(1):200-207.
6. Cipkala-Gaffin J, Talbott EO, Song MK, Bromberger J, Wilson J. Associations between psychologic symptoms and life satisfaction in women with polycystic ovary syndrome. *J Womens Health.* 2012;21(2):179-187.
7. Brutocao C, Zaiem F, Alsawas M, Morrow AS, Murad MH, Javed A. Psychiatric disorders in women with polycystic ovary syndrome: a systematic review and meta-analysis. *Endocrine.* 2018;62(2):318-325.
8. Kamathenu UK, Velayudhan A, Krishna KV, Nithya R. Social anxiety and interpersonal relationship of women with PCOD. *Med Leg Update.* 2021;21(3):523-528.
9. Deeks AA, Gibson-Helm ME, Paul E, Teede HJ. Is having polycystic ovary syndrome a predictor of poor psychological function including anxiety and depression? *Hum Reprod.* 2011;26(6):1399-1407.
10. Bazarganipour F, Ziaei S, Montazeri A, Foroozanfard F, Kazemnejad A, Faghihzadeh S. Body image satisfaction and self-esteem status among the patients with polycystic ovary syndrome. *Iran J Reprod Med.* 2013;11(10):829.
11. Fredrickson BL, Roberts TA. Objectification theory: toward understanding women's lived experiences and mental health risks. *Psychol Women Q.* 1997;21(2):173-206.
12. Feagin JR, McKinney KD. *The Many Costs of Racism.* Lanham Maryland, United States: Rowman & Littlefield Publishers; 2005.

13. Corrigan PW, Rao D. On the self-stigma of mental illness: stages, disclosure, and strategies for change. *Can J Psychiatry*. 2012;57(8): 464-469.

14. Parker R, Aggleton P. HIV and AIDS-related stigma and discrimination: a conceptual framework and implications for action. *Soc Sci Med*. 2003;57(1):13-24.

15. Kitzinger C, Willmott J. 'The thief of womanhood': women's experience of polycystic ovarian syndrome. *Soc Sci Med*. 2002;54(3): 349-361.

16. WHO Division of Mental Health. *WHO-QOL Study Protocol: The Development of the World Health Organization Quality-of-Life Assessment Instrument*. Geneva: United Nations; 1993.

17. Eftekhar T, Sohrabvand F, Zabandan N, Shariat M, Haghollahi F, Ghahghaei-Nezamabadi A. Sexual dysfunction in patients with polycystic ovary syndrome and its affected domains. *Iran J Reprod Med*. 2014;12(8):539.

18. Elsenbruch S, Hahn S, Kowalsky D, et al. Quality of life, psychosocial well-being, and sexual satisfaction in women with polycystic ovary syndrome. *J Clin Endocrinol Metab*. 2003;88(12): 5801-5807.

19. Fliegner M, Richter-Appelt H, Krupp K, Brunner F. Sexual function and socio-sexual difficulties in women with polycystic ovary syndrome (PCOS). *Geburtshilfe Frauenheilkd*. 2019;79(5):498-509.

20. Krępuła K, Bidzińska-Speichert B, Lenarcik A, Tworowska-Bardzińska U. Psychiatric disorders related to polycystic ovary syndrome. *Endokrynol Pol*. 2012;63(6):488-491.

21. Yazici K, Baz K, Yazici AE, et al. Disease-specific quality of life is associated with anxiety and depression in patients with acne. *J Eur Acad Dermatol Venereol*. 2004;18(4):435-439.

22. Khomami MB, Tehrani FR, Hashemi S, Farahmand M, Azizi F. Of PCOS symptoms, hirsutism has the most significant impact on the quality of life of Iranian women. *PLoS One*. 2015;10(4): e0123608.

23. Morshedi T, Salehi M, Farzad V, Hassani F, Shakibazadeh E. The status of relationship between coping strategies and quality of life in women with polycystic ovary syndrome. *J Educ Health Promot*. 2021;10(1):185.

24. Benson S, Hahn S, Tan S, Janssen OE, Schedlowski M, Elsenbruch S. Maladaptive coping with illness in women with polycystic ovary syndrome. *J Obstet Gynecol Neonatal Nurs*. 2010;39(1):37-45.

25. Bernadett M. Prevalence of eating disorders among women with polycystic ovary syndrome. *Psychiatr Hung*. 2016;31(2): 136-145.

26. McIntyre RS, Mancini DA, McCann S, Srinivasan J, Kennedy SH. Valproate, bipolar disorder and polycystic ovarian syndrome. *Bipolar Disord*. 2003;5(1):28-35.

27. Barber TM, Franks S. Obesity and polycystic ovary syndrome. *Clin Endocrinol*. 2021;95(4):531-541.

28. Berni TR, Morgan CL, Berni ER, Rees DA. Polycystic ovary syndrome is associated with adverse mental health and neurodevelopmental outcomes. *J Clin Endocrinol Metab*. 2018;103(6): 2116-2125.

29. Lee I, Cooney LG, Saini S, et al. Increased risk of disordered eating in polycystic ovary syndrome. *Fertil Steril*. 2017;107(3): 796-802.

30. Helvaci N, Karabulut E, Demir AU, Yildiz BO. Polycystic ovary syndrome and the risk of obstructive sleep apnea: a meta-analysis and review of the literature. *Endocr Connect*. 2017;6(7):437-445.

31. Brutocao C, Zaiem F, Alsawas M, Morrow AS, Murad MH, Javed A. Psychiatric disorders in women with polycystic ovary syndrome: a systematic review and meta-analysis. *Endocrine*. 2018;62(2):318-325.

32. Kaur I, Suri V, Rana SV, Singh A. Treatment pathways traversed by polycystic ovary syndrome (PCOS) patients: a mixed-method study. *PLoS One*. 2021;16(8):e0255830.

33. Harmancı H, Hergüner S, Toy H. Psychiatric symptoms in women with polycystic ovary syndrome. *Düşünen Adam J Psychiatry Neurol Sci*. 2013;26:157-163.

34. Lamb JD, Johnstone EB, Rousseau JA, et al. Physical activity in women with polycystic ovary syndrome: prevalence, predictors, and positive health associations. *Am J Obstet Gynecol*. 2011;204(4): 352.e1-352.e6.

35. Sharma TR. Polycystic ovarian syndrome and borderline personality disorder: 3 case reports and scientific review of literature. *J Psychiatry*. 2015;18(6):1-4.

36. Elizabeth M, Leslie NS, Critch EA. Managing polycystic ovary syndrome: a cognitive behavioral strategy. *Nurs Womens Health*. 2009;13(4):292-300.

37. Roessler KK, Glintborg D, Ravn P, Birkebaek C, Andersen M. Supportive relationships-psychological effects of group counselling in women with polycystic ovary syndrome (PCOS). *Commun Med*. 2012;9(2):125.

38. National Institute for Health and Clinical Excellence. *Generalized Anxiety Disorder and Panic Disorder in Adults: Management. Clinical Guideline [CG113]*. 2011. Last updated July 2019. Available at: http://guidance.nice.org.uk/CG113.

39. Baldwin D, Woods R, Lawson R, Taylor D. Efficacy of drug treatments for generalised anxiety disorder: systematic review and meta-analysis. *BMJ*. 2011;342:d1199.

40. Batelaan NM, Van Balkom AJ, Stein DJ. Evidence-based pharmacotherapy of panic disorder: an update. *Int J Neuropsychopharmacol*. 2012;15:403-415.

41. National Institute for Health and Clinical Excellence. *Depression: The Treatment and Management of Depression in Adults. Clinical Guideline 90*. London: National Institute for Health and Clinical Excellence; 2009.

42. Rasgon N, Elman S. When not to treat depression in PCOS with antidepressants. *Curr Psychiatry*. 2005;4:47-60.

43. Baldwin DS, Anderson IM, Nutt DJ, et al. Evidence-based pharmacological treatment of anxiety disorders, post-traumatic stress disorder and obsessive-compulsive disorder: a revision of the 2005 guidelines from the British Association for Psychopharmacology. *J Psychopharmacol*. 2014;28:403-439.

12

Polycystic Ovary Syndrome and Nonalcoholic Fatty Liver Disease

AMNA SUBHAN BUTT AND JALPA DEVI

Is There Any Link Between Polycystic Ovary Syndrome and Nonalcoholic Fatty Liver Disease?

Affecting approximately 30% of the general population, nonalcoholic fatty liver disease (NAFLD) is one of the most common causes of chronic liver disease (CLD) globally.[1] It is also a leading cause of liver transplantation not just in young adults but also in females with ethnic differences.[2,3] NAFLD includes an extensive range of liver diseases, from isolated steatosis to nonalcoholic steatohepatitis (NASH), which may progress to fibrosis, cirrhosis, and hepatocellular carcinoma (HCC).[4] The staggering rise of NAFLD calls for effective screening strategies and recognition of the population at risk to reduce the attributable risk of morbidity and mortality associated with the progression of NAFLD at an earlier stage.

Polycystic ovary syndrome (PCOS) is one of the most prevailing and complex endocrine and metabolic dysfunction disorders, affecting 6% to 20% of premenopausal females, depending on the diagnostic criteria used and the specific ethnic population.[5,6] Earlier PCOS was known as Stein-Leventhal syndrome based on the names of Drs. Stein and Leventhal, who had first described the disease in 1935. According to the Rotterdam criteria, this syndrome is characterized by clinical and/or biologic signs of hyperandrogenism (HA), oligo/anovulation, and polycystic ovarian morphology (PCOM) under B-ultrasound.[7] PCOS not only has an effect on the reproductive system, being one of the major causes of anovulatory infertility,[8] but also is linked to the body's metabolic dysfunction.

A correlation has been reported between NAFLD and PCOS.[9-12] This is probably because of the strong association with components of metabolic syndrome (MetS) that are shared by both NAFLD and PCOS (i.e., visceral obesity, hypertension, dyslipidemia, and insulin resistance [IR]).[13,14] This link is also supported by a higher prevalence of NAFLD in females suffering from PCOS.[15-18] Macut et al. elucidated that 51% of females with PCOS had NAFLD compared with 34% who did not have this syndrome.[19] Likewise, 50% of females with PCOS reported having NAFLD regardless of their body mass index (BMI).[20] Moreover, a wide range of different studies suggests that the prevalence of NAFLD among females with PCOS ranges from 34% to 70%, which is higher than the general population.[18,19,21-27]

What Is the Plausible Connection Between Polycystic Ovary Syndrome and Nonalcoholic Fatty Liver Disease?

The exact pathophysiologic link, drive, and mechanisms involved between PCOS and NAFLD still need to be explored.[18,28-32] Nevertheless, the presence of visceral obesity and IR was found to have a strong association with both entities.[33] Up to 40% to 70% of patients with PCOS have been reported to be obese or overweight[34-36] and also manifest IR along with compensatory hyperinsulinemia.[37,38] These escalate the probability of other metabolic derangements, such as hypertension, type 2 diabetes mellitus (DM), dyslipidemia, and cardiovascular diseases. HA has also been reported as a factor linked to both NAFLD and PCOS independent of IR and obesity.[15,22,34,39]

IR has been suggested as the main driver in the pathogenesis of both diseases because the frequency of IR increases with the increasing prevalence of DM, obesity, and MetS.[10,40-42] There is a bidirectional connection between IR and NAFLD augmenting the role of IR in patients with PCOS.[28] Target tissues respond to the insulin changes, with hyperinsulinemia associated with IR, which activates the pathway of progression from NAFLD to NASH.[43] Various changes occur at the cellular level, which could explain the association; for example, IR generates free fatty acids by enhancing lipolysis in visceral adipose tissues and augmenting the deposition of fat in the liver while there is a hindrance in insulin signaling because of increased lipotoxin,[44,45] mitochondrial dysfunction, and reactive oxygen species generated with lipid breakdown.[46] In the end, it activates hepatic stellate cells to release collagen and fibrinogen to develop fibrosis in the liver.[28,47,48]

IR also causes HA in PCOS patients by increasing the production of androgens from the ovary[49] and inhibiting sex hormone–binding globulin (SHBG) production, which leads to raised circulation of free androgens.[50] IR and HA are pathophysiologic links between PCOS and NAFLD.[51] A study revealed that patients with PCOS who had HA had more hepatic steatosis (HS) than both patients with PCOS who had normal androgens and females without PCOS.[22] Additionally, many studies demonstrated that only the HA component can contribute to NAFLD in PCOS females.[18,23,27,52,53] On the contrary, Macut et al. showed that the association between HA and NAFLD is not independent but via IR.[19] On a cellular and molecular level, mitochondria regulate metabolism and energy production physiologically.[54] In PCOS, they showed that mitochondrial dysfunction occurs because of IR and HA, which involves increased production of both triglycerides and cholesterol and a decrease in fatty acid β-oxidation, which boosts up HS and contributes toward the development of NAFLD.[55-62] Additionally, an inflammatory response because of lipid deposition in hepatocytes leads to progression toward NASH.[63-65]

Although genetic associations are not evident, genes that perhaps could affect both NAFLD and PCOS can be categorized into three classes: (1) *CYP17*, *CYP11A*, and *SHBG* are genes that help in androgen synthesis; (2) *IL-6*, *TNF-α*, and *TNF-R* are genes that are involved in the secretion and action of cytokines; and (3) insulin and insulin-receptor are engaged in the secretion and action of insulin.[25,28,30] The racial and ethnic differences associated with the high prevalence of NAFLD are attributed toward a genetic component: patatin-like phospholipase domain containing 3 (PNPLA3) polymorphisms.[31,40,66,67]

There is an emerging role of the microbiome in the pathophysiology of both PCOS and NAFLD.[68,69] A study showed females with this syndrome have a specific set of gut microbiota compared with those without this syndrome.[70] This needs to be explored more as modifying gut microbiota can then be investigated as a potential therapeutic target.

When to Suspect and Who to Screen

Most NAFLD patients are asymptomatic at diagnosis, but some may have nonspecific symptoms such as vague right upper quadrant (RUQ) pain, fatigue, and malaise. On physical examination, hepatomegaly is common, but its appreciation is often hampered by obesity, whereas stigmata of chronic liver disease can be found but in advanced NASH cirrhosis.[71,72] Hence, it is quite logical to suspect NAFLD if a patient presents with conditions strongly associated with NAFLD (e.g., DM or MetS). The first case of NAFLD in a woman with PCOS was reported by Brown et al. in 2005.[73] Because of significant gaps in our knowledge regarding the long-term benefits of early diagnosis and cost-effectiveness at present, routine screening for NAFLD is not recommended for patients with PCOS.[74] Nevertheless, the higher prevalence of NAFLD in females with PCOS raises a concern to study the effectiveness of screening and early treatment of NAFLD, at least in a high-risk group of PCOS. Hence, it might worthwhile sensitizing the healthcare professionals to identify and investigate for the counterpart when addressing a problem related to either PCOS or NAFLD in females in the childbearing age group.

How to Diagnose Nonalcoholic Fatty Liver Disease

NAFLD is currently a diagnosis of exclusion. It can be diagnosed after excluding significant use of alcohol (Table 12.1), other etiologies of HS, and coexisting causes of CLD, such as drugs, toxins, viral infections, nutritional and metabolic factors, autoimmune/metabolic/genetic causes of CLD, bariatric surgery, and rapid weight loss.[75] The following laboratory tests are used to diagnose NAFLD:

- NAFLD is often suspected incidentally with deranged **liver function tests (LFTs)** or fatty liver on imaging performed for other reasons. In LFTs, often serum aminotransferase levels are raised, up to 1.5 to 4 times the upper limit of normal, rarely exceeding it 10-fold. In contrast to alcoholic liver disease, the serum alanine transaminase (ALT) level is usually higher than aspartate aminotransferase (AST) in NAFLD. The alkaline phosphatase and gamma-glutamyltransferase (GGTP) levels may be elevated but less frequently. Besides the exclusion of other causes of HS, evaluation and early identification for factors that could attribute to NAFLD, such as obesity, dyslipidemia, IR, prediabetes or DM, hypothyroidism, PCOS, and sleep apnea, are recommended.[74,76]
- **Conventional ultrasonography** is widely used as a first-choice imaging modality to diagnose NAFLD. It is not only widely available, well-tolerated, and cost-effective, but it is also 85% (80%–89%) sensitive and 93% (87%–97%) specific when identifying moderate to severe HS.[76] Nevertheless, ultrasound has some limitations, including lack of assessment for the severity of liver fibrosis and

TABLE 12.1 The Amount of Alcohol Considered Significant by Various Guidelines

	Males	Females
Asia Pacific Association for the Study of Liver Diseases	>14 (140 g ethanol)	>7 standard drinks/week (70 g ethanol)
American Association for the Study of Liver Diseases	>21 standard drink on average per week	>14 standard drinks per week
European Association for the Study of Liver	>30 g/day	>20 g/day

The approximate amount of pure alcohol is 10 gm and 14 gm in one standard drink in Asia and Europe and in the USA, respectively.
From Paul, J. Recent advances in non-invasive diagnosis and medical management of non-alcoholic fatty liver disease in adult. *Egypt Liver J.* 2020;10[1]:37.

limited sensitivity in obese patients and if the steatosis is less than 20%.[77]

- Both contrast-enhanced and noncontrast **computed tomography (CT scan)** could be used to identify NAFLD by finding reduced attenuation of hepatic parenchyma compared with intrahepatic vessels, spleen, and kidney with a specificity of 100% for moderate to severe steatosis.[10,77] Limitations include high cost, lack of wide availability, exposure to radiation, and limited accuracy to detect mild steatosis.

- **Magnetic resonance imaging (MRI)** provides the most definitive qualitative and quantitative assessment of HS with a sensitivity of 76.7% to 90.0% and specificity of 87.1% to 91%. MRI has several advantages, including its ability to identify even 5% to 10% steatosis and that it is not significantly affected by demographics, histologic activity, or coexisting hepatic conditions. Nevertheless, it is costly and time-consuming and thus mostly used in clinical trials.[10]

- **Transient elastography** (also called vibration-controlled transient elastography or Fibroscan) is an ultrasound-based imaging modality that measures fat content in the liver via controlled attenuation parameter (CAP) and stiffness (fibrosis). A meta-analysis on the diagnostic accuracy of CAP illustrated the cutoffs at 248 dB/m.[10] CAP showed excellent diagnostic performance for differentiating presence and absence of HS by using a cutoff value of 241 dB/m with NAFLD but has limited value in evaluating grades of steatosis, especially in patients with high BMI (>30 kg/m²).

- ALT elevation, although common, is not specific for a severity assessment of NAFLD.[10,78,79] As a result of this, various noninvasive biomarkers have been described,[32,80-84] such as hyaluronic acid, osteopontin, type IV collagen, and matrix metalloproteinase. Moreover, another biomarker that is gaining popularity is cytokeratin-18 (CK-18); caspase-generated fragments, it shows hepatocellular apoptosis, which is a telltale sign of NASH.[50,85] Besides being costly, these novel biomarkers are not currently available for clinical use widely.

- There are noninvasive scoring systems to assess for the severity of fibrosis that include the FibroTest (FibroSure); FibroMeter; NAFLD fibrosis score; Fibrosis-4 (FIB-4); AST-to-platelet ratio (APRI); BARD (BMI, AST/ALT ratio, DM); enhanced liver fibrosis (ELF) score (TIMP-1, amino-terminal propeptide of type III procollagen [PIIINP], hyaluronic acid); NashTest; and the AST/ALT ratio. Among all, NAFLD fibrosis scores (http://gihep.com/calculators/hepatology/nafld-fibrosis-score/) and FIB-4 (http://gihep.com/calculators/hepatology/fibrosis-4-score/) and APRI are in common use.[76,86]

- **Liver biopsy** is the gold standard for diagnosis to assess the severity and prognosis of NAFLD. Nevertheless, because it is an invasive procedure, expensive, and faces interassessment variability in up to 30% of biopsies, the associated risk of complications hinders its use for screening purposes. It is recommended in selected cases (e.g., when the patient is at increased risk for having SH and/or advanced fibrosis), when competing etiologies and severity of NAFLD cannot be excluded without a liver biopsy, or for the objective assessment of outcome in clinical trials.[76]

The common factors that tend to cause NAFLD and PCOS are obesity and IR. So BMI[87] and waist circumference[88] are prognosticative factors to assess the risk of NAFLD, but now new metabolic indices have been introduced that combine both lipid and anthropometric measures, which can meticulously predict IR, prediabetes, and type 2 DM.[80,89] These are the lipid accumulation product (LAP) index, visceral adiposity index (VAI), and product of triglycerides and glucose (TyG).[90-92] An LAP index reflecting abdominal obesity is higher in females with PCOS along with MetS than their disease-free counterparts; another study showed it is an important predictor to detect NAFLD in females with PCOS.

Options We Have in the Toolbox to Treat

Currently, we do not have many pawns in our toolkit for the treatment of metabolic disorders linked with PCOS, including NAFLD. Hence, just like females without PCOS, management of NAFLD includes treatment of associated conditions (e.g., obesity, DM, MetS) and lifestyle intervention, pharmacologic therapy, and bariatric surgery or bariatric endoscopic procedures.

Lifestyle Modification

As mentioned earlier, 50% of PCOS patients are obese, having IR that leads to compensatory hyperinsulinemia and are at greater risk for type 2 DM.[93] Visceral obesity tends to be associated with raised serum sex steroids and decreased SHBG.[94] There is an increasing risk of metabolic and cardiovascular abnormalities in obese females with PCOS compared with nonobese females and those without PCOS.[95] Therefore obesity treatment should be a priority and is recommended as first-line therapy in obese females. It can be achieved by lifestyle modification to lose weight via physical activity and diet management and pharmacotherapy if indicated.[96,97] There are huge benefits to reducing weight, such as lowering adiposity, sex steroid, and insulin levels; improving ovulation and fertility; and decreasing the overall risk for cardiovascular disease (CVD).[96,98,99] A systemic review showed that aerobic exercise of moderate intensity as an aid to dietary implementation can have a tremendous impact on the improvement of endocrine and metabolic symptoms.[100] There are various studies on different diets, such as a ketogenic, low carbohydrate diet, which showed a notable improvement in their profile.[101] A meta-analysis illustrated that with monounsaturated fat, remarkable weight loss occurs and a low glycemic diet improves the menstrual cycle and causes diminution of IR.[102] To improve the HS, 3% to 5% weight loss is needed, whereas 7% to 10% weight loss is required to improve the histopathologic features of NASH. So combining a hypocaloric diet (daily reduction by 500–1000 kcal) and moderate intensity exercise is the key to maintaining the weight in the long run. Reduced visceral adiposity, hepatic steatosis, and fibrosis are linked to high-intensity interval training (HIIT), especially for those who lack time to exercise.[103] Overall moderate-intensity aerobic exercise for 150 min weekly, along with 2-3 times/week strength is quite effective. Those who cannot attend structured exercise programs would be benefited by simply reducing or breaking up sedentary time with repeated a few minutes of walking every day. However, in all cases, compliance with diet modification and regular physical activity plays a key role in achieving targets.[104]

Insulin-Sensitizing Agents

Hyperinsulinemia and IR both contribute to the development of type 2 DM, CVD, and NAFLD; therefore pharmacotherapy for managing the metabolic spectrum of PCOS should also be considered to antagonize the effects of insulin.[105]

- Thiazolidinediones: Pioglitazone, which is a peroxisome proliferator-activated receptor-gamma (PPAR-γ) agonist, regulates glucose uptake, adipogenesis, and insulin function. In randomized trials, meta-analyses, and randomized open-label studies, pioglitazone has shown promising effects on the metabolic profile of PCOS patients.[106,107] Nevertheless, there are side effects because of fluid retention and weight gain in already obese people, which is the main concern and hinders its usage.[108]
- Metformin: It belongs to the biguanide family, and the mechanism of action is via inhibition of glucose production, enhancing insulin sensitivity and glucose uptake and embellishing dyslipidemia, which is common in PCOS because of hyperinsulinemia.[109] The initial dose is 500 to 800 mg daily, and maximally it can go up to 2000 if tolerated.[110] The common adverse effects are diarrhea, abdominal bloating, and nausea and vomiting. With long-term use, it can also cause vitamin B_{12} deficiency.[111] A study comparing metformin and lifestyle modification showed a similar response of decreasing BMI, although the metformin group had decreasing androgen levels. This drug also declines BMI independent of a lifestyle intervention.[112]
- Glucagon-like peptide-1 receptor analog: This is a class with incretin mimetic activity that releases glucose-dependent insulin, especially after a meal. These include glucagon-like peptide-1 (GLP-1) and glucose-dependent insulinotropic polypeptide (GIP).[113] Liraglutide and Semaglutide have an established role in sustained body weight reduction in cases of obesity even without Type 2 Diabetes. Histological resolution of NASH with both agents has been reported in ~40% to 60% of cases. Hence, GLP-1 receptor agonists are expected to have a crucial role in managing obesity and NAFLD.[114]
- Bariatric surgery and endoscopic procedures: It helps in achieving weight loss in morbidly obese patients and also results in increasing insulin sensitivity, which leads to improvement of DM, lowering HS, cardiovascular morbidity, and other symptoms of PCOS as well.[115-118] Currently recommended for morbidly obese patients unable to lose weight via other measures.

Complications and Prognosis

Liver-Related Complication

In NAFLD with advanced fibrosis, there is an increased risk of liver-related and all-cause mortality and even in 20% of these patients, HCC develops in the absence of cirrhosis.[119-122]

Hence, because of the strong correlation with MetS, NAFLD patients with PCOS may get benefits if treated early for NAFLD.

Other Complications

NAFLD is considered the hepatic manifestation of MetS, and there is a bidirectional relationship between DM and NAFLD that is an independent predictor of disease progression, as well as with hypertension.[123,124] Dyslipidemia is one of the complications that raised the risk of atherosclerosis and leads to myocardial infarction with an incidence rate of 4.8 per 1000 person-years and cerebrovascular accidents.[121,125-128] As mentioned earlier, IR and obesity are the main drivers of NAFLD, which also lead to the development of CKD and higher mortality as well.[129,130] In a recent meta-analysis, the association of depression and neurocognitive dysfunction with NAFLD was reported.[131,132] The other complications include cholelithiasis,[133] obstructive sleep apnea,[134] osteoporosis,[135] and thyroid dysfunction.[136] The first most common cause of death is CVD and afterward extrahepatic cancers.[137]

PCOS can cause many complications (e.g., menstrual dysfunction, subfertility, endometrial adenocarcinoma, and potential vascular diseases) and also increase the risk of metabolic disorders like type 2 DM and NAFLD.[138,139] It is a lifelong disorder affecting health from infancy through postmenopause females in addition to the five times higher risk in female offspring of mothers with PCOS.[140] In addition, studies showed that in rodent models, transgenerational dysfunction of both hepatic metabolism and reproductive system is caused by prenatal sex steroid exposure, not obesity.[141,142] Offspring of PCOS females also suffer cardiometabolic and NAFLD disorder in early life, so normal BMI before conception should be a crucial target for avoiding NAFLD.[143-145] That is why it is critical to prevent DM and obesity earlier, which threaten the overall health of females with PCOS and also causes complications during pregnancy and childbirth.[146]

Conclusion

Both NAFLD and PCOS share similar risk factors and strong associations with components of MetS, especially obesity and IR. The data are limited about the effectiveness of screening all patients with PCOS. Nevertheless, early identification of NAFLD in females with PCOS who have multiple risk factors including IR and HA may help prevent disease progression and complications of cirrhosis.

References

1. Younossi Z, Tacke F, Arrese M, et al. Global perspectives on nonalcoholic fatty liver disease and nonalcoholic steatohepatitis. *Hepatology.* 2019;69(6):2672-2682.
2. Doycheva I, Issa D, Watt KD, Lopez R, Rifai G, Alkhouri N. Nonalcoholic steatohepatitis is the most rapidly increasing indication for liver transplantation in young adults in the United States. *J Clin Gastroenterol.* 2018;52(4):339-346.

3. Noureddin M, Vipani A, Bresee C, et al. NASH leading cause of liver transplant in women: updated analysis of indications for liver transplant and ethnic and gender variances. *Am J Gastroenterol.* 2018;113(11):1649-1659.

4. Sayiner M, Koenig A, Henry L, Younossi ZM. Epidemiology of nonalcoholic fatty liver disease and nonalcoholic steatohepatitis in the United States and the rest of the world. *Clin Liver Dis.* 2016;20(2):205-214.

5. Ding T, Hardiman PJ, Petersen I, Wang FF, Qu F, Baio G. The prevalence of polycystic ovary syndrome in reproductive-aged women of different ethnicity: a systematic review and meta-analysis. *Oncotarget.* 2017;8(56):96351.

6. Lim SS, Davies M, Norman RJ, Moran L. Overweight, obesity and central obesity in women with polycystic ovary syndrome: a systematic review and meta-analysis. *Hum Reprod Update.* 2012;18(6):618-637.

7. Rotterdam ESHRE/ASRM-Sponsored PCOS Consensus Workshop Group. Revised 2003 consensus on diagnostic criteria and long-term health risks related to polycystic ovary syndrome (PCOS). *Hum Reprod.* 2004;19(1):41-47.

8. Franks S. Assessment and management of anovulatory infertility in polycystic ovary syndrome. *Endocrinol Metab Clin North Am.* 2003;32(3):639-651.

9. Cerda C, Pérez-Ayuso RM, Riquelme A, Soza A, et al. Nonalcoholic fatty liver disease in women with polycystic ovary syndrome. *J Hepatol.* 2007;47(3):412-417.

10. Chalasani N, Younossi Z, Lavine JE, et al. The diagnosis and management of non-alcoholic fatty liver disease: practice guideline by the American Gastroenterological Association, American Association for the Study of Liver Diseases, and American College of Gastroenterology. *Gastroenterology.* 2012;142(7):1592-1609.

11. Gambarin–Gelwan M, Kinkhabwala SV, Schiano TD, Bodian C, Yeh HC, Futterweit W. Prevalence of nonalcoholic fatty liver disease in women with polycystic ovary syndrome. *Clin Gastroenterol Hepatol.* 2007;5(4):496-501.

12. Setji TL, Holland ND, Sanders LL, Pereira KC, Diehl AM, Brown AJ. Nonalcoholic steatohepatitis and nonalcoholic fatty liver disease in young women with polycystic ovary syndrome. *J Clin Endocrinol Metab.* 2006;91(5):1741-1747.

13. Jeanes YM, Reeves S. Metabolic consequences of obesity and insulin resistance in polycystic ovary syndrome: diagnostic and methodological challenges. *Nutr Res Rev.* 2017;30(1):97.

14. Jensen T, Wieland A, Cree-Green M, Nadeau K, Sullivan S. Clinical workup of fatty liver for the primary care provider. *Postgrad Med.* 2019;131(1):19-30.

15. Cai J, Wu C, Zhang Y, Wang Y, et al. High-free androgen index is associated with increased risk of non-alcoholic fatty liver disease in women with polycystic ovary syndrome, independent of obesity and insulin resistance. *Int J Obes.* 2017;41(9):1341-1347.

16. Carreau AM, Pyle L, Garcia-Reyes Y, et al. Clinical prediction score of nonalcoholic fatty liver disease in adolescent girls with polycystic ovary syndrome (PCOS-HS index). *Clin Endocrinol.* 2019;91(4):544-552.

17. Rocha A, Faria L, Guimarães T, et al. Non-alcoholic fatty liver disease in women with polycystic ovary syndrome: systematic review and meta-analysis. *J Endocrinol Invest.* 2017;40(12):1279-1288.

18. Wu J, Yao XY, Shi RX, Liu SF, Wang XY. A potential link between polycystic ovary syndrome and non-alcoholic fatty liver disease: an update meta-analysis. *Reprod Health.* 2018;15(1):1-9.

19. Macut D, Tziomalos K, Božić-Antić I, et al. Non-alcoholic fatty liver disease is associated with insulin resistance and lipid accumulation product in women with polycystic ovary syndrome. *Hum Reprod.* 2016;31(6):1347-1353.

20. Salva-Pastor N, Chavez-Tapia NC, Uribe M, Nuno-Lambarri N. Understanding the association of polycystic ovary syndrome and non-alcoholic fatty liver disease. *J Steroid Biochem Mol Biol.* 2019;194:105445.

21. Cussons AJ, Watts GF, Mori TA, Stuckey BG. Omega-3 fatty acid supplementation decreases liver fat content in polycystic ovary syndrome: a randomized controlled trial employing proton magnetic resonance spectroscopy. *Obstet Gynecol Surv.* 2010;65(3):175-176.

22. Jones H, Sprung VS, Pugh CJ, et al. Polycystic ovary syndrome with hyperandrogenism is characterized by an increased risk of hepatic steatosis compared to nonhyperandrogenic PCOS phenotypes and healthy controls, independent of obesity and insulin resistance. *J Clin Endocrinol Metab.* 2012;97(10):3709-3716.

23. Petta S, Ciresi A, Bianco J, et al. Insulin resistance and hyperandrogenism drive steatosis and fibrosis risk in young females with PCOS. *PLoS One.* 2017;12(11):e0186136.

24. Ramezani-Binabaj M, Motalebi M, Karimi-Sari H, Rezaee-Zavareh MS, Alavian SM. Are women with polycystic ovarian syndrome at a high risk of non-alcoholic Fatty liver disease; a meta-analysis. *Hepat Mon.* 2014;14(11):e23235.

25. Vassilatou E. Nonalcoholic fatty liver disease and polycystic ovary syndrome. *World J Gastroenterol.* 2014;20(26):8351.

26. Vassilatou E, Lafoyianni S, Vryonidou A, et al. Increased androgen bioavailability is associated with non-alcoholic fatty liver disease in women with polycystic ovary syndrome. *Hum Reprod.* 2010;25(1):212-220.

27. Vassilatou E, Vassiliadi D, Salambasis K, et al. Increased prevalence of polycystic ovary syndrome in premenopausal women with nonalcoholic fatty liver disease. *Eur J Endocrinol.* 2015;173(6):739-747.

28. Gastaldelli A. Insulin resistance and reduced metabolic flexibility: cause or consequence of NAFLD? *Clin Sci.* 2017;131(22):2701-2704.

29. Kumarendran B, O'Reilly MW, Manolopoulos KN, et al. Polycystic ovary syndrome, androgen excess, and the risk of nonalcoholic fatty liver disease in women: a longitudinal study based on a United Kingdom primary care database. *PLoS Med.* 2018;15(3):e1002542.

30. Macut D, Bjekić-Macut J, Livadas S, et al. Nonalcoholic fatty liver disease in patients with polycystic ovary syndrome. *Curr Pharm Des.* 2018;24(38):4593-4597.

31. Minato S, Sakane N, Kotani K, et al. Prevalence and risk factors of elevated liver enzymes in Japanese women with polycystic ovary syndrome. *J Clin Med Res.* 2018;10(12):904.

32. Vassilatou E, Lafoyianni S, Vassiliadi DA, et al. Visceral adiposity index for the diagnosis of nonalcoholic fatty liver disease in premenopausal women with and without polycystic ovary syndrome. *Maturitas.* 2018;116:1-7.

33. Gilbert EW, Tay CT, Hiam DS, Teede HJ, Moran LJ. Comorbidities and complications of polycystic ovary syndrome: an overview of systematic reviews. *Clin Endocrinol.* 2018;89(6):683-699.

34. Moran C, Arriaga M, Rodriguez G, Moran S. Obesity differentially affects phenotypes of polycystic ovary syndrome. *Int J Endocrinol.* 2012;2012:317241.

35. Panidis D, Macut D, Tziomalos K, et al. Prevalence of metabolic syndrome in women with polycystic ovary syndrome. *Clin Endocrinol.* 2013;78(4):586-592.

36. Yildiz BO, Knochenhauer ES, Azziz R. Impact of obesity on the risk for polycystic ovary syndrome. *J Clin Endocrinol Metab.* 2008;93(1):162-168.

37. Legro RS, Castracane VD, Kauffman RP. Detecting insulin resistance in polycystic ovary syndrome: purposes and pitfalls. *Obstet Gynecol Surv.* 2004;59(2):141-154.

38. Marshall JC, Dunaif A. Should all women with PCOS be treated for insulin resistance? *Fertil Steril.* 2012;97(1):18-22.

39. Won YB, Seo SK, Yun BH, Cho S, Choi YS, Lee BS. Non-alcoholic fatty liver disease in polycystic ovary syndrome women. *Sci Rep.* 2021;11(1):1-11.
40. Polyzos SA, Mantzoros CS. Nonalcoholic fatty future disease. *Metabolism.* 2016;65(8):1007-1016.
41. Vernon G, Baranova A, Younossi Z. Systematic review: the epidemiology and natural history of non-alcoholic fatty liver disease and non-alcoholic steatohepatitis in adults. *Aliment Pharmacol Ther.* 2011;34(3):274-285.
42. Williams CD, Stengel J, Asike MI, et al. Prevalence of nonalcoholic fatty liver disease and nonalcoholic steatohepatitis among a largely middle-aged population utilizing ultrasound and liver biopsy: a prospective study. *Gastroenterology.* 2011;140(1):124-131.
43. Pearson T, Wattis JA, King JR, MacDonald IA, Mazzatti DJ. The effects of insulin resistance on individual tissues: an application of a mathematical model of metabolism in humans. *Bull Math Biol.* 2016;78(6):1189-1217.
44. Lee HY, Birkenfeld AL, Jornayvaz FR, et al. Apolipoprotein CIII overexpressing mice are predisposed to diet-induced hepatic steatosis and hepatic insulin resistance. *Hepatology.* 2011;54(5):1650-1660.
45. Magkos F, Su X, Bradley D, et al. Intrahepatic diacylglycerol content is associated with hepatic insulin resistance in obese subjects. *Gastroenterology.* 2012;142(7):1444-1446.e2.
46. Jelenik T, Kaul K, Séquaris G, et al. Mechanisms of insulin resistance in primary and secondary nonalcoholic fatty liver. *Diabetes.* 2017;66(8):2241-2253.
47. Chalasani N, Deeg MA, Crabb DW. Systemic levels of lipid peroxidation and its metabolic and dietary correlates in patients with non-alcoholic steatohepatitis. *Am J Gastroenterol.* 2004;99(8):1497-1502.
48. Staehr P, Hother-Nielsen O, Landau BR, Chandramouli V, Holst JJ, Beck-Nielsen H. Effects of free fatty acids per se on glucose production, gluconeogenesis, and glycogenolysis. *Diabetes.* 2003;52(2):260-267.
49. Diamanti-Kandarakis E, Dunaif A. Insulin resistance and the polycystic ovary syndrome revisited: an update on mechanisms and implications. *Endocr Rev.* 2012;33(6):981-1030.
50. Yildiz BO, Azziz R. The adrenal and polycystic ovary syndrome. *Rev Endocr Metab Disord.* 2007;8(4):331-342.
51. Birkenfeld AL, Shulman GI. Nonalcoholic fatty liver disease, hepatic insulin resistance, and type 2 diabetes. *Hepatology.* 2014;59(2):713-723.
52. Kim J, Kim D, Yim J, et al. Polycystic ovary syndrome with hyperandrogenism as a risk factor for non-obese non-alcoholic fatty liver disease. *Aliment Pharmacol Ther.* 2017;45(11):1403-1412.
53. Rocha AL, Oliveira FR, Azevedo RC, et al. Recent advances in the understanding and management of polycystic ovary syndrome. *F1000Res.* 2019;8:F1000.
54. Friedman JR, Nunnari J. Mitochondrial form and function. *Nature.* 2014;505(7483):335-343.
55. Whigham LD, Butz DE, Dashti H, et al. Metabolic evidence of diminished lipid oxidation in women with polycystic ovary syndrome. *Curr Metabolomics.* 2013;1(4):269-278.
56. Garcimartín A, López-Oliva ME, Sántos-López JA, et al. Silicon alleviates nonalcoholic steatohepatitis by reducing apoptosis in aged Wistar rats fed a high–saturated fat, high-cholesterol diet. *J Nutr.* 2017;147(6):1104-1112.
57. Ju J, Huang Q, Sun J, et al. Correlation between PPAR-α methylation level in peripheral blood and atherosclerosis of NAFLD patients with DM. *Exp Ther Med.* 2018;15(3):2727-2730.
58. Kanda T, Matsuoka S, Yamazaki M, et al. Apoptosis and non-alcoholic fatty liver diseases. *World J Gastroenterol.* 2018;24(25):2661.
59. Khambu B, Yan S, Huda N, Liu G, Yin XM. Autophagy in non-alcoholic fatty liver disease and alcoholic liver disease. *Liver Res.* 2018;2(3):112-119.
60. Lee S, Kim S, Hwang S, Cherrington NJ, Ryu DY. Dysregulated expression of proteins associated with ER stress, autophagy and apoptosis in tissues from nonalcoholic fatty liver disease. *Oncotarget.* 2017;8(38):63370.
61. Shimano H, Sato R. SREBP-regulated lipid metabolism: convergent physiology—divergent pathophysiology. *Nat Rev Endocrinol.* 2017;13(12):710.
62. Stankov MV, Panayotova-Dimitrova D, Leverkus M, et al. Autophagy inhibition due to thymidine analogues as novel mechanism leading to hepatocyte dysfunction and lipid accumulation. *AIDS.* 2012;26(16):1995-2006.
63. Gao B, Tsukamoto H. Inflammation in alcoholic and nonalcoholic fatty liver disease: friend or foe? *Gastroenterology.* 2016;150(8):1704-1709.
64. Michael MD, Kulkarni RN, Postic C, et al. Loss of insulin signaling in hepatocytes leads to severe insulin resistance and progressive hepatic dysfunction. *Mol Cell.* 2000;6(1):87-97.
65. Wang J, Wu D, Guo H, Li M. Hyperandrogenemia and insulin resistance: the chief culprit of polycystic ovary syndrome. *Life Sci.* 2019;236:116940.
66. Sarkar M, Terrault N, Duwaerts CC, Tien P, Cedars MI, Huddleston H. The association of Hispanic ethnicity with nonalcoholic fatty liver disease in polycystic ovary syndrome. *Curr Opin Gynecol Obstet.* 2018;1(1):24.
67. Zhang J, Hu J, Zhang C, et al. Analyses of risk factors for polycystic ovary syndrome complicated with non-alcoholic fatty liver disease. *Exp Ther Med.* 2018;15(5):4259-4264.
68. Thackray VG. Sex, microbes, and polycystic ovary syndrome. *Trends Endocrinol Metab.* 2019;30(1):54-65.
69. Wieland A, Frank D, Harnke B, Bambha K. Systematic review: microbial dysbiosis and nonalcoholic fatty liver disease. *Aliment Pharmacol Ther.* 2015;42(9):1051-1063.
70. Jobira B, Frank DN, Pyle L, et al. Obese adolescents with PCOS have altered biodiversity and relative abundance in gastrointestinal microbiota. *J Clin Endocrinol Metab.* 2020;105(6):e2134-e2144.
71. Angulo P. Nonalcoholic fatty liver disease. *N Engl J Med.* 2002;346(16):1221-1231.
72. Matteoni CA, Younossi ZM, Gramlich T, Boparai N, Liu YC, McCullough AJ. Nonalcoholic fatty liver disease: a spectrum of clinical and pathological severity. *Gastroenterology.* 1999;116(6):1413-1419.
73. Brown AJ, Tendler DA, McMurray RG, Setji TL. Polycystic ovary syndrome and severe nonalcoholic steatohepatitis: beneficial effect of modest weight loss and exercise on liver biopsy findings. *Endocr Pract.* 2005;11(5):319-324.
74. Chalasani N, Younossi Z, Lavine JE, et al. The diagnosis and management of nonalcoholic fatty liver disease: practice guidance from the American Association for the Study of Liver Diseases. *Hepatology.* 2018;67(1):328-357. doi:10.1002/hep.29367.
75. Clark JM. The epidemiology of nonalcoholic fatty liver disease in adults. *J Clin Gastroenterol.* 2006;40:S5-S10.
76. Castera L, Friedrich-Rust M, Loomba R. Noninvasive assessment of liver disease in patients with nonalcoholic fatty liver disease. *Gastroenterology.* 2019;156(5):1264-1281.e4. doi:10.1053/j.gastro.2018.12.036.
77. Paul J. Recent advances in non-invasive diagnosis and medical management of non-alcoholic fatty liver disease in adult. *Egypt Liver J.* 2020;10(1):37. doi:10.1186/s43066-020-00043-x.
78. Ratziu V, Charlotte F, Heurtier A, et al. Sampling variability of liver biopsy in nonalcoholic fatty liver disease. *Gastroenterology.* 2005;128(7):1898-1906.
79. Sberna A, Bouillet B, Rouland A, et al. European Association for the Study of the Liver (EASL), European Association for the Study of Diabetes (EASD) and European Association for the Study of Obesity

(EASO) clinical practice recommendations for the management of non-alcoholic fatty liver disease: evaluation of their application in people with Type 2 diabetes. *Diabet Med.* 2018;35(3):368-375.

80. Amato MC, Giordano C, Galia M, et al. Visceral Adiposity Index: a reliable indicator of visceral fat function associated with cardiometabolic risk. *Diabetes Care.* 2010;33(4):920-922.

81. Angulo P, Hui JM, Marchesini G, et al. The NAFLD fibrosis score: a noninvasive system that identifies liver fibrosis in patients with NAFLD. *Hepatology.* 2007;45(4):846-854.

82. Demir M, Lang S, Nierhoff D, et al. Stepwise combination of simple noninvasive fibrosis scoring systems increases diagnostic accuracy in nonalcoholic fatty liver disease. *J Clin Gastroenterol.* 2013;47(8):719-726.

83. Harrison SA, Oliver D, Arnold HL, Gogia S, Neuschwander-Tetri BA. Development and validation of a simple NAFLD clinical scoring system for identifying patients without advanced disease. *Gut.* 2008;57(10):1441-1447.

84. Kotronen A, Peltonen M, Hakkarainen A, et al. Prediction of non-alcoholic fatty liver disease and liver fat using metabolic and genetic factors. *Gastroenterology.* 2009;137(3):865-872.

85. Sumida Y, Yoneda M, Hyogo H, et al. A simple clinical scoring system using ferritin, fasting insulin, and type IV collagen 7S for predicting steatohepatitis in nonalcoholic fatty liver disease. *J Gastroenterol.* 2011;46(2):257-268.

86. Muthiah MD, Han NC, Sanyal AJ. A clinical overview of NAFLD: a guide to diagnosis, the clinical features, and complications–What the non-specialist needs to know. *Diabetes Obes Metab.* 2022;24(suppl 2):3-14.

87. Loomis AK, Kabadi S, Preiss D, et al. Body mass index and risk of nonalcoholic fatty liver disease: two electronic health record prospective studies. *J Clin Endocrinol Metab.* 2016;101(3):945-952.

88. Motamed N, Sohrabi M, Ajdarkosh H, et al. Fatty liver index vs waist circumference for predicting non-alcoholic fatty liver disease. *World J Gastroenterol.* 2016;22(10):3023.

89. Wakabayashi I, Daimon T. A strong association between lipid accumulation product and diabetes mellitus in Japanese women and men. *J Atheroscler Thromb.* 2014;21(3):282-288.

90. Ahn N, Baumeister SE, Amann U, et al. Visceral adiposity index (VAI), lipid accumulation product (LAP), and product of triglycerides and glucose (TyG) to discriminate prediabetes and diabetes. *Sci Rep.* 2019;9(1):1-11.

91. Nusrianto R, Ayundini G, Kristanti M, et al. Visceral adiposity index and lipid accumulation product as a predictor of type 2 diabetes mellitus: the Bogor cohort study of non-communicable diseases risk factors. *Diabetes Res Clin Pract.* 2019;155:107798.

92. Roriz AKC, Passos LCS, de Oliveira CC, Eickemberg M, de Almeida Moreira P, Sampaio LR. Evaluation of the accuracy of anthropometric clinical indicators of visceral fat in adults and elderly. *PLoS One.* 2014;9(7):e103499.

93. Domecq JP, Prutsky G, Mullan RJ, et al. Lifestyle modification programs in polycystic ovary syndrome: systematic review and meta-analysis. *J Clin Endocrinol Metab.* 2013;98(12):4655-4663.

94. Kiddy D, Sharp P, White D, et al. Differences in clinical and endocrine features between obese and non-obese subjects with polycystic ovary syndrome: an analysis of 263 consecutive cases. *Clin Endocrinol.* 1990;32(2):213-220.

95. Yildirim B, Sabir N, Kaleli B. Relation of intra-abdominal fat distribution to metabolic disorders in nonobese patients with polycystic ovary syndrome. *Fertil Steril.* 2003;79(6):1358-1364.

96. Kiddy DS, Hamilton-Fairley D, Bush A, et al. Improvement in endocrine and ovarian function during dietary treatment of obese women with polycystic ovary syndrome. *Clin Endocrinol.* 1992;36(1):105-111.

97. Moran LJ, Hutchison SK, Norman RJ, Teede HJ. Lifestyle changes in women with polycystic ovary syndrome. *Cochrane Database Syst Rev.* 2011;(2):CD007506.

98. Moran LJ, Pasquali R, Teede HJ, Hoeger KM, Norman RJ. Treatment of obesity in polycystic ovary syndrome: a position statement of the Androgen Excess and Polycystic Ovary Syndrome Society. *Fertil Steril.* 2009;92(6):1966-1982.

99. Ndefo UA, Eaton A, Green MR. Polycystic ovary syndrome: a review of treatment options with a focus on pharmacological approaches. *Pharm Ther.* 2013;38(6):336-355.

100. Harrison CL, Lombard CB, Moran LJ, Teede HJ. Exercise therapy in polycystic ovary syndrome: a systematic review. *Hum Reprod Update.* 2011;17(2):171-183.

101. Mavropoulos JC, Yancy WS, Hepburn J, Westman EC. The effects of a low-carbohydrate, ketogenic diet on the polycystic ovary syndrome: a pilot study. *Nutr Metab.* 2005;2(1):1-5.

102. Moran LJ, Ko H, Misso M, et al. Dietary composition in the treatment of polycystic ovary syndrome: a systematic review to inform evidence-based guidelines. *J Acad Nutr Diet.* 2013;113(4):520-545.

103. Hamasaki H. Perspectives on interval exercise interventions for non-alcoholic fatty liver disease. *Medicines.* 2019;6(3):83. doi:10.3390/medicines6030083.

104. Carels RA, Darby LA, Rydin S, Douglass OM, Cacciapaglia HM, O'Brien WH: The relationship between self-monitoring, outcome expectancies, difficulties with eating and exercise, and physical activity and weight loss treatment outcomes. *Ann Behav Med.* 2005;30(3):182-190. doi:10.1207/s15324796abm3003_2.

105. Guzick D. Polycystic ovary syndrome: symptomatology, pathophysiology, and epidemiology. *Am J Obstet Gynecol.* 1998;179(6):S89-S93.

106. Brettenthaler N, De Geyter C, Huber PR, Keller U. Effect of the insulin sensitizer pioglitazone on insulin resistance, hyperandrogenism, and ovulatory dysfunction in women with polycystic ovary syndrome. *J Clin Endocrinol Metab.* 2004;89(8):3835-3840.

107. Xu Y, Wu Y, Huang Q. Comparison of the effect between pioglitazone and metformin in treating patients with PCOS: a meta-analysis. *Arch Gynecol Obstet.* 2017;296(4):661-677.

108. Jearath V, Vashisht R, Rustagi V, Raina S, Sharma R. Pioglitazone-induced congestive heart failure and pulmonary edema in a patient with preserved ejection fraction. *J Pharmacol Pharmacother.* 2016;7(1):41.

109. Jensterle M, Kravos NA, Ferjan S, Goricar K, Dolzan V, Janez A. Long-term efficacy of metformin in overweight-obese PCOS: longitudinal follow-up of retrospective cohort. *Endocr Connect.* 2020;9(1):44-54.

110. Duleba AJ. Medical management of metabolic dysfunction in PCOS. *Steroids.* 2012;77(4):306-311.

111. Pasquali R. Metformin in women with PCOS, pros. *Endocrine.* 2014;48(2):422-426.

112. Harborne LR, Sattar N, Norman JE, Fleming R. Metformin and weight loss in obese women with polycystic ovary syndrome: comparison of doses. *J Clin Endocrinol Metab.* 2005;90(8):4593-4598.

113. Cefalu WT. The physiologic role of incretin hormones: clinical applications. *J Am Osteopath Med.* 2010;110(suppl 32):8-14.

114. Barritt AS 4th, Marshman E, Noureddin M: Review article: role of glucagon-like peptide-1 receptor agonists in non-alcoholic steatohepatitis, obesity and diabetes-what hepatologists need to know. *Aliment Pharmacol Ther.* 2022;55(8):944-959. doi:10.1111/apt.16794.

115. Batterham RL, Cummings DE. Mechanisms of diabetes improvement following bariatric/metabolic surgery. *Diabetes Care.* 2016;39(6):893-901.

116. Maggard MA, Yermilov I, Li Z, et al. Pregnancy and fertility following bariatric surgery: a systematic review. *JAMA*. 2008;300(19):2286-2296.

117. Priyadarshini P, Singh VP, Aggarwal S, Garg H, Sinha S, Guleria R. Impact of bariatric surgery on obstructive sleep apnoea–hypopnea syndrome in morbidly obese patients. *J Minim Access Surg*. 2017;13(4):291.

118. Sacks J, Mulya A, Fealy CE, et al. Effect of Roux-en-Y gastric bypass on liver mitochondrial dynamics in a rat model of obesity. *Physiol Rep*. 2018;6(4):e13600.

119. D'Amico G, Garcia-Tsaog G, Pagliaro L. Natural history and prognostic indicators in cirrhosis: a systematic review of 118 studies. *J Hepatol*. 2006;44(1):217-231.

120. Garcia-Tsao G, Abraldes JG, Berzigotti A, Bosch J. Portal hypertensive bleeding in cirrhosis: risk stratification, diagnosis, and management: 2016 practice guidance by the American Association for the study of liver diseases. *Hepatology*. 2017;65(1):310-335.

121. Stepanova M, Rafiq N, Makhlouf H, et al. Predictors of all-cause mortality and liver-related mortality in patients with non-alcoholic fatty liver disease (NAFLD). *Dig Dis Sci*. 2013;58(10):3017-3023.

122. Younossi ZM, Stepanova M, Ong J, et al. Nonalcoholic steatohepatitis is the most rapidly increasing indication for liver transplantation in the United States. *Clin Gastroenterol Hepatol*. 2021;19(3):580-589.e5.

123. Lonardo A, Nascimbeni F, Mantovani A, Targher G. Hypertension, diabetes, atherosclerosis and NASH: cause or consequence? *J Hepatol*. 2018;68(2):335-352.

124. McPherson S, Hardy T, Henderson E, Burt AD, Day CP, Anstee QM. Evidence of NAFLD progression from steatosis to fibrosing-steatohepatitis using paired biopsies: implications for prognosis and clinical management. *J Hepatol*. 2015;62(5):1148-1155.

125. Bril F, Sninsky JJ, Baca AM, et al. Hepatic steatosis and insulin resistance, but not steatohepatitis, promote atherogenic dyslipidemia in NAFLD. *J Clin Endocrinol Metab*. 2016;101(2):644-652.

126. Siddiqui MS, Fuchs M, Idowu MO, et al. Severity of nonalcoholic fatty liver disease and progression to cirrhosis are associated with atherogenic lipoprotein profile. *Clin Gastroenterol Hepatol*. 2015;13(5):1000-1008.e3.

127. Targher G, Byrne CD, Tilg H. NAFLD and increased risk of cardiovascular disease: clinical associations, pathophysiological mechanisms and pharmacological implications. *Gut*. 2020;69(9):1691-1705.

128. Younossi ZM, Koenig AB, Abdelatif D, Fazel Y, Henry L, Wymer M. Global epidemiology of nonalcoholic fatty liver disease—meta-analytic assessment of prevalence, incidence, and outcomes. *Hepatology*. 2016;64(1):73-84.

129. Park H, Dawwas GK, Liu X, Nguyen MH. Nonalcoholic fatty liver disease increases risk of incident advanced chronic kidney disease: a propensity-matched cohort study. *J Intern Med*. 2019;286(6):711-722.

130. Wilechansky RM, Pedley A, Massaro JM, Hoffmann U, Benjamin EJ, Long MT. Relations of liver fat with prevalent and incident chronic kidney disease in the Framingham heart study: a secondary analysis. *Liver Int*. 2019;39(8):1535-1544.

131. Colognesi M, Gabbia D, De Martin S. Depression and cognitive impairment—extrahepatic manifestations of NAFLD and NASH. *Biomedicines*. 2020;8(7):229.

132. Xiao J, Lim LKE, Ng CH, et al. Is fatty liver associated with depression? A meta-analysis and systematic review on the prevalence, risk factors, and Outcomes of depression and non-alcoholic fatty liver disease. *Front Med*. 2021;8:912.

133. Loria P, Lonardo A, Lombardini S, et al. Gallstone disease in non-alcoholic fatty liver: prevalence and associated factors. *J Gastroenterol Hepatol*. 2005;20(8):1176-1184.

134. Asfari MM, Niyazi F, Lopez R, Dasarathy S, McCullough AJ. The association of nonalcoholic steatohepatitis and obstructive sleep apnea. *Eur J Gastroenterol Hepatol*. 2017;29(12):1380.

135. Chen HJ, Yang HY, Hsueh KC, et al. Increased risk of osteoporosis in patients with nonalcoholic fatty liver disease: a population-based retrospective cohort study. *Medicine*. 2018;97(42):e12835.

136. Guo Z, Li M, Han B, Qi X. Association of non-alcoholic fatty liver disease with thyroid function: a systematic review and meta-analysis. *Dig Liver Dis*. 2018;50(11):1153-1162.

137. Rafiq N, Bai C, Fang Y, et al. Long-term follow-up of patients with nonalcoholic fatty liver. *Clin Gastroenterol Hepatol*. 2009;7(2):234-238.

138. Li J, Wu Q, Wu XK, et al. Effect of exposure to second-hand smoke from husbands on biochemical hyperandrogenism, metabolic syndrome and conception rates in women with polycystic ovary syndrome undergoing ovulation induction. *Hum Reprod*. 2018;33(4):617-625.

139. Mykhalchenko K, Lizneva D, Trofimova T, et al. Genetics of polycystic ovary syndrome. *Expert Rev Mol Diagn*. 2017;17(7):723-733.

140. Risal S, Pei Y, Lu H, et al. Prenatal androgen exposure and transgenerational susceptibility to polycystic ovary syndrome. *Nat Med*. 2019;25(12):1894-1904.

141. Hogg K, Wood C, McNeilly AS, Duncan WC. The in utero programming effect of increased maternal androgens and a direct fetal intervention on liver and metabolic function in adult sheep. *PLoS One*. 2011;6(9):e24877.

142. Yan X, Dai X, Wang J, Zhao N, Cui Y, Liu J. Prenatal androgen excess programs metabolic derangements in pubertal female rats. *J Endocrinol*. 2013;217(1):119-129.

143. Ayonrinde OT, Oddy WH, Adams LA, et al. Infant nutrition and maternal obesity influence the risk of non-alcoholic fatty liver disease in adolescents. *J Hepatol*. 2017;67(3):568-576.

144. de Wilde MA, Eising JB, Gunning MN, et al. Cardiovascular and metabolic health of 74 children from women previously diagnosed with polycystic ovary syndrome in comparison with a population-based reference cohort. *Reprod Sci*. 2018;25(10):1492-1500.

145. Gunning MN, Sir Petermann T, Crisosto N, et al. Cardiometabolic health in offspring of women with PCOS compared to healthy controls: a systematic review and individual participant data meta-analysis. *Hum Reprod Update*. 2020;26(1):104-118.

146. Grieger JA, Bianco-Miotto T, Grzeskowiak LE, et al. Metabolic syndrome in pregnancy and risk for adverse pregnancy outcomes: a prospective cohort of nulliparous women. *PLoS Med*. 2018;15(12):e1002710.

13

Male Polycystic Ovary Syndrome Equivalent

AHMED SAYED METTAWI

Introduction

Polycystic ovary syndrome (PCOS) is one of the most common and well-established metabolic and endocrine disorders of females of childbearing age.[1] Up to 13% of females in the reproductive age group are estimated to be affected by the condition, although a huge proportion of them go undiagnosed (i.e., 70%).[2] The associated distressing features and complications are usually the reason why patients seek medical care; these include but are not limited to abnormal menstrual cycles, infertility, hirsutism and acne, metabolic complications (i.e., weight gain, diabetes mellitus [DM], metabolic syndrome [MetS]), and eating and mood disorders.[2]

The condition has been studied since 1935 when it was referred to as Stein-Leventhal syndrome, with polycystic ovaries being an essential component of the syndrome.[3] Over the years, the underlying pathophysiology and dysmetabolic background have been clarified to a great extent and many of the features have been agreed on (i.e., insulin insensitivity, hyperandrogenism [HA], and gonadotropin dysregulation).[1] It has been hypothesized that most cases share similar upstream aberrations (i.e., steroidogenesis or insulin abnormalities) but can differ in their downstream presentations; a polycystic ovarian morphology (PCO) would be a notable example because it only presents in 80% and can also be discovered in normal individuals.[3] Indeed, because of the broad spectrum of presentations, and to avoid confusion, many organizations sought to come up with criteria that could help clinicians reach a correct diagnosis (i.e., The National Institutes of Health [NIH], the Androgen Excess Society, and the European Society for Human Reproduction and Embryology/American Society for Reproductive Medicine [ESHRE/ASRM] or the Rotterdam consensus), ending with the most recent 2018 international PCOS guideline that built on the Rotterdam criteria (Table 13.1).[2,4] The NIH published evidence-based recommendations in their 2012 methodology workshop outlining the need to report PCOS phenotypes in research

and detailing the four phenotypes (Table 13.2).[4] It is worth noting that the diagnosis of PCOS is one of exclusion because many features overlap with other disorders (e.g., thyroid disorders, hyperprolactinemia, nonclassic congenital adrenal hyperplasia).[2]

Evidence that suggests the presence of an equivalent PCOS-like condition in males, especially in relatives of females with PCOS, has been accumulating over the years. Indeed, given that similar upstream PCOS aberrations were being observed in males, how broad the spectrum of PCOS presentation in females is, and how many authors believe that the "PCOS" naming is misleading (i.e., with "Stein-Leventhal syndrome" being a less confusing term), it is no wonder that the hypothesis that PCOS has a male equivalent has existed for long.[1,3]

The purpose of this chapter is to review the current literature that studies the equivalent PCOS condition in males, the observations found in relatives of females with PCOS, the risks associated with the condition in males, the sex differences, and the consensus statements on the topic and to provide clinical guidance on how to translate all that into useful recommendations for screening and diagnosis.

Findings in Male Relatives of Females With PCOS

Findings in male relatives (especially first-degree ones) of PCOS female patients support the hypothesis of a male PCOS equivalent. Starting off with genetic studies (from as early as 1989), the clustering and inheritance of PCOS was believed to be primarily autosomal dominant in nature and was found in association with a premature baldness trait in males, suggesting that a single gene might be responsible.[5-8] Incidentally, it seems that genetic polymorphism of the follicle-stimulating hormone (FSH) B (FSHB) gene promoter is associated with a similar background PCOS hormonal pattern in males (i.e., higher luteinizing hormone [LH] and lower FSH); FSHB is a susceptibility locus on

TABLE 13.1	**Evolution of the Diagnostic Criteria for Polycystic Ovary Syndrome Over the Years**			
Criteria and Date	NIH 1990	Rotterdam (ESHRE/ASRM) 2003	AE-PCOS Society 2006	International PCOS Evidence-Based Guidelines 2018
Items	1. Chronic anovulation/Menstrual dysfunction 2. Clinical and/or biochemical evidence of hyperandrogenism	1. Oligo- or anovulation 2. Clinical and/or biochemical evidence of hyperandrogenism 3. Polycystic ovarian morphology	1. Clinical and/or biochemical evidence of hyperandrogenism 2. Ovarian dysfunction and/or polycystic ovarian morphology	Endorses the 2003 Rotterdam criteria with emphasis that the ovarian morphology is unnecessary within 8 years postmenarche Females at-risk are monitored for fulfilling criteria over time More focus on clinical than laboratory/ultrasound assessments
Items needed for diagnosis	Both	2 out of 3	Both	Same as Rotterdam 2003 but without the polycystic ovary morphology in adolescents

AE-PCOS Society, The Androgen Excess and PCOS Society; *ESHRE/ASRM*, European Society for Human Reproduction and Embryology/American Society for Reproductive Medicine; *NIH*, National Institutes of Health; *PCOS*, polycystic ovary syndrome.
Adapted from Aversa A, la Vignera S, Rago R, et al. Fundamental concepts and novel aspects of polycystic ovarian syndrome: expert consensus resolutions. *Front Endocrinol (Lausanne)*. 2020;11(516); Teede H, Misso M, Costello M, et al. International evidence-based guideline for the assessment and management of polycystic ovary syndrome. Monash University. 2018. Monash.edu/medicine/sphpm/mchri/pcos; and NIH Evidence-Based Workshop Panel. NIH evidence-based workshop on polycystic ovary syndrome. 2012. http://prevention.nih.gov/workshops/2012/pcos/resources.aspx.

TABLE 13.2	**PCOS Various Phenotypes According to the NIH Evidence-Based Methodology Workshop[4]**		
Phenotype A	Phenotype B	Phenotype C	Phenotype D
• Hyperandrogenism • Ovulatory dysfunction • PCO morphology	• Hyperandrogenism • Ovulatory dysfunction	• Hyperandrogenism • PCO morphology	• Ovulatory dysfunction • PCO morphology

Phenotypes have subtypes with or without obesity.
NIH, National Institutes of Health; *PCO*, polycystic ovarian; *PCOS*, polycystic ovary syndrome.

chromosome 11p14.1 that was later proven to be strongly associated with PCOS and LH levels in females in the genome-wide association studies (GWAS) and such an association strongly supports the hypothesis of genetic inheritance of PCOS-like abnormalities in female patients' relatives.[9,10]

Because of the increasing interest in studying hormonal differences in male relatives of those with PCOS, a number of studies were conducted, albeit few, and their findings did identify a possible strong association between having a PCOS condition in a first-degree relative and the display of similar abnormalities. Brothers of PCOS patients do seem to exhibit the following compared with control groups: higher dehydroepiandrosterone sulfate (DHEAS) levels (and their sisters without PCOS seem to have higher DHEAS and testosterone too)[11,12]; higher basal anti-Müllerian hormone (AMH), LH, and FSH levels (fathers seem to exhibit the same abnormalities)[13]; exaggerated LH and FSH responses to gonadotropin-releasing hormone (GnRH) stimulation testing[14] (i.e., further augmenting the higher upstream defect, like gonadotropin-release defects, hypothesis). AMH levels seem to be higher in prepubertal sons of PCOS female patients.[15] Many of the studies suffer from sample size limitations that preclude further generalization of some findings (especially those pertaining to premature balding in PCOS patients' relatives).

Cardiovascular Disease and Other Risks in PCOS Patient Relatives

A growing body of evidence has been shedding light on the increased cardiovascular disease (CVD) risk in first-degree male relatives of patients with PCOS.[16,17] Taylor and colleagues attributed the reason CVD risk is not increased in females to two possibilities[17]: the abnormalities in their risk factors were not enough to raise the CVD 10-year risk (i.e., their study was calculated using the Framingham coronary heart disease [CHD] score and in reference to the National Health and Nutrition Examination Survey [NHANES] population) and/or the presence of some protective PCOS aspects (i.e., higher ovarian reserve) in females with the condition.

It has been suggested that male relatives of PCOS patients are at increased risk for metabolic disorders (i.e. obesity, DM, hypertension, and dyslipidemia),[18] although the increased risk for MetS was attributed to the increased obesity prevalence in such a population, in contrast to the independent effect of androgens on the MetS risk in females, by Coviello and colleagues in their NHANES-compared cross-sectional study.[19] In a meta-analysis by Yilmaz and colleagues, they drew the conclusion that first-degree relatives have an increased risk for MetS, hypertension, and dyslipidemia, even though they pointed out several limitations to their approach and the included studies (i.e., all were cross-sectional, in English and from PubMed only, sampling was from endocrinology/gynecologic clinics, and there was the possible use of different diagnostic criteria).[20]

Brothers of PCOS patients exhibited impaired endothelial function (i.e., measured by flow-mediated dilatation [FMD]), especially if they had a family history of DM[21]; they also had higher blood pressures and lipid profiles than controls. Kaushal and colleagues were unable to find the same FMD reduction in females with PCOS who did not have a DM family history (i.e., in contrast to the finding in the male groups).

Only a handful of studies examined the relationship between insulin resistance (IR) and having a PCOS first-degree relative. In their study, Kaushal and colleagues also demonstrated an impaired insulin sensitivity (i.e., measured by the short insulin tolerance test) in male and female relatives, and having a family history of DM only significantly impaired the sensitivity in females.[21] This result goes along with the result of a previous study by Norman and colleagues that showed that hyperinsulinemia was prevalent in almost 70% of the sample (i.e., premature baldness seemed like an important prevalent finding in males of the, albeit small-sized, sample too).[22] Yilmaz and colleagues used data of age and body mass index (BMI)–matched controls and demonstrated that first-degree relatives of PCOS patients had significantly higher IR indices (i.e., homeostatic model assessment [HOMA IR], area under the curve for insulin during the oral glucose tolerance test [AUCI, AUCG], and others) while having significantly lower insulin sensitivity ones (i.e. insulin sensitivity index [ISI], the quantitative insulin sensitivity check index [QUICKI]) and even lower serum adiponectin levels.[23]

Therefore, given the increased risk for metabolic and cardiovascular complications, a family history of a first-degree relative with PCOS should prompt the clinician to screen for/assess any present metabolic disorders. It is not yet clear, however, whether impaired fertility is associated with having a first-degree relative with PCOS.

Early-Onset Androgenic Alopecia: A Possible Male PCOS Equivalent Marker?

Background and Studied Nature of the Condition

Early-onset androgenic alopecia (AGA) (also known as premature male-pattern baldness [PMB]) could be defined as the loss of scalp hair from androgen-dependent areas (i.e., vertex and/or widow's peaks) at least at a grade III or more using the Hamilton-Norwood scale[24,25] (Fig. 13.1) before the age of 35 (with some authors advocating a cut-off age of 30; of note, both cut-offs were chosen arbitrarily[26]), possibly because of lengthier telogen phases, shorter anagen phases, and shorter hair each hair growth cycle (i.e., terminating in baldness).[1,26-28]

As mentioned previously, the findings indicating that PCOS and premature AGA share a single inheritable gene mutation[5,6] suggest that the latter sign could serve as a marker for a male PCOS-equivalent condition, especially because some authors observed a significant prevalence of premature AGA in first-degree male relatives of PCOS patients.[7,8] Notably, however, subsequent studies failed to find an observation of the same significance and attributed the relationship between premature AGA in the sample to chance; their samples of male relatives with premature AGA were so small, yet the authors still believed it was safe to state the same conclusions based on prior surveys of balding in the United States and reports suggesting that premature balding was not a reliable sign for male PCOS phenotype anymore in the UK.[11,12]

This specific male PCOS phenotype was first studied by Stárka and colleagues and their findings were later confirmed (i.e., lower sex hormone–binding globulin [SHBG] and similar sex hormonal profile) and further studied by Duskovà and colleagues.[29,30] In the latter study, the subgroup with lower SHBG, lower FSH, higher LH, and free androgen index (FAI) was found to have significantly higher IR than those, of similar age and BMI (i.e., all below 30), without the biochemical abnormalities (using the insulin tolerance test). Interestingly, SHBG was significantly lower in the PCOS hormonal pattern subgroup along with a significantly higher IR. Furthermore, the presence of no significant difference between subgroups in the frequency of the insulin gene (INS) polymorphism matches the result of previous attempts to study the relationship between premature AGA and insulin polymorphism—given the strong association between SHBG and insulin levels[31] and how insulin is believed to have a local role in hair follicle growth—thus making it more likely that other genes may be involved (as stated previously).[27,30]

Indeed, a meta-analysis of studies with a total sample of 1009 unrelated males confirmed that those with premature AGA had significantly worse hormonal and glycolipid profiles resembling those of females with PCOS with the following notable differences in the premature AGA groups: lower levels of SHBG; high levels of LH and DHEAS; higher insulin, total cholesterol, triglycerides, and low-density lipoprotein (LDL) levels; and higher HOMA indices (even in the studies using BMI-matched controls).[32] The results go along with those of the authors' (i.e., Cannarella and colleagues) future works and those of other systematic reviews as well.[28,33,34] Table 13.3 provides an excellent summary of the reported findings (biochemical and clinical) in studies of males with AGA (premature and old) and of male relatives of females with PCOS.

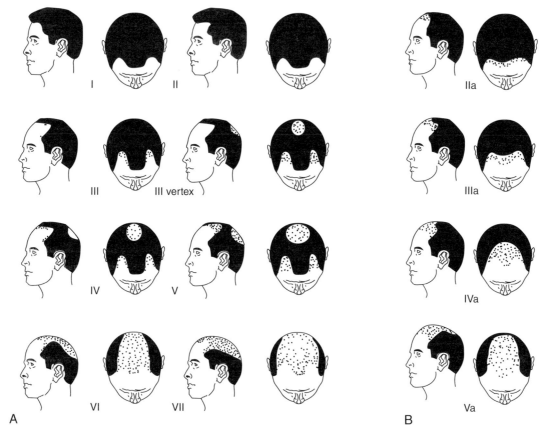

• **Fig. 13.1** Hamilton-Norwood Scale (Common and Variant Types). The left (A) shows the most common presentations of male-pattern baldness of grades I to VII and the right (B) shows the variant forms of grades II to V (IIa–Va). Type III, which is regarded by some authors as the minimum grade that defines premature androgenic alopecia (AGA), is characterized by having bilateral frontotemporal recessions extending posteriorly beyond a coronal line connecting two points lying 2 cm anterior to each external auditory meatus (there are also vertex and type A variants). For a detailed description of the other types, especially those relevant to the premature AGA definition (i.e., IV–VII), please check the main reference.[25] (From Norwood OT. Male pattern baldness: Classification and incidence. *South Med J.* 1975;68(11): 1359–1365; Figures 1 & 2.)

Sex Hormone–Binding Globulin as an Important Marker

As mentioned, a low SHBG level seems to be a frequent finding among those with early-onset AGA. Additionally, it does seem linked to higher insulin levels and glucose intolerance.[31] Although it is not widely accepted that IR contributes to the pathogenesis of AGA, it can still worsen the condition by increasing free androgens and lowering SHBG further. As such, SHBG level normalization remains an important therapeutic target (i.e., expected to normalize after losing weight or through nutritional/lifestyle interventions).[35] Notwithstanding the somewhat small sample sizes used, Arias-Santiago and colleagues concluded that a low SHBG level could serve as a marker of IR in premature AGA patients (i.e., strongly associated with higher glucose levels regardless of sex, BMI, or FAI), yet Narad and colleagues reported significantly lower SHBG levels in the premature AGA group compared with age-matched controls with similar metabolic profiles.[36,37] The subjects of the former case-controlled study were older (i.e., 45–60 years

old) than those of the latter (i.e., younger than 30 years old), which raises the hypothesis that AGA patients with low SHBG could be at risk for developing IR later in life, making it worthwhile to consider testing for it to predict the risk. This goes along with the conclusions of other authors who proposed that early-onset AGA could serve as a marker of IR regardless of BMI.[32,38]

Circulating Androgen Levels and Sex Differences

The nature of HA in studied males could be one of the sex differences in the manifestation of a PCOS-like condition. Contrary to the female equivalent, hypertestosteronemia does not seem to be a part of the male-equivalent syndrome (i.e., even when increased, it is usually within normal range) and reports of the FAI are conflicting.[30,33,39] Indeed, the level of clinical HA is usually out of proportion to the level of free testosterone; thus it is imperative to suspect that the role of other androgens (especially adrenal ones like DHEAS or even less-studied ones like the 11-oxygenated C19 steroids), and/or their peripheral conversion to stronger ones,

TABLE 13.3 Differences in Reported Findings (Clinical and/or Biochemical) Between Male Relatives of PCOS Patients, Unrelated Males With Premature AGA, and Elderly Males with AGA

Parameters	Male Relatives of Females With PCOS	Males With premature AGA	Elderly Males With AGA
Serum-free testosterone levels	–	↑	–
Serum SHBG levels	–	↓	–
Free testosterone index	–	↑	–
Serum LH levels	–	↑	–
Serum FSH levels	–	↓	–
LH/FSH ratio	–	↑	–
LH and FSH response to GnRH analogs	↑	–	–
Serum AMH levels	↑	–	–
Serum DHEAS levels	↑	↑	–
Serum 17 Alpha hydroxyprogesterone (17α-OHP)	–	↑	–
Serum adiponectin levels	↑	–	–
Serum glucose levels	–	↑	–
Serum insulin levels	↑	↑	↑
Risk for insulin resistance	↑	↑	–
Serum cholesterol levels	↑	↑	–
Risk for metabolic syndrome	–	↑	↑
Risk for type 2 diabetes mellitus	–	–	↑
Risk for endothelial dysfunction	↑	–	–
Blood pressure	↑	↑	↑
Serum aldosterone levels	–	–	↑
Serum fibrinogen levels	–	–	↑
Risk for atheromatous plaques	–	–	↑
Risk for ischemic heart disease	–	–	↑
Risk for benign prostate hyperplasia	–	–	↑
Risk for prostate cancer	–	–	↑

Table is based on work published elsewhere.[33]

↑, Increased; ↓, decreased; –, not-reported. *AGA*, androgenetic alopecia; *AMH*, anti-Müllerian hormone; *DHEAS*, dehydroepiandrosterone sulfate; *FSH*, follicle-stimulating hormone; *GnRH*, gonadotropin-realizing hormone; *LH*, luteinizing hormone; *SHBG*, sex hormone binding globulin.
Adapted from Cannarella R, Condorelli RA, Barbagallo F, la Vignera S, Calogero AE. Endocrinology of the aging prostate: current concepts. *Front Endocrinol.* 2021;12:554078; Table 1.

might be in play.[26] One interesting explanation of the difference in testosterone profiles in sexes is the likely different actions of insulin on gonadal theca and Leydig cells where it stimulates steroidogenesis in the former, thereby increasing testosterone production in females, but inhibits it in the latter, which predisposes to a less than normal testosterone in males.[40,41] There also seems to be an independent role of IR and acne regardless of HA.[42,43] More interestingly, the interplay between androgens, fat mass, and fat-free mass seem to differ slightly between sexes. Higher circulating androgens seem to cause adipocyte hypertrophy while favoring a male-pattern fat distribution (i.e., abdominal obesity)[44]; this is normally off-set in males by the higher increase in fat-free mass, which favors the metabolic profile (although protection can be lost with aging processes and can lead to sarcopenia/sarcopenic obesity).[45] The novel idea of the exposure to endocrine disruptors in the environment and its possible role in obesity and PCOS does seem like an interesting research target.[46]

As previously noted, BMI does not seem pathognomonic for PCOS even though its presence can worsen the metabolic and hormonal disturbances in place.[28,33] So a non-obese phenotype male with the syndrome could still be expected to present to clinicians, and this is in line with the finding of PCOS in slender females.[33] A slender male with premature AGA and PCOS-like hormonal alteration would be at risk for developing abdominal obesity later on in life and thus would still benefit from a healthier lifestyle earlier.[35,46]

Cannarella and colleagues managed to provide a summary of all the possible etiopathogenetic mechanisms and how they relate to each other contributing to the development of a PCOS equivalent in males, which can be found in Fig. 13.2.

Risks Associated With AGA

Cardiovascular Disease and Metabolic Syndrome Risks

Premature AGA is associated with significant cardiovascular and metabolic risks. Starting off with the association with MetS, the literature is filled with conflicting results concerning its association with AGA in males.[47-52] A meta-analysis conducted by Wu and colleagues, however, confirmed that AGA does correlate well with MetS in both sexes and in different populations (i.e., European and Asian).[53] Given that

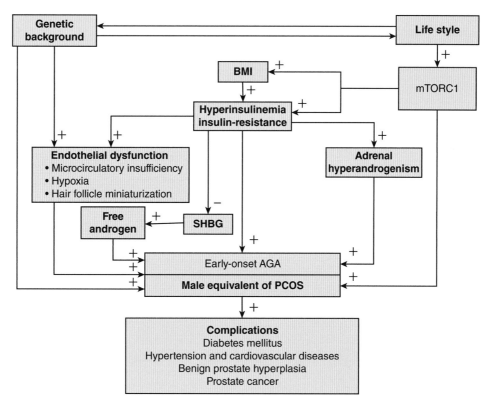

• **Fig. 13.2** Possible Pathogenetic Mechanisms Behind the Male-equivalent Polycystic Ovary Syndrome *(PCOS)* Condition and Its Complications. The figure represents an illustration of the various hypothesized mechanisms thought to be responsible for the development of the male equivalent PCOS condition. An overactive mechanistic target of rapamycin kinase *(mTORC)* signaling, presumably because of hyperalimentation and/or hyperglycemia, predisposes to obesity, insulin resistance (IR), type 2 diabetes mellitus (DM), hypertension, and cancer and can accelerate the hair growth cycle, which, together with hyperinsulinemia and the accompanying endothelial dysfunction, culminates in the development of androgenetic alopecia *(AGA)*. On the other hand, a lower sex hormone binding globulin *(SHBG)* level can lead to impaired glycemic control, and hyperinsulinemia causes adrenal hyperandrogenism, which is more prevalent among males with premature AGA (i.e., androgen receptor hyperactivation is also associated with metabolic disorders). *BMI,* Body mass index. (From Cannarella R, Condorelli RA, Mongioì LM, la Vignera S, Calogero AE. Does a male polycystic ovarian syndrome equivalent exist? J *Endocrinol Invest.* 2018;41(1):49-57; Figure 1).

a low testosterone level represents a frequent finding in premature AGA patients, their result further augments those of meta-analyses of observational studies that showed that MetS is an independent risk factor for male hypogonadism and predisposes to high CVD risk.[54,55]

Studies on CVD risk in AGA patients augments what was described in PCOS patient relatives.[1] In particular, the vertex variant of AGA seems associated the most with coronary artery disease risk (i.e., risk of myocardial infarction can be 3.4-fold higher), and the association is stronger in those with hypertension or high cholesterol levels; adjusting for confounders did not alter the risk association with vertex AGA in the physician health study (with 22,071 male physicians as subjects).[56,57] Data from the NHANES-I and the Framingham studies previously suggested that rapid progression of baldness and severe forms of AGA were highly associated with coronary artery disease, cardiovascular mortality, and all-cause mortality.[58,59] A population-based prospective cohort study with 2429 male participants later confirmed that AGA is associated with high CVD mortality

risk independent of MetS.[60] Indeed, Trieu and colleagues published a meta-analysis of 29,254 subjects with alopecia showing a positive correlation—with a dose-response relationship—between AGA and CHD risk in both sexes in addition to increased risks of MetS, hypertension, IR, and dyslipidemia.

Risk of Compromising Male Fertility

There is a need for the effect of AGA on male infertility to be further investigated (i.e., the finding of low FSH levels provided one of the hints) because the literature is scarce when it comes to such studies and results are confusing.[33] Previously, sons of females with PCOS were studied by Recabarren and colleagues and were found to have significantly higher, albeit normal, testicular volumes and AMH levels together with normal semen analysis (i.e., it could be a compensated decrease in semen production per increased number of Sertoli cells).[15] When it comes to IR and effect on male fertility, a study by Verit et al. failed to find a difference in testicular volumes or semen analysis.[61] More recently, Güngor and colleagues did find significantly worse semen parameters (i.e., volume, count, motility, and morphology) among those with Hamilton-Norwood scale scores of III or IV.[62] A subsequent study by Cannarella and colleagues showed only a significant increase in frequency of sperm apoptosis among AGA patients in addition to being at risk for having lower testicular volumes in the presence of other risk factors such as IR, lower SHBG, or higher BMI (i.e., volumes of left testes were significantly lower in the study).[34] Their conclusion that males with AGA are at risk for gonadal dysfunction in the future seems like a valid cautious one at this point until further research results are available.

Prostate-Related Risks

Existing evidence strongly points to an association between AGA and prostate disorders. Males with AGA (especially if early-onset and severe) were found to have a higher frequency of larger prostates, benign prostatic hyperplasia (BPH), prostatitis, elevated prostate-specific antigen (PSA) levels, androgen receptor gene polymorphism (SNP rs6152), high international prostate symptom scores (IPSS), and lower maximum urinary flow at an older age.[63-66] Some authors even concluded AGA could serve as an early marker for BPH, but others disagreed because the predisposition to BPH remains multifactorial in nature (with other factors

having common associations with AGA and BPH).[66,67] Interestingly, a recent meta-analysis showed that PSA levels are significantly higher in females with PCOS; the significance of the finding is yet to be further investigated.[68] In terms of prostate cancer (PCa) risk, a meta-analysis by Amoretti and colleagues showed that those with vertex AGA are at a significantly increased risk for the cancer, although the studies included had methodologic flaws including absence of information about age of presentation and some of them did not evaluate vertex balding.[69]

The aging prostate and its associated abnormalities seem to be influenced by a myriad of hormonal interactions (and the presence of comorbid conditions such as obesity, MetS, IR, and thyroid dysfunction), a detailed coverage of which was provided in a very comprehensive recent review by Cannarella and colleauges.[70] Fig. 13.3 provides an excellent summary of the various hormonal effects. The case with testosterone-mediated effects is quite the interesting one. It is a well-known fact that it plays a role in intrauterine development of the prostate by acting on androgen receptors after its conversion to the more potent dihydro-testosterone (DHT). Later in life and contrary to popular belief, testosterone's effect on prostate cell proliferation does seem to follow a saturation model with a sigmoid curve where increases in serum values up to a level of 8nmol/L can cause increases

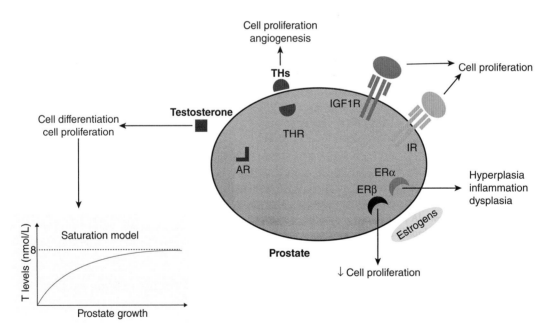

• **Fig. 13.3** Summary of the Hormonal Effects in the Prostatic Tissue. Although testosterone is essential for the development of the prostate gland during intranatal life, it does seem to follow a saturation model later in life where serum levels are well correlated with cell proliferation up to a certain point (i.e., saturation of receptors at around 8 nmol/L). Thyroid hormones do have an enhancing action through their receptors on prostate cell proliferation and angiogenesis. IR and IGF-1 interactions induce proliferations. Endogenous estrogens differ in their actions according to their type and receptors affected: 17β-estradiol (E2, a product of aromatization) and actions on ERα stimulate proliferation; actions on ERβ inhibit it. *AR*, Androgen receptor; *ERα*, estrogen receptor alpha; *ERβ*, estrogen receptor beta *IGF1*, insulin-like growth factor 1; *IGF1R*, insulin-like growth factor 1 receptor; *IR*, insulin resistance; *T*, testosterone; *THs*, thyroid hormones; *THR*, thyroid hormone receptor. (Adapted from Cannarella R, Condorelli RA, Barbagallo F, la Vignera S, and Calogero AE. Endocrinology of the aging prostate: current concepts. *Front Endocrinol.* 2021;12:554078.)

in cell proliferation and greater rises in PSA.[70] Studies on PCa and its castration-resistant subtype provide further pieces of the picture, given also the controversial nature of the topic of testosterone replacement in patients with a history of PCa. It has been suggested that other weak androgens like DHEAS or androstenedione are metabolized to the more potent DHT inside prostatic tissue, and Storbeck and colleagues postulated that the less-studied 11-oxy C19 steroids (i.e., 11keto DHT and 11Beta-hydroxy DHT) probably have similar effects on androgen receptors and concentrations to DHT.[71] Estrogen, however, has an effect that differs according to its type and the type of receptor activated: estrone (E1) and estriol (E3) are present in minimal concentrations and have little effect on the prostate; 17β-estradiol (E2), which is produced after the aromatization of testosterone by fat cells, exhibits a potent proliferation effect on prostate cells. Estrogen receptor alpha stimulates, whereas the beta ones inhibit the process and higher activation of the former than the latter results in proliferation.[70] Thyroid hormones have a stimulatory role on prostatic proliferation, but their age-related decline makes them unlikely to be contributors to the pathogenesis of BPH and other disorders.[70] Similar arguments could be made in the case of insulin-like growth factor 1 (IGF1) and its effect on prostate cell proliferation because it declines with age; nevertheless, IGF1 is elevated in DM and acromegaly, and acromegalic patients with inactive disease for more than 2 years exhibit reductions in their previously enlarged prostatic volumes.[70] MetS and its components, especially IR, are associated with BPH, and there is evidence suggesting there is a role of antidiabetic drugs, like metformin, in reducing PCa incidence and improving survival.[70]

Conclusions and Final Remarks

A male-equivalent condition for PCOS does exist, has been under study for more than a decade, and most of its features are now universally agreed on. First-degree male relatives of

females with PCOS inherit the condition or some of its features and are at similar, if not worse, cardiovascular and metabolic risks. Premature AGA is a distinct clinical feature that is accompanied by PCOS-like features and is associated with similar risks. Nevertheless, the spectrum of manifestations is quite wide (Table 13.4); not all males with premature AGA have PCOS-equivalent disorders, and even those with later-onset AGA can have a PCOS-like condition, making screening for the condition even in such a population worth it.[26,30,33] Given a prevalence of 30% for premature AGA[72] and 4% to 7% for PCOS[73] in the general population, an approximate 15% to 25% of males with premature AGA would be expected to have a PCOS-equivalent condition, supposing that both sexes have a similar prevalence of PCOS.[33] It is worth noting that the name of the condition (i.e., PCOS) confuses the general public and medical community about what it really constitutes even when speaking about the female syndrome, and it would be for the best to rename it to something more descriptive of the current understanding of the syndrome in both sexes (i.e., Stein-Leventhal can be used for the time being).

There seems to be a sex-unique perception of the clinical manifestations of the syndrome, which could partly explain the delay in recognition of the syndrome in males.[3,33] Males are far less likely to seek medical care and endocrinologic counseling for, for example, premature AGA because it could be viewed as normal for the male sex; females, however, do frequently seek counseling for menstrual abnormalities and signs of HA. Nevertheless, because the risks males with the syndrome are exposed to are substantial, one could venture to reach out to such a population using the following strategies[1,33]:

1. Screening first-degree male relatives of the presenting PCOS female patients for metabolic and cardiovascular and hormonal abnormalities
2. Monitoring bodyweight and glycolipid profiles of males with premature AGA (i.e., Hamilton-Norwood grade of III or more) starting from the second decade of life, and

Proposed Characteristic Features of the Male Equivalent of Polycystic Ovary Syndrome Per Age Group

Age	Features of the Male PCOS Equivalent
<35 years	1. Clinical signs of hyperandrogenism (early-onset AGA and/or acne and/or hypertrichosis) 2. PCOS-like hormonal pattern (increased DHEAS, AMH, 17α-OHP, FAI, decreased FSH) 3. Metabolic abnormalities (insulin-resistance, low SHBG levels, hyperglycemia, hyperinsulinemia) and/or a trend toward higher BMI values 4. A family history of PCOS
Elderly	Diabetes mellitus, cardiovascular diseases, benign prostatic hyperplasia, prostatitis, prostate cancer

The conditions listed could help the specialist to suspect the syndrome earlier in life. Similar to PCOS in females, features seem to vary with age. The syndrome predisposes to long-term complications in males too and thus is important to diagnose early.

17α-OHP, Serum 17 Alpha hydroxyprogesterone; AGA, androgenetic alopecia; AMH, anti-Müllerian hormone; BMI, body mass index; DHEAS, dehydroepiandrosterone sulfate; FAI, free androgen index; FSH, follicle-stimulating hormone; LH, luteinizing hormone; PCOS, polycystic ovary syndrome; SHBG, sex hormone–binding globulin.

From Cannarella R, Condorelli RA, Mongioì LM, la Vignera S, Calogero AE. Does a male polycystic ovarian syndrome equivalent exist? J Endocrinol Invest. 2018;41(1):49-57; Table 3.

the same can be recommended for severe AGA and vertex AGA variants regardless of age

3. Searching for the syndrome and its associated comorbidities and risks in those with the conditions listed in Table 13.4

According to a recent expert consensus, a diagnosis can be made in the presence of PCOS-like hormonal abnormalities, metabolic abnormalities, and/or higher BMI, and/or clinical evidence of HA (especially early-onset AGA) in a young patient with family history of PCOS.[1] Precise diagnostic criteria for the syndrome in males need to be thoroughly researched to come up with ones as comprehensive as the ones used in females.[26]

Finally, proper and early identification of the syndrome in males allows for the initiation of therapeutic choices that target the metabolic abnormalities to prevent complications. Similar lifestyle interventions to those prescribed to females with PCOS can be employed in males (preferably with at least a 5% body weight loss as one of the goals for those with higher BMI); these include hypocaloric and high protein diets, meal replacement, intermittent fasting, and exercise programs.[2,35] Nutraceuticals as inositols, especially Myo-inositol (MI) and D-chiro-inositol (DCI), and alpha lipoic acid have insulin-sensitizing actions and, together with vitamin D supplementation (i.e., for the deficient), serve as treatment options.[35,74] Future studies are needed to compare the different lifestyle interventions together with potential pharmacologic therapies (i.e., metformin and finasteride) and understand which is more effective for the treatment of this male syndrome's various aspects.[33,35]

References

1. Aversa A, la Vignera S, Rago R, et al. Fundamental concepts and novel aspects of polycystic ovarian syndrome: expert consensus resolutions. *Front Endocrinol (Lausanne).* 2020;11:516. doi:10.3389/fendo.2020.00516.

2. Teede H, Misso M, Costello M, et al. *International Evidence-Based Guideline for the Assessment and Management of Polycystic Ovary Syndrome.* Melbourne Australia; Monash University. 2018. Available at: monash.edu/medicine/sphpm/mchri/pcos.

3. Kurzrock R, Cohen PR. Polycystic ovary syndrome in men: Stein–Leventhal syndrome revisited. *Med Hypotheses.* 2007;68(3):480-483.

4. NIH Evidence Based Workshop Panel. *NIH Evidence Based Workshop on Polycystic Ovary Syndrome.* 2012. Available at: https://prevention.nih.gov/sites/default/files/2018-06/FinalReport.pdf

5. Carey AH, Chan KL, Short F, White D, Williamson R, Franks S. Evidence for a single gene effect causing polycystic ovaries and male pattern baldness. *Clin Endocrinol.* 1993;38(1993):653-658.

6. Carey AH, Waterworth D, Patel K, et al. Polycystic ovaries and premature male pattern baldness are associated with one allele of the steroid metabolism gene CYP17. *Hum Mol Genet.* 1994;3(10):1873-1876.

7. Lunde O, Magnus P, Sandvik L, Heglo S. Familial clustering in the polycystic ovarian syndrome. *Gynecol Obstet Invest.* 1989;28(1):23-30. doi:10.1159/000293493.

8. Govind A, Obhrai S, Clayton RN. Polycystic ovaries are inherited as an autosomal dominant trait: analysis of 29 polycystic ovary syndrome and 10 control families. *J Clin Endocrinol Metab.* 1999;84(1):38-43. doi:10.1210/jcem.84.1.5382.

9. Tüttelmann F, Laan M, Grigorova M, Punab M, Sõber S, Gromoll J. Combined effects of the variants FSHB-211G>T and FSHR 2039A>G on male reproductive parameters. *J Clin Endocrinol Metab.* 2012;97(10):3639-3647. doi:10.1210/jc.2012-1761.

10. Hayes MG, Urbanek M, Ehrmann DA, et al. Genome-wide association of polycystic ovary syndrome implicates alterations in gonadotropin secretion in European ancestry populations. *Nat Commun.* 2015;6(1):7502. doi:10.1038/ncomms8502.

11. Legro RS, Kunselman AR, Demers L, Wang SC, Bentley-Lewis R, Dunaif A. Elevated dehydroepiandrosterone sulfate levels as the reproductive phenotype in the brothers of women with polycystic ovary syndrome. *J Clin Endocrinol Metab.* 2002;87(5):2134-2138. doi:10.1210/jcem.87.5.8387.

12. Lenarcik A, Bidzińska-Speichert B, Tworowska-Bardzińska U, Krępuła K. Hormonal abnormalities in first-degree relatives of women with polycystic ovary syndrome (PCOS). *Endokrynol Pol.* 2011;62(2):129-133.

13. Torchen LC, Kumar A, Kalra B, et al. Increased antimüllerian hormone levels and other reproductive endocrine changes in adult male relatives of women with polycystic ovary syndrome. *Fertil Steril.* 2016;106(1):50-55. doi:10.1016/j.fertnstert.2016.03.029.

14. Liu DM, Torchen LC, Sung Y, et al. Evidence for gonadotrophin secretory and steroidogenic abnormalities in brothers ofwomenwith polycystic ovary syndrome. *Hum Reprod.* 2014;29(12):2764-2772.

15. Recabarren SE, Sir-Petermann T, Rios R, et al. Pituitary and testicular function in sons of women with polycystic ovary syndrome from infancy to adulthood. *J Clin Endocrinol Metab.* 2008;93(9):3318-3324. doi:10.1210/jc.2008-0255.

16. Hunter A, Vimplis S, Sharma A, Eid N, Atiomo W. To determine whether first-degree male relatives of women with polycystic ovary syndrome are at higher risk of developing cardiovascular disease and type II diabetes mellitus. *J Obstet Gynaecol.* 2007;27(6):591-596. doi:10.1080/01443610701497520.

17. Taylor MC, Kar AR, Kunselman AR, Stetter CM, Dunaif A, legro RS. Evidence for increased cardiovascular events in the fathers but not mothers of women with polycystic ovary syndrome. *Hum Reprod.* 2011;26(8):2226-2231. doi:10.1093/humrep/der101.

18. Benítez R, Sir-Petermann T, Palomino A, et al. Prevalence of metabolic disorders among family members of patients with polycystic ovary syndrome. *Rev Med Chil.* 2001;129(7):707-712. doi:10.4067/S0034-98872001000700001.

19. Coviello AD, Sam S, legro RS, Dunaif A. High prevalence of metabolic syndrome in first-degree male relatives of women with polycystic ovary syndrome is related to high rates of obesity. *J Clin Endocrinol Metab.* 2009;94(11):4361-4366. doi:10.1210/jc.2009-1333.

20. Yilmaz B, Vellanki P, Ata B, Yildiz BO. Metabolic syndrome, hypertension, and hyperlipidemia in mothers, fathers, sisters, and brothers of women with polycystic ovary syndrome: a systematic review and meta-analysis. *Fertil Steril.* 2018;109(2):356-364.e32. doi:10.1016/j.fertnstert.2017.10.018.

21. Kaushal R, Parchure N, Bano G, Kaski JC, Nussey SS. Insulin resistance and endothelial dysfunction in the brothers of Indian subcontinent Asian women with polycystic ovaries. *Clin Endocrinol (Oxf).* 2004;60(3):322-328. doi:10.1111/j.1365-2265.2003.01981.x.

22. Norman RJ, Masters S, Hague W. Hyperinsulinemia is common in family members of women with polycystic ovary syndrome. *Fertil Steril.* 1996;66(6):942-947. doi:10.1016/s0015-0282(16)58687-7.

23. Yilmaz M, Bukan N, Ersoy R, et al. Glucose intolerance, insulin resistance and cardiovascular risk factors in first degree relatives of women with polycystic ovary syndrome. *Hum Reprod.* 2005;20(9):2414-2420. doi:10.1093/humrep/dei070.

24. Hamilton JB. Patterned loss of hair in man: types and incidence. *Ann N Y Acad Sci.* 1951;53(3):708-728. doi:10.1111/j.1749-6632.1951.tb31971.x.

25. Norwood OT. Male pattern baldness: classification and incidence. *South Med J.* 1975;68(11):1359-1365. doi:10.1097/00007611-197511000-00009.

26. Stárka L, Dušková M. Remarks on the hormonal background of the male equivalent of polycystic ovary syndrome. *Prague Med Rep.* 2021;122(2):73-79. doi:10.14712/23362936.2021.8.

27. Ellis JA, Stebbing M, Harrap SB. Insulin gene polymorphism and premature male pattern baldness in the general population. *Clin Sci.* 1999;96(6):659-662.

28. Di Guardo F, Ciotta L, Monteleone M, Palumbo M. Male equivalent polycystic ovarian syndrome: hormonal, metabolic and clinical aspects. *Int J Fertil Steril.* 2020;14(2):79-83. doi:10.22074/ijfs.2020.6092.

29. Stárka L, Hill M, Poláček V. Hormonal profile in men with premature androgenic alopecia. *Sb Lek.* 2000;101(1):17-22.

30. Dusková M, Cermáková I, Hill M, Vanková M, Sámalíková P, Stárka L. What may be the markers of the male equivalent of polycystic ovary syndrome? *Physiol Res.* 2004;53(3):287-294.

31. Golden SH, Dobs AS, Vaidya D, et al. Endogenous sex hormones and glucose tolerance status in postmenopausal women. *J Clin Endocrinol Metab.* 2007;92(4):1289-1295. doi:10.1210/jc.2006-1895.

32. Cannarella R, la Vignera S, Condorelli RA, Calogero AE. Glycolipid and hormonal profiles in young men with early-onset androgenetic alopecia: a meta-analysis. *Sci Rep.* 2017;7:7801. doi:10.1038/s41598-017-08528-3.

33. Cannarella R, Condorelli RA, Mongioì LM, la Vignera S, Calogero AE. Does a male polycystic ovarian syndrome equivalent exist? *J Endocrinol Invest.* 2018;41(1):49-57. doi:10.1007/s40618-017-0728-5.

34. Cannarella R, Condorelli RA, Dall'Oglio F, et al. Increased DHEAS and decreased total testosterone serum levels in a subset of men with early-onset androgenetic alopecia: does a male PCOS-equivalent exist? *Int J Endocrinol.* 2020;2020:1942126. doi:10.1155/2020/1942126.

35. Di Guardo F, Cerana MC, D'urso G, Genovese F, Palumbo M. Male PCOS equivalent and nutritional restriction: are we stepping forward? *Med Hypotheses.* 2019;126:1-3. doi:10.1016/j.mehy.2019.03.003.

36. Arias-Santiago S, Gutiérrez-Salmerón MT, Buendía-Eisman A, Girón-Prieto MS. Sex hormone-binding globulin and risk of hyperglycemia in patients with androgenetic alopecia. *Am Acad Dermatol.* 2011;65(1):48-53. doi:10.1016/j.jaad.2010.05.002.

37. Narad S, Pande S, Gupta M, Chari S. Hormonal profile in Indian men with premature androgenetic alopecia. *Int J Trichol.* 2013;5(2):69-72. doi:10.4103/0974-7753.122961.

38. Matilainen V, Koskela P, Keinänen-Kiukaanniemi S. Early androgenetic alopecia as a marker of insulin resistance. *Lancet.* 2000;356(9236):1165-1166. doi:10.1016/s0140-6736(00)02763-x.

39. Stárka L, Čermáková I, Dušková M, Hill M, Doležal M, Poláček V. Hormonal profile of men with premature balding. *Exp Clin Endocrinol Diabetes.* 2004;112(1):24-28. doi:10.1055/s-2004-815723.

40. Ahn SW, Gang G-T, Kim YD, et al. Insulin directly regulates steroidogenesis via induction of the orphan nuclear receptor DAX-1 in testicular Leydig cells. *J Biol Chem.* 2013;288(22):15937-15946. doi:10.1074/jbc.M113.451773.

41. Cadagan D, Khan R, Amer S. Thecal cell sensitivity to luteinizing hormone and insulin in polycystic ovarian syndrome. *Reprod Biol.* 2016;16(1):53-60. doi:10.1016/j.repbio.2015.12.006.

42. Del Prete M, Mauriello M, Faggiano A, et al. Insulin resistance and acne: a new risk factor for men? *Endocrine.* 2012;42(3):555-560. doi:10.1007/s12020-012-9647-6.

43. Nagpal M, De D, Handa S, Pal A, Sachdeva N. Insulin resistance and metabolic syndrome in young men with acne. *JAMA Dermatol.* 2016;152(4):399-404. doi:10.1001/jamadermatol.2015.4499.

44. Dimitriadis GK, Kyrou I, Randeva HS. Polycystic ovary syndrome as a proinflammatory state: the role of adipokines. *Curr Pharm Des.* 2016;22(36):5535-5546. doi:10.2174/1381612822666160726103133.

45. Escobar-Morreale HF, Alvarez-Blasco F, Botella-Carretero JI, Luque-Ramírez M. The striking similarities in the metabolic associations of female androgen excess and male androgen deficiency. *Hum Reprod.* 2014;29(10):2083-2091. doi:10.1093/humrep/deu198.

46. Šimková M, Vítků J, Kolátorová L, et al. Endocrine disruptors, obesity and cytokines – How relevant are they to PCOS? *Physiol Res.* 2020;69:S279-S293. doi:10.33549/physiolres.934521.

47. Ozbas Gok S, Akin Belli A, Dervis E. Is there really relationship between androgenetic alopecia and metabolic syndrome? *Dermatol Res Pract.* 2015;2015:980310. doi:10.1155/2015/980310.

48. Su LH, Chen THH. Association of androgenetic alopecia with metabolic syndrome in men: a community-based survey. *Br J Dermatol.* 2010;163(2):371-377. doi:10.1111/j.1365-2133.2010.09816.x.

49. Yi SM, Son SW, Lee KG, et al. Gender-specific association of androgenetic alopecia with metabolic syndrome in a middle-aged Korean population. *Br J Dermatol.* 2012;167(2):306-313. doi:10.1111/j.1365-2133.2012.10978.x.

50. Mumcuoglu C, Ekmekci TR, Ucak S. The investigation of insulin resistance and metabolic syndrome in male patients with early-onset androgenetic alopecia. *Eur J Dermatol.* 2011;21(1):79-82. doi:10.1684/ejd.2010.1193.

51. Pengsalae N, Tanglertsampan C, Phichawong T, Lee S. Association of early-onset androgenetic alopecia and metabolic syndrome in Thai men: a case-control study. *J Med Assoc Thai.* 2013;96(8):947-951.

52. Banger HS, Malhotra SK, Singh S, Mahajan M. Is early onset androgenic alopecia a marker of metabolic syndrome and carotid artery atherosclerosis in young Indian male patients? *Int J Trichology.* 2015;7(4):141-147. doi:10.4103/0974-7753.171566.

53. Wu DX, Wu LF, Yang ZX. Association between androgenetic alopecia and metabolic syndrome: a meta-analysis. *Zhejiang Da Xue Xue Bao Yi Xue Ban.* 2014;43(5):597-601. doi:10.3785/j.issn.1008-9292.2014.09.016.

54. Corona G, Maseroli E, Rastrelli G, et al. Cardiovascular risk associated with testosterone-boosting medications: a systematic review and meta-analysis. *Expert Opin Drug Saf.* 2014;13(10):1327-1351.

55. Corona G, Rastrelli G, Di Pasquale G, Sforza A, Mannucci E, Maggi M. Endogenous testosterone levels and cardiovascular risk: meta-analysis of observational studies. *J Sex Med.* 2018;15(9):1260-1271. doi:10.1016/j.jsxm.2018.06.012.

56. Lesko SM, Rosenberg L, Shapiro S. A case-control study of baldness in relation to myocardial infarction in men. *JAMA.* 1993;269(8):998-1003. doi:10.1001/jama.1993.03500080046030.

57. Lotufo PA, Chae CU, Ajani UA, Hennekens CH, Manson JE. Male pattern baldness and coronary heart disease: the physicians' health study. *Arch Intern Med.* 2000;160(2):165-171. doi:10.1001/archinte.160.2.165.

58. Herrera CR, D'Agostino R, Gerstman BB, Bosco LA, Belanger AJ. Baldness and coronary heart disease rates in men from the Framingham study. *Am J Epidemiol.* 1995;142(8):828-833. doi:10.1093/oxfordjournals.aje.a117722.

59. Ford ES, Freedman DS, Byers T. Baldness and ischemic heart disease in a national sample of men. *Am J Epidemiol.* 1996;143(7):651-657. doi:10.1093/oxfordjournals.aje.a008797.

60. Su LH, Chen LS, Lin SC, Chen HH. Association of androgenetic alopecia with mortality from diabetes mellitus and heart disease. *JAMA Dermatol.* 2013;149(5):601-606. doi:10.1001/jamadermatol.2013.130.

61. Verit A, Verit FF, Oncel H, Ciftci H. Is there any effect of insulin resistance on male reproductive system? *Arch Ital Urol Androl.* 2013;86(1):5-8. doi:10.4081/aiua.2014.1.5.

62. Güngör ES, Güngör Ş, Zebitay AG. Assessment of semen quality in patients with androgenetic alopecia in an infertility clinic. *Dermatol Sin.* 2016;34(1):10-13. doi:10.1016/j.dsi.2015.06.003.

63. Oh BR, Kim SJ, Moon JD, et al. Association of benign prostatic hyperplasia with male pattern baldness. *Urology.* 1998;51(5):744-748. doi:10.1016/s0090-4295(98)00108-3.

64. Chen W, Yang CC, Chen GY, Wu MC, Sheu HM, Tzai TS. Patients with a large prostate show a higher prevalence of androgenetic alopecia. *Arch Dermatol Res.* 2004;296(6):245-249. doi:10.1007/s00403-004-0514-z.

65. Kucerova R, Bienova M, Kral M, et al. Androgenetic alopecia and polymorphism of the androgen receptor gene (SNP rs6152) in patients with benign prostate hyperplasia or prostate cancer. *J Eur Acad Dermatol Venereol.* 2015;29(1):91-96. doi:10.1111/jdv.12468.

66. Arias-Santiago S, Arrabal-Polo M, Buendía-Eisman A, et al. Androgenetic alopecia as an early marker of benign prostatic hyperplasia. *J Am Acad Dermatol.* 2012;66(3):401-408. doi:10.1016/j.jaad.2010.12.023.

67. Kaplan SA. Re: androgenetic alopecia as an early marker of benign prostatic hyperplasia. *J Urol.* 2012;188(5):1846-1847. doi:10.1016/j.juro.2012.07.079.

68. Maleki-Hajiagha A, Razavi M, Razaeinejad M, et al. Serum prostate-specific antigen level in women with polycystic ovary syndrome: a systematic review and meta-analysis. *Horm Metab Res.* 2019;51:230-242. doi:10.1055/a-0863-5779.

69. Amoretti A, Laydner H, Bergfeld W. Androgenetic alopecia and risk of prostate cancer: a systematic review and meta-analysis. *J Am Acad Dermatol.* 2013;68(6):937-943. doi:10.1016/j.jaad.2012.11.034.

70. Cannarella R, Condorelli RA, Barbagallo F, la Vignera S, Calogero AE. Endocrinology of the aging prostate: current concepts. *Front Endocrinol (Lausanne).* 2021;12:554078. doi:10.3389/fendo.2021.554078.

71. Storbeck KH, Bloem LM, Africander D, Schloms L, Swart P, Swart AC. 11β-hydroxydihydrotestosterone and 11-ketodihydrotestosterone, novel C19 steroids with androgenic activity: a putative role in castration resistant prostate cancer? *Mol Cell Endocrinol.* 2013;377(1-2):135-146. doi:10.1016/j.mce.2013.07.006.

72. Sanke S, Chander R, Jain A, Garg T, Yadav P. A comparison of the hormonal profile of early androgenetic alopecia in men with the phenotypic equivalent of polycystic ovarian syndrome in women. *JAMA Dermatol.* 2016;152(9):986-991. doi:10.1001/jamadermatol.2016.1776.

73. Azziz R, Woods KS, Reyna R, Key TJ, Knochenhauer ES, Yildiz BO. The prevalence and features of the polycystic ovary syndrome in an unselected population. *J Clin Endocrinol Metab.* 2004;89(6):2745-2749. doi:10.1210/jc.2003-032046.

74. Di Tucci C, Galati G, Mattei G, et al. The role of alpha lipoic acid in female and male infertility: a systematic review. *Gynecol Endocrinol.* 2020;37(6):497-505. doi:10.1080/09513590.2020.1843619.

14

Pharmacologic Management of PCOS: Menstrual Irregularities

FARHEEN YOUSUF AND REHANA REHMAN

Definition

The menstrual cycle is considered irregular or oligomenorrhea in the adult female who has had less than 8 menstrual cycles in a year or in whom the cycle lasts for less than 21 or more than 35 days. These females need further evaluation with regards to other features of the Rotterdam criteria.[1] In polycystic ovary syndrome (PCOS), the menstrual dysfunction usually presents as irregular, infrequent, and/or absent menstrual bleeding.[2]

PCOS should be differentiated from other causes of oligomenorrhea like hyperprolactinemia and functional hypothalamic amenorrhea. In these patients, the body mass index (BMI) is normal to low, the luteinizing hormone (LH) to follicle-stimulating hormone (FSH) ratio is normal, and there is normal to low estrogen.[3]

Incidence

The prevalence of PCOS is 2% to 13% in the general population.[4,5] The most common presentation of PCOS is menstrual irregularities in 60% to 85% of females, and 37% of females present with secondary amenorrhea.[2,6,7]

Pathophysiology

Menstrual disorders in PCOS afflict females of all age groups.[8] The pathophysiology of PCOS is discussed in detail in Chapter 5. To summarize it from the perspective of menstrual irregularities and to supplement Fig. 14.1, the following points are highlighted. A number of factors involved in the physical development of young females may cause endocrine and metabolic disorders leading to menstrual irregularities.[9] Moreover, dysfunction in the hypothalamic-pituitary-ovarian axis can also lead to these abnormalities.[10] These disorders are therefore dependent on a high blood androgen level, increase in LH:FSH ratio, and raised insulin, with a high number of follicular count, which will affect ovulation and lead to menstrual disorders.[8] It has been observed that as the age advances, there is a decrease in the antral follicular pool; hence there is a reduction in anti-Müllerian hormone (AMH) causing shorter cycles.

Effects of Gonadotropic-Releasing Hormones

Studies have shown that increased gonadotropic-releasing hormone (GnRH) pulse frequency can stimulate LH synthesis resulting in an increased LH/FSH ratio in PCOS patients. Raised LH levels are responsible for the development of reproductive and metabolic disorders and for the production of androgen in ovarian theca cells, which eventually leads to hyperandrogenemia (HA) and arrested follicle development. The peripheral sex steroids can regulate the action of GnRH neurons through a feedback effect, which is impaired in PCOS, thus forming a vicious cycle.

Neuropeptide: Kisspeptin

Located in the hypothalamus, kisspeptin is the significant upstream regulator in GnRH pulse formation. Coexpressed with neurokinin B (NKB) and dynorphin as the KNDy system, these neurons regulate GnRH pulse and LH secretion, whereby kisspeptin can excite GnRH neurons and NKB can work as a stimulatory factor while dynorphin inhibits kisspeptin production, thus modulating downstream GnRH secretion.

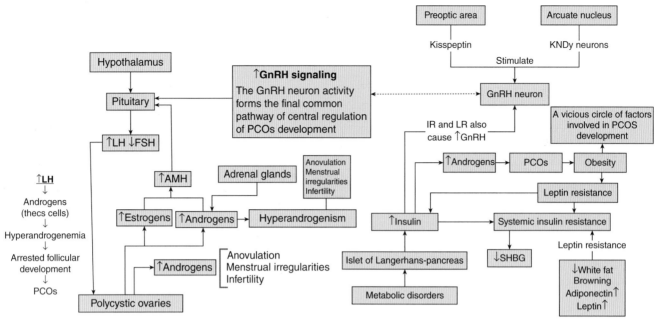

• **Fig. 14.1** The Interplay of Various Mechanisms in the Body that Lead to Menstrual Irregularities in Polycystic Ovary Syndrome *(PCOS)* Patients. *AMH,* Anti-Müllerian hormone; *FSH,* follicle-stimulating hormone; *GnRH,* gonadotropin-releasing hormone; *IR,* insulin resistance; *KNDy,* kisspeptin, neurokinin B, and dynorphin; *LH,* luteinizing hormone; *LR,* leptin resistance; *PCOs,* polycystic ovaries; *SCFA,* short-chain fatty acids; *SHBG,* sex hormone–binding globulin.

Ovarian Hormones that Regulate the Action of GnRH Neurons

PCOS patients show aberrant sex hormone levels such as HA, deviant estrogen levels, and increased AMH levels affecting ovarian dysfunction and promoting reproductive disorders in patients with PCOS.

Androgen

Androgen plays a role in both intraovarian and extraovarian mechanisms of PCOS development. It may be hyperactivated in the hypothalamus, ovary, skeletal muscle, and adipose cells mediating PCOS development.

Anti-Müllerian Hormone

AMH affects the hypothalamopituitary-ovarian (HPO) axis and impacts the ovary. AMH levels are increased because of an accumulation of small antral follicles in the ovary in PCOS patients. AMH can decrease the FSH receptor and aromatase expression in granulosa cells, thus impairing follicle growth and leading to follicular arrest in a vicious cycle.

Metabolic Regulation of GnRH Production

Insulin Resistance

Insulin resistance (IR) leads to abnormally elevated insulin levels that can promote testosterone biosynthesis in human ovarian theca cell and reduce sex hormone–binding globulin (SHBG) production. The end result is HA in patients

with PCOS. Insulin has a direct stimulating effect on LH secretion and alters reproductive functions.

At the hypothalamic level, the leptin receptor is colocalized with kisspeptin and NKB, highlighting its role in the central regulation of food intake and energy outflow and in glucose metabolism. The stimulatory effect of increased leptin levels on KNDy neurons and LH secretion promotes pathogenesis of PCOS. Leptin has a central and peripheral effect on IR that leads to obesity and metabolic changes (Zheng, 2017 #187).[10a]

Obesity

A vicious circle of accentuating relationships between obesity and insulin and leptin resistance as given in Figure 14.1 highlights their complex role in the pathogenesis of PCOS. Leptin resistance at the level of the hypothalamus results in weight gain. Increased leptin secretion by adipocytes adds to leptin resistance and promotes PCOS development. The exact role of obesity or obesity-related sympathetic activation in PCOS development is yet to established.

Implications of Menstrual Irregularities in PCOS Patients

Chronic anovulation leads to unopposed estrogen dominancy and failure to produce progesterone. It leads to endometrial cell proliferation and endometrial hyperplasia that may progress to endometrial cancers. It has been estimated that patients with PCOS have a 2.7 to 3 times increased risk of developing reproductive cancers, and 85% of endometrial cancers are because of estrogen dominance.[11] In patients with postmenstruation, endometrial thickness more than 10 mm warrant endometrial biopsy. Nonetheless the risk of ovarian cancer is reduced because of anovulation and because of prolonged use of contraceptive pills in PCOS.[12] Risk of breast cancer may increase because of obesity; however, there is no evidence of any association between PCOS and other genital cancers.[13]

Management of Menstrual Irregularities in Polycystic Ovary Syndrome

First-Line Management

Weight Reduction/Lifestyle Modifications

A holistic approach involving lifestyle modifications (LSMs), such as weight reduction with diet and exercise, should be considered in addition to pharmacologic treatment.

The Androgen Excess and PCOS Society (AEPCOS Society) stated that a reduction in body weight by 5 to 10 kg, or more than 5%, leads to improvement in biochemical disturbances and hence improves menstrual irregularities. Intake of a low caloric diet, either by cutting off fat or carbohydrates from the diet, is equally effective. Daily scheduled exercise of 30-minute duration has a synergetic effect on the reduction of weight and fat percentage of the body along with improvements in menstrual irregularities and fertility.[14]

Dileep et al. added metformin 750 to 1000 mg along with LSM in patients with mean BMI 34.7 ($\pm$ 4.3 kg/m^2) for 9 months. They found a statistically significant reduction in BMI and improvement of clinical symptoms of PCOS.[15]

In females who fail to lose weight, antiobesity drugs like Orlistat and sibutramine may be used. With the intake of these drugs along with LSMs, an additional 30% to 50% weight is lost.[14]

Bariatric surgery could be considered in females who fail to lose weight, especially if their BMI is greater than 40 kg/m^2 with comorbidities[14] (see Chapters 16 and 21).

Hormonal Treatment

Oral Contraceptive Pills

Oral contraceptive pills (OCPs) are the mainstay of treatment for regulating the menstrual cycle in those whose menstrual cycle is longer than 90 days. Management also depends on a patient's wishes and the associated characteristics/phenotype of PCOS, such as HA and IR, in addition to menstrual irregularities. This is not the drug of choice, however, for a couple who is planning to conceive.[1]

Estrogen Component of Oral Contraceptive Pills

Conjugated equine estrogen, ethinyl estradiol, and mestranol are potent synthetic estrogens; of these, estradiol valerate is preferable because it has fewer metabolic side effects. The most common estrogen in combined hormonal contraceptives (COCs) is ethinylestradiol. It sends negative feedback to gonadotrophins and enhances release of SHBG by the liver. Hence it decreases the level of LH and the free androgen index by 40% to 60%.[16]

On the other hand, it increases the risk of venous thromboembolism, further keeping in mind that PCOS is the estrogen-dominating milieu. Nevertheless, estrogen is mandatory for contraception and for regulating the cycle.[17]

Therefore to balance the pros and cons, select the estrogen as near to natural estradiol with the lowest possible dose. The optimal dose of estrogen should be less than 35 μg.[18] The higher-dose pills increase the risk of thromboembolism, whereas doses with less than 20 μg have lesser cycle control.[19]

Care should be taken in using these in females over the age of 35, those with BMI greater than 29, and smokers. This will be absolutely contraindicated in patients with active liver disease, estrogen-dependent tumors, known case of migraine with aura, and personal or family history of thromboembolism or who are positive for thrombophilia syndrome.[17,19,20]

Progesterone

The progesterone component in OCPs inhibits LH surge (and hence ovulation); in addition, it thickens the cervical mucus to inhibit sperm penetration. The type of progesterone is often divided into generations according to the era and subsequent lesser androgenic side effects. There is a wide availability of combined oral contraceptive pills (COCPs) containing second- and third-generation progesterones like levonorgestrel and gestodene, respectively. The antiandrogenic progestins include drospirenone and dienogest derivatives of 19-nortestosterone and 17alpha-spironolactone. In addition, cyproterone is a potent antiandrogenic derived from 17hydroxyprogesterone. Both drospirenone and cyproterone are considered the progesterones of choice in patients with menstrual irregularities along with features of HA.[21] Drospirenone has only 30% antiandrogenic potency compared with cyproterone acetate. The use of drospirenone surpasses cyproterone acetate because it was approved for use by the Food and Drug Administration (FDA).[22] There is a specific recommendation from the Australian and European Society of Human Reproduction and Embryology (ESHRE) PCO working group that Diantte/Diane 35 containing 35 μg of ethinyl estradiol with cyproterone acetate should not be labeled as first-line treatment because of the enhanced risk of venous thromboembolism.[23,24]

The progesterone component produces secretory changes and withdrawal bleeding. This sheds off the endometrium, hence protecting it from and preventing endometrial hyperplasia and endometrial cancer.[13]

Progesterone-Only Hormonal Treatment

In patients with a contraindication or intolerance to COCP, progesterone-only treatment can also be offered. This could be given in a cyclic manner for 21 days or intermittently in the last 14 days of the menstrual cycle. In a recent case study, cyclic oral micronized progesterone 300 mg at bedtime leads to shorter cycle, with significant improvement in premenstrual symptoms.[25,26] In the absence of robust evidence, further studies are warranted. In addition, patients should be counseled that it will not provide contraceptive benefits. For those who do not desire fertility, progesterone-only contraceptives like the progesterone-only pill (norethindrone 0.35 mg daily), injectable depot medroxyprogesterone, etonogestrel-containing implants, and levonorgestrel-containing intrauterine system (LNG IUS) would be considered with dual action of contraception and prevention of endometrial hyperplasia and cancer.[2,27,28] Nonetheless, metabolic effects of progesterone should also be taken into account.[29]

Second-Line Pharmacologic Treatment

LSM and COCPs should be combined with other agents considering individual needs and risk factors such as obesity, hyperlipidemias, hypertension, and signs of HA (Fig. 14.2).

Insulin Sensitizers

Metformin

Metformin is an insulin-sensitizing drug commonly used in patients who have high fasting insulin levels. Nevertheless, the international PCOS society recommends it in females with BMI greater than $25 kg/m^2$. A retrospective study depicts a statistically significant increase in frequency of the menstrual cycle. Continuous use of metformin for 1 year has been found to yield 11 bleeds/year.[30] Cochrane's review in 2017 exhibits improvement in menstrual frequency (odds ratio [OR] 1.72, 95% confidence interval [CI] 1.14–2.61).[31] There were two randomized controlled trials (RCTs) that compared the use of COCP with metformin in

both obese and nonobese patients; results depicted overall improvement of cholesterol, testosterone, and fasting glucose in both the groups. Because of a smaller sample size, large studies are warranted to support these findings.[32,33] Nevertheless, it commonly causes gastrointestinal disturbances, and therefore it is harder to tolerate. Other insulin-sensitizing drugs like rosiglitazone and pioglitazone are not prescribed as a routine because of their side effects and variable results.[31]

Inositol

A systematic review of 12 RCTs done by Unfer V et al. proved that the combination of Myo-ins and D-chiro-ins in a 40 to 1 ratio improved hormonal imbalance and IR. This combination further regularizes ovulation and, to some extent, menstruation, but the effects are lower compared with COCPs. The use is, however, limited for experimental purposes only.[18]

Metformin With LSM and COCP

Patients with high BMI greater than $25 kg/m^2$, high serum insulin, or impaired glucose intolerance respond better with the addition of metformin. An RCT conducted by Wei Feng compared COCP alone with a combination of COCP and metformin. The combined treatment exhibited superior results in reducing body fat, lipid profile, and fasting insulin.[34]

COCP With Antiandrogen

This treatment is reserved for patients who showed no improvement in HA after 6 months of continuous use of COCP containing cyproterone acetate along with cosmetic

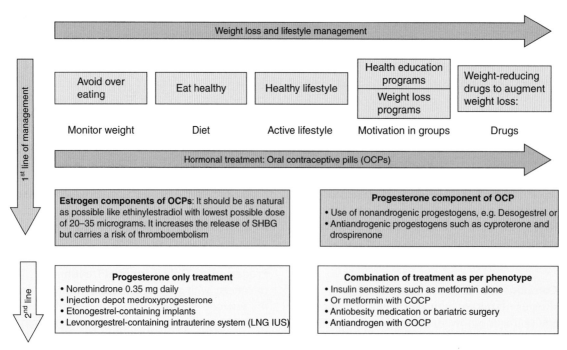

• **Fig. 14.2** Pharmacologic Management of Menstrual Irregularities in Females With Polycystic Ovary Syndrome.

treatment. Antiandrogen should not be used alone without contraception.[24]

Summary

In conclusion, the pharmacologic management of menstrual irregularities depends on personal characteristics, phenotypes, and preferences. In addition, the majority of treatments are off-label but are based on evidence. Patients should be counseled and managed appropriately under the laws of the practicing country.[1]

References

1. Teede H, Misso M, Costello M, et al. *International Evidence-Based Guideline for the Assessment and Management of Polycystic Ovary Syndrome 2018*. National Health and Medical Research Council (NHMRC), Monash University; 2018:1–198.

2. Walker K, Decherney AH, Saunders R. Menstrual dysfunction in PCOS. *Clin Obstet Gynecol*. 2021;64(1):119-125.

3. Sherif SA, Newman R, Haboosh S, et al. Investigating the potential of clinical and biochemical markers to differentiate between functional hypothalamic amenorrhoea and polycystic ovarian syndrome: a retrospective observational study. *Clin Endocrinol*. 2021;95(4):618-627.

4. Phylactou M, Clarke SA, Patel B, et al. Clinical and biochemical discriminants between functional hypothalamic amenorrhoea (FHA) and polycystic ovary syndrome (PCOS). *Clin Endocrinol*. 2021;95(2):239-252.

5. Jalilian A, Kiani F, Sayehmiri F, Sayehmiri K, Khodaee Z, Akbari M. Prevalence of polycystic ovary syndrome and its associated complications in Iranian women: a meta-analysis. *Iran J Reprod Med*. 2015;13(10):591.

6. Dewhurst J. Dewhurst's textbook of obstetrics and gynaecology. In: Edmonds K, Lees H, Bourne T, eds. *Dewhurst's Textbook of Obstetrics and Gynaecology*. 9th ed. Hoboken, NJ: John Wiley & Sons; 2012:645.

7. Taylor HS, Pal L, Sell E. *Speroff's Clinical Gynecologic Endocrinology and Infertility*. 9th ed. Philadelphia, PA: Wolters Kluwer Health/Lippincott Williams & Wilkins; 2019.

8. Zhang Y, Guo X, Ma S, et al. The treatment with complementary and alternative traditional Chinese medicine for menstrual disorders with polycystic ovary syndrome. *Evid-Based Complement Alternat Med*. 2021;2021:6678398.

9. Rajiwade SR, Sagili H, Soundravally R, Subitha L. Endocrine abnormalities in adolescents with menstrual disorders. *J Obstet Gynecol India*. 2018;68(1):58-64.

10. Rostami Dovom M, Ramezani Tehrani F, Djalalinia S, Cheraghi L, Behboudi Gandavani S, Azizi F. Menstrual cycle irregularity and metabolic disorders: a population-based prospective study. *PLoS One*. 2016;11(12):e0168402.

10a. Zhang Y, Chua Jr S. Leptin function and regulation. Comprehensive physiology. 2011 Jan 17;8(1):351-69.

11. Tokmak A, Kokanali MK, Guzel AI, Kara A, Topcu HO, Cavkaytar S. Polycystic ovary syndrome and risk of endometrial cancer: a mini-review. *Asian Pac J Cancer Prev*. 2014;15(17):7011-7014.

12. Harris H, Titus L, Cramer D, Terry K. Long and irregular menstrual cycles, polycystic ovary syndrome, and ovarian cancer risk in a population-based case-control study. *Int J Cancer*. 2017; 140(2):285-291.

13. Dumesic DA, Lobo RA. Cancer risk and PCOS. *Steroids*. 2013;78(8):782-785. doi:10.1016/j.steroids.2013.04.004.

14. Moran LJ, Pasquali R, Teede HJ, Hoeger KM, Norman RJ. Treatment of obesity in polycystic ovary syndrome: a position statement of the Androgen Excess and Polycystic Ovary Syndrome Society. *Fertil Steril*. 2009;92(6):1966-1982.

15. Dileep A, Samy MAF, Hussain N, Alabdind SZ. Effect of weight loss on symptoms of polycystic ovarian syndrome among women of reproductive age. *Dubai Med J*. 2021;l4(1):64-69.

16. Yasmin E, Balen AH. Management of polycystic ovary syndrome. *Womens Health*. 2007;3(3):355-367.

17. Dewhurst J. Dewhurst's textbook of obstetrics and gynaecology. In: Edmonds K, Lees H, Bourne T, eds. *Dewhurst's Textbook of Obstetrics and Gynaecology*. 9th ed. Hoboken, NJ: John Wiley & Sons; 2012:946.

18. Unfer V, Nestler JE, Kamenov ZA, Prapas N, Facchinetti F. Effects of inositol (s) in women with PCOS: a systematic review of randomized controlled trials. *Int J Endocrinol*. 2016;2016;1849162.

19. Yildiz BO. Oral contraceptives in polycystic ovary syndrome: risk-benefit assessment. Paper presented at the *Semin Reprod Med*. 2008;26(1):111-120.

20. Schwingl PJ, Ory HW, Visness CM. Estimates of the risk of cardiovascular death attributable to low-dose oral contraceptives in the United States. *Am J Obstet Gynecol*. 1999;180(1):241-249.

21. IARC Working Group on the Evaluation of Carcinogenic Risks to Humans, World Health Organization, International Agency for Research on Cancer. *Combined Estrogen-Progestogen Contraceptives and Combined Estrogen-Progestogen Menopausal Therapy*. Vol 91. World Health Organization; 2007.

22. Elger W, Beier S, Pollow K, Garfield R, Shi SQ, Hillisch A. Conception and pharmacodynamic profile of drospirenone. *Steroids*. 2003;68(10-13):891-905.

23. Teede HJ, Misso ML, Boyle JA, et al. Translation and implementation of the Australian-led PCOS guideline: clinical summary and translation resources from the International Evidence-based Guideline for the Assessment and Management of Polycystic Ovary Syndrome. *Med J Aust*. 2018;209:S3-S8.

24. Teede HJ, Misso ML, Costello MF, et al. Recommendations from the international evidence-based guideline for the assessment and management of polycystic ovary syndrome. *Hum Reprod*. 2018;33(9):1602-1618.

25. Briden L, Shirin S, Prior JC. The central role of ovulatory disturbances in the etiology of androgenic polycystic ovary syndrome (PCOS)—Evidence for treatment with cyclic progesterone. *Drug Discov Today Dis Models*. 2020;32:71-82.

26. Shirin S, Murray F, Hajjaran M, Goshtasebi A, Kalidasan D, Prior JC. MON-LB9 cyclic progesterone therapy in androgenic polycystic ovary syndrome (PCOS) - person-related 6-month experience changes. *J Endoc Soc*. 2020;4(suppl 1). doi:10.1210/jendso/bvaa046.2332.

27. American College of Obstetricians and Gynecologists' Committee on Practice Bulletins—Gynecology. ACOG practice bulletin No. 194: polycystic ovary syndrome. *Obstet Gynecol*. 2018;131(6): e157-e171.

28. Palshetkar N, Gudi SN. *Tackling PCOS with Hormonal Contraceptives*. FOGSI Focus Benefits Beyond Contraception. 25. https://fogsi.org/wp-content/uploads/fogsi-focus/FOGSI-Focus-Benefit-Beyond-Contraception.pdf#page=35.

29. da Silva AV, de Melo AS, Barboza RP, de Paula Martins W, Ferriani RA, Vieira CS. Levonorgestrel-releasing intrauterine system for women with polycystic ovary syndrome: metabolic and clinical effects. *Reprod Sci*. 2016;23(7):877-884. doi:10.1177/1933719115623648.

30. Jensterle M, Kravos NA, Ferjan S, Goricar K, Dolzan V, Janez A. Long-term efficacy of metformin in overweight-obese PCOS: longitudinal follow-up of retrospective cohort. *Endocr Connect.* 2020;9(1):44-54.

31. Morley LC, Tang T, Yasmin E, Norman RJ, Balen AH. Insulin-sensitising drugs (metformin, rosiglitazone, pioglitazone, D-chiro-inositol) for women with polycystic ovary syndrome, oligo amenorrhoea and subfertility. *Cochrane Database Syst Rev.* 2017;11: CD003053.

32. Morin-Papunen L, Vauhkonen I, Koivunen R, Ruokonen A, Martikainen H, Tapanainen JS. Metformin versus ethinyl estradiol-cyproterone acetate in the treatment of nonobese women with polycystic ovary syndrome: a randomized study. *J Clin Endocrinol Metab.* 2003;88(1):148-156.

33. Morin-Papunen LC, Vauhkonen I, Koivunen RM, et al. Endocrine and metabolic effects of metformin versus ethinyl estradiol-cyproterone acetate in obese women with polycystic ovary syndrome: a randomized study. *J Clin Endocrinol Metab.* 2000;85(9): 3161-3168.

34. Feng W, Jia YY, Zhang DY, Shi HR. Management of polycystic ovarian syndrome with Diane-35 or Diane-35 plus metformin. *Gynecol Endocrinol.* 2016;32(2):147-150.

15

Pharmacologic Management for Polycystic Ovary Syndrome: Hirsutism and Acne

SADIA MASOOD AND SHAYANA RUKHSAR HASHMANI

Introduction

Acne vulgaris and hirsutism are highly distressing and common issues in females presenting with polycystic ovary syndrome (PCOS). There are a variety of treatment options available for both of these conditions.[1] For hirsutism, medicines are not completely effective on terminalized hairs, and there is a need for mechanical removal of unwanted hairs. Treatment of hirsutism needs drug therapy to reduce the androgen secretion and to remove existing terminal hair. Cosmetic procedures like electrolysis and laser photothermolysis are very effective modalities for mechanical hair removal. The effective pharmacologic treatment for hirsutism is the use of antiandrogen drugs. Acne can be treated with different topical and systemic medicines. The treatment of choice depends on the severity of the acne and its impact on the quality of life of patients. The different treatment modalities include topical and systemic antibiotics, retinoids, antiandrogen drugs, and androgen suppression by oral contraceptives.[2,3]

Treatment of Hirsutism

Hair growth is a slow cyclical process. Hirsutism is a common problem, the effect of which is often underestimated. It takes many months to see the clinical response of the drugs used to treat hirsutism, and it may take more than a year to observe the full benefits.[4] In addition, treatment for hirsutism is symptomatic; after discontinuation of treatment, there is a reversal of changes in hair growth, especially in hyperandrogenic individuals.[5] Nevertheless, treatments should be kept for a longer period and attention should be given to the safety of the patients. Hair terminalization is an irreversible process, and the drugs are not completely effective against terminalized hair, and hair removal is usually necessary.[6] There are various treatment options available, which, when tailored to an individuals clinical profile, can achieve good results. Non pharmacologic treatment techniques should be used in combination with pharmacologic therapy for hirsutism.

Cosmetic and Direct Hair Removal Measures

Direct hair removal can be achieved using nonpermanent techniques. These measures consist of shaving, depilatory agents, waxing, and threading. Bleaching hair in the affected areas to be a similar color to the skin is a form of camouflage. These measures are temporary and can be repeated whenever needed. They may cause irritation of the skin, but they are relatively inexpensive and also effective, and safe.

Photoepilation includes laser and intense pulsed light therapy. It removes dark hair quickly through photothermolysis by selectively damaging the pigmented part of the hair follicle. Several treatment cycles are necessary, with treatment intervals depending on the body region being treated. Laser treatments are far less unpleasant and give a considerably quicker response than electrolysis.[7]

Electrolysis is the favored method of treatment for lightly pigmented hair because the light source of the laser only destroys the anagen hair follicles with dark bulb areas. The major adverse effects of laser and intense pulsed light therapy include postinflammatory pigmentation, folliculitis, reactivation of herpes simplex, and paradoxic hypertrichosis.

These complications can be avoided by using a long pulse-duration; a long-wavelength laser delivered with the proper skin cooling device is the preferable photoepilation mode.[7]

Electrolysis can permanently remove the hair because it works by weakening the dermal papilla and eventually causes complete destruction. Electrolysis uses a fine-needle insertion into individual follicles to destroy the hair follicle through current (galvanic electrolysis), a high-frequency alternating current (thermolysis), or a blend of the two. Major disadvantages of the technique are scarring, folliculitis, and hyperpigmentation. Because of the discomfort and expense, it is generally used for treating limited body areas.

Medical Therapy

Topical Therapy

Eflornithine is a U.S. Food and Drug Administration (FDA)–approved topical agent used for the reduction of unnecessary facial hair in females. It is an irreversible inhibitor of an enzyme ornithine decarboxylase, which catalyzes the rate-limiting step for follicular polyamine synthesis, which is essential for growth of hair. It takes approximately 6 to 8 weeks to see the clinical effects and should be used frequently to prevent the growth. It is a useful adjunct to photoepilation and provides a rapid response.[8]

Systemic Therapy

Combination Oral Contraceptives

A combination of estrogen and progestin therapy in the form of a combined oral contraceptive (COC) is the first-line endocrine therapy for acne and hirsutism. The combination of estrogen-progestin suppresses the hypothalamic-pituitary-ovarian axis, which helps to reduce the excess androgen secretion by the ovary. It helps to regulate the menstrual cycles and decreases acne and hirsutism. COCs are packaged such that the active ingredients are taken once daily for 21 successive days.[9] The choice of COC agent depends on the clinical findings and cost considerations of the individual patient.

Antiandrogens Receptor Antagonist

Antiandrogenic therapy in combination with a COC reduces hirsutism, and the response rate has individual variation. Antiandrogens inhibit the androgen-induced conversion of vellus to terminal hairs that reduce the growth of hairs.[10] Nevertheless, because of the prolonged growth cycle of hair follicles, the maximum effects of these agents cannot be appreciated for 9 to 12 months. The contraceptive measure should be prescribed while taking antiandrogen therapy, and the optimal contraception choice in this setting is a COC because it is the best treatment for the irregular menstruation that is often caused by antiandrogens. Antiandrogens have a minor impact on the metabolic abnormalities associated with PCOS. There are several different antiandrogens available.

Spironolactone

Spironolactone is an aldosterone antagonist that possesses antiandrogenic properties, which is used to treat hirsutism. Traditionally it is used as a diuretic for the management of hypertension. It affects the hair follicle by competing for androgenic receptors and displacing dihydrotestosterone at the cytosol and nuclear receptors. It is the safest and most effective available antiandrogen drug. In combination with COCs, it lowers the extent of hirsutism.

Start Spironolactone at a low dose and gradually build up to maximum therapeutic dose. Approximately 9 to 12 months of treatment is needed to attain the desired effect because of the prolonged hair growth cycle. The dose can be gradually reduced after 1 year of treatment. Electrolyte and liver function tests should be monitored after the start of treatment. Side effects include transient diuresis, fatigue, polydipsia, menorrhagia, breast tenderness, and gastrointestinal (GI) bleeding; however, no long-term issues have been identified.[11]

Cyproterone Acetate

Cyproterone acetate was the first androgen receptor antagonist used for the treatment of hirsutism. The antiandrogenic effects of cyproterone acetate are caused by the competitive displacement of dihydrotestosterone from its receptor and a decrease in 5-alpha-reductase activities in the skin.

Pregestational activity causes gonadotropin suppression and also the suppression of ovarian testosterone secretions. It is a progestin with an antiandrogenic activity used to treat hirsutism. Its prolonged use can induce amenorrhea because of its progestogenic properties. Drug regulatory agencies in Europe have limited its use as "second-line" therapy because of an increased risk of hepatotoxicity.[12]

Flutamide

It is a selective antiandrogen with efficacy similar to cyproterone. It may induce ovulation in patients with PCOS, although its usefulness for patients who want to conceive is restricted because of the risk of feminization of the male fetus.[13] Amenorrhea, decreased libido, decreased appetite, and dry skin are the common adverse effects. Hepatotoxicity is an uncommon yet significant documented adverse effect.[14] As a result, flutamide is often reserved for resistant cases of hirsutism, and individuals using this medicine should check their liver functions on a regular basis.[15]

Finasteride

It interferes with androgen action by competitively inhibiting the 5-alpha-reductase that blocks the conversion of testosterone to dihydrotestosterone. It is slightly less effective than spironolactone for the treatment of females with hirsutism. Transient GI upset, headaches, and an unexpected rise in total testosterone are common side effects.

Treatment of Acne Vulgaris

Early and effective treatment of acne is really important because scarring and inflammation can lead to long-term psychosocial and physical complications.[16] Facial scarring affects a majority of acne patients and the severity of scarring is related to the type and duration of acne. The goals of acne treatment are to:

- reduce sebum production,
- control the overproduction of keratin,
- reduce production of *Propionibacterium acnes, and*
- control the inflammatory acne.

Topical and systemic drugs can be used to treat acne. These treatment modalities are chosen according to the type and severity of skin condition. Topical treatments usually affect all the key factors responsible for acne development, except for sebum production, whereas systemic therapies affect all the steps responsible for acne production.

Topical Therapy

Topical Retinoids

Topical retinoids include isotretinoin (tazarotene), all-trans retinoic acid (tretinoin), and adapalene. Retinoids reduce the abnormal growth and development of keratinocytes in the pilosebaceous unit. The reversal of hypercornification within the follicular canal and the induction of the follicular epithelium unplugs the hair follicle. Adapalene and tazarotene are more effective than tretinoin and rarely produce skin irritation. Topical tretinoin application can cause skin irritation and photosensitivity. It can be controlled by initiation with the lowest-strength creams (0.025% cream). Moreover, the use of sunscreen is highly recommended.[17]

Topical Antibiotics

Topical antibiotics including clindamycin and benzyl peroxide (BPO) are better than placebo in the treatment of inflammatory acne. Their use in acne as a single therapy is not advocated because of the risk of bacterial resistance. BPO is a powerful antimicrobial agent that destroys the ductal and surface *P. acnes* and yeasts. After application on the skin, it decomposes in the sebaceous follicles and releases free oxygen radicals that have anti-inflammatory and bactericidal activity. BPO can cause allergic contact dermatitis, which is rare with other topical agents. Topical antibiotics can be used alternately or in combination with topical retinoid, and these combinations are better than monotherapy.[18]

Topical Dapsone

In two placebo-controlled trials, 5% topical dapsone gel was used to improve acne severity, but no comparison trials against other active drugs have been conducted to determine the potential benefit of this unique preparation.[19]

Azelaic Acid

Azelaic acid reduces the production of comedones by normalizing the keratinocytes differentiation in the follicular infundibulum. It is available as a 20% topical cream. It is not sebosuppressive but reduces the numbers and function of *P. acnes*. It is recommended for mild to moderate papulopustular acne.[20]

Systemic Therapy

Systemic Antibiotic

Oral antibiotics are commonly prescribed drugs and are usually prescribed for extensive truncal and facial acne and moderate facial acne that do not respond to topical therapies. Oral antibiotics bring a more rapid clinical response than topical therapies but can cause GI disturbances. Cyclines (oxytetracycline, tetracycline, doxycycline, minocycline, lymecycline) are the antibiotics of choice. Because of reports of potentially serious adverse effects including drug hypersensitivity syndrome (DHS), diffuse exanthematous skin eruption, pulmonary eosinophilia, drug-induced lupus, and hepatitis, minocycline is not recommended as first-line therapy. Macrolides (erythromycin, azithromycin, or clindamycin) are also used for acne but have fallen out of favor because of the emergent *P. acne* antibiotic-resistant strains. Azithromycin can be used in intermittent dosing schedules (250 mg thrice weekly), which have been found to be effective in acne because of their long half-life. In acne patients, antibiotic resistance is a common problem, so topical agents should be added, antibiotics should only be prescribed when necessary, and the treatment duration should be short.[21]

Hormonal Therapy

Estrogens and Progestins

Oral contraceptives potentially improve acne. COCs generally contain estrogen (most commonly ethinyloestradiol) and progestin. Estrogen increases the synthesis of sex hormone–binding globulins (SHBG) that enhance the binding of testosterone and decrease levels of free circulating testosterone.

Androgen Receptor Blockers

Androgen receptor blockers suppress sebum and provide potential benefit to acne. Co-cyprindiol (Estelle-35 and Dianette) is an oral contraceptive that improves acne. It is as effective as oral tetracycline given over 6 months. It has a wide risk of deep venous thrombosis embolism, and recent recommendations suggest that when the acne is improved, co-cyprindiol preparation should be replaced with a COC that contains a lower dose of estrogen.[10]

Spironolactone

Spironolactone is effective in acne treatment. The common side effects are fluid retention, breast tenderness, menstrual irregularity, and melasma in rare cases. Pregnancy should be avoided because of the risk of fetal anomalies in the male baby.

Oral Isotretinoin

Oral isotretinoin (13-cis-retinoic acid) is a synthetic vitamin A analog. It is the most common and effective therapy for acne, which produces long-term remission and improvement in acne patients. It decreases the sebum production, reduces *P. acnes* proliferation, inhibits the formation of comedones, and possesses anti-inflammatory properties. Isotretinoin is the treatment of choice for severe acne that has failed to respond to conventional therapies. The conventional dosage of isotretinoin is 1 mg/kg/day, which is effective in most cases of acne. Nevertheless, because of its adverse side effects, it is recommended that isotretinoin should be reserved for severe disease that have failed to respond to other treatments. Detailed counseling of patients should be done regarding teratogenicity and contraception advice. Common adverse effects include dryness of the mucous membranes, conjunctivitis, headache, fatigue, superficial palmoplantar peeling, the elevation of serum triglycerides, and transient abnormalities in liver function tests. The common mucocutaneous adverse effects are dose-dependent and can be managed well by modifying the dose and regularly using good emollients. In addition, regular monitoring of liver function tests and triglycerides is important.[22]

Oral Zinc

Two double blind trials found that zinc gluconate had a substantial improvement on inflammatory acne lesions. A comparison with minocycline 100 mg/day revealed that the acne is improved up to 63% compared with 32% with elemental zinc 30 mg/day.

Devices and Physical Modalities for Treating Active Acne

Light cautery or hyfrecation has been demonstrated to benefit patients with numerous macrocomedones.[2] The hyfrecation or cautery should be adjusted as low as possible to prevent any discomfort. The treatment of every skin lesion usually takes a few seconds and leaves postinflammatory pigmentation or mild scarring. For macrocomedones, this treatment modality is more successful than topical retinoid therapy.

Visible light therapy is another good treatment modality. One study comparing red blue light phototherapy with BPO for mild to moderate papulopustular acne found that this modality was superior to BPO. It is only recommended at a low dose for the treatment of mild to severe papulopustular acne.[1]

Lasers and photodynamic therapy destroy *P. acnes* by targeting porphyrins produced by them. It also suppresses different proinflammatory cytokines. A comprehensive analysis of 16 RCTs and three controlled trials evaluating photodynamic therapy and laser light sources for acne treatment found that most light sources help treat inflammatory acne lesions in the short term, whereas photodynamic therapy provides the most consistent outcomes (up to 68% improvement, methyl aminolevulinate, aminolaevulinic acid, and red light). Pain, erythema, crusting, edema, pigmentary changes, and pustular eruptions may occur as a result of light treatment.[23]

Conclusion

Acne and hirsutism are both common and bothersome symptoms of PCOS. It is obvious that antiandrogen medications can slow the growth of hairs in many hyperandrogenic individuals. These medications are ineffective against terminalized hair, necessitating the use of cosmetic procedures to remove these hairs.[24] In the management of existing hirsutism, oral contraceptives are not very effective. Cyproterone acetate and spironolactone are the first-line antiandrogen medications used to treat hirsutism.[24] The treatment of hirsutism is long-term, and the safety of the patient should be a major consideration when selecting a treatment modality. Topical or systemic therapies might be used depending on the severity of the acne. The first-line therapies are topical treatments. Nevertheless, systemic antibiotics and retinoids should be prescribed in the case of severe acne or in people who do not respond to topical therapy. Systemic retinoids are identified as the most effective therapy for moderate to severe type of acne. Antiandrogen medications and oral contraceptives may be beneficial adjuncts to these treatments.

References

1. Teede HJ, Misso ML, Costello MF, et al. Recommendations from the international evidence-based guideline for the assessment and management of polycystic ovary syndrome. *Hum Reprod.* 2018;33(9):1602-1618.
2. Zaenglein A.L., Pathy A.L., Schlosser B.J., Alikhan, A., et al. Guidelines of care for the management of acne vulgaris. *J Am Acad Dermatol.* 2016;74(5):945-973.
3. Lookingbill, D. P., Chalker, D. K., Lindholm, J. S., Katz, H. I., et al. Treatment of acne with a combination clindamycin/benzoyl peroxide gel compared with clindamycin gel, benzoyl peroxide gel and vehicle gel: combined results of two double-blind investigations. *J Am Acad Dermatol.* 1997;37(4):590-595
4. Aktar R, Gunes Bilgili S, Yavuz IH, et al. Evaluation of hirsutism and hormonal parameters in acne vulgaris patients treated with isotretinoin. *Int J Clin Pract.* 2021;75(3):e13791.
5. Yoost J, Savage A. Screening and management of the hyperandrogenic adolescent. *Obstet Gynecol.* 2019;134(4):E106-E114.
6. DeUgarte CM, Woods KS, Bartolucci AA, Azziz R. Degree of facial and body terminal hair growth in unselected black and white women: toward a populational definition of hirsutism. *J Clin Endocrinol Metab.* 2006;91(4):1345-1350.
7. Haedersdal M, Wulf H. Evidence-based review of hair removal using lasers and light sources. *J Eur Acad Dermatol Venereol.* 2006;20(1):9-20.
8. Wolf Jr JE, Shander D, Huber F, et al. Randomized, double-blind clinical evaluation of the efficacy and safety of topical eflornithine HCl 13.9% cream in the treatment of women with facial hair. *Int J Dermatol.* 2007;46(1):94-98.

9. Adeniji AA, Essah PA, Nestler JE, Cheang KI. Metabolic effects of a commonly used combined hormonal oral contraceptive in women with and without polycystic ovary syndrome. *J Womens Health*. 2016;25(6):638-645.

10. Stegeman BH, de Bastos M, Rosendaal FR, et al. Different combined oral contraceptives and the risk of venous thrombosis: systematic review and network meta-analysis. *BMJ*. 2013;347:f5298.

11. Brown J, Farquhar C, Lee O, Toomath R, Jepson RG. Spironolactone versus placebo or in combination with steroids for hirsutism and/or acne. *Cochrane Database Syst Rev*. 2009;(2):CD00194.

12. van der Spuy ZM, Le Roux PA. Matjila MJ. Cyproterone acetate for hirsutism. *Cochrane Database Syst Rev*. 2003;2003(4):CD001125.

13. De Zegher F, Ibáñez L. Therapy: low-dose flutamide for hirsutism: into the limelight, at last. *Nat Rev Endocrinol*. 2010;6(8):421-422.

14. Manso G, Thole Z, Salgueiro E, Revuelta P, Hidalgo A. Spontaneous reporting of hepatotoxicity associated with antiandrogens: data from the Spanish pharmacovigilance system. *Pharmacoepidemiol Drug Saf*. 2006;15(4):253-259.

15. Barth JH, Cherry CA, Wojnarowska F, Dawber RP. Cyproterone acetate for severe hirsutism: results of a double-blind dose-ranging study. *Clin Endocrinol*. 1991;35(1):5-10.

16. Hart R, Doherty DA. The potential implications of a PCOS diagnosis on a woman's long-term health using data linkage. *J Clin Endocrinol Metab*. 2015;100(3):911-919.

17. Katsambas, A.D., Stefanaki, C., Cunliffe, W. J., et al. Guidelines for treating acne. *Clinics in dermatology*. 2004; 22(5):439-444.

18. Worret WI, Fluhr JW. Acne therapy with topical benzoyl peroxide, antibiotics and azelaic acid. *J Dtsch Dermatolo Ges*. 2006;4(4):293-300.

19. Draelos ZD, Carter E, Maloney JM, et al. Two randomized studies demonstrate the efficacy and safety of dapsone gel, 5% for the treatment of acne vulgaris. *J Am Acad Dermatol*. 2007;56(3):439.e1-439.e10.

20. Graupe K, Cunliffe WJ, Gollnick HP, Zaumseil RP. Efficacy and safety of topical azelaic acid (20 percent cream): an overview of results from European clinical trials and experimental reports. *Cutis*. 1996;57(suppl 1):20-35.

21. Leyden J, Thiboutot DM, Shalita AR, et al. Comparison of tazarotene and minocycline maintenance therapies in acne vulgaris: a multicenter, double-blind, randomized, parallel-group study. *Arch Dermatol*. 2006;142(5):605-612.

22. Acmaz G, Cınar L, Acmaz B, et al. The effects of oral isotretinoin in women with acne and polycystic ovary syndrome. *Biomed Res Int*. 2019;2019:2513067.

23. Mathew ML, Karthik R, Mallikarjun M, Bhute S, Varghese A. Intense pulsed light therapy for acne-induced post-inflammatory erythema. *Indian Dermatol Online J*. 2018;9(3):159-164.

24. Franik G, Bizoń A, Włoch S, Kowalczyk K, Biernacka-Bartnik, Madej P. Hormonal and metabolic aspects of acne vulgaris in women with polycystic ovary syndrome. *Eur Rev Med Pharmacol Sci*. 2018;22(14):4411-4418.

16

Pharmacologic Management for Polycystic Ovary Syndrome: Weight Loss

SARAH NADEEM AND ASMA ALTAF HUSSAIN MERCHANT

Significance of Weight in Polycystic Ovary Syndrome

Polycystic ovary syndrome (PCOS) is a syndrome with primary manifestations of irregular menstrual cycles and hyperandrogenism. The 2003 Rotterdam consensus workshop modified previous guidelines for the diagnosis of PCOS.[1] Based on the Rotterdam criteria, PCOS diagnosis can be made if a female has two out of the following three criteria (after secondary diagnoses are excluded, as PCOS is a diagnosis of exclusion):

- Oligomenorrhea/anovulation
- Hyperandrogenism (clinical and/or biochemical evidence of hyperandrogenism):
  - Clinical: Hirsutism, acne, and/or acanthosis nigricans
  - Biochemical: Elevated testosterone levels, free testosterone level is more sensitive than total testosterone levels), and/or elevated androstenedione and/or dehydroepiandrosterone sulfate (DHEA-S)
- Polycystic ovaries on ultrasound ($\geq$12 follicles of 2–9 mm in diameter in one ovary or ovarian volume >10 cc) with exclusion of other etiologies (congenital adrenal hyperplasia, androgen-secreting tumors, Cushing syndrome)

The majority (50%–80%) of patients diagnosed with PCOS are clinically either overweight (body mass index [BMI] 25–30 kg/m^2) or obese (BMI greater than 30 kg/m^2).[2,3] For all females aged 25 to 35, including those with PCOS, optimal weight is defined as a BMI of less than 24 kg/m^2. In a meta-analyses, in over 35-year-old PCOS patients, the pregnancy rate was seen to significantly decrease at the BMI cut-off point of 18–20 kg/m^2 (OR = 0.6969, 95% CI [0.4947,0.9817]). In over 35-year-old non-PCOS patients, there are no significant cut-off points between BMI and the pregnancy rate.[4] Worldwide as the prevalence of obesity increases, there has also been a sharp increase in obesity prevalence in patients with PCOS, from 51% in the 90s to 74% in the decades since.[5] Nevertheless, it is important to note that there exists a small percentage of females with BMI of less than or equal to 25 kg/m^2 who fulfill the diagnostic criteria of PCOS. This phenomenon is known as "lean PCOS" and has an overall prevalence of 1.5% to 6.6%,[6] depending on different ethnicities. Patients with lean PCOS have a lower risk of developing insulin resistance (IR), type 2 diabetes mellitus (T2DM), and other comorbidities.

There are several mechanisms that contribute to the development of obesity longitudinally in a patient with PCOS (Fig. 16.1). The resultant obesity predisposes to an increased risk of related comorbidities, such as prediabetes, T2DM, hypertension, and obstructive sleep apnea. The most pervasive feature of PCOS remains IR, which contributes to multiple manifestations. Hyperinsulinemia leads to the development of metabolic syndrome in PCOS with downregulation of insulin receptors, increased free fatty acids and intracellular lipid concentration, and the modification of its own action via circulation of tumor necrosis factor-alpha (TNF-α) and interleukin-6 (IL-6).

Achieving and maintaining an optimum healthy weight is a major component of PCOS management with resultant improved insulin sensitivity and reduced symptoms of hyperandrogenism and anovulation.

Weight Management

Weight management refers to the entire spectrum of weight loss, prevention of further weight gain, and maintenance of this balance. A 5% to 10% reduction in weight has been shown to have beneficial outcomes in psychological, reproductive, and metabolic aspects of a patient's life who is diagnosed with PCOS.[7] Different modalities of weight loss exist, which include dietary and lifestyle modifications, pharmacologic, and surgical interventions (Table 16.1).

Lifestyle Modification Strategies

Lifestyle modifications encompass three main areas: diet, physical activity, and behavioral coaching.[8] Several longitudinal

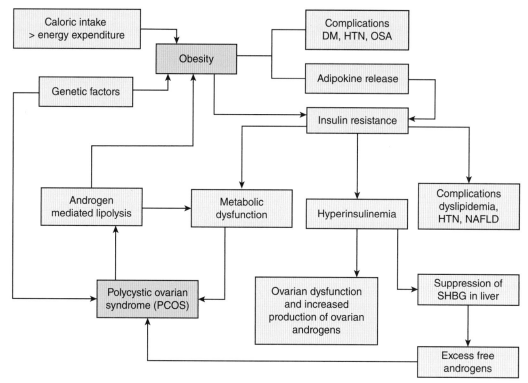

• **Fig. 16.1** Pathogenesis and Mechanisms Associated With Polycystic Ovary Syndrome and Obesity. *DM,* Diabetes mellitus; *HTN,* hypertension; *NAFLD,* nonalcoholic fatty liver disease; *OSA,* obstructive sleep apnea; *SHBG,* sex hormone–binding globulin.

TABLE 16.1 Pharmacologic and Surgical Interventions for Weight Loss in Polycystic Ovary Syndrome

Pharmacologic Interventions for Weight Loss		
Intervention		
01	Glucagon-like Peptide 1 (GLP-1) Agonists	Liraglutide; Food and Drug Administration (FDA)-approved
		Semaglutide; FDA-approved
02	Sympathomimetic/Anticonvulsant	Phentermine/topiramate extended release (ER); FDA-Approved
03	Opioid Antagonist/Antidepressant	Naltrexone ER/bupropion ER; FDA-approved
04	Lipase Inhibitor	Orlistat; FDA-approved
05	Serotonin 5-HT$_{2c}$ Agonist	Lorcaserin Not recommended, off market because of malignancy risk

Surgical Interventions for Weight Loss	
Type of Bariatric Surgery	**Examples**
01	Restrictive (Decreases stomach's natural capacity, thereby restricting food intake and reducing weight)	1. Horizontal gastroplasty 2. Vertical banded gastroplasty 3. Silastic ring vertical gastroplasty 4. Adjustable gastric banding
02	Malabsorptive (Reroutes the intestine to bypass a significant portion of small intestine, leading to decreased nutrient absorption, which contributes to increase in weight)	1. Jejunoileal bypass 2. Biliopancreatic diversion 3. Duodenal switch 4. Long-limb gastric bypass
03	Mixed: Restrictive and malabsorptive (Reduces the size of the stomach along with bypassing majority of small intestine)	1. Roux-en-Y gastric bypass procedure (RYGB)

studies have demonstrated that these interventions collectively can help achieve 10% of weight loss and maintain it for at least 1 year, with caloric restriction being the mainstay of weight loss and maintenance of this reduction through a sustained activity/exercise plan.[9] Weight reduction of as little as 5% of total body weight through lifestyle modifications can result in significant metabolic, reproductive, and psychological benefits.[5] A major challenge to long-term maintenance of weight loss is absence of preplanned goals and continuous behavioral coaching, hence requiring more focus in the weight reduction process.

Dietary Management

Weight loss is primarily achieved by creating a caloric deficit. This holds true for all, including patients with PCOS. There are no scientific data for a specific PCOS diet, but any dietary plans that cause a calorie deficiency will yield weight loss.

Goal setting is vital before initiation of a specific dietary plan to personalize it for the individual and make it achievable. A reduction of 500 to 1000 kcal/day from the patient's normal diet can work toward achieving a loss of 0.5 to 1 kg per week. Slow but maintained dietary changes are required, including smaller portion sizes, replacing sugar-containing beverages with water, increasing the intake of whole-grain cereals, and decreasing unsaturated fats or complex carbohydrates in the diet.[10]

Females on very low-calorie diets (providing 800 calories or less per day with weekly weight losses averaging approximately 1 to 2.5 kg per week) see greater initial weight loss than other forms of calorie restriction but need to be monitored by healthcare professionals to prevent micronutrient deficiencies.[10] To achieve maximum weight loss with better long-term outcomes, combination of physical exercise is vital with caloric restriction.

Physical Activity

The role of physical activity in weight loss is majorly centered on maintaining the reduced weight. To reduce obesity in the general population, the Physical Activity Guidelines for Americans recommend a moderate intensity aerobic activity of 150 to 300 minutes once per week or a vigorous intensity aerobic activity of 75 to 150 minutes once within a week.[11] Coventry Dieticians at the National Health Services Trust recommends 30 minutes of moderate physical activity for 5 days a week for adults.[12] Similar guidelines can be extended to PCOS patients who can achieve their designated goals of weight through a combination of a moderate to vigorous intensity physical workouts with dietary restrictions.

Patients with PCOS have impaired lipolysis, which contributes to weight gain. Some recent studies have shown that lipolytic impairment can be partially reversed with aerobic exercise leading to a decrease in weight.[13] Furthermore, aerobic exercise has favorable effects on IR and on cardiovascular (CV) disease (CVD) risk. Strength training is quite beneficial for patients with PCOS as well; this includes yoga, Pilates, and progressive resistance training (PRT), which is a method of strength training aimed at increasing muscle mass by increasing the overload to facilitate adaptation. PRT has been studied specifically in patients with PCOS, showing a reduction in overall body fat percentage and waist circumference and improvement in muscle strength, along with decreased hyperandrogenism.[14] Yoga and Pilates in PCOS patients have demonstrated significant reduction in abdominal and hip circumference.[15]

Randomized controlled trials (RCTs) have shown that a combination of diet therapy, such as a reduced carbohydrate diet, and regular exercise have significantly larger sustained effects on weight reduction in PCOS compared with exercise alone. A combination of these interventions have also demonstrated a greater reduction in IR and hyperandrogenism symptoms.[10]

Behavior Modification

Behavior-modification therapy aims at enabling obese patients with PCOS to recognize, understand, and accordingly alter their practices involving nutrition and activity to have favorable outcomes.[10] A systematic review of limited literature on behavior modification interventions highlights the benefit of combining several modalities of these interventions.[7] The key recommendations extracted from this review recommend:

- Self-monitoring with regular measuring of one's weight and diet
- Setting of realistic goals and outcomes using the SMART model (specific, measurable, achievable, realistic, and timely)
- Understanding and differentiating the components of weight reduction and weight management
- Restructuring cognition by encouraging positive thoughts
- Recognizing barriers to healthy behavior, followed by an in-depth analysis of its possible solutions
- Surrounding oneself with encouraging people
- Taking help from professionals (experts in cognitive behavioral therapy [CBT] and other behavior-modifying therapies) when required

Pharmacologic Interventions

Pharmacologic interventions should be considered as initial therapy in patients with PCOS who are either only obese (BMI >30.0 kg/m^2) or are overweight (BMI 25–30 kg/m^2) with an underlying weight-related comorbidity such as hypertension, T2DM, dyslipidemia, sleep apnea, arthritis, or hyperuricemia. In the last few decades, newer medications working through diverse mechanisms have become available for weight reduction in obese and overweight individuals, and the same can be used for patients with PCOS meeting the weight indications for use.

The five drugs currently approved by the Food and Drug Administration (FDA) for chronic weight management include subcutaneous liraglutide, subcutaneous semaglutide, the oral combination of phentermine and topiramate, oral orlistat, and the oral combination of naltrexone and bupropion.[16] Metformin and lorcaserin are *not* recommended.

Metformin

As per most current scientific data, metformin is *not* recommended to be used as a pharmacologic agent for weight loss in patients with PCOS. It is indicated for use in patients with clinical features or biochemical evidence of IR, prediabetes, and/or diabetes. Traditionally, metformin has been used for symptomatic management in patients with PCOS with their primary effect on increasing insulin sensitivity and prevention of the development of T2DM, with controversial evidence regarding its effect on weight.[17] Its side effects, although mild, include gastrointestinal intolerance and risk of vitamin B_{12} deficiency.[18]

Lorcaserin

Lorcaserin should *not* be used for weight loss. It previously had a weight loss indication but is now no longer approved because of its higher risk for developing pancreatic, colorectal, and lung cancer in patients.[19]

Proven pharmacologic options for weight loss in PCOS patients are discussed in detail in the following sections.

Glucagon-Like Peptide-1 Agonists (Liraglutide and Semaglutide)

Glucagon-like peptide-1 (GLP-1) is one of the major peptide hormones responsible for regulation of food intake. Upon release, it increases glucose-dependent insulin secretion with a reduction in the release of glucagon in addition to decreasing appetite and delaying gastric emptying. Exenatide was the first clinically used GLP-1 analog in the United States in 2005 to be approved as a glucose regulating medication with CV risk reduction benefits.[20] Since 2014, GLP-1 agonists have been approved as weight loss agents as well, having an appetite regulation effect through both peripheral and central nervous system pathways.[21] Peripherally, it slows gastric emptying, leading to decreased antral motility and increased pyloric tone, which stimulates vagal afferent signals to medulla and hypothalamus to induce satiety. Centrally, these analogs, especially liraglutide, have been shown to stimulate proopiomelanocortin (POMC) neurons directly and inhibit neuropeptide-Y and Agouti-related peptide neurons of the arcuate nucleus, resulting in appetite suppression. Besides improving glucose homeostasis, GLP-1 agonists enhance satiety, decrease gut motility, and reduce body weight.[21]

Liraglutide is the first GLP-1 analog approved for the indication of weight loss alone even in nondiabetics, at the dose of 3 mg once daily subcutaneous injection. Definitive evidence has shown that liraglutide, in addition to lifestyle modifications, leads to a mean reduction in body weight of 4.9% to 7.4%.[16] Compared with metformin and orlistat, it has been shown to have fewer side effects with a significant dose-related weight reduction.

Semaglutide is a long acting GLP-1 analog that was approved by the FDA for once-weekly subcutaneous administration in 2017 for use in diabetic patients. Oral semaglutide was approved in September of 2019 for use as adjunct to diet and exercise to improve glycemic control in adults with T2DM and, most recently, in June 2021, semaglutide (2.4 mg once weekly subcutaneously) was approved for chronic weight management in adults with obesity or who are overweight with at least one weight-related condition (such as high blood pressure, T2DM, or high cholesterol), in addition to a reduced calorie diet and increased physical activity. Following a combination of all these interventions has been shown to have a mean reduction in body weight of 9.6% to 16%.[16]

Trials evaluating the efficacy of semaglutide in PCOS have shown significant weight reduction with additional benefit of decreased CVD risk.[18] After 104 weeks of weekly subcutaneous administration of 0.5 mg and 1.0 mg semaglutide in a trial, it reduced mean body weight by 3.6 kg and 4.9 kg, respectively.[22] Similarly, oral semaglutide was superior to subcutaneous liraglutide for weight reduction in another 26-week trial where the participants were also prescribed a stable maximum tolerated dose of oral metformin.[23] The PIONEER 2 Trial also showed superiority of 14 mg of its oral dose daily over 25 mg daily dose of empagliflozin (sodium-glucose cotransporter-2) with 4.8 kg weight reduction over a loss of 3.8 kg, respectively, after 52 weeks.[24]

The most common side effects of both liraglutide and semaglutide include nausea and vomiting. A disadvantage identified with the use of liraglutide is its subcutaneous administration; oral semaglutide is hence preferred, which is currently not approved for nondiabetic patients and has strict guidelines of being administered in the early morning on an empty stomach, at least 30 minutes before intake of any food or beverage.[25] Other adverse but rare complications include pancreatitis for liraglutide and excessive thyroxine levels if semaglutide is taken with thyroxine. All GLP1-agonists have been found to show an increased risk of thyroid C-cell tumors in rodents; no human case has been associated, but use of GLP1- agonists is generally avoided in patients with a higher risk of thyroid C-cell tumors.[26]

Combination of Phentermine and Topiramate

A combination of phentermine and topiramate is FDA-approved for weight loss. Monotherapy with each of these agents is possible; however, the combination is shown to have a reduced side effect profile because of its extended release (ER) formula. Pharmacologically related to amphetamine, phentermine acts centrally as an appetite suppressant through a possible release of catecholamines in the hypothalamus.[27] Topiramate is a sulfamate-substituted monosaccharide, commonly used as an antiepileptic and now shown to have a positive weight loss effect of approximately 10.2 to 10.8 kg in 56 weeks.[28,29] There are several proposed mechanisms for topiramate's mechanism of action attributing to weight loss, with proposed theories on having both a central and systemic distribution of activity. In rats being examined for weight loss, it was shown to have effects on neuropeptide-Y and its Y1 and Y5 receptors, corticotrophin-releasing hormone, and type-II glucocorticoid receptors, which suppresses appetite and increases satiety, leading to weight reduction.[27]

Phentermine/Topiramate ER is taken orally once daily in the morning. Four different doses of phentermine and ER topiramate are available: (1) starting dose (3.75 mg/23 mg), (2) recommended dose (7.5 mg/46 mg), (3) transition dose (11.25 mg/69 mg), and (4) top dose (15 mg/92 mg). After initiation, the weight should be evaluated after 12 weeks; if the weight loss is less than 3%, the therapy can either be discontinued or, using the transition dose for 14 days, be converted to top dose.[10] If the weight loss is less than 5% after use of top dose, however, it should be discontinued after taking it on alternate days for 1 week because abrupt disuse can precipitate seizures.[16] The overall mean reduction in body weight with phentermine/topiramate and lifestyle modifications have shown to be 9.8% to 10.9 %. The EQUIP trial, a 56-week RCT, compared the effects of phentermine/topiramate controlled release (CR) with a placebo using 4-week postrandomization titration period, followed by 52 weeks at the randomized treatment dose.[28] Doses of 3.75/23 mg and 15/92 mg were more effective than placebo over the course of 52 weeks in addition to a suggestively higher body weight loss percentage compared with other marketed drugs. CONQUER, another 56-week RCT, used 7.5/46 mg and 15/92 mg of phentermine/topiramate CR and also showed more weight loss than the placebo.[29] As a follow-up, the SEQUEL trial was conducted for the evaluation of this drug's long-term efficacy for an extended period of 52 weeks.[30] At week 108, there were dose-related weight loss rates observed within the participants (1.8% for placebo, 9.3% for 7.5/46 mg, and 10.7% for 15/92 mg) with the latter causing a significant decrease in triglyceride, high-density lipoprotein cholesterol, and low-density lipoprotein cholesterol levels compared with the placebo, making it one of the most effective drugs for weight loss in PCOS.

The most commonly reported side effects include paresthesia, dry mouth, and constipation.[29] This medication is contraindicated in pregnancy; in patients with glaucoma; in hyperthyroidism; in patients receiving treatment or within 14 days after treatment with monoamine oxidase inhibitors; and in patients with hypersensitivity or idiosyncrasy to sympathomimetic amines, topiramate, or any of the inactive ingredients in the medication.

Combination of Naltrexone and Bupropion

The FDA approved the combination of naltrexone and bupropion ER in September 2014. It is available in a combination dose of 16 mg/180 mg twice daily to be efficient in having a mean weight loss of 3.7% to 8.1% if paired with lifestyle modifications.

Naltrexone is an opioid antagonist, having its effects on μ, δ, and κ opiate receptors with maximum antagonistic effect on μ opiate receptors.[31] It has shown to block the inhibition feedback mechanism of β endorphin on hypothalamic POMC cells, which, in turn, secrete melanocyte-stimulating hormone (MSH). Because MSH works as an appetite regulator by indicating satiety to the brain, its continuous MSH secretion results in appetite reduction. Bupropion is a dopamine and norepinephrine reuptake inhibitor and, being similar to amphetamine, it works as an appetite suppressor through its action on the hypothalamus.[31]

The first clinical trial based on these dosages in addition to a balanced diet and 180 minutes exercise per week showed a statistically significant difference in the number of participants who achieved a 5% reduction in their total body weight, with an average weight loss of 4.2% after 56 weeks.[32] Another trial having a similar population with same duration and baseline lifestyle interventions showed a dose-dependent weight loss of 3.7% and 4.8% with 16 mg/360 mg and 32 mg/360 mg of naltrexone slow release (SR)/bupropion SR, respectively.[33] Within the diabetic population, this combination indicates a weight loss of 3.2% in addition to a controlled diet and physical activity.[34]

The most common side effects with naltrexone ER/bupropion ER are reported to be nausea, constipation, headache, dizziness, and dry mouth. Because bupropion works as an antidepressant, it can also precipitate suicidal thoughts and behaviors.[35] It is absolutely contraindicated in opiate abusers, with relative contraindications in uncontrolled hypertension and ischemic heart disease because of bupropion's tendency to further exacerbate these symptoms, and in both hepatic and renal dysfunction because of their potentially drug-induced damage.[31]

Orlistat

Orlistat 120 mg orally was approved as a prescription product by the FDA in 1999 for obesity management in conjunction with a reduced caloric diet and to reduce the risk of regaining weight after prior weight loss. It works by altering lipid digestion by binding irreversibly to pancreatic and gastric lipases, thus resulting in decreased absorption of dietary lipids. Through this mechanism, orlistat has been shown to have a chronic maintenance effect on the reduced weight with improved lipid profile and glycemic index. The overall mean weight loss using orlistat with lifestyle modifications ranges from 4.6% to 10.2 %.[16] Its prescribed dose for the obese general population is 120 mg orally three times daily within an hour of ingesting a fatty meal. Nevertheless, if any meal has been skipped, its subsequent dose can be omitted.

A meta-analysis reviewed the effect of orlistat on several parameters of PCOS, concluding a significant decrease in BMI/weight in overweight/obese women with PCOS.[36] Additionally, it has also shown to have a favorable impact, similar to metformin, on improving testosterone levels, IR, and lipid profile with better tolerated side effects of nausea and epigastric pain. Another review of RCTs showed orlistat to be effective in achieving at least 5% weight loss of the total body weight compared with a placebo after 52 weeks of use.[37] Side effects of orlistat include increased flatulence with discharge and fatty/oily stools with possible fecal incontinence, which greatly limits compliance. Because of these side effects, it is contraindicated in pregnancy, chronic malabsorption syndrome, and cholestasis.[16]

Bariatric Surgery

Bariatric surgery is the most effective way to achieve weight loss in obese patients. According to the National Institute of Health (NIH)'s National Institute of Diabetes and Digestive and Kidney Diseases (NIDDK), weight-loss surgery is recommended for patients who either have a BMI of 40 kg/m² or greater, BMI of 35 kg/m² or greater associated with a comorbidity such as T2DM, sleep apnea, or heart disease, or a BMI of 30 kg/m² or greater with T2DM difficult to manage with lifestyle modifications and pharmacologic therapy.[38] The three main types of bariatric surgeries include restrictive (horizontal gastroplasty, vertical banded gastroplasty, silastic ring vertical gastroplasty, and adjustable gastric banding), malabsorptive (jejunoileal bypass, biliopancreatic diversion, duodenal switch, and long limb gastric bypass) and those with a combination of both these types (Roux-en-Y gastric bypass procedure [RYGB]).[9] The hypothesis associated with reduced weight postsurgery revolves around increased satiety and a decline in hunger because of hormonal regulation of neuroendocrine mechanisms and gut chemicals (ghrelin).

Recent advances in bariatric surgery have made it less invasive with an efficient result in weight loss that often leads to a secondary treatment for metabolic comorbidities. This has made the surgical option for weight reduction increasingly popular as highlighted in the International Federation for the Surgery of Obesity and Metabolic Disorders (IFSO) Global Registry Report 2019.[39] The report commented on an almost twofold increase in the volume of bariatric surgeries with an increase of 439,256 bariatric procedures from 2018 to 2019 as per records of 61 countries, with the most common being RYGB, sleeve gastrectomy procedures (horizontal gastrectomy), one anastomosis gastric bypass procedures, and gastric banding procedures (Fig. 16.2).

Several studies have evaluated the outcome of bariatric surgery on metabolic aspects of PCOS. Evidence shows RYGB to be superior to sleeve gastrectomy in achieving a higher weight loss; however, no RCT has been conducted to establish this relationship. In a study assessing weight loss in women with PCOS after biliopancreatic bypass or a laparoscopic RYGB, an average of 41 kg weight loss was achieved with improved symptoms of decreased hirsutism, testosterone levels, and regulation of menstrual cycles.[18,40] Another retrospective study concluded about 56.7% weight loss at 12 months in patients with PCOS who underwent RYGB, along with a decrease in Hb A$_{1c}$ of 3% in 3 months.[18,41] Recent studies support the efficacy of bariatric surgery on weight loss and other androgenic features in PCOS; up to 25 kg weight loss has been reported at 6-month follow-up, which has shown to increase to an overall weight loss ranging from 34 to 93.6 kg at 1 year, a possible 100% menstrual cycle regularity and less than 50% reduction in hirsutism consistent until at least 1 year after surgery.[42,43]

Other than bariatric surgery, FDA has also approved the use of several noninvasive weight-loss/management devices such as temporary placement of intragastric balloon systems (aimed at increasing satiety by occupying space), gastric

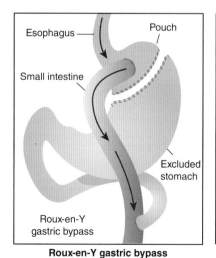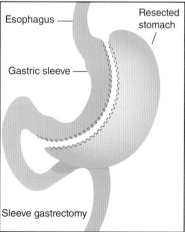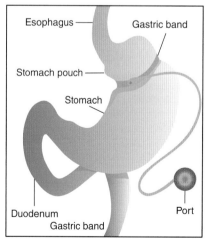

Roux-en-Y gastric bypass
Combination of restrictive and malabsorptive bariatric surgery with bypassing of most of stomach and small intestine; most commonly performed

Sleeve gastrectomy
Restrictive bariatric surgery with approximately 80% stomach removed; 2nd most commonly performed

Adjustable gastric banding
Restrictive bariatric surgery with a silicone band in proximal stomach to restrict food intake; 3rd most commonly performed

• **Fig. 16.2** Most Common Bariatric Surgical Procedures for Weight Loss. (Gandhi D., Boregowda U., Sharma P., et al., A review of commonly performed bariatric surgeries: Imaging features and its complications. Clinical Imaging. 2021; 72: 122-135.)

emptying systems (drain a part of the stomach contents postmeal to prevent absorption), oral removable palatal space occupying device (to aid in limiting bite size), and ingested, transient, space-occupying device (ingested material aimed at occupying the space within the stomach).[44] Each of these devices have its own set of risks and benefits; hence appropriate patient selection is extremely vital for such interventions to achieve the best possible output.

References

1. Rotterdam ESHRE/ASRM-Sponsored PCOS Consensus Workshop Group. Revised 2003 consensus on diagnostic criteria and long-term health risks related to polycystic ovary syndrome (PCOS). *Hum Reprod.* 2004;19(1):41-47.
2. Anagnostis P, Paparodis R, Bosdou J, et al. The major impact of obesity on the development of Type 2 Diabetes (T2D) in women with PCOS: a systematic review and meta-analysis of observational studies [Abstract]. *J Endocr Soc.* 2021;5(suppl 1):A746-A747.
3. *Obesity Raises Type 2 Diabetes Risk in Women with PCOS.* Endocrine.org. 2021. Available at: https://www.endocrine.org/news-and-advocacy/news-room/featured-science-from-endo-2021/obesity-raises-type-2-diabetes-risk-in-women-with-pcos, in press.
4. Wang F, Dai W, Yang X, Guo Y, Sun Y. Analyses of optimal body mass index for infertile patients with either polycystic or nonpolycystic ovary syndrome during assisted reproductive treatment in China. *Sci Rep.* 2016;6(1):34538.
5. Teede H, Misso M, Costello M, et al. Recommendations from the international evidence-based guideline for the assessment and management of polycystic ovary syndrome. *Clin Endocrinol.* 2018;89(3):251-268.
6. Pourmatroud E. Lean women with polycystic ovary syndrome. In: Agrawal NK, Singh K, eds. *Debatable Topics in PCOS Patients.* London: IntechOpen; 2017.
7. Brennan L, Teede H, Skouteris H, Linardon J, Hill B, Moran L. Lifestyle and behavioral management of polycystic ovary syndrome. *J Womens Health.* 2017;26(8):836-848.
8. Jameson J. *Harrison's Endocrinology.* 4th ed. New York: McGraw-Hill Education; 2017.
9. Gardner D, Shoback D, Greenspan F. *Greenspan's Basic & Clinical Endocrinology.* 10th ed. Cenveo Publisher Services; 2018.
10. Melmed S, Polonsky K, Larson P, Kronenberg H. *Williams Textbook of Endocrinology.* 13th ed. New Delhi: Elsevier; 2016.
11. Piercy K, Troiano R. Physical activity guidelines for Americans from the US department of health and human services. *Circ Cardiovasc Qual Outcomes.* 2018;11(11):e005263.
12. NHS. *Weight Management: Advice for Asian People.* England: NHS Trust; 2017.
13. Abazar E, Mardanian F, Forozandeh D, Taghian F. Effects of aerobic exercise on plasma lipoproteins in overweight and obese women with polycystic ovary syndrome. *Adv Biomed Res.* 2015;4(1):68.
14. Kogure G, Miranda-Furtado C, Pedroso D, et al. Effects of progressive resistance training on obesity indices in polycystic ovary syndrome and the relationship with telomere length. *J Phys Act Health.* 2019;16(8):601-607.
15. Mohseni M, Eghbali M, Bahrami H, Dastaran F, Amini L. Yoga effects on anthropometric indices and polycystic ovary syndrome symptoms in women undergoing infertility treatment: a randomized controlled clinical trial. *Evid Based Complement Alternat Med.* 2021;2021:5564824.
16. Karam N, Nathan J. *A Review of FDA-Approved Medications for Chronic Weight Management.* Drug Topics; 2021. Available from: https://www.drugtopics.com/view/a-review-of-fda-approved-medications-for-chronic-weight-management.
17. Lashen H. Review: Role of metformin in the management of polycystic ovary syndrome. *Ther Adv Endocrinol Metab.* 2010;1(3):117-128.
18. Abdalla M, Deshmukh H, Atkin S, Sathyapalan T. A review of therapeutic options for managing the metabolic aspects of polycystic ovary syndrome. *Ther Adv Endocrinol Metab.* 2020;11:204201882093830.
19. NIH. *LiverTox: Clinical and Research Information on Drug-Induced Liver Injury.* Bethesda (MD): National Institute of Diabetes and Digestive and Kidney Diseases; 2012. Available from: https://www.ncbi.nlm.nih.gov/books/NBK548834/.
20. Rodbard H. The clinical impact of GLP-1 receptor agonists in type 2 diabetes: focus on the long-acting analogs. *Diabetes Technol Ther.* 2018;20(suppl 2):S233-S241.
21. Crane J, McGowan B. The GLP-1 agonist, liraglutide, as a pharmacotherapy for obesity. *Ther Adv Chronic Dis.* 2016;7(2):92-107.
22. Marso SP, Bain SC, Consoli A, et al. Semaglutide and cardiovascular outcomes in patients with type 2 diabetes. *N Engl J Med.* 2016;375(19):1834-1844.
23. Pratley R, Amod A, Hoff S, et al. Oral semaglutide versus subcutaneous liraglutide and placebo in type 2 diabetes (PIONEER 4): a randomised, double-blind, phase 3a trial. *Lancet.* 2019;394(10192):39-50.
24. Rodbard H, Rosenstock J, Canani L, et al. Oral Semaglutide versus empagliflozin in patients with type 2 diabetes uncontrolled on metformin: the PIONEER 2 trial. *Diabetes Care.* 2019;42(12):2272-2281.
25. Hughes S, Neumiller JJ. Oral semaglutide. *Clin Diabetes.* 2020;38(1):109-111.
26. Chiu W, Shih S, Tseng C. A review on the association between glucagon-like peptide-1 receptor agonists and thyroid cancer. *Exp Diabetes Res.* 2012;2012:924168.
27. Cosentino G, Conrad AO, Uwaifo GI. Phentermine and topiramate for the management of obesity: a review. *Drug Des Devel Ther.* 2011;7:267-278.
28. Allison DB, Gadde KM, Garvey WT, et al. Controlled-release phentermine/topiramate in severely obese adults: a randomized controlled trial (EQUIP). *Obesity (Silver Spring).* 2012;20(2):330-342.
29. Gadde KM, Allison DB, Ryan DH, et al. Effects of low-dose, controlled-release, phentermine plus topiramate combination on weight and associated comorbidities in overweight and obese adults (CONQUER): a randomised, placebo-controlled, phase 3 trial. *Lancet.* 2011;377(9774):1341-1352.
30. Garvey WT, Ryan DH, Look M, et al. Two-year sustained weight loss and metabolic benefits with controlled-release phentermine/topiramate in obese and overweight adults (SEQUEL): a randomized, placebo-controlled, phase 3 extension study. *Am J Clin Nutr.* 2012;95(2):297-308.
31. Tek C. Naltrexone HCI/bupropion HCI for chronic weight management in obese adults: patient selection and perspectives. *Patient Prefer Adherence.* 2016;10:751-759.
32. Wadden TA, Foreyt JP, Foster GD, et al. Weight loss with naltrexone SR/bupropion SR combination therapy as an adjunct to behavior modification: the COR-BMOD trial. *Obesity (Silver Spring).* 2011;19(1):110-120.
33. Greenway FL, Fujioka K, Plodkowski RA, et al. Effect of naltrexone plus bupropion on weight loss in overweight and obese

adults (COR-I): a multicentre, randomised, double-blind, placebo-controlled, phase 3. *Lancet*. 2010;376(9741):595-605.

34. Hollander P, Gupta AK, Plodkowski R, et al. Effects of naltrexone sustained-release/bupropion sustained-release combination therapy on body weight and glycemic parameters in overweight and obese patients with type 2 diabetes. *Diabetes Care*. 2013;36(12): 4022-4029.

35. Ornellas T, Chavez B. Naltrexone SR/Bupropion SR (Contrave): a new approach to weight loss in obese adults. *P T*. 2011;36(5): 255-262.

36. Graff SK, Mario FM, Ziegelmann P, Spritzer PM. Effects of orlistat vs. metformin on weight loss-related clinical variables in women with PCOS: systematic review and meta-analysis. *Int J Clin Pract*. 2016;70(6):450-461.

37. Khera R, Murad MH, Chandar AK, et al. *Association of pharmacological treatments for obesity with weight loss and adverse events: a systematic review and meta-analysis. JAMA*. 2016;315(22): 2424-2434.

38. NIH. *Potential Candidates for Weight-Loss Surgery | NIDDK*. National Institute of Diabetes and Digestive and Kidney Diseases; 2021. Available at: https://www.niddk.nih.gov/health-information/weight-management/bariatric-surgery/potential-candidates.

39. IFSO. *IFSO Registry | International Federation for the Surgery of Obesity and Metabolic Disorders*. Ifso.com; 2021. Available at: https://www.ifso.com/ifso-registry.php.

40. Escobar-Morreale HF, Botella-Carretero JI, Alvarez-Blasco F, Sancho J, San Millán JL. The polycystic ovary syndrome associated with morbid obesity may resolve after weight loss induced by bariatric surgery. *J Clin Endocrinol Metab*. 2005;90(12):6364-6369.

41. Eid GM, Cottam DR, Velcu LM, et al. Effective treatment of polycystic ovarian syndrome with Roux-en-Y gastric bypass. *Surg Obes Relat Dis*. 2005;1(2):77-80.

42. Christ JP, Falcone T. Bariatric surgery improves hyperandrogenism, menstrual irregularities, and metabolic dysfunction among women with polycystic ovary syndrome (PCOS). *Obes Surg*. 2018;28(8):2171-2177.

43. Singh D, Arumalla K, Aggarwal S, Singla V, Ganie A, Malhotra N. Impact of bariatric surgery on clinical, biochemical, and hormonal parameters in women with polycystic ovary syndrome (PCOS). *Obes Surg*. 2020;30(6):2294-2300.

44. *Weight-Loss and Weight-Management Devices*. U.S. Food and Drug Administration; 2021. Available at: https://www.fda.gov/medical-devices/products-and-medical-procedures/weight-loss-and-weight-management-devices#loss.

17

Role of Insulin Sensitizers in the Management of Polycystic Ovary Syndrome

OWAIS RASHID AND MAHWISH FATIMA

Introduction

Hyperinsulinemia and insulin resistance (IR) are considered major culprits behind the pathophysiology of polycystic ovary syndrome (PCOS). Hyperinsulinemia and IR cause chronic anovulation, hyperandrogenemia, metabolic dysfunction, and its associated comorbidities by influencing endocrine glands (ovaries, adrenals, pituitary) and peripheral tissues (adipose, liver, and muscle) in a variety of ways. Based on these inferences, a number of insulin sensitizers have been evaluated to see if they could be a treatment option for patients with PCOS. Coupled with lifestyle modification, insulin sensitizers are used to reduce insulin levels and ameliorate IR, which eventually leads to improved endocrine and metabolic function associated with PCOS.

The hypothesis behind using insulin sensitizers in most patients with PCOS is that nearly all obese females with PCOS and more than half of PCOS patients with normal weight present with IR and show fasting or stimulated hyperinsulinemia to some extent.

Mechanism of Insulin Sensitizers in PCOS

Various mechanisms highlighting the favorable effects of insulin sensitizers involve a reduction in insulin levels leading to an increase in sex hormone–binding globulin (SHBG), thus decreasing the availability of both free and circulating androgens to peripheral tissues. Improved insulin sensitivity and decreased insulin concentration enhance the fertility chances in both infertile and subfertile females with PCOS. Decreased insulin levels cause a reduction in bound and free androgen, which improves most of the signs and symptoms of hyperandrogenemia. By improving IR and decreasing insulin levels with insulin sensitizers, there is improvement in glucose intolerance that helps in delaying the onset of type 2 diabetes mellitus (T2DM) and progression of metabolic syndrome, along with its related cardiovascular (CV) risk.

Insulin Sensitizers in Polycystic Ovary Syndrome

The following agents are primarily used as insulin sensitizers in the management of PCOS:
1. Metformin
2. Thiazolidinediones
3. Glucagon-like peptide-1 receptor agonists (GLP-1 RA)
4. Inositols
5. Alpha-lipoic acid

Metformin

In 1994 metformin was the first antidiabetes drug used in patients with PCOS to try to discover the role of IR in the pathogenesis of the syndrome.[1]

Metformin has reformed the treatment approaches of numerous metabolic disorders in the past four decades. Among the other categories of insulin-lowering drugs, metformin is known to be the most investigated drug in short- and long-term treatment regimens. Nevertheless, strong evidence is still lacking, and there is a dire need to further explore this old drug in various ways for patients with PCOS.[2]

Mechanism of Action

Metformin acts on a variety of tissues that cause reproductive and metabolic abnormalities in PCOS such as the liver, adipose tissues, skeletal muscle, and the ovary. It decreases hepatic gluconeogenesis, reduces lipogenesis, and enhances uptake of glucose in the liver, adipose tissues, skeletal muscles, and ovaries.

Metformin is supposed to produce direct and indirect effects on the ovary for the production of androgen. Initiating metformin therapy in patients with PCOS resulted in reduction of cytochrome P450 17A1 (*CYP17A1*) activity, leading to a decrease in serum insulin levels. Additionally, metformin causes inhibition of ovarian steroidogenesis forthrightly, and for this, mitochondrial complex I inhibition has been involved as one of the potential mechanisms of action. Metformin may also reduce the level of androgen via inhibition of 3β-hydroxysteroid dehydrogenase/Δ^5-Δ^4 isomerase type 2.

The clinical response to metformin treatment is, at times, highly variable among different PCOS phenotypes, and a number of genetic factors have been implicated as a possible reason. Nevertheless, large-scale genome-wide studies are needed to identify markers for these variable responses.

Clinical Effects

Effect on Androgens
Metformin, by lowering insulin levels, results in a decrease in testosterone levels in nearly 20% to 25% of females with PCOS,[2] and this decrease in testosterone is more prominent in nonobese patients with PCOS. Nevertheless, some other potential mechanisms for lowering testosterone levels are also reported. Some studies reported lowering of testosterone within a span of 48 hours of initiation of metformin therapy, even before producing any substantial change in insulin sensitivity and other metabolic components. Evidence suggests that metformin produces significant effects on the free androgen index, total testosterone, and SHBG levels. Some studies have shown that metformin reduces testosterone levels in females with PCOS despite the fact that no improvement was observed in insulin sensitivity as assessed by the commonly sampled intravenous glucose tolerance test. These effects of metformin may vary among various PCOS phenotypes.

Menstrual Irregularity and Clinical Hyperandrogenism
Although metformin lowers testosterone levels, its use in PCOS is not always associated with improvements of irregular menstruation or clinical hyperandrogenism. Evidence suggests that metformin therapy only produces slight improvement in menstrual pattern with substantial heterogeneity.[3] Additionally, metformin has not appeared as potent therapy for improving the symptoms of clinical hyperandrogenism like acne or hirsutism. Therefore metformin is not endorsed as the first choice of drug for management of irregular menstruation and clinical hyperandrogenism in PCOS.

Fertility and Live Birth Rate
Metformin use in PCOS may improve the ovulation rate, pregnancy rate, and fertility rate; however, it does not improve miscarriage rate and live birth rate per pregnancy. Compared with clomiphene citrate, metformin has not

shown significant differences in terms of ovulation induction, multiple pregnancies, or live birth. Therefore it is not recommended as the treatment of choice for anovulatory infertility in PCOS.[4]

Insulin Insensitivity and Hyperinsulinemia
Burghan originally described the relationship between PCOS and hyperinsulinemia. During the OGTT test, he compared the responses of insulin among females with and without PCOS. He found similar glucose responses among both groups, whereas insulin responses were significantly higher in patients with PCOS. Later, various research studies using the gold standard hyperinsulinemic–euglycemic clamp technique demonstrated insulin-mediated glucose disposal reduction in females with PCOS in contrast with a group of reproductively normal females matched for age and body mass index (BMI). Based on the evidence, metformin has been titled as an insulin sensitizer in patients with PCOS.[5]

Metformin appears to reduce fasting insulin levels in patients with PCOS but with significant heterogeneity. This effect is more pronounced in nonobese females.[5] There is no evidence that the combination of metformin and oral contraceptives produce any impact on insulin levels in patients with PCOS.[5] Therefore the clinical significance of metformin therapy in PCOS for improving insulin sensitivity shows high variability and depends on the metabolic attributes and PCOS phenotype.

Glucose Intolerance
Recent guidelines on the management of PCOS recommend metformin as first-line medication for the treatment of patients with T2DM or impaired glucose tolerance who do not benefit from lifestyle interventions. Studies that explore the effect of metformin on diabetes risk, particularly in patients with PCOS, have not been conducted yet. Nevertheless, considering the fact that these patients are at very high risk for developing diabetes, it has been suggested that metformin may provide greater benefit in individuals with higher metabolic risk, including those with diabetes risk factors, impaired glucose tolerance, or high-risk ethnic groups.[5]

Body Weight and Composition
The effect of metformin on body composition and weight loss is disputed. Use of metformin for 6 months at a daily dose of 1500 mg produced no impact on BMI and only a minimal reduction in waist-to-hip ratio (WHR), but it produces beneficial effects on BMI and central obesity when coupled with lifestyle modification. The use of metformin alone is not related to any reduction in BMI. The effect of metformin on visceral versus subcutaneous fat deposits has not been examined well. Evidence suggests that when metformin is combined with a low calorie diet in PCOS patients, it results in a moderate effect on body weight and central obesity. To establish the use of metformin in this regard, however, further studies are required.[5]

Dyslipidemia and Cardiovascular Disease

There is a high risk of CV disease in patients with PCOS because of the presence of IR and its associated metabolic consequences, namely T2DM, metabolic syndrome, and dyslipidemia. Nevertheless, the definite prevalence of CV events in PCOS is not known. Evidence on whether metformin therapy improves dyslipidemia and CV risk in patients with PCOS is of low certainty and future well-designed, large prospective randomized clinical trials are required to address these uncertainties.

Dose and Side Effects

Metformin doses of 500 mg/day to 1000 mg/day are generally advised to reduce side effects and enhance compliance. Extended release preparations can be helpful in minimizing side effects as well.[2]

Gastrointestinal (GI) upsets (e.g., diarrhea, dyspepsia, flatulence, nausea) are the commonest adverse effects of metformin. They occur in around 10% to 50% of patients but are generally transient and settle in a couple of days to a week. To reduce the side effects, it is advisable to start therapy with a low dose of 500 mg with a gradual increase in 1 to 2 weeks or to administer metformin along with food.[2]

Vit-B12 malabsorption caused by metformin therapy is rare. It is mainly linked with dose, aging, and duration of treatment. Metformin-related lactic acidosis and megaloblastic anemia are extremely rare. It can be safely prescribed until the estimated glomerular filtration rate drops below 30 mL/min. Nevertheless, reduction in dose is recommended at 45 mL/min. Contraindication includes alcohol abuse because metformin and alcohol are incompatible and concomitant use results in hypoglycemia and lactic acidosis.

In most countries, metformin is regarded as an off-label indication for the management of PCOS, but its use is not strictly restricted if healthcare professionals inform patients and discuss its effects.[2]

Thiazolidinediones

Troglitazone, the first and foremost thiazolidinedione (TZD), was approved in 1997 as an antihyperglycemic agent. Later, in 2000, it was withdrawn from the market because of its hepatotoxic effect.[6] Presently, two TZDs are available: pioglitazone and rosiglitazone. International agencies restricted the use of rosiglitazone because of its cardiotoxic profile, although it is considered hepatoprotective.[6]

Mechanism of Action

TZD selectively binds to the peroxisome proliferator-activated receptors, a group of nuclear transcription factors. It is mostly expressed in pancreatic cells, vascular endothelium, adipocytes, and macrophages and, in less proportion, in the heart and skeletal muscle tissue. Mechanisms of action involve stimulation of fatty acid uptake and deposit in subcutaneous adipose tissue and increased secretion of adiponectin from adipose tissue; as a result, insulin sensitivity increases specifically in the liver. TZD inhibits hepatic gluconeogenesis, improves dyslipidemia, and boosts anti-arteriosclerotic and anti-inflammatory effects.

Metabolic and Endocrine Effects

Pioglitazone and rosiglitazone are the most widely investigated TZDs in patients with PCOs. TZDs play a significant role in decreasing fasting and postprandial glycemic levels. Pioglitazone is supposed to positively regulate the ovarian androgen synthesis; it affects the ovarian steroid hormone metabolism in cultured granulosa cells in a variety of ways, such as (1) progesterone biosynthesis upregulation, (2) testosterone inhibition, and (3) estradiol (E2) production via insulin-independent and dependent pathways.

Evidence suggests that in PCOS, pioglitazone improves the menstrual cycle, whereas it does not produce any effect in endocrine (testosterone, SHBG), metabolic (fasting insulin), and anthropometric (BMI, WHR) outcomes.[2] Compared with metformin, rosiglitazone showed promising results in patients with PCOS in levels of total testosterone, dehydroepiandrosterone sulfate (DHEAS), follicular-stimulating hormone, and luteinizing hormone, whereas metformin showed better results in free testosterone, estradiol, and androstenedione levels. Considering the fasting glucose, insulin, or homeostasis model assessment of IR, treatment with metformin and rosiglitazone exhibited insignificant differences.[2]

Side Effects

TZDs cause weight gain, fatigue, diarrhea, edema, anemia, and congestive heart failure; pioglitazone, specifically, enhances risk of bladder cancer and osteoporosis. Additionally, both pioglitazone and rosiglitazone have been placed in category C for pregnancy. Both drugs produce similar effects in terms of weight gain, fluid retention, and bone fractures.

Further, the combination therapy of TZD and metformin is not advisable when the desired outcome is weight loss, and this combination is contraindicated if pregnancy is to be planned.

Glucagon-Like Peptide 1 Agonists

Mechanism of Action

Glucagon-like peptide 1 (GLP-1) receptor agonists are antidiabetic drugs that are incretin mimetics. Incretins, including glucose-dependent insulin-tropic peptide (GIP) and GLP-1, are gut hormones released from enteroendocrine cells upon ingestion of food. GLP-1 agonists produce action via stimulating the secretion of insulin, inhibiting the secretion of glucagon, and suppressing the intake of food and appetite. Besides improving glucose homeostasis, GLP-1 agonists are capable of reducing weight, improving dyslipidemia, and moderately decreasing blood pressure. Their weight-lowering effect helps in improving a number of risk factors of metabolic syndrome, such as BMI, glucose intolerance, T2DM, nonalcoholic fatty liver disease, and steatohepatitis. Decrease in weight also improves hyperinsulinemia and IR. Based on these encouraging results, a number of different preparations of GLP-1 agonists have been tried and tested in PCOS in the past decade. First, exenatide was investigated in patients with PCOS in 2008. After that, various studies on liraglutide showed weight loss, decreased hyperandrogenism, and improved menstruation.

Various preparations of GLP-1 agonists are available. Historically, all available GLP-1 preparations are in the form of injectable doses and are administered via the subcutaneous route because the oral route showed poor bioavailability. Liraglutide and lixisenatide are taken as single-dose, daily injections, whereas dulaglutide, semaglutide, and albiglutide can be administered either twice a day or once a week. Semaglutide, an oral preparation, has recently been approved by the Federal Drug Administration (FDA). Trial and investigation on taspoglutide, a novel GLP-1 analog, has been suspended because it caused GI tract–related side effects and hypersensitivity.

Metabolic Effects and Endocrine Effects

Evidence suggests that exenatide and liraglutide significantly reduced weight in obese females with PCOS if used alone or when combined with metformin. They produced weight reduction in terms of BMI and waist circumference. Some studies have reported a decrease in androgen levels with improvement in menstruation.[7] IR index (homeostatic model assessment [HOMA]) and testosterone level also improved after treatment with a GLP-1 agonist. Nearly all of these outcomes have been linked to reduction in weight associated with GLP-1 agonists.

Nevertheless, the majority of studies evaluating the effect of GLP-1 agonists in PCOS are considered weak because of the small sample size and poor generalization because only obese and overweight patients with PCOS were enrolled. In a nutshell, GLP-1 agonists might help in improving metabolic outcomes in PCOS patients, but their role in fertility is still experimental[2] (Tables 17.1 and 17.2).

Side Effects

The most common side effects of GLP-1 agonists include GI symptoms (e.g., nausea, vomiting, diarrhea), headache, dizziness, and weakness. Nausea and vomiting are usually transient and resolve in a week or two. Other common adverse effects of these drugs include injection site reactions, headache, and nasopharyngitis. Compliance to

TABLE 17.1   Endocrine Outcomes of Insulin Sensitizers in Polycystic Ovary Syndrome

	Menstruation	Ovulation Rate	Hyperandrogenism
Metformin	Improved	Improved	Slightly reduced
Thiazolidinediones	Improved	Unchanged or slightly improved	Unchanged or slightly reduced
Glucagon-like peptide-1 receptor agonists (GLP-1 RA)	Improved[a]		Improved[a]
Inositols		Improved[a]	
Alpha-lipoic acid	Improved[a]		

[a]Little evidence of effect.

TABLE 17.2   Metabolic Outcomes of Insulin Sensitizers in Polycystic Ovary Syndrome

	Glucose Intolerance	Body Weight	Insulin Sensitivity
Metformin	Improved	Unchanged or slightly reduced	Improved
Thiazolidinediones	Improved	Unchanged or slight gain	Improved
Glucagon-like peptide-1 receptor agonists (GLP-1 RA)	Improved	Weight loss	Improved[b]
Inositols		No effect	Improved[a]
Alpha-lipoic acid			Improved[a]

[a]Little evidence of effect.
[b]Limited evidence of effect.

treatment may be affected by the cost of medication and parenteral route of administration.

Miscellaneous Agents

Inositols, particularly myoinositol (MI) and D-chiro-inositol (DCI), favor the formation of insulin second messengers, possibly leading to a decrease in IR. Evidence suggests that DCI helps in improving the rate of ovulation but has no effect on BMI, WHR, or blood pressure. Besides displaying some effect on serum SHBG levels, fasting glucose, fasting insulin, and lipids (total cholesterol, triglycerides), DCI did not show any effect on hormonal parameters. Therefore international guidelines on the management of PCOS recommend cautious use of inositol, and they are considered as experimental therapy in patients with PCOS.

Alpha-lipoic acid (ALA) is a biologic antioxidant being investigated as an insulin sensitizer. Based on the strong association of oxidative stress and IR, ALA was historically investigated in T2DM patients. Data have shown that ALA may enhance insulin sensitivity in peripheral tissues and help in improving glucose homeostasis in diabetes patients.

Use of ALA is considered a unique treatment in PCOS. Its effect has been investigated in both lean and overweight females. After a dose of 400 mg once daily, ALA produced improvement in triglycerides, insulin sensitivity, menstrual frequency, and liver function parameters. Various studies reported the effect of different preparations containing ALA and specifically ALA in combination with MI. When metformin at a dose of 3 gm per day was compared with a combination therapy of ALA, MI, and metformin (1.7g/day), better responses were observed in the BMI, hyperandrogenism, and HOMA index.[2]

Comparative Studies Among Various Insulin Sensitizers

Data on comparison of use of various insulin sensitizers in PCOS are scarce; however, as far as endocrine outcomes are concerned, significant results were not observed upon comparing metformin with TZD or inositol. With respect to metabolic outcome, when metformin was compared with TZD, it showed effective results on triglycerides in people who were at high risk for metabolic syndrome, but the opposite effects were noticed when these two drugs were compared on HOMA index and fasting insulin. Negligible differences on metabolic outcomes were found when comparing metformin with inositol.[2]

Conclusion

Management of PCOS remains a challenge for a physician because no single treatment regime has proven to be efficacious or has been able to address the variable pathophysiology and phenotypes of PCOS. Plenty of insulin sensitizers have been investigated and proposed, but they are still far from being an absolute indication of PCOS. Metformin is the only insulin sensitizing agent that has shown promising results in patients with PCOS. Nevertheless, it is regarded as off-label. The other available options (TZD, inositols, ALA, and GLP-1 agonists) are mostly experimental, and data show huge variation in terms of combination therapies, dose, and target subjects. Despite their promising clinical outcomes in a few studies, all agents are deemed to be experimental in patients with PCOS.

References

1. He L, Wondisford FE. Metformin action: concentrations matter. *Cell Metab.* 2015;21(2):159-162.
2. Romualdi D, Versace V, Lanzone A. What is new in the landscape of insulin-sensitizing agents for polycystic ovary syndrome treatment. *Ther Adv Reprod Health.* 2020;14. doi:10.1177/2633494120908709.
3. Tang T, Lord JM, Norman RJ, Yasmin E, Balen AH. Insulin-sensitising drugs (metformin, rosiglitazone, pioglitazone, D-chiro-inositol) for women with polycystic ovary syndrome, oligo amenorrhoea and subfertility. *Cochrane Database Syst Rev.* 2012;(5):CD003053.
4. Sam S, Ehrmann DA. Metformin therapy for the reproductive and metabolic consequences of polycystic ovary syndrome. *Diabetologia.* 2017;60(9):1656-1661.
5. Miller RA, Chu Q, Xie J, Foretz M, Viollet B, Birnbaum MJ. Biguanides suppress hepatic glucagon signalling by decreasing production of cyclic AMP. *Nature.* 2013;494(7436):256-260.
6. Nanjan M, Mohammed M, Kumar BP, Chandrasekar M. Thiazolidinediones as antidiabetic agents: a critical review. *Bioorg Chem.* 2018;77:548-567.
7. Lamos EM, Malek R, Davis SN. GLP-1 receptor agonists in the treatment of polycystic ovary syndrome. *Expert Rev Clin Pharmacol.* 2017;10(4):401-408.

Reading List

He L, Wondisford FE. Metformin action: concentrations matter. *Cell Metab.* 2015;21(2):159-162.

Kim LH, Taylor AE, Barbieri RL. Insulin sensitizers and polycystic ovary syndrome: can a diabetes medication treat infertility? *Fertil Steril.* 2000;73(6):1097-1098.

Lamos EM, Malek R, Davis SN. GLP-1 receptor agonists in the treatment of polycystic ovary syndrome. *Expert Rev Clin Pharmacol.* 2017;10(4):401-408.

Nanjan MJ, Mohammed M, Kumar BP, Chandrasekar MJN. Thiazolidinediones as antidiabetic agents: a critical review. *Bioorg Chem.* 2018;77:548-567.

Pasquali R, Gambineri A. Insulin-sensitizing agents in polycystic ovary syndrome. *Eur J Endocrinol.* 2006;154(6):763-775.

Romualdi D, Versace V, Lanzone A. What is new in the landscape of insulin-sensitizing agents for polycystic ovary syndrome treatment. *Ther Adv Reprod Health.* 2020;14. doi:10.1177/2633494120908709.

Sam S, Ehrmann DA. Metformin therapy for the reproductive and metabolic consequences of polycystic ovary syndrome. *Diabetologia.* 2017;60(9):1656-1661.

Stracquadanio M, Ciotta L. *Metabolic Aspects of PCOS.* Heidelberg, NY: Springer; 2015.

Tang T, Lord JM, Norman RJ, Yasmin E, Balen AH. Insulin-sensitising drugs (metformin, rosiglitazone, pioglitazone, D-chiro-inositol) for women with polycystic ovary syndrome, oligo amenorrhoea and subfertility. *Cochrane Database Syst Rev.* 2012;(5):CD003053.

Xing C, Li C, He B. Insulin sensitizers for improving the endocrine and metabolic profile in overweight women with PCOS. *J Clin Endocrinol Metab.* 2020;105(9):2950-2963.

Zhao H, Xing C, Zhang J, He B. Comparative efficacy of oral insulin sensitizers metformin, thiazolidinediones, inositol, and berberine in improving endocrine and metabolic profiles in women with PCOS: a network meta-analysis. *Reprod Health.* 2021; 18(1):171.

18

Cardiovascular Risk Reduction in Polycystic Ovary Syndrome

PIRBHAT SHAMS, INTISAR AHMED, AND ZAINAB SAMAD

Background

Cardiovascular disease (CVD) is the most frequent cause of death in females.[1] Patients with the polycystic ovarian syndrome (PCOS) have a ubiquitous prevalence of traditional risk factors for CVD, including metabolic syndrome (MetS). PCOS is associated with dyslipidemia, obesity, and diabetes mellitus (DM).[2] Additionally, studies have found increased markers of subclinical CVD in patients with PCOS, such as coronary calcium (CAC), C-reactive protein (CRP), and endothelial dysfunction.[3] This is largely based on observational studies. There is a lack of large prospective studies exploring the causal relationship between PCOS and incident CVD, including acute coronary syndrome and ischemic stroke.

Establishing a CVD risk profile in patients with PCOS presents a useful window for CVD prevention.[4] Females with PCOS should have an early risk stratification for useful prevention outcomes. Although the association between CVD risk enhancers and PCOS is established, it is uncertain if this association translates into a direct risk of clinical and subclinical CVD.[4] In this chapter, we shall review CVD risk factors and their management in patients with PCOS.

Cardiovascular Risk Factors in Polycystic Ovary Syndrome

Hypertension, diabetes, and obesity are some of the major CVD risk factors in patients with PCOS.[5] Metabolic and hormonal derangements are the hallmark of PCOS. This plays a vital role in the pathogenesis of hypertension, DM, dyslipidemia, and other CVD risk enhancers.[6]

Hypertension and Polycystic Ovary Syndrome

Hypertension is a major established risk factor for CVD. Although there are no large population-based studies to support this association, small observational studies have reported a higher prevalence of hypertension in young females with PCOS compared with the matched controls.[7]

Hypertension in PCOS may not be related to body mass index (BMI) and obesity.[8] Joham et al. demonstrated in a large cohort that hypertension was more common in females of reproductive age with PCOS than those without PCOS. On subgroup analysis, there was an association of hypertension with BMI in non-PCOS patients, but not in PCOS patients, pointing toward the relation between PCOS and hypertension, independent of BMI.[8]

Although the pathogenesis of hypertension in PCOS is multifactorial, aldosterone is the pivotal factor in the development of hypertension. Young patients with PCOS have a higher level of aldosterone compared with healthy females.[9] Hyperandrogenism (HA) in PCOS patients can potentially contribute to hypertension. In an experimental study, by an unclear mechanism, giving androgen to ovariectomized female rats increased blood pressure in a dose-dependent manner. This effect was not observed when the renin-angiotensin system (RAS) was blocked.[10]

Increased androgens have been associated with increased expression of angiotensinogen. Studies have shown higher renin and prorenin levels in patients with PCOS and oligo-menorrhea.[11] This explains the possible role of androgen in the pathogenesis of hypertension in PCOS patients via the RAS pathway. Chen et al. studied the relationship between androgens and hypertension in 150 young PCOS patients and found that after adjustment for BMI and dyslipidemia, both systolic ($p = .0008$) and diastolic ($p = .0018$) blood pressures (SBP and DBP, respectively) were strongly related to free androgen index (FAI). Females in the highest SBP quartile also had higher FAI levels than females in the lower (0.0006) and lowest SBP quartile (0.019).[12]

Likewise, endothelin-1, a marker of vasculopathy, is another possible mediator for PCOS-related hypertension. Patients with PCOS have higher endothelin-1 levels than controls ($p < .02$).[13] Hyperinsulinemia has also been proposed as a risk factor for hypertension because of autonomic imbalance, sodium retention, and impaired nitric oxide production.[7]

Obesity, Metabolic Syndrome, and Polycystic Ovary Syndrome

Obesity is commonly present in PCOS patients. As many as 80% of PCOS patients are obese or overweight. Females with PCOS have a higher waist to hip ratio compared with the age-matched healthy population.[14] In a systemic review and meta-analysis of a population of more than 14,000 from 34 studies, there was a higher prevalence of central obesity in PCOS patients (risk ratio [RR] 1.73) compared with females without PCOS. This was independent of age and geographic distribution.[15] MetS and PCOS might share a common pathogenesis. The overlap in presence of traditional risk factors, such as central obesity, dyslipidemia, insulin resistance (IR), hypertension, and elevated fasting blood glucose, points toward a common pathway.[16]

Ehrmann et al. looked at the prevalence of MetS in 394 PCOS patients, which was 33.4%. The prevalence did not differ between racial/ethnic groups with as many as 50% of Asians, 34% of Caucasians, 26% of African Americans, and 31% of Hispanics having symptoms of MetS. The presence of MetS in this cohort of PCOS patients was associated with higher SBP and DBP, higher BMI, a greater waist circumference, and a bigger waist-to-hip ratio compared with PCOS patients without MetS.

Obesity in PCOS is likely because of IR and elevated insulin levels.[15] Hyperinsulinemia increases the synthesis of steroids in ovaries and inhibits the production of androgen-binding globulins in the liver. The resulting increase in free androgens leads to visceral fat accumulation and weight gain.[17]

MetS is a cluster of cardiometabolic risk factors, including increased waist circumference, increased triacyl-glycerides, low high-density lipoprotein carbohydrates (HDL-C), hypertension, and elevated blood glucose.[18] A meta-analysis of more than 6000 females from 15 studies has shown that females with PCOS are more likely to have MetS (odds ratio [OR] 2.8) compared with those without PCOS.[19] IR and hyperinsulinemia hence play a central role in the pathogenesis of MetS and its clinical manifestations.[20]

Insulin Resistance, Diabetes Mellitus, and Polycystic Ovary Syndrome

More than one-third of patients with PCOS have impaired glucose tolerance (IGT) tests and at least 7% to 10% have DM.[19,21] Patients with PCOS have an increased risk of developing DM irrespective of age and BMI.[22] Moreover, the prevalence of PCOS is higher in diabetic young females compared with the nondiabetic population.[23]

The expert consensus is that PCOS is a risk factor for DM, which is an established risk factor for CVD. This is because females with PCOS have increased IR regardless of their BMI.[24] A meta-analysis showed that PCOS patients had lower insulin sensitivity (IS) compared with controls (mean effect -27%, 99% confidence interval [CI] ± 6%). Nevertheless, the IS was further reduced by 15% in patients with larger BMI and by 10% in patients with lower sex hormone–binding globulin (SHBG).[24]

IR and the pathogenesis of DM in PCOS are very well described in the literature. A defect in the insulin signaling pathway and impaired phosphorylation of insulin receptors, as well as its substrate, are the major contributors to IR and DM.[25] Other factors include decreased level of glucose transporter in adipose tissues, impaired clearance of insulin from the liver and mitochondrial dysfunction, and activation of serine kinases.[25]

Dyslipidemia and Polycystic Ovary Syndrome

Dyslipidemia, especially higher levels of low-density lipoproteins (LDL), is strongly associated with CVD.[26] Most common lipid abnormalities in women with PCOS include increased levels of triglycerides (TG) and LDL and reduced levels of HDL. A meta-analysis of more than 30 has shown that females with PCOS had 26 mg/dL higher TG levels, 12.6 mg/dL higher LDL-C, and 6 mg/dL lower HDL-C levels compared with the age-matched females without PCOS.[27] Dyslipidemia in PCOS patients is mainly because of IR, obesity, and HA.[28]

Polycystic Ovary Syndrome and Cardiovascular Diseases

PCOS encompasses several metabolic abnormalities that serve as major risk factors for CVD. Nevertheless, there are limited data on the direct association of clinical CVD with PCOS. The increased risk of CVD in PCOS is inferential and based on the atherosclerotic CVD (ASCVD) risk factors present in females with PCOS.[29]

Clinical Cardiovascular Disease

A large population-based study from Denmark studied more than 70,000 females and followed them for more than 10 years. The study showed that PCOS patients had a hazard ratio (HR) of 1.7 for developing clinical CVD compared with the age-matched control group.[30] In patients with PCOS, the median age of CVD diagnosis was 35 years. Obesity, DM, and infertility were associated with an increased incidence of CVD.[30]

A large population-based study of 25,000 females from Australia reported a higher incidence of ischemic heart disease and cerebrovascular diseases in the PCOS group compared with age-matched controls, with an adjusted HR of 2.8 and 2.5, respectively.[31] In a meta-analysis of five studies, the PCOS group had two times higher risk of CVD after adjusting for BMI.[32] Another meta-analysis by Luqian Zhao et al. showed that PCOS females had a higher incidence of CVD (OR 1.30).[33]

Another meta-analysis of eight studies showed that PCOS had an elevated risk of cerebrovascular accidents (OR 1.36). On adjusting for BMI, however, this difference became statistically nonsignificant (OR 1.24 [95% CI 0.98–1.59]).[34]

Subclinical Cardiovascular Disease

Several researchers have studied the markers of subclinical CVD in patients with PCOS. These include coronary calcium score, intima-media thickness, inflammatory markers such as CRP, and endothelin-1, a marker of vascular endothelial dysfunction.

A study by Rose C. Cristian et al. reported an increased prevalence of coronary calcium scores in females with PCOS compared with matched controls.[35] Another study showed that after adjusting for age and BMI, individuals with PCOS had a higher coronary calcium score than those without PCOS.[36]

A meta-analysis demonstrated that females with PCOS have significantly elevated mean carotid intima-media thickness (CIMT) compared with the non-PCOS group, placing them at a higher risk of clinical CVD.[37] The higher CIMT in patients with PCOS could be explained by central obesity; elevated levels of insulin, inflammatory markers, TG, and LDL-C; and lower levels of HDL-C.[38,39]

Another meta-analysis of more than 45 studies of around 5000 females reported that the PCOS group had significantly higher levels of CRP and homocysteine levels compared with the non-PCOS group.[40] The meta-analysis further demonstrated that females with PCOS have elevated levels of plasminogen activator inhibitor-1, endothelin-1, and vascular endothelial growth factor.[40] Several research studies have reported endothelial dysfunction in PCOS. These studies have further shown that endothelial dysfunction coexists with elevated levels of inflammatory markers, including CRP, which provides indirect evidence that chronic inflammation causes endothelial dysfunction and promotes atherosclerosis.[36,41]

Cardiovascular Risk Management in Polycystic Ovary Syndrome

CVD risk reduction in patients with PCOS revolves around efficient management of traditional risk factors and a basic understanding at both the physician's and patient's ends of a heightened risk for CVD. Optimal identification and management of CVD risk in PCOS require a multidisciplinary team that focuses on early metabolic screening and intervention, nutritional and exercise guidance, and behavioral and psychological support. Realizing the greater prevalence of CVD risk factors in PCOS patients, an individualized approach should be used to stratify patients for CVD at each healthcare encounter. Every encounter presents an opportunity to identify high-risk patients and counsel them for a healthier lifestyle. Experts now believe that the key potential therapeutic target to reduce CVD risk in PCOS patients is insulin-glucose metabolism and managing the incident risk of DM, which represents a central risk factor for CVD.

The consensus statement by the Androgen Excess and Polycystic Ovary Syndrome Society (AE-PCOS) recommends stratifying patients based on their risk profile into the "at-risk" category and the "at high-risk" category.[42] The at-risk category is defined by the presence of obesity, tobacco addiction, hypertension, dyslipidemia, any evidence of subclinical vascular disease or IGT, and family history positive for premature CVD. On the other hand, PCOS patients with established MetS or type 2 DM, and overt renovascular disease fall into the high-risk category.[42]

The following strategies can be focused on considering recent literature on CVD:

- All patients should undergo BMI and waist circumference measurements to assess abdominal obesity in every healthcare encounter.
- In consensus with the American Heart Association (AHA) guidelines for CVD prevention in females, a complete lipid profile should be done every 2 years or earlier (if weight gain occurs).[43] Target LDL level should be less than 130 mg/dL in females with PCOS but with no additional CVD risk factors. All "at high-risk" patients should get their LDL-C levels to less than 70 to 100 mg/dL.
- All patients should be screened for IGT. IGT screening using a 2-hour post 75 g oral glucose challenge should be done every 2 years or sooner in high-risk patients. The focus should be on females with a BMI of more than 30 kg/m² or those with advanced renovascular disease. Patients with positive IGT tests should undergo annual screening for type 2 DM. The endorsed Hb A_{1c} cutoff remains at 6.5% for these patients.
- Blood pressure should be checked at each encounter to detect early-onset hypertension. The target BP is 120/80 mm Hg or lower.
- Patients with PCOS should be advised for intensive lifestyle modification. This would decrease the risk of conversion from IGT to type 2 DM.[44]
- Physicians prescribing combined oral contraceptives (COC) for menstrual irregularity should be cognizant of the elevated risk of CVD associated with COCs.[45,46]
- Use of metformin results in a reduction in IGT and a favorable effect on lipid profile. This can both indirectly and theoretically improve long-term cardiovascular outcomes.
- Strong psychosocial support is required to encourage adherence to lifestyle changes and combat depression. Literature suggests a weaker adherence to lifestyle changes in patients with depression and type 2 DM.[47]

- Guideline-directed medical therapy is indicated for hypertension and dyslipidemia to achieve target levels.

Primary Prevention Strategies for Cardiovascular Disease Risk Reduction in Patients With Polycystic Ovary Syndrome

Lifestyle Changes

Lifestyle change is the first-line treatment in PCOS patients. It encompasses weight loss, smoking cessation, recommended daily exercise, and dietary modification. Weight loss results in an expected improvement in CVD risk.[48] Patients should aim for 500 to 1000 kcal/day reduction and derive less than 30% of calories from fat and less than 10% from saturated fat. At the very least, moderately intense exercise for 30 minutes is recommended. Overweight patients should aim for 5% to 10% weight loss initially and 10% to 20% ultimately in the long run and a waist circumference target of less than 80 to 88 cm.

Medical Therapy

Medical therapy encompasses insulin sensitizers, a cholesterol-lowering medication, and antihypertensive medications.

Conclusion

PCOS patients have a higher prevalence of traditional risk factors for CVD, and IR significantly contributes to the pathogenesis of these risk factors. Although central obesity has been reported to potentiate atherosclerosis, PCOS patients have an elevated risk of CVD irrespective of BMI. Additionally, the prevalence of subclinical ASCVD is reportedly higher in PCOS compared with controls. Nevertheless, there are limited data on the direct association of PCOS with clinical ASCVD (myocardial infarction and stroke). Population-based studies are required to establish the direct association of PCOS with clinical CVD. Lifestyle modifications, including a healthy diet, physical activity, weight reduction, and smoking cessation, reduce the CVD risk in PCOS. All patients with PCOS should be regularly screened and treated for ASCVD risk factors and encouraged to have a healthy lifestyle.

References

1. Centre for Disease Control and Prevention. Women and Heart Disease. 2022. https://www.cdc.gov/heartdisease/women.
2. Zhu T, Cui J, Goodarzi MO. Polycystic ovary syndrome and risk of type 2 diabetes, coronary heart disease, and stroke. *Diabetes.* 2021;70(2):627-637.
3. Diamanti-Kandarakis E, Alexandraki K, Piperi C, et al. Inflammatory and endothelial markers in women with polycystic ovary syndrome. *Eur J Clin Invest.* 2006;36(10):691-697.
4. Osibogun O, Ogunmoroti O, Michos ED. Polycystic ovary syndrome and cardiometabolic risk: opportunities for cardiovascular disease prevention. *Trends Cardiovasc Med.* 2020;30(7):399-404.
5. Young L, Cho L. Unique cardiovascular risk factors in women. *Heart.* 2019;105(21):1656-1660.
6. Osibogun O, Ogunmoroti O, Michos ED. Polycystic ovary syndrome and cardiometabolic risk: opportunities for cardiovascular disease prevention. *Trends Cardiovasc Med.* 2020;30(7):399-404.
7. Marchesan LB, Spritzer PM. ACC/AHA 2017 definition of high blood pressure: implications for women with polycystic ovary syndrome. *Fertil Steril.* 2019;111(3):579-587.e1.
8. Joham AE, Boyle JA, Zoungas S, Teede HJ. Hypertension in reproductive-aged women with polycystic ovary syndrome and association with obesity. *Am J Hypertens.* 2015;28(7):847-851.
9. Cascella T, Palomba S, Tauchmanovà L, et al. Serum aldosterone concentration and cardiovascular risk in women with the polycystic ovarian syndrome. *J Clin Endocrinol Metab.* 2006;91(11):4395-4400.
10. Reckelhoff JF. Gender differences in the regulation of blood pressure. *Hypertension.* 2001;37(5):1199-1208.
11. Uncu G, Sözer MC, Develioğlu O, Cengiz C. The role of plasma renin activity in distinguishing patients with polycystic ovary syndrome (PCOS) from oligomenorrheic patients without PCOS. *Gynecol Endocrinol.* 2002;16(6):447-452.
12. Chen MJ, Yang WS, Yang JH, Chen CL, Ho HN, Yang YS. Relationship between androgen levels and blood pressure in young women with polycystic ovary syndrome. *Hypertension.* 2007;49(6):1442-1447.
13. Diamanti-Kandarakis E, Spina G, Kouli C, Migdalis I. Increased endothelin-1 levels in women with polycystic ovary syndrome and the beneficial effect of metformin therapy. *J Clin Endocrinol Metab.* 2001;86(10):4666-4673.
14. Sam S. Obesity and polycystic ovary syndrome. *Obes Manag.* 2007;3(2):69-73.
15. Lim SS, Davies MJ, Norman RJ, Moran LJ. Overweight, obesity and central obesity in women with polycystic ovary syndrome: a systematic review and meta-analysis. *Hum Reprod Update.* 2012;18(6):618-637.
16. Third Report of the National Cholesterol Education Program (NCEP) expert panel on detection, evaluation, and treatment of high blood cholesterol in adults (Adult Treatment Panel III) final report. *Circulation.* 2002;106(25):3143-3421.
17. Rachoń D, Teede H. Ovarian function and obesity-interrelationship, impact on women's reproductive lifespan and treatment options. *Mol Cell Endocrinol.* 2010;316(2):172-179.
18. Grundy SM, Cleeman JI, Daniels SR, et al. Diagnosis and management of the metabolic syndrome: an American Heart Association/National Heart, Lung, and Blood Institute Scientific Statement. *Circulation.* 2005;112(17):2735-2752.
19. Moran LJ, Misso ML, Wild RA, Norman RJ. Impaired glucose tolerance, type 2 diabetes and metabolic syndrome in polycystic ovary syndrome: a systematic review and meta-analysis. *Hum Reprod Update.* 2010;16(4):347-363.
20. Lim SS, Kakoly NS, Tan JWJ, et al. Metabolic syndrome in polycystic ovary syndrome: a systematic review, meta-analysis, and meta-regression. *Obes Rev.* 2019;20(2):339-352.
21. Salley KE, Wickham EP, Cheang KI, Essah PA, Karjane NW, Nestler JE. Glucose intolerance in polycystic ovary syndrome-a position statement of the Androgen Excess Society. *J Clin Endocrinol Metab.* 2007;92(12):4546-4556.
22. Kakoly NS, Earnest A, Teede HJ, Moran LJ, Joham AE. The impact of obesity on the incidence of type 2 diabetes among women

with polycystic ovary syndrome. *Diabetes Care*. 2019;42(4): 560-567.

23. Sirmans SM, Pate KA. Epidemiology, diagnosis, and management of polycystic ovary syndrome. *Clin Epidemiol*. 2013;6:1-13.

24. Cassar S, Misso ML, Hopkins WG, Shaw CS, Teede HJ, Stepto NK. Insulin resistance in polycystic ovary syndrome: a systematic review and meta-analysis of euglycaemic-hyperinsulinaemic clamp studies. *Hum Reprod*. 2016;31(11):2619-2631.

25. Anagnostis P, Tarlatzis BC, Kauffman RP. Polycystic ovarian syndrome (PCOS): long-term metabolic consequences. *Metabolism*. 2018;86:33-43.

26. Weitgasser R, Ratzinger M, Hemetsberger M, Siostrzonek P. [LDL-cholesterol and cardiovascular events: the lower the better?]. *Wien Med Wochenschr*. 2018;168(5-6):108-120.

27. Wild RA, Rizzo M, Clifton S, Carmina E. Lipid levels in polycystic ovary syndrome: systematic review and meta-analysis. *Fertil Steril*. 2011;95(3):1073-1079.e1-11.

28. Diamanti-Kandarakis E, Papavassiliou AG, Kandarakis SA, Chrousos GP. Pathophysiology and types of dyslipidemia in PCOS. *Trends Endocrinol Metab*. 2007;18(7):280-285.

29. Wild RA. Polycystic ovary syndrome: a risk for coronary artery disease? *Am J Obstet Gynecol*. 2002;186(1):35-43.

30. Glintborg D, Rubin KH, Nybo M, Abrahamsen B, Andersen M. Cardiovascular disease in a nationwide population of Danish women with polycystic ovary syndrome. *Cardiovasc Diabetol*. 2018;17(1):37.

31. Corrigenda. *J Clin Endocrinol Metab*. 2015;100(6):2502.

32. de Groot PC, Dekkers OM, Romijn JA, Dieben SW, Helmerhorst FM. PCOS, coronary heart disease, stroke and the influence of obesity: a systematic review and meta-analysis. *Hum Reprod Update*. 2011;17(4):495-500.

33. Zhao L, Zhu Z, Lou H, et al. Polycystic ovary syndrome (PCOS) and the risk of coronary heart disease (CHD): a meta-analysis. *Oncotarget*. 2016;7(23):33715-33721.

34. Zhou Y, Wang X, Jiang Y, et al. Association between polycystic ovary syndrome and the risk of stroke and all-cause mortality: insights from a meta-analysis. *Gynecol Endocrinol*. 2017;33(12):904-910.

35. Christian RC, Dumesic DA, Behrenbeck T, Oberg AL, Sheedy PF II, Fitzpatrick LA. Prevalence and predictors of coronary artery calcification in women with polycystic ovary syndrome. *J Clin Endocrinol Metab*. 2003;88(6):2562-2568.

36. Talbott EO, Zborowski JV, Rager JR, Boudreaux MY, Edmundowicz DA, Guzick DS. Evidence for an association between metabolic cardiovascular syndrome and coronary and aortic calcification among women with polycystic ovary syndrome. *J Clin Endocrinol Metab*. 2004;89(11):5454-5461.

37. Meyer ML, Malek AM, Wild RA, Korytkowski MT, Talbott EO. Carotid artery intima-media thickness in polycystic ovary syndrome: a systematic review and meta-analysis. *Hum Reprod Update*. 2012;18(2):112-126.

38. Cascella T, Palomba S, De Sio I, et al. Visceral fat is associated with cardiovascular risk in women with polycystic ovary syndrome. *Hum Reprod*. 2008;23(1):153-159.

39. Saha S, Sarkar C, Biswas SC, Karim R. Correlation between serum lipid profile and carotid intima-media thickness in polycystic ovarian syndrome. *Indian J Clin Biochem*. 2008;23(3):262-266.

40. Toulis KA, Goulis DG, Mintziori G, et al. Meta-analysis of cardiovascular disease risk markers in women with polycystic ovary syndrome. *Hum Reprod Update*. 2011;17(6):741-760.

41. Diamanti-Kandarakis E, Alexandraki K, Piperi C, et al. Inflammatory and endothelial markers in women with polycystic ovary syndrome. *Eur J Clin Invest*. 2006;36(10):691-697.

42. Wild RA, Carmina E, Diamanti-Kandarakis E, et al. Assessment of cardiovascular risk and prevention of cardiovascular disease in women with the polycystic ovary syndrome: a consensus statement by the Androgen Excess and Polycystic Ovary Syndrome (AE-PCOS) Society. *J Clin Endocrinol Metab*. 2010;95(5):2038-2049.

43. Mosca L. Guidelines for prevention of cardiovascular disease in women: a summary of recommendations. *Prev Cardiol*. 2007;10(suppl 4):19-25.

44. Knowler WC, Barrett-Connor E, Fowler SE, et al. Reduction in the incidence of type 2 diabetes with lifestyle intervention or metformin. *N Engl J Med*. 2002;346(6):393-403.

45. Kaminski P, Szpotanska-Sikorska M, Wielgos M. Cardiovascular risk and the use of oral contraceptives. *Neuro Endocrinol Lett*. 2013;34(7):587-9. PMID: 24464000.

46. Roach RE, Helmerhorst FM, Lijfering WM, Stijnen T, Algra A, Dekkers OM. Combined oral contraceptives: the risk of myocardial infarction and ischemic stroke. *Cochrane Database of Systematic Reviews*. 2015(8).

47. Sumlin LL, Garcia TJ, Brown SA, et al. Depression and adherence to lifestyle changes in type 2 diabetes: a systematic review. *Diabetes Educ*. 2014;40(6):731-744.

48. McCartney CR, Marshall JC. CLINICAL PRACTICE. polycystic ovary syndrome. *N Engl J Med*. 2016;375(1):54-64.

19

Management of Subfertility in Polycystic Ovary Syndrome

SUMAIRA NAZ AND AZRA AMERJEE

Introduction

Polycystic ovary syndrome (PCOS) is the most common endocrine disorder and affects approximately 20% females of reproductive age.[1,2] This syndrome has a heterogeneous presentation, with clinical or biochemical hyperandrogenism (HA), ovulatory dysfunction, and polycystic ovarian morphology (PCOM) on ultrasound[3,4] (Table 19.1).

PCOS is a multifactorial disorder with the involvement of different factors, including genetic, hormonal, neuroendocrine, and environmental factors.[5,6] Hyperinsulinemia is the hallmark of PCOS and is associated with insulin resistance (IR), increased androgens, and luteinizing hormone (LH) secretion, contributing to hormonal, metabolic, and reproductive effects of the syndrome.[7] PCOS belongs to the World Health Organization (WHO) anovulation group II,

which encompasses normogonadotrophic hypogonadism and, based on National Institutes of Health (NIH) 2012 criteria, ovulatory dysfunction is observed in PCOS phenotypes A, B, and D[8] (Table 19.2).

These females usually present with menstrual irregularities ranging from oligomenorrhea to amenorrhea and infertility. Not all patients with PCOS have difficulty becoming pregnant. Nevertheless, infertility is prevalent in 75% to 80% of patients because of anovulation.[9,10]

Physiologic Principles of Gonadotrophin Ovarian Stimulation

At birth, there are around 1 to 2 million primordial follicles in each ovary.[11,12] The number reduces gradually to 3000 follicles at the time of puberty. Under an unknown stimulus, these primordial follicles progress to primary, secondary, and then small antral follicles. This initial development (gonadotrophin responsive) takes about 70 to 80 days and during this phase, small follicles of 2 to 5 mm in diameter become responsive to low levels of gonadotrophins. Once the follicles reach the antral stage, they become follicle-stimulating hormone (FSH) dependent and eligible for cyclical recruitment (gonadotrophin dependent). At puberty,

TABLE 19.1	Diagnostic Criteria of Polycystic Ovary Syndrome[4]	
Criterion	**Description**	
Androgen excess	Clinical[a] & /or biochemical hyperandrogenism[b]	
Ovarian dysfunction	Oligo/anovulation and/or polycystic ovarian morphology[c]	
Exclusion	Other causes of Androgen excess or other ovulatory disorders[d]	

[a]Such as hirsutism
[b]Hyperandrogenemia such as elevated levels of total or free testosterone
[c]Defined by either the number of intermediate-sized follicles (>8–12 follicles between 2–9 mm in diameter) and/ or increased ovarian volume (e.g., > 10 mL3) Associated with irregular menstrual cycles (> 35 days apart or with short duration of < 21 day)
[d]Including, but not limited to 21-Hydroxylase deficiency, nonclassical adrenal hyperplasia, thyroid dysfunction, hyperprolactinemia, neoplastic androgen secretion, or drug-induced androgen excess.
Adapted from Azziz R. Diagnostic criteria for polycystic ovary syndrome: A reappraisal. *Fertil Steril.* 2005;83(5):1343–1346.

TABLE 19.2	The National Institutes of Health Criteria 2012 Classifies Polycystic Ovary Syndrome into Four Phenotypes[8]	
1	Phenotype A	Hyperandrogenism + ovulatory dysfunction + polycystic ovarian morphology (PCOM)
2	Phenotype B	hyperandrogenism + ovulatory dysfunction
3	Phenotype C	hyperandrogenism + PCOM
4	Phenotype D	ovulatory dysfunction + PCOM

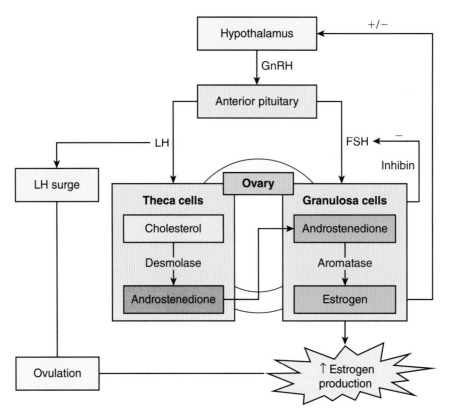

• **Fig. 19.1** The Hypothalamic Pituitary Axis, Two Cells-Two Gonadotrophins Concept, and Hormonal Interplay. *FSH*, Follicle-stimulating hormone; *GnRH*, gonadotrophin-releasing hormone; *LH*, luteinizing hormone.

maturation of the hypothalamic–pituitary system stimulates FSH secretion to levels that trigger ovulatory cycles. Ovarian follicular development from the small antral stage to a preovulatory follicle requires the combined actions of two gonadotrophins (i.e., FSH and LH). In the first half of the follicular phase, FSH predominates, and LH leads the events in the second half of this phase. Normally, LH acts on ovarian theca cells and activates the LH receptor to promote androgen production, and FSH acts on the ovarian granulosa cells to transform the androgens to estrogens (Fig. 19.1).

Follicle-Stimulating Hormone Threshold/ Window Concept

During the menstrual cycle, FSH levels start rising gradually in the late luteal phase and allow recruitment of a pool of small antral follicles (i.e., rescued from atresia) to undergo further growth (Fig. 19.2). During the early to mid-follicular phase, the rise in FSH above a particular serum level (FSH threshold) for a limited duration is called the FSH window. Once there is a leading follicle with a diameter of 9 to 10 mm, the FSH level falls below the threshold (see Fig. 19.2). The granulosa cells of the dominant follicle, under influence of FSH, acquire LH receptors and further development of the preovulatory follicle becomes

LH dependent (Fig. 19.3). The rest of the follicles undergo atresia because of the low levels of FSH. This threshold/window concept is important for monofollicular development. If FSH window is widened and FSH levels are maintained above the threshold for a longer duration, multifollicular development occurs, whereas rise for a shorter duration above the threshold results in unifollicular ovulation.

Luteinizing Hormone Role in Folliculogenesis

Optimal follicular development is also dependent on minimal exposure to LH levels. During the late follicular phase, rising LH levels promote follicular atresia, help the dominant follicle to maintain its growth, and induce unifollicular ovulation. The LH threshold is important for folliculogenesis because too high levels, as observed in PCOS patients, can impede follicular development and lead to premature luteinization, whereas low levels result in insufficient androgen and estrogen synthesis, impaired folliculogenesis, and lead to inadequate endometrial proliferation (Fig. 19.4).

Anti-Müllerian Hormone and Folliculogenesis

Another important modulator of folliculogenesis is anti-Müllerian hormone (AMH), a member of the growth

Gonadotrophins dependent follicular growth & FSH window concept

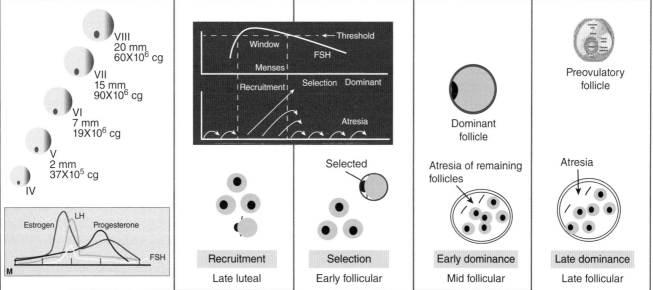

• **Fig. 19.2** Gonadotrophin-Dependent Follicular Growth and the Follicle-Stimulating Hormone Window. *FSH*, Follicle-stimulating hormone; *LH*, luteinizing hormone. (From http://slideplayer.com/slide/575035/)

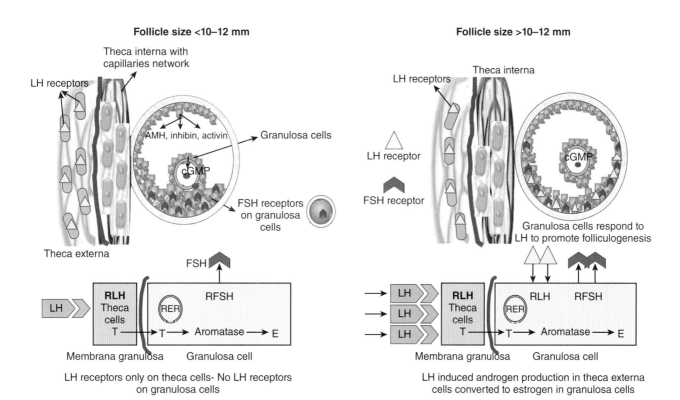

Acquisition of LH receptors in granulosa cells and LH support for follicle maturation
T=Testosterone, E=Estrogen, RFSH=Receptors for Follicular Stimulating Hormone, RLH=Receptors for Luteinizing Hormone, RER=Rough Endoplasmic Reticulum

• **Fig. 19.3** Acquisition of Luteinizing Hormone (LH) Receptors. *FSH*, Follicle-stimulating hormone. (Adapted from https://clinicalgate.com/getting-ready-for-pregnancy/ and Slide player Regulation of Menstrual Cycle: by CEM FICICIOGLU, M.D, Ph.D, AA, MBA)

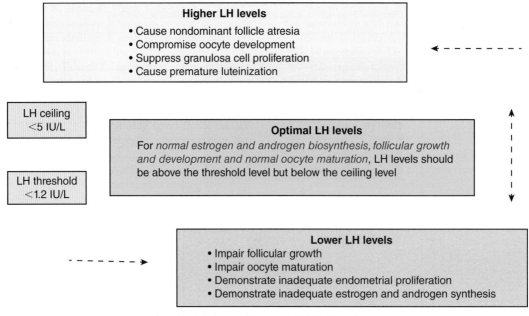

• **Fig. 19.4** Luteinizing Hormone *(LH)* Ceiling Concept.

factor receptor beta (GFR-β) superfamily. AMH is mainly produced by the granulosa cells of preantral and small antral follicles of up to 4 mm. It acts as a "safeguard of the ovarian follicular pool" and leads to reduction in FSH receptors and aromatase expression. Furthermore, AMH prevents progressive folliculogenesis and the progression of earlier resting follicles into active follicles.[13,14] Once the follicles attain a size greater than 8 mm, AMH influence is reduced, and these follicles become more sensitive to FSH action (Fig. 19.5). This shift promotes increased estrogen secretion from the growing follicle and leads to selection of the dominant follicle and subsequent ovulation.[14]

Pathophysiology: The Effect of Polycystic Ovary Syndrome on Fertility

For more information, see the chapter-07 on PCOS and subfertility: ovulation dysregulation, and fertility problems.

The pathophysiology of PCOS entails disruption of the hypothalamic–pituitary-ovarian axis (HPO), amplification of insulin secretion and androgen levels, and alteration in ovarian function.[15] PCOS can influence fertility in different ways. Reduced fertility potential in these patients is attributed to chronic anovulation and to altered endometrial receptivity. In PCOS, there is an imbalance of LH and FSH, along with elevated levels of androgens and

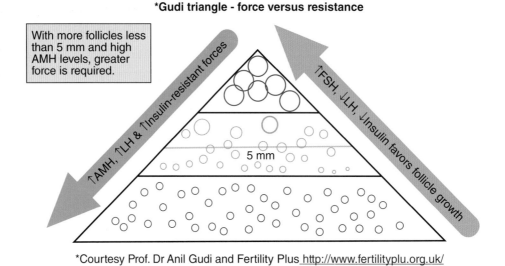

*Courtesy Prof. Dr Anil Gudi and Fertility Plus http://www.fertilityplu.org.uk/

• **Fig. 19.5** Force overcomes resistance. *AMH,* Anti-Müllerian hormone.

TABLE 19.3	What's Going Wrong in Polycystic Ovary Syndrome?
Abnormal gonadotropin secretion	• Increased amplitude of gonadotropin-releasing hormone (GnRH) pulses[20] • Hypersecretion of LH; particularly evident in the lean PCOS phenotype • Intrinsic deficiency of FSH action • Raised Kisspeptin levels[21]
Insulin resistance	• Hyperinsulinemia • Hyperandrogenism (including in utero exposure to hyperandrogenism)[21,22]
Abnormal steroidogenesis	• Increased ovarian production of androgens and estrogens[16] • Follicles are more resistant to FSH action, culminating in disruption of follicular maturation and ovulation, and inhibition of aromatase expression • Large cohort of small follicles arrest in development (but are capable of responding to exogenous FSH)
Affected endometrial receptivity	The endometrial environment appears to be altered in females with PCOS with changes in[16,23]: • Progesterone sensitivity • Adhesion molecules • Cytokines • Inflammatory cascades • Oxidative status
Effect of micronutrients (deficiencies and disturbed metabolism)	• Vitamin D deficiency • Disturbed folate metabolism through alterations in the methylenetetrahydrofolate reductase gene[16]

Adapted from Azziz R, Carmina E, Chen Z, et al. Polycystic ovary syndrome. Nature Rev Dis Primers. 2016:11;2(1):1-8.

insulin.[11,15] This triad of hormonal changes with low levels of vitamin D enhances AMH expression and contributes to ovulatory dysfunction.[16,17] High AMH levels result in inhibition of aromatase expression, affect FSH release, and increase follicular resistance to FSH action.[18,19] Eventually, follicular development is hampered, and their growth gets arrested at a diameter of 4 to 8 mm. Because a dominant follicle does not develop, ovulation and thereby fertilization of egg by sperm does not occur, ultimately leading to infertility. Even if ovulation occurs, hormonal imbalance affects endometrial lining and interferes with implantation of the fertilized egg (Table 19.3).

Investigations of Infertility Patients in Polycystic Ovary Syndrome

PCOS is often characterized by raised LH levels and serum fasting serum insulin and reversed LH–FSH ratio. Nevertheless, the confirmation of diagnosis is based on exclusion of other causes of anovulation, including thyroid disease, 21-hydroxylase deficiency, hyperprolactinemia, Cushing syndrome, and androgen-producing neoplasms. The following investigations should be considered in patients with PCOS who are trying to conceive:

- Hormone profile, including serum testosterone, thyroid-stimulating hormone (TSH), prolactin, and day 3 FSH levels to investigate oligomenorrhea/anovulation.
- Ultrasound for evaluation of PCOM and follicular tracking.[24,25]
- Semen analysis in all patients with PCOS before ovulation induction therapy.[26]

- In females older than 35 years of age and when clinical history is indicative of tubal or uterine pathology, a hysterosalpingogram should be performed along with semen analysis before starting ovulation induction.[24,26]
- An AMH assessment is currently not recommended for screening of PCOS and PCOM because of the absence of standardization and correct cutoff levels for different available assays.[27,16] Emerging evidence favors that estimation of AMH may be useful in predicting ovarian follicle counts and response to treatment.[28,29] AMH level greater than 5 ng/mL has a specificity of 97% and sensitivity higher than the current criteria for PCOM.[29] AMH may help provide a guide for the appropriate regimen before ovarian stimulation in in-vitro fertilization (IVF) patients and to minimize the risk of ovarian hyperstimulation syndrome (OHSS).[30]

Principles of Management of Anovulatory Infertility in Polycystic Ovary Syndrome

To date, there is no pharmacological therapy that provides a definite cure for PCOS, but treatment strategies are available that ameliorate its clinical symptoms and improve metabolic and reproductive effects. In PCOS, anovulation is mainly responsible for infertility; therefore successful restoration of ovulation can help majority of patients to attain conception. After optimizing health, correction of ovulatory dysfunction is carried out with the intention of inducing normal ovulatory cycles. This can be achieved by augmentation of FSH levels that act as a driving force to shift follicular growth from the androgenic to estrogenic milieu. Care should be taken when using force because a large cohort of small follicles is arrested in development. This driving force should be sufficient enough to overcome resistant forces and to allow unifollicular ovulation but should not exceed to a level of hyperstimulation (see Fig. 19.5). The AMH level can guide to an extent; if its levels are high, more resistance can be expected. Furthermore, chronic anovulation in PCOS is associated with hyperinsulinemia, HA, and obesity, and these metabolic abnormalities should also be taken into consideration for effective improvement in ovulatory function. Therefore to restore ovulatory dysfunction, fertility management is based on three principles:

- Improving IR through lifestyle modifications, such as diet, exercise, and weight reduction, and insulin-sensitizing agents
- Increasing FSH levels through the use of oral antiestrogens (e.g., letrozole, clomiphene citrate [CC]), parenteral gonadotrophin therapy, or IVF
- Reducing high LH levels through laparoscopic ovarian surgery

Before starting infertility treatment for PCOS, the following prerequisites should be considered (Table 19.4).

Management Therapies

Fertility management for PCOS involves the combination of nonpharmacologic, pharmacologic, and surgical interventions[25] (Algorithm 19.1). Nonpharmacologic therapy involves lifestyle changes; pharmacologic therapies include oral ovulation–inducing agents, such as clomiphene citrate and letrozole, and exogenous gonadotrophins. They also include a combination of first- and second-line therapies and insulin-sensitizing agents, such as metformin and inositol. Surgical therapy involves laparoscopic ovarian surgery, including ovarian drilling and transvaginal hydrolaparoscopy (THL). IVF is considered for cases that do not respond to conventional ovulation induction methods.[31] In vitro maturation (IVM) is a promising alternative to conventional IVF for young females with PCOS.[32]

Improving Insulin Resistance

Lifestyle Modifications and Weight Loss

In PCOS patients, cycle irregularity and anovulation correlate with a patient's body mass index (BMI). At least half of the patients diagnosed with PCOS are obese (BMI > 30 kg/m²). Because of the difficult visualization of ovaries on ultrasound scans, treatment monitoring is often challenging in obese PCOS patients. This increases the risk of missing multiple follicular development and multiple pregnancy.[26]

Lifestyle modification is considered the first-line intervention for PCOS patients with BMI ≥25 kg/m², before initiation of any fertility treatment. Ideally, ovulation inducing treatment should be deferred until the BMI is less than 35 kg/m² in morbidly obese patients. However, for younger females with normal ovarian reserve, weight reduction to BMI less than 30 kg/m² is preferable.[33] Lifestyle recommendations include dietary modifications, regular physical exercise, and weight reduction strategies, including pharmacologic therapy and surgery. Even 5% to 10% weight loss helps to achieve ovulation induction and improved response to all forms of fertility treatment. Before prescribing a pharmacologic treatment for weight loss, the safety of the drugs during early pregnancy should be considered.[25]

Metformin, an insulin-sensitizing drug, is not in itself a weight reducing therapy; however, when combined with lifestyle modification, it may improve body weight.[34] Antiobesity drugs provide only short-term benefits. In morbidly obese patients, if weight reduction is not achieved with conventional methods, bariatric surgery should be considered. Indications for bariatric surgery for PCOS patients are similar to the general population (BMI ≥40kg/m²).[35] For those with comorbidities, such as diabetes mellitus (DM), lower levels of BMI (35 kg/m²) should be considered.[26] Bariatric surgery helps achieve appreciable weight loss postoperatively and improves total and free serum testosterone levels. Furthermore, resolution of hirsutism and ovulatory dysfunction has been observed in as many as 53% and 96% of females, respectively.[36]

TABLE 19.4	Prerequisites Before Starting Infertility Treatment in Polycystic Ovary Syndrome Patients[24,25]

Key Points:

- Pregnancy should be excluded in patients with amenorrhea or oligomenorrhea before starting treatment.
- Optimization of health is recommended before commencing ovulation inducing therapy (e.g., weight reduction in obese females).
- Adequate dietary intake of vitamin D and folic acid supplementation should be ensured.
- The aim of ovulation induction is to restore mono-ovulation.
- In polycystic ovary syndrome (PCOS), patient education, counseling, lifestyle advice, and psychological wellbeing need to be considered along with pharmacologic therapy.
- Pharmacologic treatment should be recommended keeping in mind the patient's personal characteristics, preferences, and values.
- Benefits, adverse effects, and contraindications should be considered before prescribing treatment.
- Multiple follicles development should be avoided because of adverse consequences: ovarian hyperstimulation syndrome and multiple pregnancy.
- Letrozole and metformin are off-label drugs for ovulation induction. Nevertheless, their use in PCOS is evidence-based and permitted in many countries.

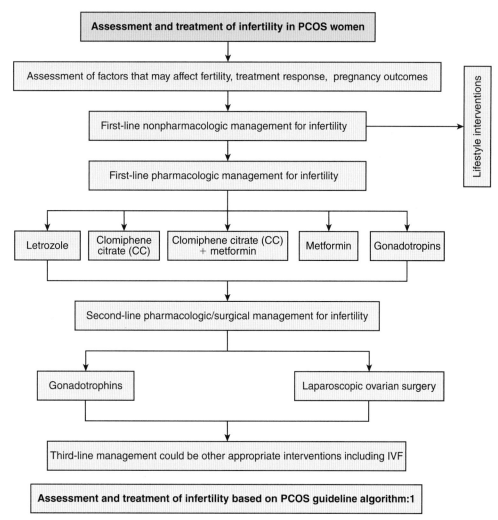

• **ALGORITHM 19.1** Treatment for Infertility Management in Polycystic Ovary Syndrome *(PCOS)* Patients. *IVF,* In vitro fertilization.

Insulin-Sensitizing Agents

Metformin

Metformin helps to improve fertility rates[37] by reducing insulin levels, facilitating normal gonadotropin-releasing hormone (GnRH) and gonadotropin release.[38] Because of the slow onset of action, clinical effects of metformin may become evident only after weeks of treatment.[39] In PCOS patients, metformin alone is less effective than clomiphene citrate (CC); however, it can be used as a first-line pharmacologic therapy when no other treatment option is available. Compared with CC, its effect appears to be BMI dependent. Metformin is more effective in nonobese females, whereas in obese females, it results in a decrease in live birth rates.[39] Metformin is the most commonly recommended adjuvant therapy for CC-resistant patients. Combined metformin and CC therapy could be used as a first-line pharmacologic therapy in anovulatory obese patients with PCOS because it increases the ovulation and pregnancy rate with no effect on the live birth rate.[39] There is insufficient evidence available to recommend metformin as an add-on therapy with letrozole or laparoscopic ovarian drilling (LOD).[40]

Metformin should be considered as an adjunct therapy to gonadotrophin and IVF treatment because it significantly reduces the incidence of OHSS.[41]

The recommended dose for metformin is 1500 mg to 2500 mg daily for 4 to 60 weeks.[26] Metformin is safe for long-term use; however, ongoing treatment needs consideration at intervals because its use may result in low vitamin B_{12} levels. Side effects such as nausea, vomiting, and other gastrointestinal disturbances[25] may affect its use. Nevertheless, a gradual increase in dose with increments of 500 mg in 1 to 2 weeks and use of extended-release preparations can improve compliance for metformin. Lactic acidosis is a rare complication of metformin. Metformin is excreted by the kidney, and before starting its use, a serum creatinine of less than 1.4 mg/dL should be confirmed.

Myoinositol

Inositol is an emerging insulin-sensitizing therapy for patients with PCOS. The two most commonly used inositol isomers are myoinositol (MI) and D-chiro inositol (DCI).[42] These isomers operate on different pathways: MI exerts ovarian and nonovarian actions, whereas DCI has nonovarian insulin-sensitizing effects. Both forms are considered more effective in PCOS when used as a combined form at ratio that corresponds to the plasma physiologic ratio (MI: DCI of 40:1).[43] Inositol acts as an intracellular messenger and regulates hormones like TSH, FSH, and insulin.[44] Studies have highlighted inositol's role in human reproduction.[43] Pundir et al.[45] found that inositol therapy helps to improve ovulation rate and the frequency of menstrual cycles. Patients with PCOS may have altered inositol metabolism, and thus administration of inositol helps to improve insulin sensitivity (IS), ameliorates metabolic effects, and leads to improved embryo quality and fertilization rate.[42] Similarly, in PCOS patients undergoing IVF treatment, inositol use has shown promising results. Currently no evidence is available for its effect on improvements in pregnancy, miscarriages, and live birth rates. The recommended dose is 2 to 4 g for MI and 1000 to 1200 mg for DCI per day.[46] Inositol can be used alone or in combination with other therapies; however, its use is considered experimental.

Other Insulin-Reducing Therapies

Thiazolidinediones (TZDs; e.g., pioglitazone and rosiglitazone) are prescribed as second-line management options in PCOS patients. Treatment with TZDs is considered effective for patients who are obese or have hyperinsulinemia.[47]

Exenatide, a glucagon-like peptide-1 (GLP-1) receptor agonist reduces IR and is effective in the management of type 2 DM. It improves IS and helps to reduce body weight. In obese PCOS patients, this drug improves menstruation, reduces weight, and decreases androgen levels. Compared with metformin, exenatide improves IS and pregnancy rate to a higher degree. Combined therapy of metformin and GLP-1 receptor agonists is considered more effective than monotherapy for the management of metabolic and reproductive irregularities of PCOS. Further studies are required to explore the effectiveness of GLP1 analogs in obese PCOS females.[48]

Improving Follicle-Stimulating Hormone/Luteinizing Hormone Levels

First-Line Therapy

Clomiphene Citrate

CC has been used as the first-line pharmacologic treatment for ovulation induction in PCOS females because of its relatively low cost, easy use, fewer side effects, minimal monitoring requirements, and availability of evidence-based data on drug safety.[49]

Mechanism of Action. CC is a selective estrogen receptor modulator that competitively binds to endogenous estrogen receptor binding sites in endocrine glands (hypothalamus, pituitary, and ovaries). CC has both estrogen agonist and antagonist properties; however, the clinical effects of CC are mainly because of its antagonist action.[50,51] The prolonged binding of CC to estrogen receptors at the hypothalamus level eliminates the negative feedback loop for endogenous estrogens and estradiol. This results in increased secretion of GnRH. Rising GnRH release increases the plasma levels of LH and FSH and promotes follicular maturation and ultimately ovulation[37] (Fig. 19.6).

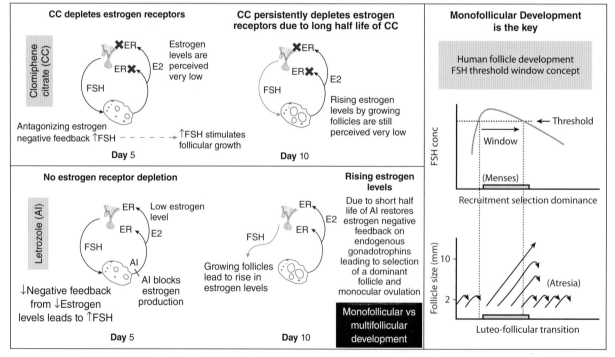

• **Fig. 19.6** A Comparison of the Mode of Action of Clomiphene Citrate Versus Letrozole in Follicular Development. *AI,* Aromatase Inhibitor: *ER,* Estrogen receptor; *FSH,* follicle-stimulating hormone. (From Yang A-M, Cui N, Sun Y-F and Hao G-M (2021) Letrozole for Female Infertility. Front. Endocrinol. 12:676133. doi: 10.3389/fendo.2021.676133 and B.C.J.M Fauser, A.M van Heusden, Manipulation of human ovarian function: physiological concepts and clinical consequences. Endocr Rev, 18 (1997), p. 71-106.)

Selection of Patients. CC can be prescribed for anovulatory PCOS patients with normal FSH and estradiol (E2) levels. Factors such as phenotype A, obesity, hyperinsulinemia, elevated androgen levels, high LH, and old age affect the outcome with CC treatment.[52,53] Similarly, CC-treated patients with elevated AMH levels have low ovulation and pregnancy rates compared with patients with low AMH levels. Elevated AMH levels correlate with the increased pool of arrested intermediate follicles and reflect resistance (see Fig. 19.5). Hence use of serum AMH levels can predict ovarian response to CC, using 3.4 ng/mL as the cutoff level.[54]

Dose. The starting dose for CC is 50 mg per day for 5 days from day 2 to 5 of the natural cycle or after withdrawal bleeding with progesterone treatment. Ovulation usually occurs 5 to 10 days after the last day of treatment. If ovulation is not achieved, the dose is gradually increased to 150 mg/day.[8] If ovulation occurs, the same dose is continued for three to six cycles. Higher doses (200 mg) improve efficacy but do not provide additional benefit. If exaggerated response occurs with 50 mg/day, then dose should be reduced to 25 mg/day.[55]

Monitoring. The ultrasound monitoring of ovulation is recommended at least for the first cycle during day 12 to 14 (or 7 days after the last dose) to adjust the dose for successive cycles.[24] This also helps in follicular tracking and provides information regarding endometrial thickness. The response is considered appropriate when there is one leading follicle of 18 to 25 mm and endometrial thickness is greater than 7 mm. Functional ovarian cysts may appear during treatment with CC. They usually resolve spontaneously within one menstrual cycle. Treatment should be withheld until the cysts resolve.

Ovulation Trigger and Luteal Phase Support. Use of human chorionic gonadotropin (hCG) as an ovulatory trigger is not recommended during CC treatment cycles. Its use does not improve reproductive outcomes.[56] Nevertheless, hCG can be considered during monitored cycles on individual basis. If recommended, hCG (5000–10,000 USP IU) can be administered when an appropriate response is observed on transvaginal scan. Luteal phase support is not required during CC treatment with hCG[57]; it can be considered if endometrial thickness is less than 6 mm on the transvaginal scan.

Efficacy of Clomiphene Citrate. Use of CC is associated with ovulation rates of 75% to 80% and pregnancy rates of up to 22% per cycle. The discrepancy of around 40% between the ovulation rate and the pregnancy rate is mainly related to the hypoestrogenic effect of CC on the endometrium and cervical mucus. Treatment with clomiphene should be limited to six cycles in responsive females.[55,58] The pregnancy rate reaches up to 50% to 60%, but thereafter CC efficacy falls significantly.[59]

Safety of Clomiphene Citrate. The twin and triplet pregnancy rates are 5% to 7% and 0.3%, respectively, and the risk of OHSS is minimal (less than 1%); therefore regular cycle monitoring is not required with CC. CC is considered a safe drug, and the reported rate of congenital abnormalities (genetic and structural) is 3.9%, which is comparable to spontaneously conceived pregnancies.[60] Use of CC for more than 12 cycles has been associated with a risk for borderline ovarian malignancy and breast carcinoma, but no causal relationship has been proven.[11]

Side effects of CC include hot flushes, visual disturbances including diplopia (in which case the drug should be stopped immediately), abdominal distention, mood swings, breast tenderness, distention, and nausea. CC should be avoided in patients with ovarian cysts, uncontrolled thyroid disorder, and impaired liver functions.[61]

Clomiphene Citrate Resistance and Failure. After the maximum dose of 150 mg/day for three cycles, failure to ovulate is considered clomiphene resistance; approximately 15% to 40% of PCOS patients do not respond to CC.[62] Clomiphene failure is considered when pregnancy is not achieved after six ovulatory cycles. For CC resistant and failure cases, other metabolic and infertility factors should be evaluated. To improve response, alternative therapies and second-line treatments should be considered.

Extended use of CC with a 150-mg dose for 10 days is a safe and effective option but is associated with lower pregnancy rates.[63] Metformin use with CC helps to improve ovulation and clinical pregnancy rates, and this treatment should be considered before proceeding with more aggressive treatment options.[25] Combined use of CC with glucocorticoids has also been reported in CC-resistant patients with raised levels of dehydroepiandrosterone sulfate (DHEA-S). Prednisolone (5 mg daily) or dexamethasone (0.5–2.0 mg daily) can be used from day 5 to 14 of the menstrual period for 3 to 6 cycles in responsive patients. This combined treatment improves ovulation rates; however, it is not recommended as routine practice.[11]

In CC resistant cases, combined treatment of CC with letrozole has been used and results are promising with improved ovulation and pregnancy rates and reduced risks at a lower cost.[52,64]

Aromatase Inhibitors

Letrozole and anastrozole are third-generation aromatase inhibitors that are used for ovulation induction in females with PCOS. Letrozole is comparatively more effective than anastrozole with higher pregnancy rates.

Letrozole is considered as an off-label drug for anovulatory infertility in many countries. Emerging evidence from the European Society of Human Reproduction & Embryology and American Society for Reproductive Medicine 2018 consensus guideline and WHO support the use of letrozole as a first-line pharmacologic treatment for ovulation induction. CC can be used as first-line therapy in settings where letrozole is not available, or its use is not permitted, or cost affects treatment choice.[25,65] Besides this, letrozole has shown better results for ovulation and pregnancy rates than gonadotrophins when used for CC resistant cases.[66]

Mechanism of Action. Letrozole acts locally on aromatase enzyme and blocks conversion of androgen to estrogen in ovarian follicle, peripheral tissue, and the brain. Because of its dual effect, letrozole blocks the conversion of androstenedione to estrone and testosterone to estradiol and prevents systemic biosynthesis of estrogen. Low levels of estrogen generate positive feedback on the HPO axis and enhance release of GnRH, which stimulates FSH production. Rising levels of FSH promote folliculogenesis and improve follicle maturation, followed by ovulation[15,67] (see Fig. 19.6).

Dose. The dose of letrozole ranges from 2.5 mg to 7.5 mg per day depending on the response to treatment. It is administered from day 3 to 7 of the menstrual cycle for 5 days. Use of a single high dose (20 mg) administered on day 3 has also been reported with promising effects. Treatment with letrozole is usually recommended for six ovulatory cycles. There is insufficient data for use of luteal phase support for letrozole treatment.[68,69,57]

Comparison of Letrozole and Clomiphene Citrate. Females with PCOS are significantly more likely to ovulate and have a live birth after use of letrozole compared with CC, the previous first-line agent. The likelihood of live birth is increased up to 40% to 60% with letrozole compared with CC. Similarly, failure to ovulate (letrozole resistance) is lower with letrozole versus CC.[17,69]

As mentioned in Table 19.5, CC has a half-life of 5 to 7 days. Its prolonged half-life results in the depletion of estrogen receptors and disrupts the HPO axis for a long duration. Prolonged elevation of FSH levels can cause multifollicular growth and increase the risk for multiple pregnancies. In comparison to CC, the half-life of letrozole is only 2 days,[42,17] and it does not affect estrogen receptors. Because of its short half-life, the central feedback mechanism remains intact. The growing dominant follicle increases estrogen levels, and through central negative feedback,[67] estrogen suppresses FSH production and leads to unifollicular ovulation with small follicle atresia. This effect provides a unique safety benefit to letrozole and prevents risk of OHSS and multiple pregnancy risk.[26,67,70]

CC causes thinning of the endometrial lining and affects cervical mucus,[48] whereas letrozole does not cause estrogen receptor antagonism. This explains the lack of antiestrogenic effect of letrozole on the endometrium and cervical mucus. The prevalence of anomalies observed with letrozole or CC is less than 5% (the expected anomaly rate with spontaneous pregnancy is 5%–8%). The reported risk of teratogenicity is similar with CC and letrozole.[17,46]

Hot flushes are less common with letrozole than CC, but fatigue and dizziness are more common with letrozole. Compared with CC, letrozole has a unique benefit of promoting ovulation in obese patients with PCOS.[17]

Combined use of letrozole with gonadotropin regimens leads to a lesser gonadotropin requirement; pregnancy rates are also comparable to that achieved with gonadotropins alone. The role of aromatase inhibitors in assisted reproductive treatments (ARTs) remains to be proven.[67]

Tamoxifen

Tamoxifen is an antiestrogenic anticancer agent used in females with breast cancer. It is used as an alternative option for ovulation induction in those who fail to or do not respond to CC. Tamoxifen has a similar action to CC; however, it has beneficial effects on cervical mucus and the endometrium. It is, however, not as effective as CC and is not used as a first-line therapy.[71] The dose of tamoxifen is 20 mg twice daily for 5 days, and it results in ovulation in 70% to 80% of patients with a pregnancy rate of 35% to 40%.[72]

Second-Line Therapy

Gonadotrophins

Exogenous gonadotropins are usually offered as a second-line therapy for patients who are nonresponsive or resistant to first-line ovulation-inducing agents.[25] Nevertheless, FSH may be used as a first-line infertility treatment for older patients with PCOS.[25] Gonadotrophin therapy is used with the intention to achieve mono ovulation in anovulatory PCOS patients whereas, for females with normal ovulatory function their use helps to attain multifollicular ovulation.[73]

Prerequisites for Therapy. Gonadotrophin therapy should only be advised by experts who have the requisite training and experience. Before starting treatment, other infertility factors such as uterine cavity abnormalities (myomas, adhesions), tubal blockade, endometriosis, and semen

TABLE 19.5 Comparison of Clomiphene and Letrozole

Parameters	Clomiphene	Letrozole
Mechanism of Action	Selective estrogen receptor modulator	Aromatase inhibitor
Half life	Long, 5–7 days	Short, 45 hours
Antiestrogenic effects	Thin endometrium & altered cervical mucus	Thick endometrium & favorable cervical mucus
Uterine blood flow	Decreased	Increased
Miscarriages	Possibly high	Less incidence
Ovarian hyperstimulation syndrome risk	High	Low
Multiple pregnancy	High	Low
Teratogenicity	Similar	

abnormalities should be ruled out. Similarly, an evaluation should be done to exclude high prolactin and thyroid levels.

Mechanism of Action. Gonadotropins (LH and FSH) are naturally produced by the pituitary gland and play a vital role in follicular growth and ovulation. In PCOS patients, although CC and letrozole are favored as first-line therapy because of their easier administration and cost effectiveness compared with the gonadotropins, use of gonadotropins may yield greater effects for infertility treatment.[74]

Choice of Gonadotrophins. Gonadotropins are available in urinary and recombinant forms. Both preparations are equally effective and have the same level of efficacy in inducing ovulation and no difference in the risk of OHSS and multiple pregnancy.[24,75] Theoretically, because of the high endogenous LH levels, the preferred gonadotropin preparation for patients with PCOS is the one that does not contain LH. Nevertheless, preparations that contain both FSH and LH as well as pure FSH preparations have been successfully used for ovulation induction in patients with PCOS.

Gonadotrophin Protocol For PCOS Patients. Anovulatory patients with PCOS have an increased number of small antral follicles. These growth arrested follicles do not ovulate in response to dysfunctional endogenous FSH. Nevertheless, with administration of exogenous FSH, these follicles can show an exuberant response, and lead to multifollicular development. To avoid the hyper-responsiveness of the polycystic ovaries, the conventional high-dose (150 IU) stepwise protocol is not recommended for PCOS patients and has been replaced by low-dose treatment regimens (Fig. 19.7).[76] The low-dose regimens can be used in a step-up, step-down, or sequential fashion.

The Chronic Low-Dose, Step-Up Protocol. The chronic low-dose, step-up protocol is considered as the preferred method for ovulation induction in patients with PCOS.[77,69] Low-dose administration with gradual dose increments allows FSH to rise

gradually just above the FSH threshold, and this helps to avoid excessive response and the associated risks of OHSS and multiple pregnancies. This approach starts with a small daily dose of FSH (typically 37.5–75 IU), which is continued without any dose change usually for 14 days. Dose is then increased every 5 to 7 days in small increments of 25 to 37.5 IU until a dominant follicle is observed during monitoring. This protocol provides best results with monofollicular ovulation of 70% and pregnancy rates of 20% per cycle (40% per patient) and reduces the risk of multiple pregnancies and OHSS to 5% and less than 1%, respectively. Nevertheless, the long duration of treatment is a problem, and attempts have been made to reduce cycle duration from the initial 14 days to 7 days. Results have shown similar success rates, but with a slightly higher rate of multiple pregnancy for the 7-day period[70] (Fig. 19.8).

The Step-Down Protocol. This protocol mimics the physiologic FSH threshold/window concept.[78] Treatment starts with a high dose of FSH (150 IU FSH/day) that continues until the appropriate ovarian response is achieved (Fig. 19.8). The dose is then reduced by 37.5 IU in two steps. Initially, the dose is reduced when one follicle of 10 mm is observed and by the same amount every 3 days if follicular growth proceeds. The dose is reduced gradually to 75 IU/day, which is then continued until the day of hCG injection. This regimen is as successful as the chronic low-dose, step-up protocol in achieving monofollicular development, with reduced duration of treatment. Nevertheless, extensive follicular monitoring is usually required because of frequent dose adjustments

The Sequential Protocol. This protocol is a combination of the step-up and step-down regimens and starts with an initial step-up protocol. Once a dominant follicle appears, a step-down regimen is followed.

Monitoring of the Treatment. Treatment with gonadotropin is recommended only for six ovulatory cycles. During treatment cycles, serial ultrasound monitoring is required to

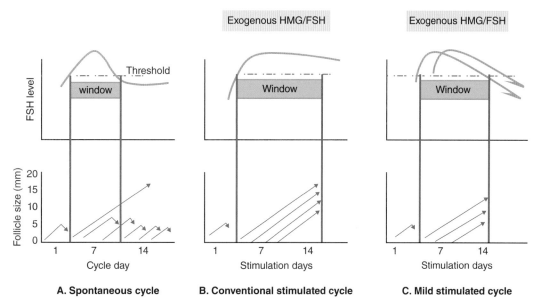

• **Fig. 19.7** Follicle-Stimulating Hormone (*FSH*) Window Concept With Gonadotropin Stimulation. *HMG,* Human menopausal gonadotropin. (From Macklon NS, Stouffer RL, Giudice LC, Fauser BC: The science behind 25 years of ovarian stimulation for in vitro fertilization. Endocr Rev 27[2]:170–207, 2006.)

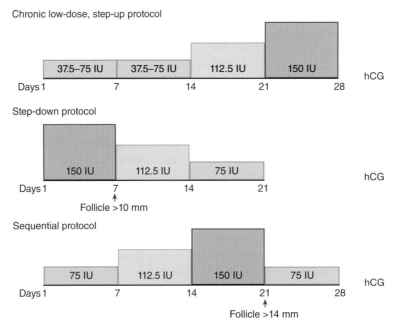

• **Fig. 19.8** Gonadotropin Protocols for Polycystic Ovary Syndrome Patients. *hCG*, Human chorionic gonadotropin. (Adapted from Amer S. Gonadotropin induction of ovulation. Obstet Gynaecol Reprod Med. 2007; 17 (7): 205-10.)

determine follicular growth and development in response to gonadotropin stimulation. The mono-ovulatory cycle is defined when there is a single follicle of 16 mm with no other follicle greater than 12 mm. Therefore the overall number of follicles is considered, and all follicles greater than 10 mm should be documented. Cycle cancellation is considered in the presence of more than three follicles that are greater than 14 mm and with serum estradiol levels of more than 15,000 pmol/L. hCG administration should be withheld in the presence of more than two follicles 16 mm or greater or more than one follicle equal to or greater than 16 mm and two additional follicles 14 mm or greater to minimize the risk of multiple pregnancies and OHSS.[25,79,15]

Luteal phase support is recommended for treatment with gonadotrophins because it improves clinical pregnancy and live birth rates. Gonadotrophin use affects LH secretion from the hypothalamus, and this affects progesterone release from the corpus luteum, leading to a short luteal phase. Progesterone supplements and hCG both can be used. Nevertheless, use of progesterone supplements is recommended because of side effects (OHSS) associated with hCG administration. Progesterone vaginal preparations are preferable to oral forms because of low cost and fewer side effects.[57] Combined use of metformin with gonadotrophins can be considered because it improves ovulation, pregnancy, and live birth rates and helps to reduce risk of OHSS.

Gonadotrophin Treatment Cycle

- With the onset of periods, the first day is considered with the start of menstrual flow.
- Baseline transvaginal scan is performed on cycle days 2 or 3 to rule out underlying ovarian cysts.
- If ultrasound is normal, treatment starts from day 2 of the cycles with a relatively low dose of gonadotrophins (37.5–75 IU/day).
- Daily injections are typically given subcutaneous (SC) or intramuscularly (IM) at the same time each day in the evening (5:00 – 8:00 PM).
- Sonograms and estradiol levels (every 2–3 days) are scheduled in the morning (8:00 – 10:00 AM).
- Ultrasonography provides an assessment of follicular development and is generally performed after the first 4 to 5 days of treatment and at intervals of 1 to 3 days thereafter based on the response of the therapy and protocol used.
- The stimulation phase of treatment usually lasts for 7 to 14 days.
- All follow-up appointments after cycle day 8 are arranged based on the size of the largest measured follicle.
- Once a mature follicle has developed, generally measuring 16 to 18 mm in mean diameter, human chorionic gonadotropin (hCG) is administered in a dose of 5,000–10,000 IU IM or SC.
- Although there are no specific guidelines for optimal timing, the ovulatory stimulus can be administered when at least one, and ideally, no more than two follicles greater than 16 to 18 mm in mean diameter are observed.
- Ovulation can be expected to occur between 24 and 48 hours after injection of hCG. Consequently, intercourse within that interval can help maximize the likelihood of conception.
- Intrauterine insemination is preferably indicated with gonadotropin therapy and planned approximately 24 to 36 hours after the injection.
- Progesterone use should be considered for luteal phase support.

Counseling of the Patient. Before starting treatment with gonadotropins, counseling of the patient is important. This should encompass a discussion regarding treatment plan, cost, and response of therapy and the associated risk of higher-order multiple pregnancies and OHSS.[80] Strict cycle cancellation criteria is agreed on with the patient before proceeding with treatment. Different people respond to gonadotrophins at different rates, and even the same person will not respond to therapy in the same way during each cycle. Therefore adjustment of gonadotrophin dosage and intensive monitoring is required to achieve a successful treatment response. With gonadotrophin therapy, there are typical pregnancy rates of 15% to 20% per cycle and the spontaneous miscarriage rate is 20% to 25%, which is slightly higher than for spontaneous conceptions. Gonadotrophin therapy does not, however, increase risk for congenital abnormalities.[11]

Combined Oral and Parenteral Ovulation Induction Treatments. The combination of CC with gonadotrophins is in use for ovulation induction in CC resistant PCOS. Emerging studies also support the combined administration of letrozole and gonadotrophins. Letrozole plus gonadotrophins provides better results with a greater ovulation rate, lesser cancellation rate, and better endometrial thickness than letrozole alone and fewer risks than CC plus gonadotrophins (Algorithm 19.2). Nevertheless, there is a greater risk for multiple pregnancies with this treatment regimen.[81] The combination of letrozole and CC with gonadotrophin has also been attempted and may be appropriate for patients who are sensitive to gonadotrophins.[82]

Risks of Gonadotropin Treatment. Although gonadotropin therapy is highly effective in inducing ovulation, it is associated with significant risks of multiple pregnancy and OHSS.[11,27]

Multiple Pregnancy. There has been a substantial rise in multiple pregnancies in recent years because of the use of gonadotropins for ovulation induction, controlled ovarian hyperstimulation, and ARTs. Multiple pregnancies are considered high risk because of associated pregnancy complications, thereby compromising perinatal outcome with increased neonatal morbidity and mortality.

To minimize the risk of multiple pregnancy, treatment should aim to induce mono-ovulation in all anovulatory females. Careful monitoring of the cycle should be done, and cycle cancellation should be considered when there are excessive maturing follicles.

Ovarian Hyperstimulation Syndrome. OHSS is a potentially life-threatening complication associated with gonadotropin treatment. Approximately 1% of patients develop severe OHSS after ovulation induction with gonadotropins. It is characterized by fluid shift from the intracellular to extracellular compartment, leading to intravascular volume depletion, hypovolemia, and hemoconcentration.

The exact mechanism of OHSS is unknown; however, hCG, either exogenous or endogenous, is considered the main triggering factor. Possibly, hCG activates the release of certain vasoactive mediators (e.g., vascular endothelial growth factor [VEGF]) from the ovary. These factors generate a cascade of events in the body leading to the pathophysiologic consequences of OHSS. Furthermore, in PCOS patients, the large pool of intermediate size follicles is sensitive to exogenous FSH and once stimulated leads to high levels of estrogen. Elevated serum estradiol mediates the effect of hCG on the vascular system. Besides this, improving levels of insulin potentiates gonadotropin actions on granulosa cells and theca cells. Finally, overexpression of VEGF from polycystic ovaries increases the vascular permeability. This results in a fluid shift from the intracellular to extracellular compartment, leading to intravascular volume depletion, hypovolemia, and hemoconcentration.

There are two patterns of OHSS, early and late, depending on the source of hCG. Early OHSS is induced by

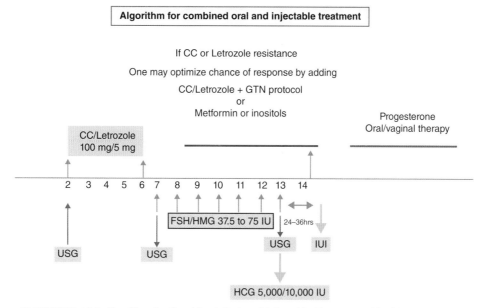

• **ALGORITHM 19.2** Algorithm for Combined Oral and Injectable Treatment. *CC*, Clomiphene citrate; *GTN*, gonadotrophin; *IUI*, intrauterine insemination; *USG*, ultrasonography.

exogenous hCG, and symptoms occur within 3 to 7 days of its administration. Late OHSS is caused by endogenous (placental) hCG arising from the trophoblast of the early pregnancy and symptoms appear 12 to 17 days after hCG administration. OHSS may be mild, moderate, or severe. It is normally self-limiting and resolves spontaneously within several days. Late OHSS may worsen and persist for a longer duration because of ongoing pregnancy.

Thin lean PCOS patients receiving high doses of gonadotropins and who have had previous episodes of the syndrome are considered high risk for OHSS. A large number of intermediate-sized ovarian follicles, high estradiol levels (2500 pg/mL), and hCG use for luteal support all increase the risk for OHSS.

When the risk of OHSS is suspected during gonadotropin stimulation, withholding hCG should be considered. An alternative approach is coasting without further gonadotropin stimulation and delaying hCG administration for 1 to 3 days until estradiol levels plateau or decline. Progesterone rather than hCG should be used for luteal support if necessary. Low-dose stimulation protocols should be considered for patients with a previous history of OHSS.

Malignancy. In nulliparous females, use of fertility drugs may be associated with an increased incidence of borderline serous ovarian tumors but not with invasive cancers. Nevertheless, no causal relationship between gonadotropin treatment and ovarian cancer has been seen. Recent larger studies have not supported this risk.[11]

Surgical Ovulation Induction

Laparoscopic Ovarian Drilling (LOD). LOD is an alternative to gonadotrophin therapy in CC resistant patients. This procedure has replaced the more damaging technique of ovarian wedge resection. LOD is particularly useful for PCOS patients who have not responded to first-line fertility treatment or need a laparoscopic pelvic assessment and who cannot follow gonadotrophin therapy because of frequent monitoring. Young patients and those with persistently elevated LH levels are more likely to benefit from LOD,[42] whereas those with obesity, high androgen levels, or long duration of infertility are more likely to be resistant. LOD has no advantages over CC as a first-line treatment[83,84]; however, it has shown similar efficacy to gonadotrophins in the treatment of CC resistant PCOS.[85]

Method. LOD is performed under general anesthesia, using a 10-mm traditional endoscope through the subumbilical port, and with two additional trocars. Commonly employed methods for LOD include monopolar or bipolar electrocautery and laser with comparable results.[85] The number of ovarian punctures may vary depending on the ovarian volume. A greater number of punctures has been associated with more trauma to ovarian tissue and an increased risk of premature ovarian failure. Based on Adam Balen and Armer's technique, drilling should be performed preferably at four sites, avoiding the ovarian cortex, to a depth of 4 mm, for 4 seconds, and at 40 W to minimize ovarian trauma. Postprocedure instillation of isotonic solution into the peritoneal cavity also prevents heat injury to ovaries and reduces the risk of adhesions. There is no major difference in outcomes with LOD performed on one or both ovaries,[86] but unilateral interventions are preferred to reduce the incidence of adverse effects. Up to 86% ovulation and pregnancy rates are achieved with LOD.[42]

Mechanism of Action. LOD directly destroys ovarian tissue including follicles and surrounding stroma, which reduces AMH levels and production of androgens. This helps to reduce the levels of LH and testosterone[87] and promotes increased release of FSH, thus supporting follicular growth and ovulation.[72] In, addition, it improves the LH/FSH ratio, reduces androstenedione and DHEA-S levels, and increases SHBG[88,89] (Fig. 19.9). Other

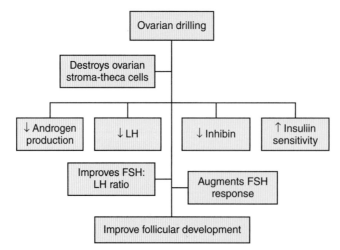

Mechanism of action: laparocopic ovarian drilling

• **Fig. 19.9** Mechanism of Action of Laparoscopic Ovarian Drilling. *LH,* Luteinizing hormone. (Julie Collée, Marie Mawet, Linda Tebache, Michelle Nisolle & Géraldine Brichant (2021) Polycystic ovarian syndrome and infertility: overview and insights of the putative treatments, Gynecological Endocrinology, 37:10, 869-874, DOI: 10.1080/09513590.2021.1958310)

consequences of a LOD procedure include decreased inhibin levels and increased production of several growth factors (insulin-like growth factor-I) because of thermal stimulus to the ovary. These changes augment FSH activity and lead to follicular development.[90] LOD also reduces ovarian and stroma volume and increases IS.[91] These changes also improve responsiveness to exogenous FSH stimulation.

Side Effects. LOD may be associated with postoperative complications including bleeding, infections, and a small risk of postoperative adhesions. Because the effect of LOD on ovarian function is not permanent, with time menstrual irregularities may reoccur.[42,92] In addition, there is a theoretical risk of reduction in ovarian reserve, and this needs consideration during counseling of the patient. An overenthusiastic approach should be avoided during the procedure because it can cause extensive ovarian damage and lead to premature menopause. With a safer approach and advanced techniques, however, this risk can be minimized.

Advantages of Laparoscopic Ovarian Drilling. Ultrasound monitoring is not required for LOD because it induces mono-follicular development.[81] LOD is associated with a reduced risk of multiple pregnancies and OHSS compared with other ovulation induction therapies.[93] With LOD, ovulation and pregnancy rates vary from 30% to 80% and 60%, respectively.[94] The choice of technique may also influence the efficacy of LOD. Giampaolino et al. reported ovulation and pregnancy rates of 82.9% and 70%, respectively, in the 6 months after THL.[92]

Besides its efficacy in terms of the pregnancy rate, LOD also has long-term benefits. Studies have shown that after the procedure, an improvement in symptoms of PCOS can persist for up to 20 years. This long-term efficacy is not achieved with the other treatment options (except for lifestyle modifications when they are followed over a long period). In a retrospective study in 2020, Debras et al. showed that LOD helps in the achievement of spontaneous pregnancy and has a long-term effect for appropriately selected patients.[92]

Predictors of Success. Approximately 30% of PCOS patients fail to respond to LOD. Treatment is considered unsuccessful when amenorrhea and anovulation persist until 8 weeks after the procedure.[94] Factors that enhance the efficacy of LOD are high LH concentration (>10 UI/L), infertility duration (<3 years), age younger than 35 years, and low antral follicle count (<50).[95] Factors that are associated with poor response to LOD[92] are described in Table 19.6.

In approximately 50% of LOD-treated patients, adjuvant therapy will be required.[26] If ovulation is not detected, oral ovulation-inducing drugs can be used after 12 to 24 weeks, and gonadotrophin therapy can be considered 6 months after the procedure.

Transvaginal Hydrolaparoscopy (THL). THL is a new emerging procedure that can be performed under spinal anesthesia.[42] THL is performed with instillation of saline solution within the peritoneal cavity. The endoscope has an angle of 30 degrees and permits better examination of the entire

TABLE 19.6	Factors Associated With Poor Response to Laparoscopic Ovarian Drilling

- Duration of infertility greater than 3 years
- Low basal LH levels <10 IU/L
- Testosterone level >4.5 nmo1/L
- High basal anti-Müllerian hormone (AMH) >7.7 ng/mL
- High body mass index (BMI; >35kg/m²)
- Insulin resistance

Debras E, Fernandez H, Neveu M-E, Deffieux X, Capmas P. Ovarian drilling in polycystic ovarian syndrome. Long-term pregnancy rate. *Euro J Obstet Gynaecol Reprod Biol.* 2019.

pelvic cavity. It also allows for evaluation of the fimbriae and fallopian tubes at the same time by using salpingoscopy.[96]

The safety of the procedure is influenced by the choice of technique. Compared with laparoscopy, THL is quicker, reduces the risk of adhesions, and is associated with less postoperative pain.[96] These benefits could be because of intraperitoneal installation of saline, a shorter time duration, use of bipolar diathermy, and minimal bleeding because of lower manipulation of the ovaries than during an LOD. THL is also an appropriate approach for obese patients. Finally, the learning curve with THL is shorter than with laparoscopy.[97]

There is small risk of rectal perforation (0.5%) associated with this technique.[98] This is usually managed conservatively with antibiotics. In such cases, a second-look laparoscopy will be needed to confirm recovery. Other techniques, including laparoscopic ovarian multineedle intervention and ultrasound-guided transvaginal ovarian drilling, are under trial.

Intrauterine Insemination (IUI). IUI is indicated for patients with unexplained infertility, mild endometriosis, or mild male factor.[24] For patients with PCOS, IUI can be considered as an add-on treatment option for females who have had an unsuccessful two to three cycles of ovulation induction with oral,[99] combined oral, and parenteral therapy or parenteral treatment alone[81] and if there is associated male factor infertility.[100] IUI is performed after 24 to 36 hours of hCG trigger in a stimulated cycle. Reported pregnancy rates for IUI combined with gonadotrophins are around 11% to 20%.[55]

Third-Line Management

In Vitro Fertilization

IVF is considered third-line management for anovulatory infertility in PCOS patients.[89] This mode of treatment is not directly advised as an option and is recommended when the second-line treatment options have failed or there is another associated infertility factor, including male factor, tubal blockade, and endometriosis. Furthermore, egg freezing can be considered in young PCOS females who have concerns about fertility potential.[25,15]

IVF, for patients with PCOS, presents multiple challenges ranging from a poor to an exaggerated response, affected egg to follicle ratio, impaired fertilization and poor blastocyst formation, and increased risk of OHSS (5%–10%) and multiple pregnancies (10%). To avoid these complications, a patient-tailored approach should be considered. Ovarian stimulation for these patients should be planned carefully keeping in mind the antral follicle count, AMH and LH levels. IVF treatment involves low-dose gonadotropin stimulation combined with GnRH agonist and antagonist use.[101] For PCOS patients, GnRH antagonist short protocol is preferred over GnRH agonist long protocol. For antagonist treatment cycles, GnRH agonist is considered a trigger rather than hCG for final oocyte maturation.[102] In those who are at a high risk for OHSS, elective freezing of embryos is recommended. Similarly, metformin use (1500–2550 mg) as an adjuvant therapy before and during stimulated cycles helps to improve pregnancy rates and reduces the risk of OHSS.[25]

IVM is an emerging ART that helps to avoid the IVF-associated risk of OHSS in young females with PCOS. This treatment is considered cost effective because it involves gonadotrophin stimulation for a short duration, and a trigger injection is not required.[25] Furthermore, oocytes are retrieved at an earlier stage when follicles are 10 to 11 mm in size compared with conventional IVF. This early intervention helps to minimizes gonadotrophin stimulation. The further maturation process of retrieved immature oocytes (meiosis and maturation to metaphase II) occurs in vitro. At the final maturation stage, the hCG trigger is given and ovum

pick is done after 36 hours followed by the intracytoplasmic sperm injection procedure. However, pregnancy rates associated with the procedure are low[101,103] (Algorithm 19.3).

Conclusion

Lifestyle modification is a first-line intervention for obese patients with PCOS and is a preventive strategy for females with normal BMI. The first-line pharmacologic treatment for ovulation induction is letrozole. CC can be used as first-line therapy in settings where letrozole is not available, or its use is not permitted, or cost affects treatment choice. Metformin combined with CC is more effective in obese females than CC alone and metformin alone. Inositol has shown promising results in IVF treatment, but its use is considered experimental. Gonadotrophins are used as second-line treatment for ovulation induction in CC resistant PCOS patients. These are more effective than CC in elderly females with PCOS, and can be considered as a first-line therapy in the presence of monitoring facilities and counseling of patient on cost and associated risks of multiple pregnancy and OHSS. In PCOS nonobese patients with a high LH concentration, short infertility duration, and young age at conceiving, LOS is effective as a second-line therapy. IVF can be considered in cases where all other treatment options for improving ovulation are ineffective (Algorithm 19.4 and Table 19.7).

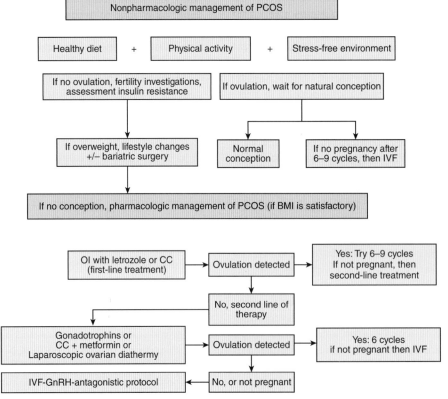

• **ALGORITHM 19.3** Fertility Treatment in Polycystic Ovary Syndrome (*PCOS*) Females. *BMI*, Body mass index; *CC*, clomiphene citrate; *GnRH*, gonadotrophin-releasing hormone; *IVF*, in vitro fertilization; *OI*, ovulation induction. (Adapted and simplified for book chapter from: Balen AH., et al. The management of anovulatory infertility in women with polycystic ovarian syndrome; ana analysis of evidence to support the development of global WHO guidance. Hum Reprod Update 2016.)

IVF treatment for PCOS women

ART cycles
↓
Antagonist protocol
↓
Low starting dose
↓
Careful monitoring of the cycle
↓
Agonist trigger
↓
SET after modified LPS
↓
Consider egg freezing
↓
An algorithm 4: IVF treatment in women with PCOS [25]

• **ALGORITHM 19.4** In Vitro Fertilization *(IVF)* Treatment for Polycystic Ovary Syndrome *(PCOS)* Females. *ART,* Assisted reproductive treatment; *LPS,* Luteal Phase Support; *SET,* Selective Embryo Transfer.

TABLE 19.7 Summary: Management of Anovulatory Infertility in Polycystic Ovary Syndrome

Lifestyle intervention is recommended as the first-line treatment.

Bariatric surgery is considered if BMI ≥35 kg/m² and lifestyle therapy has failed.

Letrozole is the drug of choice: Both CC and Letrozole can be used as first-line pharmacotherapy for OI.

Both metformin and myoinositol improve follicular milieu and hence fertilization rate but have no effect on live birth rates.

CC + metformin can be used in *CC* resistant cases.

Low-dose gonadotrophins therapy and LODs can be used as second-line management.

For those who fail to respond to life style modifications and OI therapy, or who have additional infertility factors, IVF can be used with the GnRH antagonistic protocol. IVM is an upcoming technique as a third-line management.

If a GnRH-agonist protocol is used, metformin as an adjunct may reduce the risk of OHSS.

BMI, Body mass index; *GnRH,* gonadotrophin-releasing hormone; *GT,* gonadotropin; *IVF,* in vitro fertilization; *IVM,* in vitro maturation; *LBR,* live birth rate; *LOD,* laparoscopic ovarian drilling; *OHSS,* ovarian hyperstimulation syndrome; *OI,* ovulation induction.

References

1. Azziz R, Carmina E, Dewailly D, et al. Positions statement: criteria for defining polycystic ovary syndrome as a predominantly hyperandrogenic syndrome: an Androgen Excess Society guideline. *J Clin Endocrinol Metab.* 2006;91(11):4237-4245.
2. Bozdag G, Mumusoglu S, Zengin D, et al. The prevalence and phenotypic features of polycystic ovary syndrome: a systematic review and meta-analysis. *Hum Reprod.* 2016;31(12):2841-2855.
3. Escobar-Morreale HF. Polycystic ovary syndrome: definition, aetiology, diagnosis, and treatment. *Nat Rev Endocrinol.* 2018; 14(5):270.
4. Azziz R. Diagnostic criteria for polycystic ovary syndrome: a reappraisal. *Fertil Steril.* 2005;83(5):1343-1346. doi:10.1016/j.fertnstert.2005.01.085.
5. Minocha N. Polycystic ovarian disease or polycystic ovarian syndrome: how to identify and manage—a review. *Arch Pharm Pract.* 2020;11(2):102-106.
6. Dennett CC, Simon J. The role of polycystic ovary syndrome in reproductive and metabolic health: overview and approaches for treatment. *Diabetes Spectr.* 2015;28(2):116-120. Available at: https://doi.org/10.2337/diaspect.28.2.116.
7. Witchel SF, Oberfield SE, Peña AS. Polycystic ovary syndrome: pathophysiology, presentation, and treatment with emphasis on adolescent girls. *J Endocr Soc.* 2019;3(8):1545-1573.
8. Fauser B, Tarlatzis B, Rebar R, Legro R, Balen A. Consensus on women's health aspects of polycystic ovary syndrome (PCOS): the Amsterdam ESHRE. Paper presented at: ASRM-sponsored 3rd PCOS Consensus Workshop Group. *Fertil Steril.* 2011;97:28.
9. Lizneva D, Gavrilova-Jordan L, Walker W, Azziz R. Androgen excess: investigations and management. *Best Pract Res Clin Obstet Gynaecol.* 2016;30:1-21. Available at: https://doi.org/10.1016/j.bpobgyn.2016.05.003.
10. Melo AS, Ferriani RA, Navarro PA. Treatment of infertility in women with polycystic ovary syndrome: approach to clinical practice. *Clinics.* 2015;70(11):765-769.
11. Taylor HS, Pal L, Seli E. Regulation of the menstrual cycle. In: *Speroff's Clinical Gynecologic Endocrinology and Infertility.* Philadelphia: Lippincott Williams & Wilkins; 2019:137-173.
12. Lew R. Natural history of ovarian function including assessment of ovarian reserve and premature ovarian failure. *Best Pract Res Clin Obstet Gynaecol.* 2019;55:2-13.
13. Pellatt L, Rice S, Mason HD. Anti-Müllerian hormone and polycystic ovary syndrome: a mountain too high? *Reproduction.* 2010;139:825-833.
14. Pellatt L, Rice S, Dilaver N, et al. Anti-Müllerian hormone reduces follicle sensitivity to follicle-stimulating hormone human granulosa cells. *Fertil Steril.* 2011;96:1246-1251.
15. Mascarenhas M, Balen AH. Treatment update for anovulation and subfertility in polycystic ovary syndrome. *Curr Opin Endocr Metab Res.* 2020;12:53-58.
16. Conway G, Dewailly D, Diamanti-Kandarakis E, et al. The polycystic ovary syndrome: a position statement from the European Society of Endocrinology. *Eur J Endocrinol.* 2014;171(4):P1-P29.
17. Bhide P, Homburg R. Anti-Müllerian hormone, and polycystic ovary syndrome. *Best Prac Res Clin Obstet Gynaecol.* 2016;37:38-45.
18. Seifer D, Tal R. *Anti-Mullerian Hormone: Biology, Role in Ovarian Function and Clinical Significance. Obstetrics and Gynaecology Advances.* Nova Science Publishers, Inc.; 2016.
19. Wang F, Niu W, Kong H, Guo YH, Sun Y. The role of AMH and its receptor SNP in the pathogenesis of PCOS. *Mol Cell Endocrinol.* 2017;439:363-368.

20. Porter DT, Moore AM, Cobern JA, et al. Prenatal testosterone exposure alters GABAergic synaptic inputs to GnRH and KNDy neurons in a sheep model of polycystic ovarian syndrome. *Endocrinology.* 2019;160:2529-2542.

21. de Assis Rodrigues NP, Laganà AS, Zaia V, et al. The role of Kisspeptin levels in polycystic ovary syndrome: a systematic review and meta-analysis. *Arch Gynecol Obstet.* 2019;300:1423-1434.

22. Homburg R. Androgen circle of polycystic ovary syndrome. *Hum Reprod.* 2009;24:1548-1555.

23. Ferreira SR, Motta AB. Uterine function: from normal to polycystic ovarian syndrome alterations. *Curr Med Chem.* 2018;25:1792-1804.

24. National Institute for Health and Care Excellence. *Fertility: Assessment and Treatment for People with Fertility Problems. CG156.* London: NICE; 2013. Available at: http://www.nice.org.uk/CG156.9.

25. Teede HJ, Misso ML, Costello MF, et al. Recommendations from the international evidence-based guideline for the assessment and management of polycystic ovary syndrome. *Hum Reprod.* 2018;33(9):1602-1618.

26. Balen AH. Polycystic ovary syndrome (PCOS). *Obstet Gynaecol.* 2017;19(2):119-129.

27. Dewailly D, Lujan ME, Carmina E, et al. Definition and significance of polycystic ovarian morphology: a task force report from the Androgen Excess and Polycystic Ovary Syndrome Society. *Hum Reprod Update.* 2014;20(3):334-352.

28. Escobar-Morreale HF. Polycystic ovary syndrome: definition, aetiology, diagnosis, and treatment. *Nat Rev Endocrinol.* 2018; 14(5):270.

29. Christiansen SC, Eilertsen TB, Vanky E, Carlsen SM. Does AMH reflect follicle number similarly in women with and without PCOS? *PLoS One.* 2016;11(1):e0146739.

30. Grisendi V, La Marca A. Individualization of controlled ovarian stimulation in vitro fertilization using ovarian reserve markers. *Minerva Ginecol.* 2017;69(3):250-258.

31. Costello MF, Misso ML, Wong J, et al. The treatment of infertility in polycystic ovary syndrome: a brief update. *Aust N Z J Obstet Gynaecol.* 2012;52:400-403.

32. Walls ML, Hunter T, Ryan JP, Keelan JA, Nathan E, Hart RJ. In vitro maturation as an alternative to standard in vitro fertilization for patients diagnosed with polycystic ovaries: a comparative analysis of fresh, frozen and cumulative cycle outcomes. *Hum Reprod.* 2015;30:88-96.

33. Balen AH, Anderson R. Impact of obesity on female reproductive health. British Fertility Society, Police and Practice Guidelines. *Hum Fertil.* 2007;10:195-206.

34. Naderpoor N, Shorakae S, de Courten B, Misso ML, Moran LJ, Teede HJ. Metformin and lifestyle modification in PCOS: systematic review and meta- analysis. *Hum Reprod Update.* 2015;21:560-574.

35. Azziz R, Carmina E, Dewailly D, et al. The Androgen Excess and PCOS Society criteria for the polycystic ovary syndrome: the complete task force report. *Fertil Steril.* 2009;91(2):456-488.

36. Ali SS, Rehman R. Polycystic ovary syndrome and subfertility. In: *Subfertility.* Amsterdam: Elsevier Inc.; 2021:115-134.

37. Pasquali R. Contemporary approaches to the management of polycystic ovary syndrome. *Ther Adv Endocrinol Metab.* 2018;9:123-134.

38. Goodman NF, Cobin RH, Futterweit W, Glueck JS, Legro RS, Carmina E. American Association of Clinical Endocrinologists, American College of Endocrinology, and Androgen Excess and PCOS Society disease state clinical review: guide to the best practices in the evaluation and treatment of polycystic ovary syndrome-part 1. *Endocr Pract.* 2015;21(11):1291-1300.

39. Nestler JE. Metformin in the treatment of infertility in PCOS: an alternative perspective. *Fertil Steril.* 2008;90:14-16.

40. Morley LC, Tang T, Yasmin E, Norman RJ, Balen AH. Insulin-sensitising drugs (metformin, rosiglitazone, pioglitazone, D-chiro-inositol) for women with polycystic ovary syndrome, oligo amenorrhoea and subfertility [Internet]. *Cochrane Database Syst Rev.* 2017. Available at: https://www.cochranelibrary.com/cdsr/doi/10.1002/14651858.CD003053.pub6/full.

41. Tso LO, Costello MF, Albuquerque LET, Andriolo RB, Macedo CR. Metformin treatment before and during IVF or ICSI in women with polycystic ovary syndrome. *Cochrane Database Syst Rev.* 2014;2014:CD006105.

42. Collée J, Mawet M, Tebache L, Nisolle M, Brichant G. Polycystic ovarian syndrome and infertility: overview and insights of the putative treatments. *Gynecol Endocrinol.* 2021;37(10):869-874. doi:10.1080/09513590.2021.1958310.

43. Facchinetti F, Bizzarri M, Benvenga S, et al. Results from the international consensus conference on myo-inositol and d-chiro-inositol in obstetrics and gynecology: the link between metabolic syndrome and PCOS. *Eur J Obstet Gynecol Reprod Biol.* 2015;195:72-76.

44. Baillargeon JP, Iuorno MJ, Jakubowicz DJ, Apridonidze T, He N, Nestler JE. Metformin therapy increases insulin-stimulated release of D-chiro-inositol-containing inositolphosphoglycan mediator in women with polycystic ovary syndrome. *J Clin Endocrinol Metab.* 2004;89(1):242-249.

45. Pundir J, Psaroudakis D, Savnur P, et al. Inositol treatment of anovulation in women with polycystic ovary syndrome: a meta-analysis of randomised trials. *BJOG.* 2018;125(3):299-308.

46. Atay V, Cam C, Muhcu M, Cam M, Karateke A. Comparison of letrozole and clomiphene citrate in women with polycystic ovaries undergoing ovarian stimulation. *J Int Med Res.* 2006;34(1):73-76.

47. Stout DL, Fugate SE. Thiazolidinediones for treatment of polycystic ovary syndrome. *Pharmacotherapy.* 2005;25:244-252.

48. Sanchez-Garrido MA, Tena-Sempere M. Metabolic dysfunction in polycystic ovary syndrome: pathogenic role of androgen excess and potential therapeutic strategies. *Mol Metab.* 2020;35:100937.

49. Practice Committee of the American Society for Reproductive Medicine. Use of clomiphene citrate in infertile women: a committee opinion. *Fertil Steril.* 2013;100:341-348.

50. Clark JH, Markaverich BM. The agonistic and antagonistic effects of short acting estrogens: a review. *Pharmacol Ther.* 1983; 21(3):429-453.

51. Use of clomiphene citrate in infertile women: a committee opinion. *Fertil Steril.* 2013;100:341-348.

52. Ege S, Bademkıran MH, Peker N, Tahaoğlu AE, Çaça FNH, Özçelik SM. A comparison between a combination of letrozole and clomiphene citrate versus gonadotropins for ovulation induction in infertile patients with clomiphene citrateresistant polycystic ovary syndrome—a retrospective study. *Ginekol Pol.* 2020;91(4):185-188.

53. Shokeir T, El-Kannishy G. Rosiglitazone as treatment for clomiphene citrate-resistant polycystic ovary syndrome: factors associated with clinical response. *J Womens Health (Larchmt).* 2008;17(9):1445-1452.

54. Mahran A, Abdelmeged A, El-Adawy AR, Eissa MK, Shaw RW, Amer SA. The predictive value of circulating anti-Müllerian hormone in women with polycystic ovarian syndrome receiving clomiphene citrate: a prospective observational study. *J Clin Endocrinol Metab.* 2013;98(10):4170-4175.

55. Thomas S, Sudharshini S. Polycystic ovarian syndrome: treatment options for infertility. *Curr Med Issues*. 2016;14(4):87.

56. George K, Kamath MS, Nair R, Tharyan P. Ovulation triggers in anovulatory women undergoing ovulation induction. *Cochrane Database Syst Rev*. 2014;31(1):CD006900. Available at: https://www.cochranelibrary.com/cdsr/doi/10.1002/14651858.CD006900.pub3/abstract.

57. Hill MJ, Whitcomb BW, Lewis TD, et al. Progesterone luteal support after ovulation induction and intrauterine insemination: a systematic review and meta-analysis. *Fertil Steril*. 2013;100(5):1373-1380.

58. Thessaloniki ESHRE/ASRM-Sponsored PCOS Consensus Workshop Group. Consensus on infertility treatment related to polycystic ovary syndrome. *Hum Reprod*. 2008;23:462-477.

59. Dickey RP, Taylor SN, Lu PY, et al. Effect of diagnosis. Age, sperm quality and number of preovulatory follicles on the outcome of multiple cycles of clomiphene citrate-intrauterine insemination. *Fertil Steril*. 2002;78:1088-1095.

60. Sharma S, Ghosh S, Singh S, et al. Congenital malformations among babies born following letrozole or clomiphene for infertility treatment. *PLoS One*. 2014;9(10):e108219.

61. Mbi Feh MK, Wadhwa R. Clomiphene. In: *StatPearls [Internet]*. Treasure Island, FL: StatPearls Publishing; 2021.

62. Abu Hashim H, Foda O, Ghayaty E. Combined metforminclomiphene in clomiphene-resistant polycystic ovary syndrome: a systematic review and meta-analysis of randomized controlled trials. *Acta Obstet Gynecol Scand*. 2015;94:921-930.

63. Omara MA, El Khouly NI, Salama HT, Solyman AE. Extended use of clomiphene citrate in induction of ovulation in polycystic ovary syndrome with clomiphene citrate resistance. *Egypt J Hosp Med*. 2021;82(3):567-573.

64. Mejia RB, Summers KM, Kresowik JD, Van Voorhis BJ. A randomized controlled trial of combination letrozole and clomiphene citrate or letrozole alone for ovulation induction in women with polycystic ovary syndrome. *Fert Steril*. 2019;111(3):571-578.

65. Balen AH, Morley LC, Misso M, et al. The management of anovulatory infertility in women with polycystic ovary syndrome: an analysis of the evidence to support the development of global WHO guidance). *Hum Reprod Update*. 2016;22(6):687-708. doi:10.1093/humupd/dmw025.

66. Dawood AS, Abdelghaffar SD, Borg HM. Letrozole versus gonadotropins for ovulation induction in clomiphene citrate resistance: a randomized controlled study. *Ann Gynecol Obstet*. 2021;5(1):127-132.

67. Holzer H, Casper RR, Tulandi T. A new era in ovulation Induction. *Fertil Steril*. 2006;85(2):277-284.

68. Mitwally MF, Casper RF. Single-dose administration of an aromatase inhibitor for ovarian stimulation. *Fertil Steril*. 2005;83:229-231.

69. Legro RS, Brzyski RG, Diamond MP, et al. Letrozole versus clomiphene for infertility in the polycystic ovary syndrome. *N Engl J Med*. 2014;371:119-129.

70. Franik S, Kremer JA, Nelen WL, Farquhar C. Aromatase inhibitors for subfertile women with polycystic ovary syndrome. *Cochrane Database Syst Rev*. 2014;(2):CD010287.

71. Badawy A, Gibreal A. Clomiphene citrate versus tamoxifen for ovulation induction in women with PCOS: a prospective randomized trial. *Eur J Obstet Gynecol Reprod Biol*. 2011;159:151-154.

72. Steiner AZ, Terplan M, Paulson RJ. Comparison of tamoxifen and clomiphene citrate for ovulation induction: a meta-analysis. *Hum Reprod*. 2005;20:1511-1515.

73. Royal Collegue of Obstetricians and Gynaecologists. *Long-Term Consequences of Polycystic Ovary Syndrome: Green-Top Guideline no. 33*. 2014. Available at: https://www.rcog.org.uk/globalassets/documents/guidelines/gtg_33.pdf.

74. Homburg R, Hendriks ML, Konig TE, et al. Clomifene citrate or low-dose FSH for the first-line treatment of infertile women with anovulation associated with polycystic ovary syndrome: a prospective randomized multinational study. *Hum Reprod*. 2012;27:468-473.

75. Weiss NS, Kostova E, Nahuis M, et al. Gonadotrophins for ovulation induction in women with polycystic ovary syndrome. *Cochrane Database Syst Rev*. 2019;(1):CD010290. doi:10.1002/14651858.CD010290.pub3.

76. Melo AS, Ferriani RA, Navarro PA. Treatment of infertility in women with polycystic ovary syndrome: approach to clinical practice. *Clinics*. 2015;70:765-769.

77. Dafopoulos K, Tarlatzis BC. Hormonal treatments in the infertile women. In: Petraglia F, Fauser B, eds. Female Reproductive Dysfunction. Endocrinology. Springer, Cham; 2020:247-261.

78. Della Corte L, Foreste V, Barra F, et al. Current and experimental drug therapy for the treatment of polycystic ovarian syndrome. *Expert Opin Investig Drugs*. 2020;29(8):819-830. Available at: https://doi.org/10.1080/13543784.2020.1781815.

79. Sood A, Mathur R. Ovarian hyperstimulation syndrome. *Obstet Gynaecol Reprod Med*. 2020;30(8):251-255. Available at: https://doi.org/10.1016/j.ogrm.2020.05.004.

80. Du DF, Li MF, Li XL. Ovarian hyperstimulation syndrome: a clinical retrospective study on 565 inpatients. *Gynecol Endocrinol*. 2020;36(4):313-317.

81. El-Sayed Abd El-Maksoud A, Zakaria El-Sheikha K, El-Sayed Ibrahim A. Comparison between letrozole alone versus letrozole-gonadotrophins combination in versus clomiphene citrate–gonadotrophins combination in ovarian induction for PCOS patient undergoing intrauterine insemination. *Al Azhar Med J*. 2021;50(1):253-264.

82. Xi W, Liu S, Mao H, Yang Y, Xue X, Lu X. Use of letrozole and clomiphene citrate combined with gonadotropins in clomiphene-resistant infertile women with polycystic ovary syndrome: a prospective study. *Drug Des Devel Ther*. 2015;9:6001-6008.

83. Amer SA, Li TC, Metwally M, Emarh M, Ledger WL. Randomized controlled trial comparing laparoscopic ovarian diathermy with clomiphene citrate as a first-line method of ovulation induction in women with polycystic ovary syndrome. *Hum Reprod*. 2009;24(1):219-225.

84. Abu Hashim H, Foda O, Ghayaty E, Elawa A. Laparoscopic ovarian diathermy after clomiphene failure in polycystic ovary syndrome: is it worthwhile? A randomized controlled trial. *Arch Gynecol Obstet*. 2011;284(5):1303-1309.

85. Farquhar C, Brown J, Marjoribanks J. Laparoscopic drilling by diathermy or laser for ovulation induction in anovulatory polycystic ovary syndrome. *Cochrane Database Syst Rev*. 2012;(6):CD001122.

86. Roy KK, Baruah J, Moda N, Kumar S. Evaluation of unilateral versus bilateral ovarian drilling in clomiphene citrate resistant cases of polycystic ovarian syndrome. *Arch Gynecol Obstet*. 2009;280(4):573-578.

87. Lebbi I, Ben Temime R, Fadhlaoui A, Feki A. Ovarian drilling in PCOS: is it really useful? *Front Surg*. 2015;2:30.

88. Gjonnaess H. Polycystic ovarian syndrome treated by ovarian electrocautery through the laparoscope. *Fertil Steril*. 1984;41(1):20-25.

89. Ott J, Mayerhofer K, Nouri K, Walch K, Seemann R, Kurz C. Perioperative androstenedione kinetics in women undergoing laparoscopic ovarian drilling: a prospective study. *Endocrine.* 2014;47(3):936-942.

90. Felemban A, Tan SL, Tulandi T. Laparoscopic treatment of polycystic ovaries with insulated needle cautery: a reappraisal. *Fertil Steril.* 2000;73:266-269.

91. Saleh AM, Khalil HS. Review of nonsurgical and surgical treatment and the role of insulin-sensitizing agents in the management of infertile women with polycystic ovary syndrome. *Acta Obstet Gynecol Scand.* 2004;83:614-621.

92. Debras E, Fernandez H, Neveu ME, Deffieux X, Capmas P. Ovarian drilling in polycystic ovary syndrome: long term pregnancy rate. *Eur J Obstet Gynecol Reprod Biol X.* 2019;4:100093.

93. Bordewijk EM, Ng KY, Rakic L, et al. Laparoscopic ovarian drilling for ovulation induction in women with anovulatory polycystic ovary syndrome. *Cochrane Database Syst Rev.* 2020;2:CD001122.

94. Seow KM, Juan CC, Hwang JL, Ho LT. Laparoscopic surgery in polycystic ovary syndrome: reproductive and metabolic effects. *Semin Reprod Med.* 2008;26(1):101-110.

95. Practice Committee of American Society for Reproductive Medicine. Diagnostic evaluation of the infertile female: a committee opinion. *Fertil Steril.* 2012;98(2):302-307. doi:10.1016/j.fertnstert.2012.05.032.

96. Giampaolino P, Morra I, Tommaselli GA, Di Carlo C, Nappi C, Bifulco G. Post-operative ovarian adhesion formation after ovarian drilling: a randomized study comparing conventional laparoscopy and transvaginal hydrolaparoscopy. *Arch Gynecol Obstet.* 2016;294(4):791-796.

97. Giampaolino P, De Rosa N, Della Corte L, et al. Operative transvaginal hydrolaparoscopy improve ovulation rate after clomiphene failure in polycystic ovary syndrome. *Gynecol Endocrinol.* 2018;34(1):32-35.

98. Ezedinma NA, Phelps JY. Transvaginal hydrolaparoscopy. *JSLS.* 2012;16(3):461-465.

99. Nguyen TT, Doan HT, Quan LH, Lam NM. Effect of letrozole for ovulation induction combined with intrauterine insemination on women with polycystic ovary syndrome. *Gynecol Endocrinol.* 2020;36(10):860-863.

100. Giudice LC. Endometrium in PCOS: implantation and predisposition to endocrine CA. *Best Pract Res Clin Endocrinol Metab.* 2006;20:235-244.

101. Walls ML, Hart RJ. In vitro maturation. *Best Pract Res Clin Obstet Gynaecol.* 2018;53:60-72.

102. Thakre N, Homburg R. A review of IVF in PCOS patients at risk of ovarian hyperstimulation syndrome. *Expert Rev Endocrinol Metab.* 2019;14(5):315-319.

103. Walls ML, Hunter T, Ryan JP, Keelan JA, Nathan E, Hart RJ. In vitro maturation as an alternative to standard in vitro fertilization for patients diagnosed with polycystic ovaries: a comparative analysis of fresh, frozen and cumulative cycle outcomes. *Hum Reprod.* 2015;30:88-96.

20

Management of Associated Risks of Pregnancy in Polycystic Ovary Syndrome

LUMAAN SHEIKH, ZAHEENA SHAMSUL ISLAM, AND NIDA NAJMI

Polycystic ovary syndrome (PCOS) is one of the most common endocrinologic disorders in females of childbearing age, affecting 5% to 20% of females.[1-3] It is associated with Hyper Androgenism (HA), ovulatory dysfunction, and characteristic ultrasonographic morphology of polycystic ovaries in one or both ovaries.[4] The pathophysiology of PCOS is multifactorial. There is an underlying genetic predisposition, combined with excess adiposity and hormonal dysregulation because of excess androgen, hyperinsulinemia, and elevated luteinizing hormone levels.[5]

During pregnancy, physiologic Insulin Resistance (IR) leads to a compensatory hyperinsulinemia in the latter half of the pregnancy. This physiologic IR is necessary to restrict use of maternal glucose and increase its availability to the growing fetus. This process is facilitated by the pregnancy hormones, including Estradiol (E2), Progesterone (P2), Prolactin, Cortisol, Human Chorionic Gonadotropin, Placental Growth Hormone, and Human Placental Lactogen. The last two of these hormones are mainly responsible for IR in pregnancy.[6]

HA and IR are the characteristic features of patients with PCOS. These features are not restricted to obese females. Thin females with PCOS can also have inherent IR. Obesity further adds to the already existent IR in patients with PCOS because of the presence of excess adipose tissue. As the female enters pregnancy, this baseline IR is further aggravated. Hence risk of pregnancy complications is increased. Pregnant patients with PCOS are at higher risk of spontaneous miscarriage, Gestational Diabetes Mellitus (GDM), Pregnancy Induced Hypertension (PIH), preterm birth (PTB), and a small-for-gestational-age (SGA) fetus. The extent of the incidence of GDM, PIH, preeclampsia, and cesarean section (CS) varies among studies but is reproducibly increased even when data are adjusted for body

mass index (BMI).[1,7] Therefore PCOS can have profound effects on a female's physical and mental health with important implications for reproductive outcomes. Management of metabolic and reproductive problems relating to pregnancy forms the cornerstone of management of PCOS.

Possible Underlying Mechanism of Pathophysiologic Changes in Females With PCOS During Pregnancy

PCOS Phenotypes

IR is the hallmark of PCOS and occurs independently of adiposity; however, it is further worsened by adiposity. Thus the risk is altered according to the different phenotypes and has a linear correlation with BMI. Some studies report that a combination of HA and IR and/or hyperinsulinemia may result in an increased risk of complications in pregnancy in patients with PCOS, such as miscarriages,[8] intrauterine growth restriction,[9,10] GDM, PIH, preeclampsia, PTB, and antepartum hemorrhage,[11-13] by altering normal placental implantation.[8] Even with different diagnostic criteria for PCOS, it is well established that regardless of phenotype, patients with PCOS need to be screened and managed for adverse pregnancy outcomes equivalently.[14]

Effects of Insulin Resistance

IR and hyperinsulinemia, the hallmarks of HA, occur in more than half of patients with PCOS.[15] During pregnancy, a combination of PIH and preexisting IR increases the risk for development of GDM.[1] Although some studies fail to show this association, other have shown a clear relationship.[12,16,17] IR leads to vasoconstriction, which plays a role in the development of hypertensive disorders of pregnancy (HDP).[18] It also promotes prothrombotic and profibrotic effects and has an augmented blood pressure response to the sodium intake.[19] This combined effect results in the development of preeclampsia.[16] Similarly the vascular dysfunction secondary to IR is associated with an increased risk of PTB and fetal growth disorders, such as large for gestational age (LGA) and SGA birth.[20]

Effects of Obesity and Gestational Weight Gain

Around 61% of patients with PCOS are overweight or obese.[21] Adverse pregnancy outcomes are directly related to prepregnancy BMI.[22] PCOS is the most important predictor of GDM if BMI is greater than 25 kg/m².[23]

Effect of Inflammation

HA is thought to be responsible for creating a chronic low-grade inflammatory milieu in the tissues of PCOS patients.[11,20] This leads to an increase in inflammatory markers such as white blood cells count, C-reactive protein, inflammatory cytokines (i.e., interleukin-6 [IL-6]) and interleukin-8 [IL-8]), and cellular adhesion molecules (i.e., soluble endothelial leukocyte adhesion molecule-1 [sE-selectin], soluble intercellular adhesion molecule-1 [sICAM-1], and soluble vascular cell adhesion molecule-1 [sVCAM-1]).[12,24] The exact mechanism and its association with poor pregnancy outcomes in PCOS is not clear.

Effect of Infertility and Multiple Pregnancy

The vast majority of patients with PCOS are able to conceive spontaneously; however, more than three-fourth of patients with PCOS require assistance or treatment for infertility.[25] A significant number of these females require use of assisted reproductive techniques (ART), varying from 17% to 40%.[26] Literature review suggests a higher risk of adverse pregnancy outcomes, such as PTB, low birth weight (LBW), congenital abnormalities, GDM, and HDP, even in a spontaneously conceived pregnancy in a subfertile female.[27,28] ART is associated with a high rate of adverse pregnancy outcomes including PTB, LBW, SGA fetuses, perinatal mortality, and congenital malformations.[29] Thus the risk of adverse pregnancy outcomes in PCOS associated with subfertility is further increased over this baseline risk, possibly because of factors such as fertility treatment and multiple pregnancies.

Risks Associated With Pregnancy in Polycystic Ovary Syndrome

Early Pregnancy Loss

Patients with PCOS face fertility issues because of anovulation. With progress in ART, conception rates have greatly improved in PCOS. There is some inconsistent evidence on whether PCOS patients are at greater risk for early pregnancy loss (first trimester miscarriage). The potential causes for early pregnancy loss include altered endometrial environment and subsequent reduction in implantation success because of hyperinsulinemia and concurrent HA. The risk was found to be 2.9-fold higher in pregnancies with PCOS compared with females without PCOS.[22] Nevertheless, BMI and ART are the major confounders because both are independent risk factors for miscarriage.[30,31] Hyperinsulinemia aggravated by obesity in PCOS is shown to be associated with increased levels of plasminogen activator inhibitor-1, a powerful inhibitor of fibrinolysis and a potential factor involved in pregnancy loss.[30] Moreover, many prospective and retrospective cohort studies have shown a significantly increased risk of miscarriage.[32,33]

Gestational Diabetes Mellitus

GDM commonly complicates pregnancy with PCOS. Different meta-analyses concluded a significantly higher risk for GDM.[1,7,22,34] In one study, a GDM rate of 40% to 50% was diagnosed in pregnancies.[35] When studies matched PCOS and non-PCOS females for age and BMI, risk for GDM was found to be higher in PCOS females with BMI ranging from normal to overweight,[12,17] but risk of GDM was similar in females with BMI greater than 30 kg/m².[32]

Hypertensive Disease in Pregnancy

Pregnant patients with PCOS have an up-to-fourfold increased risk of developing hypertensive disorders, including gestational hypertension and preeclampsia.[7,34] Based on the available data, the prevalence of gestational hypertension and preeclampsia is estimated as 10% to 30% and 8% to 15%, respectively, among pregnant patients with PCOS. Higher incidence of multiple pregnancies because of use of ART in PCOS is a potential confounder. Vascular dysfunction because of hyperinsulinemia can be one major contributor for HDP in PCOS.[7,36]

Preterm Birth

The relationship between PCOS and PTB is not directly linked. Various studies have reported a higher incidence of PTB in PCOS patients. Use of ovulation induction drugs in patients with PCOS can lead to multiple pregnancy, which itself is directly associated with PTB and SGA fetuses. Meta-analysis on adverse outcomes in PCOS females by Boomsma et. al have clearly shown a significantly higher chance of PTB,[1] although, in this meta-analysis, there was no difference in the incidence of multiple pregnancies in patients with PCOS versus the normal population. Results of studies included in this meta-analysis showed statistically significant heterogeneity. Moreover, none of the studies stratified preterm delivery for its cause. Hence other confounders such as iatrogenic indication for delivery because of placental insufficiency, hypertension, or diabetes contributed to preterm delivery as well. Another meta-analysis demonstrated no effect of PCOS on PTB.[34] Naver et al. confirmed an increased risk of preterm delivery in HA females with PCOS.[37] This finding does not correlate with the results of the most recent meta-analysis by Qin et al., which suggested no such association.[34]

Small for Gestational Age Fetus

The evidence in relation to the SGA fetus in PCOS women is also variable. Although Boomsma et al. have reported no significant association of SGA with PCOS, another meta-analysis conducted a few years later showed a nearly twofold increase in the risk of SGA in PCOS patients.[1,7] Other studies have reported an association of PCOS with LGA fetuses, which is possibly confounded by the presence of maternal hyperinsulinemia and GDM. This association was more pronounced in PCOS patients who were obese compared with the nonobese controls.[38] This may be because of a complex interplay between HA, IR, and hyperinsulinemia.[9,10]

Data regarding the risk of CS in pregnancies with PCOS are inconclusive. Some studies have shown significantly higher CS rates, whereas others have similar rates compared with pregnancies without PCOS.[22,39] The risk of admission to a neonatal intensive care unit of newborns of mothers with PCOS was also increased in meta-analyses. A possible explanation may be increased PTB with subsequent complications, such as respiratory distress syndrome.[40] Similarly, the rate of perinatal mortality is also found to be increased because of the higher rate of multiple pregnancies and PTB.

Management of Pregnancy Complications in Polycystic Ovary Syndrome Patients

PCOS is one of the most common endocrine disorders in females in the reproductive age group and has significant implications. Women with PCOS should have preconception counseling about the metabolic, psychological, and reproductive consequences of PCOS, and advice should be given regarding the impact of lifestyle, obesity, and age on fertility.[26] The effect of PCOS on reproductive outcomes should be emphasized. These women should be advised about the importance of planned pregnancy and optimization of health before planning pregnancy. In the preconception visit and first antenatal visit, risk of GDM should be discussed and screening should be offered. PCOS has also been included as a risk factor by the American Diabetes Association for screening of type 2 diabetes in the pregnant population at the first prenatal visit.[41] Optimal euglycemia control could enhance successful pregnancy outcomes in pregnancies with PCOS. Folic acid supplementation should be advised. Smoking cessation if applicable should be recommended.

Lifestyle Modifications

The role of lifestyle management is crucial as a vital and first-line treatment strategy for patients with PCOS.[15] Multidisciplinary interventions, including dietary, exercise, and behavioral management, to aim for appropriate BMI are essential. A prepregnancy weight loss (5%–10% of body weight) is associated with improved pregnancy outcomes in women with PCOS, especially with greater benefits when pregnancy is embarked on immediately after the weight loss.[42,43] All obese pregnant females should be counseled about the beneficial effects of dietary and/or physical activity during pregnancy on the gestational weight gain.[44] The Institute of Medicine recommends BMI-specific gestational weight gain.[45] Women should be encouraged to consume appropriate amounts of vegetables, fruit, cereal foods, protein foods, dairy foods, and alternatives and to limit the consumption of foods containing saturated fat, refined carbohydrates, and added salt and sugars, as well as reduce alcohol consumption. Certain foods such as fish with high mercury levels should be avoided. Although these recommendations are not specific for patients with PCOS, a modest prepregnancy weight loss, keeping healthy with moderate physical activity and consumption of healthy food to maintain gestational weight gain according to the prepregnancy BMI, can improve the reproductive outcomes in these high-risk cases.

Metformin

Metformin has been used for decades in the management of diabetes, even during pregnancy, because it is a well-recognized, affordable, and safe oral hypoglycemic drug, which crosses the placenta.[47] However, data regarding its efficacy specifically in PCOS are limited. A systematic review has shown no protective effect on the rate of miscarriage when used preconception compared with placebo.[48] Nevertheless, some studies have shown protection against GDM and preeclampsia when used during pregnancy.[49] A meta-analysis failed to confirm this finding.[51] Similarly, some protective effect was shown against preterm delivery.[50] Lower gestational weight gain is also associated with metformin use.[51] There are still limited data to establish this protective relationship. Although the medicine is nonteratogenic, long-term effects on the offspring are not known, and therefore its use in PCOS females without GDM is not recommended.

Myoinositol

Myoinositol is a naturally occurring cyclitol, present in tissue cells of animal and plant with an insulin-like properties and having an altered metabolism in IR and diabetes.[52] The data regarding its effectiveness have shown no benefit on miscarriage rate, though low incidence of GDM in patients with a parent with type 2 diabetes mellitus was noted.[53] Its role is still unclear in pregnancies with PCOS.

Conclusion

In conclusion, pregnant women should be educated about the increased chances of adverse pregnancy outcomes associated with IR and hyperandrogenic state of PCOS. Optimization of prepregnancy health, need to closely monitor for maternal and fetal wellbeing during pregnancy, and timely provision of preventive and therapeutic interventions can assure favorable obstetric outcomes in women with PCOS.

References

1. Boomsma CM, Eijkemans MJ, Hughes EG, Visser GH, Fauser BC, Macklon NS. A meta-analysis of pregnancy outcomes in women with polycystic ovary syndrome. *Hum Reprod Update.* 2006;12:673-683.
2. March WA, Moore VM, Willson KJ, Phillips DI, Norman RJ, Davies MJ. The prevalence of polycystic ovary syndrome in a community sample assessed under contrasting diagnostic criteria. *Hum Reprod.* 2010;25:544-551.
3. Fauser BC, Tarlatzis BC, Rebar RW, et al. Consensus on women's health aspects of polycystic ovary syndrome (PCOS): the Amsterdam ESHRFJASRM-Sponsored 3rd PCOS Consensus Workshop Group. *Fertil Steril.* 2012;97:28-38.
4. Azziz R, Carmina E, Chen Z, et al. Polycystic ovary syndrome. *Nat Rev Dis Primers.* 2016;2:16057.
5. Homburg R. Polycystic ovary syndrome. *Best Pract Res Clin Obstet Gynaecol.* 2008;22(2):261-274.
6. Kamalanathan S, Sahoo JP, Sathyapalan T. Pregnancy in polycystic ovary syndrome. *Indian J Endocrinol Metab.* 2013;17(1):37-43.
7. Kjerulff LE, SanchezRamos L, Duffy D. Pregnancy outcomes in women with polycystic ovary syndrome: a meta analysis. *Am J Obstet Gynecol.* 2011;204:558.e16.
8. Al-Biate MA. Effect of metformin on early pregnancy loss in women with polycystic ovary syndrome. *Taiwan J Obstet Gynecol.* 2015;54:266-269.
9. Sir-Petermann T, Hitchsfeld C, Maliqueo M, et al. Birth weight in offspring of mothers with polycystic ovarian syndrome. *Hum Reprod.* 2005;20:2122-2126.
10. Mumm H, Jensen DM, Sorensen JA, et al. Hyperandrogenism and phenotypes of polycystic ovary syndrome are not associated with differences in obstetric outcomes. *Acta Obstet Gynecol Scand.* 2015;94:204-211.
11. Lovvik TS, Wikstrom AK, Neovius M, Stephansson O, Roos N, Vanky E. Pregnancy and perinatal outcomes in women with polycystic ovary syndrome and twin births: a population-based cohort study. *BJOG.* 2015;122:1295-1302.
12. Palomba S, Falbo A, Chiossi G, et al. Low-grade chronic inflammation in pregnant women with polycystic ovary syndrome: a prospective controlled clinical study. *J Clin Endocrinol Metab.* 2014;99:2942-2951.
13. Wolf M, Sandler L, Hsu K, Vossen-Smirnakis K, Ecker JL, Thadhani R. First-trimester C-reactive protein and subsequent gestational diabetes. *Diabetes Care.* 2003;26:819-824.
14. Kollmann M, Klaritsch P, Martins WP, et al. Maternal and neonatal outcomes in pregnant women with PCOS: comparison of different diagnostic definitions. *Hum Reprod.* 2015;30:2396-2403.
15. Teede H, Deeks A, Moran L. Polycystic ovary syndrome: a complex condition with psychological, reproductive and metabolic manifestations that impacts on health across the lifespan. *BMC Med.* 2010;8:41.
16. Bjercke S, Dale PO, Tanbo T, Storeng R, Ertzeid G, Abyholm T. Impact of insulin resistance on pregnancy complications and outcome in women with polycystic ovary syndrome. *Gynecol Obstet Invest.* 2002;54:94-98.
17. Nouh AA, Shalaby SM. The predictive value of uterine blood flow in detecting the risk of adverse pregnancy outcome in patients with polycystic ovary syndrome. *Middle East Fertil Soc J.* 2011;16:284-290.
18. Aktun HL, Yorgunlar B, Acet M, Aygun BK, Karaca N. The effects of polycystic ovary syndrome on gestational diabetes mellitus. *Gynecol Endocrinol.* 2016;32:139-142.
19. Zhou M-S, Schulman IH, Zeng Q. Link between the renin–angiotensin system and insulin resistance: implications for cardiovascular disease. *Vasc Med.* 2012;17:330-341.
20. Bennett SN, Tita A, Owen J, Biggio JR, Harper LM. Assessing White's classification of pregestational diabetes in a contemporary diabetic population. *Obstet Gynecol.* 2015;125:1217.
21. Lim SS, Davies MJ, Norman RJ, Moran LJ. Overweight, obesity and central obesity in women with polycystic ovary syndrome: a systematic review and meta-analysis. *Hum Reprod Update.* 2012;18:618-637.
22. Yu HF, Chen HS, Rao DP, Gong J. Association between polycystic ovary syndrome and the risk of pregnancy complications: a PRISMA-compliant systematic review and meta-analysis. *Medicine.* 2016;95:e4863.
23. Turhan NO, Seckin NC, Aybar F, Inegol I. Assessment of glucose tolerance and pregnancy outcome of polycystic ovary patients. *Int J Gynaecol Obstet.* 2003;81:163-168.
24. Diamanti-Kandarakis E, Paterakis T, Alexandraki K, et al. Indices of low-grade chronic inflammation in polycystic ovary syndrome and the beneficial effect of metformin. *Hum Reprod.* 2006;21:1426-1431.
25. Hudecova M, Holte J, Olovsson M, Sundström Poromaa I. Long-term follow-up of patients with polycystic ovary syndrome: reproductive outcome and ovarian reserve. *Hum Reprod.* 2009;24:1176-1183.
26. Joham AE, Teede HJ, Ranasinha S, Zoungas S, Boyle J. Prevalence of infertility and use of fertility treatment in women with polycystic ovary syndrome: data from a large community-based cohort study. *J Womens Health.* 2015;24:299-307.
27. Zhu JL, Obel C, Bech BH, Olsen J, Basso O. Infertility, infertility treatment and fetal growth restriction. *Obstet Gynecol.* 2007;110:1326.
28. Zhu JL, Basso O, Obel C, Bille C, Olsen J. Infertility, infertility treatment, and congenital malformations: Danish national birth cohort. *BMJ.* 2006;333:679.
29. Qin JB, Wang H, Sheng X, Xie Q, Gao S. Assisted reproductive technology and risk of adverse obstetric outcomes in dichorionic twin pregnancies: a systematic review and meta-analysis. *Fertil Steril.* 2016;105:1180-1192.
30. Homburg R. Pregnancy complications in PCOS. *Best Pract Res Clin Endocrinol Metab.* 2006;20:281-292.
31. Wang JX, Davies MJ, Norman RJ. Polycystic ovarian syndrome and the risk of spontaneous abortion following assisted reproductive technology treatment. *Hum Reprod.* 2001;16:2606-2609.
32. Elkholi DG, Nagy HM. The effects of adipocytokines on the endocrino-metabolic features and obstetric outcome in pregnant obese women with polycystic ovary syndrome. *Middle East Fertil Soc J.* 2014;19:293-302.
33. Li HW, Lee VC, Lau EY, Yeung WS, Ho PC, Ng EH. Cumulative live-birth rate in women with polycystic ovary syndrome or isolated polycystic ovaries undergoing in-vitro fertilisation treatment. *J Assist Reprod Genet.* 2014;31:205-211.

34. Qin JZ, Pang LH, Li MJ, Fan XJ, Huang RD, Chen HY. Obstetric complications in women with polycystic ovary syndrome: a systematic review and meta-analysis. *Reprod Biol Endocrinol.* 2013;11:56.

35. Veltman Verhulst SM, van Haeften TW, Eijkemans MJ, de Valk HW, Fauser BC, Goverde AJ. Sex hormonebinding globulin concentrations before conception as a predictor for gestational diabetes in women with polycystic ovary syndrome. *Hum Reprod.* 2010;25:31233128.

36. de Vries MJ, Dekker GA, Schoemaker J. Higher risk of preeclampsia in the polycystic ovary syndrome: a case control study. *Eur J Obstet Gynecol Reprod Biol.* 1998;91-95.

37. Naver KV, Grinsted J, Larsen SO, et al. Increased risk of preterm delivery and pre-eclampsia in women with polycystic ovary syndrome and hyperandrogenaemia. *BJOG.* 2014;121:575-581.

38. Roos N, Kieler H, Sahlin L, Ekman-Ordeberg G, Falconer H, Stephansson O. Risk of adverse pregnancy outcomes in women with polycystic ovary syndrome: population-based cohort study. *Br Med J.* 2011;343:d6309.

39. Mikola M, Hiilesmaa V, Halttunen M, Suhonen L, Tiitinen A. Obstetric outcome in women with polycystic ovarian syndrome. *Hum Reprod.* 2001;16:226-229.

40. Fridstrom M, Nisell H, Sjoblom P, Hillensjo T. Are women with polycystic ovary syndrome at an increased risk of pregnancyinduced hypertension and/or preeclampsia? *Hypertens Pregnancy.* 1999;18:73-80.

41. American Diabetes Association. Standards of medical care in diabetes—2011. *Diabetes Care.* 2011;34:S11-S61.

42. Moran LJ, Hutchison SK, Norman RJ, Teede HJ. Lifestyle changes in women with polycystic ovary syndrome. *Cochrane Database Syst Rev.* 2011;7:CD007506.

43. Legro RS, Dodson WC, Kunselman AR, et al. Benefit of delayed fertility therapy with preconception weight loss over immediate therapy in obese women with PCOS. *J Clin Endocrinol Metab.* 2016;101:2658-2666.

44. Agha M, Agha RA, Sandell J. Interventions to reduce and prevent obesity in pre-conceptual and pregnant women: a systematic review and meta-analysis. *PLoS One.* 2014;9:e95132.

45. NICE. *Weight Management Before, During and After Pregnancy (ed. N. I. o. C. Excellence).* London, UK: NICE; 2010.

46. Kominiarek Michelle A, Priya Rajan. Nutrition Recommendations in Pregnancy and lactation. The Medical Clinics of North America. 2016;100(6):1199–1215. doi:10.1016/j.mcna.2016.06.004. In this issue.

47. Vanky E, Zahlsen K, Spigset O, Carlsen SM. Placental passage of metformin in women with polycystic ovary syndrome. *Fertil Steril.* 2005;83:1575-1578.

48. Palomba S, Falbo A, Orio Jr F, Zullo F. Effect of preconceptional metformin on abortion risk in polycystic ovary syndrome: a systematic review and meta-analysis of randomized controlled trials. *Fertil Steril.* 2009;92:1646-1658.

49. Khattab S, Mohsen IA, Aboul Foutouh I, et al. Can metformin reduce the incidence of gestational diabetes mellitus in pregnant women with polycystic ovary syndrome? Prospective cohort study. *Gynecol Endocrinol.* 2011;27:789-793.

50. Vanky E, Stridsklev S, Heimstad R, et al. Metformin versus placebo from first trimester to delivery in polycystic ovary syndrome: a randomized, controlled multicenter study. *J Clin Endocrinol Metab.* 2010;95:E448-E455.

51. Croze ML, Soulage CO. Potential role and therapeutic interests of myo-inositol in metabolic diseases. *Biochimie.* 2013;95:1811-1827.

52. Pundir J, Psaroudakis D, Savnur P, et al. Inositol treatment of anovulation in women with polycystic ovary syndrome: a meta-analysis of randomised trials. *BJOG.* 2018;125:509-510.

53. D'Anna R, Scilipoti A, Giordano D, et al. myo-Inositol supplementation and onset of gestational diabetes mellitus in pregnant women with a family history of type 2 diabetes: a prospective, randomized, placebo-controlled study. *Diabetes Care.* 2013;36:854-857.

21
Importance of Lifestyle Modifications

BHAGWAN DAS AND TEHSEEN FATIMA

Introduction

The importance of lifestyle modification in the management of polycystic ovary syndrome (PCOS) cannot be overemphasized because it has been recommended as the first step in the management of PCOS.[1-6] Robust evidence exists regarding the effectiveness of lifestyle interventions such as modifications in diet, caloric restriction, exercise training regimens, and behavioral changes, both in isolation and in combination, in improving the PCOS disease spectrum. Nevertheless, a uniform guideline regarding optimal dietary and exercise strategies and clear-cut targets and endpoints are still lacking. This often reflects as a void in patients' and healthcare providers' knowledge regarding the optimal management of their condition through lifestyle interventions,[7,8] which may hinder desirable treatment outcomes.

We aimed in this chapter to review the existing evidence regarding the impact of lifestyle modification on the biochemical, metabolic, cardiovascular, and reproductive health of patients with PCOS.

How Lifestyle Interventions Work

Pathophysiology/Mechanism

Insulin resistance (IR) and hyperandrogenism (HA) are the hallmarks of PCOS.[5] Intrinsic IR has been found to be a contributor to multiple manifestations of the PCOS spectrum in both overweight/obese and lean patients with PCOS.[2,9] Hyperinsulinemia causes increased production of androgens in more than one way. Increased insulin levels decrease the hepatic production of sex hormone–binding globulins (SHBG), leading to higher circulating levels of free androgen. This is further exacerbated by obesity, especially abdominal adiposity, which leads to a vicious/self-perpetuating cycle of increased androgen production leading to increased abdominal adipose tissue and vice versa.[10] This HA manifests as menstrual irregularities, anovulation, acne, and hirsutism in patients with PCOS. IR, hyperinsulinemia, and overweight/obesity also increase the risk for metabolic syndrome (MetS), impaired glucose metabolism, and dyslipidemia, which are all risk factors for cardiovascular disease (CVD).

Lifestyle interventions, such as dietary modification, exercise, and behavioral therapy, benefit the PCOS spectrum mainly through weight loss. Significant clinical improvement is seen with around 5% to 10% weight loss.[11] Weight loss causes improved insulin sensitivity and reduces the metabolic risks associated with PCOS, such as MetS, dyslipidemia, impaired glucose metabolism, and risk of CVD. In addition to having a notable impact on the quality of life and psychosocial wellbeing of patients with PCOS, lifestyle interventions increase the chances of being able to have a natural birth as well,[11,12] as shown in Fig. 21.1.

Diet Modification

Diet modification remains the major method for weight loss in PCOS, as it is in the general population. Currently, there is no uniform guideline regarding the specific configuration of an ideal diet for patients with PCOS. Multiple randomized controlled trials (RCTs) comparing different diet plans, such as a diet rich in protein versus a high carbohydrate diet and high protein with a normal protein diet, did not show any superiority of one type of diet over the other.[1] Overall, evidence favors diets leading to weight loss by caloric restriction. Obese or overweight females are advised to aim for a reduction of approximately 30% or 500 to 750 kcal/day in total caloric intake to achieve adequate weight loss.[11] Emphasis should be on making healthy eating habits a lifestyle rather than a short-term notion. The diet plan should be individualized and tailored according to the patients' nutritional requirements, baseline body weight, and energy expenditure level. Patient preferences and choices, cultural diversity, and adaptability to patients' resources should be considered when laying out individual nutrition plans. Avoidance of unnecessary nutrient deprivation when developing a nutrition plan is crucial.[11]

Diets with a low glycemic index specifically have a positive impact on PCOS features, although the data are limited.[13,14] This effect is likely mediated through slower absorption of glucose, consequently reducing insulin levels. A diet rich in fibers also has a positive effect on PCOS, likely through weight loss, because of early satiety and thus decreased food intake.[13,14] An interesting finding has been an inverse relationship of dietary fiber intake with PCOS features such as

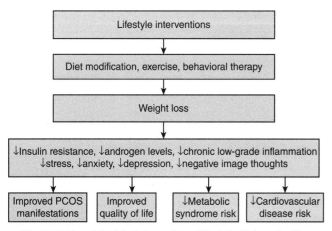

• **Fig. 21.1** How Lifestyle Interventions Work in Polycystic Ovary Syndrome *(PCOS)*.

IR, fasting insulin levels, postprandial glucose levels, triglyceride, and testosterone levels. High-density lipoprotein (HDL) levels were positively correlated with dietary fiber.[13-15] As this finding comes from small data sets, further research is needed to infer a definite recommendation.

A low carbohydrate diet, a diet in which less than 45% of the calorie content is derived from carbohydrates, has shown significant improvement in body mass index (BMI), IR, and circulating insulin levels, total cholesterol, and low-density lipoprotein (LDL) cholesterol.[16,17] Additionally, a low carbohydrate/low-fat diet, which is defined as one containing less than 45% carbohydrates and less than 35% of fat, has specifically shown a significant increase in follicle-stimulating hormone (FSH) and SHBG levels and decreased levels of serum testosterone in patients with PCOS.[16] The effects of low carbohydrates were further enhanced when practiced for longer than 4 weeks. The beneficial effects of these diets are brought about by decreased insulin levels and improved sensitivity, which then decreases androgen levels through effects on ovaries and adrenals. Hyperinsulinemia is the key factor in inhibiting follicular development and ovulation, through a direct effect on ovaries and an increased ratio of luteinizing hormone (LH) to FSH.[18] Decreased insulin levels and increased FSH levels improve menstrual cyclicity and ovulation rates, fertility, and hirsutism.[19-21]

Exercise

There are extensive and consistent data about the beneficial effects of exercise on metabolic, hormonal, and psychosocial features of PCOS. The recommendations made in clinical practice are largely derived by evidence from systematic reviews and meta-analyses; however, no unified guidelines regarding the optimal type, duration, and intensity of exercise intervention exist.

Numerous diverse exercise models have been studied and reported in the literature to have benefitted patients with PCOS. A recent meta-analysis examined studies regarding various aerobic exercise programs ranging from 12 weeks' to 6 months' duration, at least 3 days a week, with each session lasting for 30 to 60 minutes of moderate to vigorous intensity exercise. The results for all programs consistently showed improved fasting insulin levels and insulin sensitivity.[22]

Another meta-analysis, which separated studies of exercise along with diet from exercise alone, concluded that exercise along with diet, as well as exercise alone, improves the plasma levels of SHBG, FSH, androstenedione, testosterone, and the Ferriman-Gallwey score for hirsutism in females with PCOS.[23] Lower insulin and androgen levels and resumption of ovulation in obese or overweight females with PCOS in response to regular exercise with or without diet were also reported by Hakimi.[24] In all studies examined in this meta-analysis, the exercise intervention was unique. Exercise has also been shown as an independent factor to improve IR and ovulation.[25] Aerobic exercise directly improves insulin sensitivity by ameliorating different pathophysiologic pathways associated with IR, such as reduction of adipokines, oxidative stress, and inflammatory responses, and improvement in the signal transduction of insulin via different cellular and molecular pathways.[26] Improvement in serum triglycerides, total cholesterol, HDL, LDL, and lipoprotein profile as an independent effect of exercise has also been suggested in the literature, although the data are limited and should be cautiously interpreted.[27,28]

Recently, some age-specific exercise recommendations have been proposed by the international evidence-based guidelines to prevent weight gain in patients with PCOS.[11] According to these guidelines, for a female between 18 and 64 years of age, a minimum of 75 minutes per week of vigorous intensities or 150 minutes per week of moderately intense physical activity or an identical combination of both, including muscle-strengthening activities on two nonconsecutive days per week, is recommended. In adolescents, a minimum of 60 minutes of moderately to vigorously intense physical activity per day, including muscle and bone-strengthening activities, is recommended at least three times per week. The guidelines recommend that physical activity should be done in bouts of at least 10 minutes or around 1000 steps, with an aim of spending at least 30 minutes daily on most days. For weight loss, they recommend a minimum of 150 minutes per week of vigorously intense or 250 minutes per week of moderately intense activities or an identical combination of these two along with muscle-strengthening activities involving major muscle groups on two nonconsecutive days per week.[11]

Cultural, personal, and family preferences should be considered when devising structured exercise plans. It is important to address the psychosocial aspect of the PCOS spectrum. Compared with controls, patients with PCOS are more likely to have reduced self-esteem, anxiety, and depression.[29] Physical activity has been shown to improve emotional wellbeing, decrease anxiety and depression, and improve mood in the general population.[30] Lifestyle modification, including diet and exercise, has also shown improvement in depression and self-esteem in patients with PCOS.[31] Further research is needed to elucidate the independent effect of exercise on psychosocial health and quality of life in patients with PCOS.

Behavioral Strategies

Patients with PCOS often struggle with psychosocial issues, such as anxiety, depression, disordered eating, and negative body image.[32,33] These may often present as a barrier to the effective management of PCOS. Motivational and emotional barriers, such as lack of an immediate reward and depression, decrease patient compliance to lifestyle intervention.[34]

In addition, these psychological issues have also been reported to have some link with dysregulation of the hypothalamic-pituitary-adrenal axis, leading to chronic low-grade inflammation, a mild increase in cortisol, IR, HA, and overall worsening of PCOS manifestations,[35,36] as shown in Fig. 21.2.

Because of this huge effect on the overall disease spectrum, it is very important for healthcare providers to identify and address such factors.

Strategies such as increased contact frequency with care providers, social support, improved motivation, realistic goal setting, and periodic self-monitoring have all shown to be effective at increasing adherence to lifestyle interventions.[37,38] Cognitive-behavioral interventions should be considered to increase patient support, engagement, adherence, retention, and maintenance of a long-term healthy lifestyle.[11]

Vitamin D

Vitamin D deficiency is a common entity among patients with PCOS.[39] Several studies have demonstrated that low levels of vitamin D are associated with increased IR, hirsutism, HA, irregularities in ovulation and menstrual cycles, lower pregnancy success, overweight/obesity, and elevated future risk for CVD.[39,40] There is some evidence that vitamin D supplementation can improve menstrual dysfunction and IR in patients with PCOS.[40,41] Improvement in fasting insulin, serum triglycerides, SHBG, total testosterone, and free androgen index (FAI) has been demonstrated as a result of vitamin D supplementation, although the data are limited.[42,43] Further research is needed in this area before specific recommendations can be made regarding the routine use of vitamin D in the treatment of PCOS.

Environmental Endocrine Disruptors

Exposure to environmental endocrine disruptors (EEDs) has also been documented to have a significant impact on the overall disease spectrum of PCOS.[44] EEDs have been reported to cause a disturbance in hormonal regulation at multiple levels, such as increase in estrogen, HA, weight gain, hyperinsulinemia, and impaired glucose metabolism.[44-46] EEDs, like smoking, snoring, usage of indoor decoration, and plastic tableware have an association with menstrual irregularities.[47]

In addition to the aforementioned associations, exposure to bisphenol A has also been known to affect fertility.[48]

Nevertheless, the exact effects of these EEDs remain to be studied, but based on the available literature, it can be concluded that in addition to lifestyle modifications, patients with PCOS should also be advised to have reduced exposure to EEDs.

Summary

Lifestyle interventions remain the first-line treatment for PCOS. Beneficial effects of dietary modifications, exercise, and weight loss on IR, menstrual irregularities, ovulation, and HA and improvement in cardiovascular risk factors have been consistently demonstrated in the literature. Further

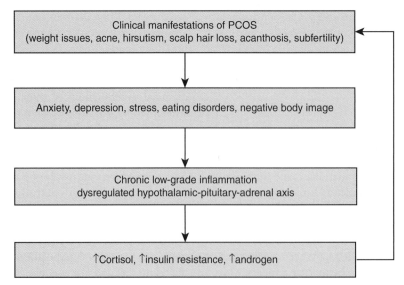

• **Fig. 21.2** The Vicious Cycle Between Polycystic Ovary Syndrome *(PCOS)* Manifestations and Psychological Issues.

research is needed to develop explicit recommendations, and standardized, structured lifestyle intervention models, which are both realistic and sustainable, to improve the quality of care in patients with PCOS.

References

1. Moran LJ, Tassone EC, Boyle J, et al. Evidence summaries and recommendations from the international evidence-based guideline for the assessment and management of polycystic ovary syndrome: lifestyle management. *Obes Rev.* 2020;21(10):e13046. doi:10.1111/obr.13046.

2. Goodman NF, Cobin RH, Futterweit W, Glueck JS, Legro RS, Carmina E. American Association of Clinical Endocrinologists, American College of Endocrinology, and Androgen Excess and PCOS Society Disease State Clinical Review: guide to the best practices in the evaluation and treatment of polycystic ovary syndrome – part 2. *Endocr Pract.* 2015;21(12):1415-1426. doi:10.4158/Ep15748.Dscpt2.

3. Legro RS, Arslanian SA, Ehrmann DA, et al. Diagnosis and treatment of polycystic ovary syndrome: an Endocrine Society clinical practice guideline. *J Clin Endocrinol Metab.* 2013;98(12):4565-4592. doi:10.1210/jc.2013-2350.

4. Hoeger KM, Dokras A, Piltonen T. Update on PCOS: consequences, challenges, and guiding treatment. *J Clin Endocrinol Metab.* 2021;106(3):e1071-e1083. doi:10.1210/clinem/dgaa839.

5. Ibáñez L, Oberfield SE, Witchel S, et al. An international consortium update: pathophysiology, diagnosis, and treatment of polycystic ovarian syndrome in adolescence. *Horm Res Paediatr.* 2017;88(6):371-395. doi:10.1159/000479371.

6. Teede H, Misso M, Costello M, et al. *On behalf of the International PCOS Network. International Evidence Based Guideline for the Assessment and Management of Polycystic Ovary Syndrome.* Melbourne, Australia: Monash University; 2018.

7. Gibson-Helm M, Tassone EC, Teede HJ, Dokras A, Garad R. The needs of women and healthcare providers regarding polycystic ovary syndrome information, resources, and education: a systematic search and narrative review. *Semin Reprod Med.* 2018;36(1):35-41. doi:10.1055/s-0038-1668086.

8. Gibson-Helm M, Teede H, Dunaif A, Dokras A. Delayed diagnosis and a lack of information associated with dissatisfaction in women with polycystic ovary syndrome. *J Clin Endocrinol Metab.* 2017;102(2):604-612. doi:10.1210/jc.2016-2963.

9. Stepto NK, Cassar S, Joham AE, et al. Women with polycystic ovary syndrome have intrinsic insulin resistance on euglycaemic-hyperinsulaemic clamp. *Hum Reprod.* 2013;28(3):777-784. doi:10.1093/humrep/des463.

10. Alzanati N. *Polycystic Ovarian Syndrome and Adipose Tissue: Contribution of Peripheral Androgen Synthesis to Hyperandrogenism in Polycystic Ovarian Syndrome.* University of Nottingham; 2017. https://eprints.nottingham.ac.uk/39390/.

11. Teede HJ, Misso ML, Costello MF, et al. Recommendations from the international evidence-based guideline for the assessment and management of polycystic ovary syndrome. *Hum Reprod.* 2018;33(9):1602-1618. doi:10.1093/humrep/dey256.

12. Costello MF, Misso ML, Balen A, et al. Evidence summaries and recommendations from the international evidence-based guideline for the assessment and management of polycystic ovary syndrome: assessment and treatment of infertility. *Hum Reprod Open.* 2019;2019(1):hoy021. doi:10.1093/hropen/hoy021.

13. Eslamian G, Baghestani AR, Eghtesad S, Hekmatdoost A. Dietary carbohydrate composition is associated with polycystic ovary syndrome: a case-control study. *J Hum Nutr Diet.* 2017;30(1):90-97. doi:10.1111/jhn.12388.

14. Cutler D. *The Impact of Lifestyle on the Reproductive, Metabolic, and Psychological Well-Being of Women with Polycystic Ovary Syndrome (PCOS).* University of British Columbia; 2019. https://dx.doi.org/10.14288/1.0378929.

15. Aly JM, Decherney AH. Lifestyle modifications in PCOS. *Clin Obstet Gynecol.* 2021;64(1):83-89. doi:10.1097/grf.0000000000000594.

16. Zhang X, Zheng Y, Guo Y, Lai Z. The effect of low carbohydrate diet on polycystic ovary syndrome: a meta-analysis of randomized controlled trials. *Int J Endocrinol.* 2019;2019:4386401. doi:10.1155/2019/4386401.

17. de Luis DA, Izaola O, Aller R, de la Fuente B, Bachiller R, Romero E. Effects of a high-protein/low carbohydrate versus a standard hypocaloric diet on adipocytokine levels and insulin resistance in obese patients along 9 months. *J Diabetes Complications.* 2015;29(7):950-954. doi:10.1016/j.jdiacomp.2015.06.002.

18. Jonard S, Dewailly D. The follicular excess in polycystic ovaries, due to intra-ovarian hyperandrogenism, may be the main culprit for the follicular arrest. *Hum Reprod Update.* 2004;10(2):107-117. doi:10.1093/humupd/dmh010.

19. Crosignani PG, Colombo M, Vegetti W, Somigliana E, Gessati A, Ragni G. Overweight and obese anovulatory patients with polycystic ovaries: parallel improvements in anthropometric indices, ovarian physiology and fertility rate induced by diet. *Hum Reprod.* 2003;18(9):1928-1932. doi:10.1093/humrep/deg367.

20. Thomson RL, Buckley JD, Brinkworth GD. Exercise for the treatment and management of overweight women with polycystic ovary syndrome: a review of the literature. *Obes Rev.* 2011;12(5):e202-e210. doi:10.1111/j.1467-789X.2010.00758.x.

21. Marzouk TM, Sayed Ahmed WA. Effect of dietary weight loss on menstrual regularity in obese young adult women with polycystic ovary syndrome. *J Pediatr Adolesc Gynecol.* 2015;28(6):457-461. doi:10.1016/j.jpag.2015.01.002.

22. Shele G, Genkil J, Speelman D. A systematic review of the effects of exercise on hormones in women with polycystic ovary syndrome. *J Funct Morphol Kinesiol.* 2020;5(2):35. doi:10.3390/jfmk5020035.

23. Haqq L, McFarlane J, Dieberg G, Smart N. Effect of lifestyle intervention on the reproductive endocrine profile in women with polycystic ovarian syndrome: a systematic review and meta-analysis. *Endocr Connect.* 2014;3(1):36-46. doi:10.1530/ec-14-0010.

24. Hakimi O, Cameron LC. Effect of exercise on ovulation: a systematic review. *Sports Med.* 2017;47(8):1555-1567. doi:10.1007/s40279-016-0669-8.

25. Harrison CL, Lombard CB, Moran LJ, Teede HJ. Exercise therapy in polycystic ovary syndrome: a systematic review. *Hum Reprod Update.* 2011;17(2):171-183. doi:10.1093/humupd/dmq045.

26. Yaribeygi H, Atkin SL, Simental-Mendía LE, Sahebkar A. Molecular mechanisms by which aerobic exercise induces insulin sensitivity. *J Cell Physiol.* 2019;234(8):12385-12392. doi:10.1002/jcp.28066.

27. Kite C, Lahart IM, Afzal I, et al. Exercise, or exercise and diet for the management of polycystic ovary syndrome: a systematic review and meta-analysis. *Syst Rev.* 2019;8(1):1-28.

28. Brown AJ, Setji TL, Sanders LL, et al. Effects of exercise on lipoprotein particles in women with polycystic ovary syndrome. *Med Sci Sports Exerc.* 2009;41(3):497-504. doi:10.1249/MSS.0b013e31818c6c0c.

29. Sayyah-Melli M, Alizadeh M, Pourafkary N, et al. Psychosocial factors associated with polycystic ovary syndrome: a case control study. *J Caring Sci*. 2015;4(3):225-231. doi:10.15171/jcs.2015.023.

30. Guszkowska M. [Effects of exercise on anxiety, depression and mood]. *Psychiatr Pol*. 2004;38(4):611-620.

31. Jiskoot G, Dietz de Loos A, Beerthuizen A, Timman R, Busschbach J, Laven J. Long-term effects of a three-component lifestyle intervention on emotional well-being in women with polycystic ovary syndrome (PCOS): a secondary analysis of a randomized controlled trial. *PLoS One*. 2020;15(6):e0233876. doi:10.1371/journal.pone.0233876.

32. Alur-Gupta S, Chemerinski A, Liu C, et al. Body-image distress is increased in women with polycystic ovary syndrome and mediates depression and anxiety. *Fertil Steril*. 2019;112(5):930-938.e1. doi:10.1016/j.fertnstert.2019.06.018.

33. Cooney LG, Lee I, Sammel MD, Dokras A. High prevalence of moderate and severe depressive and anxiety symptoms in polycystic ovary syndrome: a systematic review and meta-analysis. *Hum Reprod*. 2017;32(5):1075-1091. doi:10.1093/humrep/dex044.

34. Lim S, Smith CA, Costello MF, MacMillan F, Moran L, Ee C. Barriers and facilitators to weight management in overweight and obese women living in Australia with PCOS: a qualitative study. *BMC Endocr Disord*. 2019;19(1):106. doi:10.1186/s12902-019-0434-8.

35. Rudnicka E, Suchta K, Grymowicz M, et al. Chronic low grade inflammation in pathogenesis of PCOS. *Int J Mol Sci*. 2021;22(7):3789. doi:10.3390/ijms22073789.

36. Wang F, Zhang ZH, Xiao KZ, Wang ZC. Roles of hypothalamic-pituitary-adrenal axis and hypothalamus-pituitary-ovary axis in the abnormal endocrine functions in patients with polycystic ovary syndrome. *Zhongguo Yi Xue Ke Xue Yuan Xue Bao*. 2017;39(5):699-704. doi:10.3881/j.issn.1000-503X.2017.05.017.

37. Greaves CJ, Sheppard KE, Abraham C, et al. Systematic review of reviews of intervention components associated with increased effectiveness in dietary and physical activity interventions. *BMC Public Health*. 2011;11:119. doi:10.1186/1471-2458-11-119.

38. Brennan L, Teede H, Skouteris H, Linardon J, Hill B, Moran L. Lifestyle and behavioral management of polycystic ovary syndrome. *J Womens Health (Larchmt)*. 2017;26(8):836-848. doi:10.1089/jwh.2016.5792.

39. He C, Lin Z, Robb SW, Ezeamama AE. Serum vitamin D levels and polycystic ovary syndrome: a systematic review and meta-analysis. *Nutrients*. 2015;7(6):4555-4577. doi:10.3390/nu7064555.

40. Thomson RL, Spedding S, Buckley JD. Vitamin D in the aetiology and management of polycystic ovary syndrome. *Clin Endocrinol (Oxf)*. 2012;77(3):343-350. doi:10.1111/j.1365-2265.2012.04434.x.

41. Miao CY, Fang XJ, Chen Y, Zhang Q. Effect of vitamin D supplementation on polycystic ovary syndrome: a meta-analysis. *Exp Ther Med*. 2020;19(4):2641-2649. doi:10.3892/etm.2020.8525.

42. Menichini D, Facchinetti F. Effects of vitamin D supplementation in women with polycystic ovary syndrome: a review. *Gynecol Endocrinol*. 2020;36(1):1-5. doi:10.1080/09513590.2019.1625881.

43. Zhao JF, Li BX, Zhang Q. Vitamin D improves levels of hormonal, oxidative stress and inflammatory parameters in polycystic ovary syndrome: a meta-analysis study. *Ann Palliat Med*. 2021;10(1):169-183. doi:10.21037/apm-20-2201.

44. Gore AC, Chappell VA, Fenton SE, et al. EDC-2: The endocrine society's second scientific statement on endocrine-disrupting chemicals. *Endocr Rev*. 2015;36(6):E1-E150. doi:10.1210/er.2015-1010.

45. Wang Y, Zhu Q, Dang X, He Y, Li X, Sun Y. Local effect of bisphenol A on the estradiol synthesis of ovarian granulosa cells from PCOS. *Gynecol Endocrinol*. 2017;33(1):21-25. doi:10.1080/09513590.2016.1184641.

46. Kandaraki E, Chatzigeorgiou A, Livadas S, et al. Endocrine disruptors and polycystic ovary syndrome (PCOS): elevated serum levels of bisphenol A in women with PCOS. *J Clin Endocrinol Metab*. 2011;96(3):E480-E484. doi:10.1210/jc.2010-1658.

47. Zhang B, Zhou W, Shi Y, Zhang J, Cui L, Chen ZJ. Lifestyle and environmental contributions to ovulatory dysfunction in women of polycystic ovary syndrome. *BMC Endocr Disord*. 2020;20(1):19.

48. Pivonello C, Muscogiuri G, Nardone A, et al. Bisphenol A: an emerging threat to female fertility. *Reprod Biol Endocrinol*. 2020;18(1):22. doi:10.1186/s12958-019-0558-8.

22

Role of Complementary and Alternative Medicine in Polycystic Ovary Syndrome

RIDA SIDDIQUE AND MALIK HASSAN MEHMOOD

Introduction

Polycystic ovary syndrome (PCOS) is an endocrine disorder resulting in abnormal menstruation, weight gain, hirsutism, and obesity, usually accompanied by insulin resistance (IR) and metabolic disorders.[1] The development of PCOS and its complications are because of the mutual interplay of endocrine, genetic, and environmental factors.[2] In the current era, because of unhealthier lifestyles, unbalanced eating habits, and abrupt psychological and socioeconomic pressures, a rise of 5% to 10% in the incidence of PCOS has been reported worldwide.[1,2] In Pakistan, recorded prevalence is 15.7% to 37%, affecting around 10% of reproductive-aged females, because of urbanization.[3] The majority of the patients are not well educated and are ignorant about the expression of clinical symptoms of PCOS; thus it remains difficult to track the disease in a timely fashion. This leads to the establishment of complications.[4]

Etiology

The etiology of PCOS is still unclear but is linked with hirsutism and menstrual dysfunction.[5] Clinical manifestations of PCOS include hirsutism, irregular menstrual cycles, obesity, acne, and alteration of sympathetic nerve activity.[6] Its diagnosis can be confirmed using the Rotterdam diagnostic criteria. Criteria for diagnosis of PCOS include ovulatory dysfunction and hyperandrogenism (HA) with specific disorders such as androgen-secreting neoplasms, adrenal hydroxylase deficiency, and hyperprolactinemia. PCOS is diagnosed by physical examination, blood tests, and ultrasound.[7]

The prime dysfunction involved in PCOS is of varied origin.[8,9] It also includes extraovarian factors involving modified ovarian behavior. The most prominent clinical feature defining PCOS is menstrual cycle disturbance because of oligo/anovulation.[10] HA and morphologic distribution of the ovaries can lead to the development of polycystic ovaries.[11] Polycystic ovaries can exist in patients without prior signs and symptoms. Nevertheless, the tendency of weight gain in females with polycystic ovaries may lead to expression of the onset of this disease. Being a multifactorial disease, different components of PCOS symptoms are associated with different genetic variants.[12] Serum concentrations of luteinizing hormone (LH) are found 95% elevated in patients with PCOS. Elevated LH results in a reduced chance of conception and an increased chance of miscarriage. High levels of LH secretions in such females contribute to increased levels of androgen (male hormones, such as testosterone), which, along with low levels of follicle-stimulating hormone (FSH), can cause poor egg development leading to infertility (because of the inability to ovulate).[13] Hirsutism and acne are expressed clinically because of HA in PCOS,[14] but the exact presence and prevalence of these symptoms is still up for debate. Although some studies show conflict with the necessary evidence, biochemical HA has a more accurate contribution in relation to PCOS.[15,16] Serum testosterone concentration, if greater than 4.8 nmol/L, becomes evidence of the expression of PCOS, provided that Cushing syndrome, congenital adrenal hyperplasia, and androgen-secreting tumors of the ovary and adrenals have been excluded.[17] Therefore free androgen index (FAI) measured by equilibrium dialysis, ammonium sulfate precipitation, and sex hormone–binding globulin (SHBG) methods is used to assess HA.[18]

Hyperandrogenism

HA in patients suffering from PCOS results in deregulation of steroidogenesis. The initial step involves the conversion of cholesterol to pregnenolone, which undergoes

171

17 alpha hydroxylation followed by conversion to dehydroepiandrosterone (DHEA), resulting in the formation of testosterone.[19] Theca interna of the ovarian follicle and zona fasciculate of the adrenal cortex are responsible for 50% of the production of testosterone by biochemical metabolism using enzymes under the control of LH in ovaries and adrenocorticotropic hormone (ACTH) in the adrenal cortex.[20] Intraovarian androgen contributes to normal follicular growth and to the production of estradiol. LH acts on theca interna cells of the ovary to secrete androgen, which, in turn, gets converted to estrogens by aromatase when FSH acts on the granulosa cells. Abnormal regulation in PCOS results in follicular atresia because of poor maturation of follicles and abnormal estrogen formation, thus affecting reproduction.[21] Another study further confirmed the relative production of androstenedione, testosterone, and estradiol when exogenous gonadotropin-releasing hormone (GnRH) was given to patients with PCOS. Thus as a result of dysregulation of androgen synthesis within the ovary, the ovary becomes hyperresponsive to gonadotrophins, leading to increased estrogen concentration.[22]

Hyperinsulinemia

Hyperinsulinemia is another characteristic feature of PCOS resulting from the higher degree of IR that has been reported in almost all PCOS patients; in particular, IR was more profound in the South Asian population.[23] Hyperinsulinemia because of IR is irrespective of body mass index (BMI) and obesity and results in worsening of anovulation and HA because of the inhibition of insulin-like growth factor 1 (IGF-1) and insulin-like growth factor 1 binding protein (IGFB1) by the liver resulting in increased bioavailability of IGF1 and IGF2, thus impairing follicular maturation and increased steroidogenesis by increasing the action of LH on theca interna cells.[24-25]

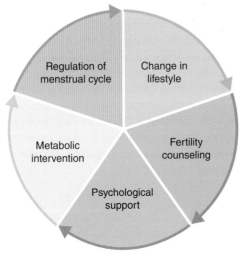

• **Fig. 22.1** Steps of Polycystic Ovary Syndrome Management.

Treatment Modalities

As per the disease basis and its clinical features, different treatment modalities are exercised for PCOS, including weight management, regular exercise, improvement in IR, attenuation of androgen levels, regulation of menstrual cycle, and induction of ovulation, as shown in Fig. 22.1.

Conventional Treatment Approaches

Metformin, specialized proresolving mediators, human bone marrow mesenchymal stem cells, and angiotensin-converting enzyme inhibitors are involved in the treatment of PCOS.[26-29] PCOS involves a continuous level of inflammatory markers (i.e., C-reactive protein [CRP], interleukin-1 [IL-1], and IL-6) that represent chronic inflammation. Selective progesterone receptor modulators are found to have a beneficial role in chronic inflammatory disease while clinical trials are still continued.[27] Lisinopril has been experimented with in letrozole-induced rodent PCOS and has been found to inhibit plasminogen activator inhibitor-1, thus modifying the letrozole behavior. Nevertheless, its use has been under further investigation.[29] The adverse effects of metformin include asthenia, diarrhea, flatulence, weakness, and myalgia. It also causes gastrointestinal complaints and hypoglycemia and, rarely, lactic acidosis. Lisinopril causes heart failure, hypotension, and cough. Prolonged use also causes an increase in creatinine level and hyperkalemia. The side effects of these drugs limit their role in long-term treatments. Complementary and alternative medicines (CAMs) with fewer side effects can play a beneficial role in the treatment of PCOS.

Complementary Approaches

Despite such conventional treatment approaches, associated challenges include poor patient compliance, adverse drug reactions, and limited success.[30] Therefore there is a dire need to find effective and patient-compliant alternative treatment modalities for PCOS. CAM, an alternative treatment approach, is independent of Western medicine but has widespread use in healthcare systems globally. Extensive literature has highlighted the efficacy and acceptance of CAM to counter PCOS.[31] CAM therapy differs in different parts of the world as per their indigenous practices and resources; for example, in China, Chinese herbal medicine, acupuncture, and Qigong have been used to address PCOS effectively.[32] In Pakistan, medicinal herbs of the northern areas, nuts, and indigenous functional food and meditation therapies are popular ways to treat various chronic disorders, including PCOS, as shown in Fig. 22.2.

Complementary and Alternative Medicine

CAM, an alternative therapy independent of Western medicine, has been used extensively in healthcare systems

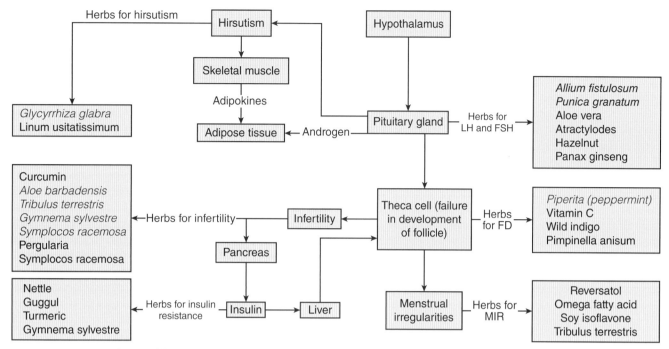

• **Fig. 22.2** Mechanism of Action of Different Remedies on Polycystic Ovary Syndrome. *FD*, Follicle development; *FSH*, follicle-stimulating hormone; *LH*, luteinizing hormone; *MIR*, Menstrual irregularities.

worldwide.[33-35,36] Numerous studies suggest that the use of CAM, including acupuncture, Chinese herbal medicine, Tai Chi, yoga, and Qigong, can also effectively treat PCOS with fewer adverse reactions.[36] Based on this, the purpose of this review is to provide more accurate evidence for the treatment of PCOS by CAM and to analyze its underlying mechanisms.[37]

Conventional therapy is effective in the treatment of PCOS, but prolonged usage can cause side effects. Patients with PCOS can use an alternative therapy to manage their infertility problems. Hence the current scientific research focuses on evidence-based results of preclinical evaluation to summarize the importance of herbal medicines in PCOS.[38]

Role of Phytoconstituents and Vitamins in the Management of PCOS

Resveratrol

Resveratrol is a natural polyphenol (phytoconstituent) found in nuts, berries, and grapes that has antioxidant, cardioprotective, and anti-inflammatory properties.[39] It can also be used as a therapeutic agent to treat PCOS-related infertility, decreased ovarian reserve, and obesity.[40,41] Because of its antideciduogenic properties, its administration should be avoided in pregnancy and in the luteal phase.[42] It also inhibits cellular retinoic acid-binding protein 2 (CRABP2-RAR) expressions to combat the process of decidual genes that encode IGF-1 and prolactin.[43] Clinical studies have shown that by using resveratrol, the abortion rate is increased and the rate of pregnancy is reduced. It has

also been documented that supplementation of resveratrol failed to increase insulin sensitivity.[44]

Flavones and Flavonoids

Naringenin is a popular flavanone derived from different plant species and grapefruit.[45] Literature demonstrates its protective role in PCOS with anti-inflammatory and cytoprotective effects.[46] Its administration decreases estradiol and testosterone levels in patients, increases the enzyme concentration in reactive oxygen species scavenging, and has a beneficial effect on weight gain in females with PCOS.[47,48] Rutin, another flavonoid, has also been used to treat PCOS.[49]

Vitamin C

Vitamin C, known as ascorbic acid, plays an effective role in the growth of cells in the body and has an important impact because of its antioxidant properties as well.[50] Vitamin C requires constant dietary intake because it is water soluble and thus excreted in urine. Olaniyan et al. investigated vitamin C–associated metabolic changes in Wister rats having polycystic ovaries and found that the levels fluctuate with the events of the menstrual cycle. The levels decrease just before ovulation and increase with the postovulatory rise in temperature. The role of ascorbic acid in the menstrual cycle includes facilitation of ovulation, depicted by its uptake in the preovulatory phase, and stimulation of progesterone and oxytocin production associated with its high concentration in the growth of follicles and corpus luteum.[51] The property of collagen synthesis facilitates the repair of ovarian tissue in the postovulatory phase. Deficiency of vitamin C impairs the aforementioned functions and leads to the development of PCOS.[52]

Vitamin E

Physiologic levels can be maintained through vitamin E because it is fat soluble, released in minute quantities, and stored in the liver.[53] It is an antioxidant, so it neutralizes free radicals and enhances the renewal of cells.[54] Because of its antioxidant and anticoagulant properties, it can improve the thickness of the endometrium in patients with idiopathic infertility.[55] Although treatment with coenzyme Q10 and vitamin E reduced SHBG levels in patients with PCOS and reduced plasma testosterone levels, it has also been demonstrated that short-term vitamin E supplementation can be given to induce ovulation in patients with PCOS. Use of vitamin E will also help reduce oxidative stress and the dosage of human menopausal gonadotropin (HMG) hormone.[56]

Vitamin D

Vitamin D is a secosteroid with progesterone-like action.[57] It is used to promote the mineralization of bone and maintain calcium homeostasis.[58] Two hydroxylation steps are required for vitamin D to become active; it first yields calcidiol {25-hydroxycholecalciferol or 25(OH)D}, which is a prehormone, followed by the hormone calcitriol 1,25-dihydroxycholecalciferol {1,25(OH)2D}.[59] Vitamin D deficiency is observed in inflammation, PCOS, decreased fertility, IR, and dyslipidemia.[60] The combined effect of calcium and vitamin D with metformin was studied on gonadotropins, in patients with PCOS and those having menstrual abnormalities, where vitamin D and calcium supplements support the metformin effect in patients with PCOS and vitamin D deficiency without having a significant impact on the IGF1 system and gonadotropins.[61] It has also been noted that vitamin D supplements have no positive effect on BMI, DHEA sulfate, and triglyceride or high-density-lipoprotein (HDL) cholesterol levels.[62] Nevertheless, studies have shown that vitamin D supplements reduce HA and IR in patients with PCOS. Some studies documented that supplementation of vitamin D can decrease the levels of glucose in plasma an hour after the oral glucose tolerance test, resulting in greater endometrial thickness and thus increasing the chances of conception in females who have normal vitamin D levels.[63] Vitamin D increases the synthesis of androgens and follicles in patients with PCOS by decreasing the effects of advanced glycation endproducts.[64]

Fatty Acid

Omega-3 is a polyunsaturated fatty acid that is derived from fatty fish like herring, salmon, tuna, bluefish, and mackerel.[65]

Among polyunsaturated fatty acids, docosahexaenoic acid (DHA) and eicosatetraenoic acid (EPA) are biologically active.[66] It has antioxidant, insulin-sensitizing, antiobesity, and anti-inflammatory properties. It is known to increase the sensitivity of insulin by increasing anti-inflammatory adiponectin secretion and decreasing the production of inflammatory cytokines, such as IL-6 and tumor necrosis factor-alpha (TNF-α).[67] Obesity and IR can lead to hypertension, diabetes, and dyslipidemia after 40 years of age.[68]

In a study by Sadeghi and colleagues, it was demonstrated that in patients with PCOS, IR was not improved by supplementing omega-3 fatty acid. Nevertheless, it increases HDL and low density lipoproteins (LDL), waist circumference, triglycerides, and menstrual cycle regularity in non-PCOS patients.[69] Moreover, the study of Yang et al. showed that IR was related to the supplementation of omega-3 fatty acids causing an increase in LDL, total cholesterol, and triglycerides. It increases insulin sensitivity by decreasing proinflammatory cytokines and increasing anti-inflammatory adipokine production.[70] Nevertheless, in patients with PCOS, the inflammatory state is decreased because of increased levels of adiponectin and reduced levels of CRP.[71]

Daily intake of omega-3 fatty acids is 0.5% to 2% of the body requirement, whereas the minimum requirement of EPA:DHA is 500mg/day and 2000 to 4000mg/day in people with altered levels of triglycerides. Side effects of omega-3 fatty acids include intestinal gas, gut discomfort, headache, nausea, and diarrhea. Nevertheless, it is contraindicated in patients on anticoagulant and antiplatelet therapy and is given with caution in pregnancy because of its interference with drugs and side effects. Therefore EPA administration is avoided in pregnancy because of its interference with arachidonic acid, which is required at a fetal stage for the growth process.[72] Keeping in view its high calorific value, it should be used carefully in obese patients to avoid harmful effects on cardiometabolic-related alterations in patients with PCOS.[73]

Role of Medicinal Herbs in the Management of PCOS

Wild Indigo (*Tephrosia purpurea*)

Tephrosia purpurea is used as a medicine for the treatment of disorders of the female reproductive system and inflammatory disorders. It can be demonstrated that the extract of *Tephrosia purpurea* is used to enhance the ovulation process in rats in whom letrozole was used to induce PCOS. This treatment was used to normalize hormonal levels of steroids and the estrous cycle. FSH and LH being secreted from the pituitary gland were not affected, and the action of *Tephrosia purpurea* was limited to the ovaries. To check fertility in rats, they were mated to confirm pregnancy.[74]

Aniseed (*Pimpinella anisum*)

Pimpinella anisum is used as a traditional medicine in Iran. It contains estragole, methyl chavicol, anethol, anisaldehyde, and eugenol. It is used for treating epilepsy and seizures and can also be used as an antipyretic, antifungal, antibacterial agent for stimulating the effect of the digestive system. The oil extract of *Pimpinella anisum* when used in the dosage of 200 mg/kg and 400 mg/kg decreases PCOS signs in the ovarian tissue of rats.[75]

Pergularia (*Pergularia daemia*)

Pergularia daemia contains triterpenes, steroidal compounds, saponins, alkaloids, and cardenolides. It is used as an antidiabetic and as a hepatoprotective and antifertility agent. In rats where PCOS was induced by testosterone propionate, the combined effect of metformin and *Pergularia daemia* was found to be effective compared with treatment with metformin when used alone. Progesterone, estradiol, testosterone, FSH, and LH plasma levels were measured. The effects of obesity in PCOS-induced rats can be demonstrated. Their results showed that the treatment of coronary heart disease and obesity in PCOS can be used to prevent atherosclerosis in rats. Therefore it is an effective treatment for lowering serum cholesterol levels and PCOS.[76]

Aloe Vera (*Aloe barbadensis*)

Aloe vera has been traditionally used to control hypertension, diabetes, and some digestive and skin problems, including skin cancers and burns. Some researchers used aloe vera for managing PCOS in rats. First, letrozole was used to induce PCOS in rats and later aloe vera was used to control it for 2 months. Later, rats were made pregnant and sacrificed at a late stage of gestation to check for regulatory proteins and hormonal status. Assays were taken; results showed that aloe vera was directly involved in modulating the action of some of the main receptors, including the LH receptor, aromatase receptor, and androgen receptor. This proved that for PCOS phenotypic persons, aloe vera is a good preconceptive agent.[77]

Atractylodes (*Atractylodes macrocephala* Koidz)

Atractylodes macrocephala Koidz (AMK) were used to assess activity in the HA model of PCOS rats. The HA state was induced by testosterone propionate. AMK is a herb used for medicinal purposes to treat PCOS.

During the research, five groups of animals were used; PCOS was induced via testosterone propionate. Enzyme-linked immunosorbent assays measuring total testosterone (TT), SHBG, androstenedione, FSH, LH, and anti-Müllerian hormone were used. Polymerase chain reaction and biochemistry measured the expression of FSH and aquaporin-9. Extract of AMK helped to alleviate PCOS by improving the estrous cycle and reducing the plasma levels of TT and androstenedione. It also reduced the FSH receptor expression and increased aquaporin-9 expression in the ovaries of rats.[78]

Guggul (*Commiphora wightti*)

The effects of *Commiphora wightti* were studied by Kavitha et al. in an experiment on four groups of rats where DHEA was used to induce PCOS. These animals were additionally given metformin and *Commiphora wightti*. The levels of serum glucose and steroids were evaluated. The results demonstrated that the *Commiphora wightti* has a greater role in alleviating symptoms in DHEA-induced PCOS by reducing the morphologic abnormalities in ovarian follicles.[79]

Mistletoe Fig

The effects of *Ficus deltoidea* were studied on organs of reproduction in letrozole-induced PCOS in six groups of rats who were treated with different concentrations of clomiphene citrate used as a standard. Ovaries and uterus were collected at the end of the treatment period, and their weight was evaluated. Histopathology revealed that the tissues treated with the substance showed fewer cystic follicles. It decreased the ovarian wet weight and increased uterine wet weight. Another study showed these leaves to have good effects against ovarian and uterine-induced PCOS.[80]

Licorice (*Glycyrrhiza glabra*)

Licorice is well known for its antimicrobial and hypoglycemic effects. Glabridin and isoflavone are two natural compounds derived from licorice that demonstrate estrogen activities. They are very effective in weight loss and, when used for the treatment of hirsutism with spironolactone, can protect the volume depletion caused by spironolactone and potentiate its antiandrogenic property.[81]

Peppermint (*Mentha piperita*)

Peppermint (Family: Labiatae) is well known for its antimicrobial, antitumor, anti-inflammatory, and antiallergic properties. It also lowers free testosterone levels in the blood because of its antiandrogenic effect. Therefore it has been used as an alternative therapy in the treatment of PCOS.[82]

Ginseng (*Panax ginseng*)

Ginseng is used in herbal medicine as a tonic and is a well-known plant for its antiaging properties. It has been found to normalize LH levels in PCOS, thus improving ovulation disturbances by normalizing endocrine function.[83]

Puncture vine (*Tribulus terrestris*)

Puncture vine has experimentally been shown as an excellent herb for fertility in PCOS. It has been found to improve follicular growth, ovulation, and regulation of the menstrual cycle by improving steroidal hormonal levels. Therefore it is known as an excellent ovarian stimulant.[84]

Gymnema (*Gymnema sylvestre*)

Gymnema sylvestre (Asclepiadaceae) is well known for its glucose and lipid-lowering properties. It is experimentally found to be very beneficial in the treatment of diabetes mellitus (DM) because of its property of treating the root cause of IR and lowering serum triglycerides levels that are prevalent with the disease.[85]

Lodh Tree (*Symplocos racemosa*)

Symplocos racemosa belongs to the Symplocaceae family. In letrozole PCOS rat models, the Lodh tree has been found to improve testosterone, estrogen, and progesterone levels. Thus it has an effective antiandrogenic role in the treatment of PCOS that improves subfertility. It has also been found to normalize ovarian tissue levels, thus improving ovarian function in PCOS.[86]

Chaste Tree (*Vitex negundo*)

The Chaste tree belongs to the Verbenaceae family. It is well known for its antimicrobial, anti-inflammatory, and analgesic properties. It is also used in gynecologic disorders for its antiandrogenic and estrogenic properties. It has shown multiple benefits when given to letrozole-induced PCOS experimental rats. It has been found to improve FSH, LH, hyperglycemia, hyperlipidemia, menstrual cycle irregularities, and serum sex steroid profile.[87]

Licogliflozin

Hyperinsulinemia in PCOS leads to increased androgenesis. Licogliflozin is a sodium-glucose 1 and 2 cotransporter inhibitor that ameliorates IR in type 2 DM and hyperinsulinemia. A study conducted on its efficacy revealed that it significantly reduces hyperinsulinemia and androgen levels.[88]

(L.) Roxb. (*Caesalpinia bonduc*)

Caesalpinia bonduc has been used for many years in India to reduce fever and inflammation. Now its effectiveness is depicted to correct the dysregulation of menstrual cycle in PCOS.[89]

Humanin

Humanin is a mitochondrial-derived peptide. A study revealed that humanin supplementation, when given to rats with PCOS, attenuated fasting glucose and insulin levels, thus decreasing IR. Its role is also depicted by a decrease in humanin concentration in follicular fluid of polycystic ovaries. Moreover, it stimulates the signaling pathway of exercise, helping in reducing weight, which ameliorates symptoms.[90]

Role of Functional Foods in the Management of PCOS

Soy Isoflavone (*Glycine max*)

Glycine max (soybean) contains isoflavones, which are used for the treatment of menopausal females as an alternative hormonal therapy. Rajan et al.[91] studied physical, endocrinologic, and metabolic parameters in rats in which letrozole was used to induce PCOS. The characteristic ovarian changes in rats were studied by histopathologic studies. Soy isoflavones have shown beneficial effects in clinical and biochemical parameters and PCOS.

Turmeric (Curcumin)

Curcumin is an essential part of curcuma longa rhizomes. It is used as a food additive and possesses anti-inflammatory, antihyperlipidemic, hypoglycemic, and antioxidant properties. Properties of curcumin were evaluated in five groups of rats with letrozole-induced PCOS. Curcumin and clomiphene citrate were compared by evaluating lab results of fasting blood glucose, glycosylated hemoglobin, and lipid profile. Catalase and superoxide dismutase activity determine the antioxidant property of curcumin. Results revealed that curcumin is directly involved in reducing fasting glucose and glycosylated hemoglobin levels. Curcumin is beneficial in the treatment of letrozole-induced PCOS.[92]

Onion (*Allium fistulosum*)

Allium fistulosum is well used in Asia as a traditional medicine in addition to food. *Allium fistulosum*–extracted therapy was found to cure ovulation disruption by normalizing LH and FSH levels. It has also been found to normalize follicular growth and ovarian cysts.[93]

Flaxseed (*Linum usitatissimum*)

Flaxseeds are sourced from dietary lignin. Flaxseeds have been found to be an effective remedy for hirsutism, HA that normalizes excess testosterone levels in PCOS, and hyperlipidemia. Apart from this, it has also been found to improve ovarian follicular growth, decrease ovarian volume, and regulate the menstrual cycle.[94]

Pomegranate (*Punica granatum*)

Pomegranates belong to the Punicaceae family. This fruit is rich in folic acid, thiamine, vitamin C, organic acid, and saturated and unsaturated fatty acids. In experimental PCOS-induced animal rats, it has been found to normalize hormonal imbalance and decrease the complications associated with PCOS.[95]

Cinnamon (*Cinnamomum zeylanicum*)

Cinnamon belongs to the Lauraceae family and potentiates the glucose uptake of insulin. It also controls glycogen synthesis. It has shown a profound hypoglycemic effect in an experimental study of patients with PCOS. It contains procyanidins and phenols, which sensitize insulin by potentiating the insulin signaling pathway. In another experiment, it has been found to normalize the menstrual cycle regularity and improve metabolic dysfunction in PCOS.[96]

Role of Nuts Intake in the Management of PCOS

Hazelnut

Hazelnut oil was used to assess its activity in letrozole-induced PCOS by Demirel. Some of the parameters assessed were serum FSH, LH, estradiol, testosterone, progesterone, lipid, leptin, and glucose in addition to antioxidant activity and phytosterol content of the oil. Results were impressive, showing HDL concentration high with glucose and leptin concentration low in the treatment group. The oil has tocopherols, sitosterols, squalene, campesterol, and stigmasterol. It is effective in PCOS.[97]

Walnut

Consumption of almond and walnut as a source of monounsaturated fatty acids and polyunsaturated fatty acids (PUFA) was studied respectively and their effects were compared in patients with PCOS. It was demonstrated that the consumption of walnuts had a significant increase in the concentration of lipoic acid and alpha-lipoic acid; however, the serum concentration of EPA and DHA remained unchanged. The group of PCOS patients consuming walnut showed raised serum concentration of SHGB and adiponectin, whereas concentration of LDL cholesterol and Apo lipoprotein H levels were decreased.[98]

Almond

In PCOS patients, the serum concentration of amino acids, SHBG, and adiponectin were increased, whereas the FAI value was decreased, suggesting that an increase in adiponectin level had no effect on insulin sensitivity. There was no significant change in the serum concentration of proinflammatory cytokines (IL-6 and IL-1) and CRPs. It was concluded that walnut consumption as a source of PUFA may significantly improve the hormonal and lipid profile in PCOS patients and decrease the risk of cardiovascular diseases. Nut intake exerted beneficial effects on plasma lipids and androgens in PCOS as shown in Fig. 22.2.[98]

References

1. Sneha S. Effect of high levels of testosterone on cardiovascular risk in polycystic ovary syndrome (PCOS). *Int J Res Rev.* 2020;7(7):285-289.
2. Hachey LM, Kroger-Jarvis M, Pavlik-Maus T, Leach R. Clinical implications of polycystic ovary syndrome in adolescents. *Nurs Womens Health.* 2020;24(2):115-126.
3. Haq N, Khan Z, Riaz S, et al. Prevalence and knowledge of polycystic ovary syndrome (PCOS) among female science students of different public universities of Quetta, Pakistan. *Imp J Interdiscip Res.* 2017;35(6):385-392.
4. Anjum N, Zohra S, Arif A, et al. Prevalence of metabolic syndrome in Pakistani women with polycystic ovarian syndrome. *Pak J Biochem Mol Biol.* 2013;46(3):97-100.
5. Hamza DH, Hassan SA. Polycystic ovary syndrome and some hormonal and physiological changes: a review. *Eur Asian J BioSci.* 2020;14(2):5149-5156.
6. Ibáñez L, Oberfield SE, Witchel S, et al. An international consortium update: pathophysiology, diagnosis, and treatment of polycystic ovarian syndrome in adolescence. *Horm Res Paediatr.* 2017;88:371-395.
7. Azziz R, Kintziger K, Li R, et al. Recommendations for epidemiologic and phenotypic research in polycystic ovary syndrome: an androgen excess and PCOS society resource. *Hum Reprod.* 2019;34(11):2254-2265.
8. Rosenfield RL, Ehrmann DA. The pathogenesis of polycystic ovary syndrome (PCOS): the hypothesis of PCOS as functional ovarian hyperandrogenism revisited. *Endocr Rev.* 2016;37(5):467-520.
9. Shukla P, Mukherjee S. Mitochondrial dysfunction: an emerging link in the pathophysiology of polycystic ovary syndrome. *Mitochondrion.* 2020;52:24-39.
10. Hart R, Hickey M, Franks S. Definitions, prevalence and symptoms of polycystic ovaries and polycystic ovary syndrome. *Best Pract Res Clin Obstet Gynaecol.* 2004;18(5):671-683.
11. Asghari R, Shokri V, Rezaei H, et al. Alteration of TGFB1, GDF9, and BMPR2 gene expression in preantral follicles of an estradiol valerate-induced polycystic ovary mouse model can lead to anovulation, polycystic morphology, obesity, and absence of hyperandrogenism. *Korean J Fertil Steril.* 2021;48(3):245-254.
12. Soumya V. Polycystic ovary disease (PCOD)-an insight into rodent models, diagnosis and treatments. *J Clin Med Img.* 2021;5(11):1-13.
13. Kabil Kucur S, Kurek Eken M, Sanli I, et al. Predictive value of serum and follicular fluid chemerin concentrations during assisted reproductive cycles in women with polycystic ovary syndrome. *Gynecol Endocrinol.* 2021;37(9):814-818.
14. Amin S, Nabi M, Andrabi SM, et al. Androgen receptor coregulator long non coding RNA CTBP1-AS is associated with polycystic ovary syndrome in Kashmiri women. *Endocrine.* 2022;75(2):614-622.
15. Escobar-Morreale HF. Polycystic ovary syndrome: definition, aetiology, diagnosis and treatment. *Nat Rev Endocrinol.* 2018;14(5):270-284.
16. Laven JS, Imani B, Eijkemans MJ, Fauser BC. New approaches to PCOS and other forms of anovulation. *Obstet Gynecol Surv.* 2002;57:755-767.
17. Ferk P, Perme MP, Teran N, Gersak K. Androgen receptor gene (CAG) n polymorphism in patients with polycystic ovary syndrome. *Fertil Steril.* 2008;90(3):860-863.

18. Keevil BG, Adaway J. Assessment of free testosterone concentration. *J Steroid Biochem Mol Biol.* 2019;190:207-211.
19. Rosenfield RL. Ovarian and adrenal function in polycystic ovary syndrome. *Endocrinol Metab Clin North Am.* 1999;28(2):265-293.
20. Zeng X, Xie YJ, Liu YT, Long SL, Mo ZC. Polycystic ovarian syndrome: correlation between hyperandrogenism, insulin resistance and obesity. *Clinica Chimica Acta.* 2022;502:214-221.
21. Hsueh AJ, Adashi EY, Jones PB, Welsh Jr TH. Hormonal regulation of the differentiation of cultured ovarian granulosa cells. *Endocr Rev.* 1984;5(1):76-127.
22. White DW, Leigh A, Wilson C, et al. Gonadotrophin and gonadal steroid response to a single dose of a long-acting agonist of gonadotrophin-releasing hormone in ovulatory and anovulatory women with polycystic ovary syndrome. *Clin Endocrinol.* 1995;42: 475-481.
23. Ezeh U, Ida Chen YD, Azziz R. Racial and ethnic differences in the metabolic response of polycystic ovary syndrome. *Clin Endocrinol.* 2020;93(2):163-172.
24. Di Bari F, Catalano A, Bellone F, Martino G, Benvenga S. Vitamin D, bone metabolism, and fracture risk in polycystic ovary syndrome. *Metabolites.* 2021;11(2):116.
25. Speelman DL. Nonpharmacologic management of symptoms in females with polycystic ovary syndrome: a narrative review. *Int J Osteopath Med.* 2019;119(1):25-39.
26. Paris VR, Walters KA. Humanin: a potential treatment for PCOS? *Endocrinology.* 2021;162(8);bqab085.
27. Regidor PA, Mueller A, Sailer M, Gonzalez Santos F, Rizo JM, Moreno Egea F. Chronic inflammation in PCOS: the potential benefits of specialized pro-resolving lipid mediators (SPMs) in the improvement of the resolutive response. *Int J Mol Sci.* 2021; 22(1):384.
28. Chugh RM, Park HS, El Andaloussi A, et al. Mesenchymal stem cell therapy ameliorates metabolic dysfunction and restores fertility in a PCOS mouse model through interleukin-10. *Stem Cell Res Ther.* 2021;12(1):388.
29. Coskun B, Ercan CM, Togrul C, et al. Effects of lisinopril treatment on the pathophysiology of PCOS and plasminogen activator inhibitor-1 concentrations in rats. *Reprod Biomed Online.* 2021;42(1):16-25.
30. Naz S, Anjum N, Gul I A Community based cross sectional study on prevalence of polycystic ovarian syndrome (PCOS) and health related quality of life in Pakistani females. Research square. 2020:1–8.
31. Gale N. The sociology of traditional, complementary and alternative medicine. *Sociol Compass.* 2014;8(6):805-822.
32. Pan SY, Gao SH, Zhou SF, Tang MK, Yu ZL, Ko KM. New perspectives on complementary and alternative medicine: an overview and alternative therapy. *Altern Ther Health Med.* 2012;18(4):20-36.
33. Ben-Nun L. Treatment of infertility.
34. Hamza DH, Hassan SA. Polycystic ovary syndrome and some hormonal and physiological changes: a review. *Eur Asian J BioSci.* 2020;14(2):5149-5156.
35. Ibáñez L, Oberfield SE, Witchel S, et al. An international consortium update: pathophysiology, diagnosis, and treatment of polycystic ovarian syndrome in adolescence. *Horm Res Paediatr.* 2017;88:371-395.
36. Park YL, Canaway R. Integrating traditional and complementary medicine with national healthcare systems for universal health coverage in Asia and the Western Pacific. *Health Syst Reform.* 2019;5(1):24-31.
37. Jia LY, Feng JX, Li JL, et al. The complementary and alternative medicine for polycystic ovary syndrome: a review of clinical

application and mechanism. *Evid Based Complement Alternat Med.* 2021;2021:5555315.
38. Devaki R. *Preclinical Evaluation of Siddha Poly-Herbal Formulation Ashuwathi Chooranam for its Naturally Curing PCOS. Doctoral Dissertation.* Chennai: Government Siddha Medical College; 2017.
39. Farkhondeh T, Folgado SL, Pourbagher-Shahri AM, Ashrafizadeh M, Samarghandian S. The therapeutic effect of resveratrol: Focusing on the Nrf2 signaling pathway. *Biomed Pharmacother.* 2020;127:110234.
40. Zhang T, Zhou Y, LI L, et al. SIRT1, 2, 3 protect mouse oocytes from postovulatory aging. *Aging (Albany NY).* 2016;8(4):685.
41. Cabello E, Garrido P, Morán J, et al. Effects of resveratrol on ovarian response to controlled ovarian hyperstimulation in ob/ob mice. *Fertil Steril.* 2015;103(2):570-579.
42. Ortega I, Duleba AJ. Ovarian actions of resveratrol. *Ann N Y Acad Sci.* 2015;1348(1):86-96.
43. Iervolino M, Lepore E, Forte G, Laganà AS, Buzzaccarini G, Unfer V. Natural molecules in the management of polycystic ovary syndrome (PCOS): an analytical review. *Nutrients.* 2021; 13(5):1677.
44. Benrick A, Maliqueo M, Miao S, et al. Resveratrol is not as effective as physical exercise for improving reproductive and metabolic functions in rats with dihydrotestosterone-induced polycystic ovary syndrome. *Evid Based Complement Alternat Med.* 2013;2013:964070.
45. Hong Y, Yin Y, Tan Y, Hong K, Zhou H. The flavanone, naringenin, modifies antioxidant and steroidogenic enzyme activity in a rat model of letrozole-induced polycystic ovary syndrome. *Med Sci Monit.* 2019;25:395.
46. Mihanfar A, Nouri M, Roshangar L, Khadem-Ansari MH. Polyphenols: natural compounds with promising potential in treating polycystic ovary syndrome. *Reprod Biol.* 2021;21(2):100500.
47. Wawrzkiewicz-Jałowiecka A, Kowalczyk K, Trybek P, et al. In search of new therapeutics—molecular aspects of the PCOS pathophysiology: genetics, hormones, metabolism and beyond. *Int J Mol Sci.* 2020;21(19):7054.
48. Hong Y, Yin Y, Tan Y, Hong K, Zhou H. The flavanone, naringenin, modifies antioxidant and steroidogenic enzyme activity in a rat model of letrozole-induced polycystic ovary syndrome. *Med Sci Monit.* 2019;25:395.
49. Jahan S, Munir F, Razak S, et al. Ameliorative effects of rutin against metabolic, biochemical and hormonal disturbances in polycystic ovary syndrome in rats. *J Ovarian Res.* 2016;9(1):1-9.
50. Pehlivan FE. Vitamin C: an antioxidant agent. *Vitamin C.* 2017; 2:23-35.
51. Olaniyan OT, Femi A, Iliya G, et al. Vitamin C suppresses ovarian pathophysiology in experimental polycystic ovarian syndrome. *Pathophysiology.* 2019;26(3-4):331-341.
52. Bendich A, Machlin LJ, Scandurra O, Burton GW, Wayner DD. The antioxidant role of vitamin C. *Adv Free Radic Biol Med.* 1986;2(2):419-444.
53. Chandrasekhar U. *Unit-7 Fat-Soluble Vitamins: Vitamin A, D, E, and K.* New Delhi: Indira Gandhi National Open University; 2021.
54. Ebhohimen IE, Okanlanwon TS, Osagie AO, Izevbigie ON. Vitamin E in Human Health and Oxidative Stress Related Diseases. *Diseases and Health Aspects.* IntechOpen. 2021.
55. Cicek N, Eryilmaz OG, Sarikaya E, Gulerman C, Genc Y. Vitamin E effect on controlled ovarian stimulation of unexplained infertile women. *J Assist Reprod Genet.* 2012;29(4):325-328.
56. Izadi A, Ebrahimi S, Shirazi S, et al. Hormonal and metabolic effects of coenzyme Q10 and/or vitamin E in patients with

polycystic ovary syndrome. *J Clin Endocrinol Metab.* 2019;104(2):319-327.

57. Monastra G, De Grazia S, De Luca L, Vittorio S, Unfer V. Vitamin D: a steroid hormone with progesterone-like activity. *Eur Rev Med Pharmacol Sci.* 2018;22(8):2502-2512.

58. Goltzman D, Miao D, Panda DK, Hendy GN. Effects of calcium and of the Vitamin D system on skeletal and calcium homeostasis: lessons from genetic models. *J Steroid Biochem Mol Biol.* 2004;89:485-489.

59. Holick MF. Vitamin D deficiency. *N Engl J Med.* 2007;357(3): 266-281.

60. Iervolino M, Lepore E, Forte G, Laganà AS, Buzzaccarini G, Unfer V. Natural molecules in the management of polycystic ovary syndrome (PCOS): an analytical review. *Nutrients.* 2021;13(5):1677.

61. Kadoura S, Alhalabi M, Nattouf AH. Effect of calcium and vitamin D supplements as an adjuvant therapy to metformin on menstrual cycle abnormalities, hormonal profile, and IGF-1 system in polycystic ovary syndrome patients: a randomized, placebo-controlled clinical trial. *Adv Pharmacol Sci.* 2019;2019: 9680390.

62. Iervolino M, Lepore E, Forte G, Laganà AS, Buzzaccarini G, Unfer V. Natural molecules in the management of polycystic ovary syndrome (PCOS): an analytical review. *Nutrients.* 2021; 13(5):1677.

63. Lerchbaum E, Rabe T. Vitamin D and female fertility. *Curr Opin Obstet Gynecol.* 2014;26(3):145-150.

64. Merhi Z, Buyuk E, Cipolla MJ. Advanced glycation end products alter steroidogenic gene expression by granulosa cells: an effect partially reversible by vitamin D. *Mol Hum Reprod.* 2018;24(6):318-326.

65. Oliver L, Dietrich T, Marañón I, Villarán MC, Barrio RJ. Producing omega-3 polyunsaturated fatty acids: a review of sustainable sources and future trends for the EPA and DHA market. *Resources.* 2020;9(12):148.

66. Watanabe Y, Tatsuno I. Omega-3 polyunsaturated fatty acids focusing on eicosapentaenoic acid and docosahexaenoic acid in the prevention of cardiovascular diseases: a review of the state-of-the-art. *Expert Rev Clin Pharmacol.* 2021;14(1):79-93.

67. Monk JM, Turk HF, Liddle DM, et al. n-3 polyunsaturated fatty acids and mechanisms to mitigate inflammatory paracrine signaling in obesity-associated breast cancer. *Nutrients.* 2014;6(11): 4760-4793.

68. Bellver J, Rodríguez-Tabernero L, Robles A, et al. Polycystic ovary syndrome throughout a woman's life. *J Assist Reprod Genet.* 2018;35(1):25-39.

69. Sadeghi A, Djafarian K, Mohammadi H, Shab-Bidar S. Effect of omega-3 fatty acids supplementation on insulin resistance in women with polycystic ovary syndrome: meta-analysis of randomized controlled trials. *Diabetes Metab Syndr.* 2017;11(2): 157-162.

70. Yang K, Zeng L, Bao T, Ge J. Effectiveness of omega-3 fatty acid for polycystic ovary syndrome: a systematic review and meta-analysis. *Reprod Biol Endocrinol.* 2018;16(1):1-13.

71. Tosatti JA, Alves MT, Cândido AL, Reis FM, Araújo VE, Gomes KB. Influence of n-3 fatty acid supplementation on inflammatory and oxidative stress markers in patients with polycystic ovary syndrome: a systematic review and meta-analysis. *Br J Nutr.* 2021;125(6):657-668.

72. Tu Wei-Chun. Effects of Dietary Alpha Linolenic Acid on Biosynthesis of N-3 Long Chain Polyunsaturated Fatty Acids in Animals (Doctoral Dissertation). 2011.

73. Sheehan MT. Polycystic ovarian syndrome: diagnosis and management. *Clin Med Res.* 2004;2(1):13-27.

74. Thakor AP, Patel AJ. Normalizing of estrous cycle in polycystic ovary syndrome (PCOS) induced rats with *Tephrosia purpurea* (Linn.) Pers. *J Appli Nat Sci.* 2014;6(1):197-201.

75. Mahood RAH. Effects of *Pimpinella anisum* oil extract on some biochemical parameters in mice experimentally induced for human polycystic ovary syndrome. *J Biotec Res Cent.* 2012;6: 67-73.

76. Bhuvaneshwari S, Poornima R, Averal HI. Comparative study of *Pergularia daemia* and *Citrullus colocynthis* in polycystic ovarian syndrome induced albino wistar rats. *Int J Multidisc Res Dev.* 2015;2(9):207-212.

77. Radha MH, Laxmipriya NP. The role of Aloe Barbadensis Mill. as a possible pre-conceptive herb for the management of polycystic ovarian syndrome: a rodent model study. *Austin J Reprod Med Infertil.* 2016;3(2):1040.

78. Zhou J, Qu F, Barry JA, et al. An atractylodes macrocephala koidz extract alleviates hyperandrogenism of polycystic ovarian syndrome. *Int J Clin Exp Med.* 2016;9(2):2758-2767.

79. Kavitha A, Babu AN, Kumar MS, Kiran SV. Evaluation of effects of *Commiphora wightii* in dehydroepiandrosterone (DHEA) induced polycystic ovary syndrome (PCOS) in rats. *Pharma Tutor.* 2016;4(1):47-55.

80. Suhaimi NA, Nooraain H, Nurdiana S. Effects of *Ficus deltoidea* Ethanolic leaves extract on female reproductive organs among Letrozole-induced polycystic ovarian syndrome rats. *J Sci Res Dev.* 2016;3(4):8-14.

81. Yang H, Kim HJ, Pyun BJ, Lee HW. Licorice ethanol extract improves symptoms of polycystic ovary syndrome in Letrozole-induced female rats. *Integr Med Res.* 2018;7(3):264-270.

82. Amoura M, Lotfy ZH, Neveen E, Khloud, A. Potential effects of *Mentha piperita* (peppermint) on Letrozole-induced polycystic ovarian syndrome in female albino rat. *Int J.* 2015;3(10):211-226.

83. Choi JH, Jang M, Kim EJ, et al. Korean Red Ginseng alleviates dehydroepiandrosterone-induced polycystic ovarian syndrome in rats via its antiinflammatory and antioxidant activities. *J Ginseng Res.* 2020;44(6):790-798.

84. Saiyed A, Jahan N, Makbul SAA, Ansari M, Bano H, Habib SH. Effect of combination of *Withania somnifera* Dunal and *Tribulus terrestris* Linn on letrozole induced polycystic ovarian syndrome in rats. *Integr Med Res.* 2016;5(4):293-300.

85. Sudhakar P, Suganeswari M, Pushkalai PS, Haripriya S. Regulation of estrous cycle using combination of Gymnema sylvestre and Pergularia daemia in estradiol valerate induced PCOS rats. *Asian J Res Pharm Sci.* 2018;8(1):4-8.

86. Jadhav M, Menon S, Shailajan S. Anti-androgenic effect of *Symplocos racemosa* Roxb. Against letrozole induced polycystic ovary using rat model. *J Coast life Med.* 2013;1(4):309-314.

87. Kakadia N, Patel P, Deshpande S, Shah G. Effect of *Vitex negundo* L. seeds in letrozole induced polycystic ovarian syndrome. *J Tradit Complement Med.* 2019;9(4):336-345.

88. Tysoe O. Licogliflozin effective in PCOS treatment. *Nat Rev Endocrinol.* 2021;17(10):577.

89. Kandasamy V, Balasundaram U. *Caesalpinia bonduc* (L.) Roxb. As a promising source of pharmacological compounds to treat poly cystic ovary syndrome (PCOS): a review. *J Ethnopharmacol.* 2021;279:114375.

90. Paris VR, Walters KA. Humanin: a potential treatment for PCOS? *Endocrinology.* 2021;162(8);bqab085.

91. Rajan RK, Balaji B. Soy isoflavones exert beneficial effects on letrozole-induced rat polycystic ovary syndrome (PCOS) model

through anti-androgenic mechanism. *Pharm Biol.* 2017;55(1): 242-251.

92. Reddy PS, Begum N, Mutha S, Bakshi V. Beneficial effect of Curcumin in Letrozole induced polycystic ovary syndrome. *Asian Pac J Reprod.* 2016;5(2):116-122.

93. Lee YH, Yang H, Lee SR, Kwon SW, Hong EJ, Lee HW. Welsh onion root *(Allium fistulosum)* restores ovarian functions from letrozole induced-polycystic ovary syndrome. *Nutrients.* 2018;10(10):1430.

94. Jelodar G, Masoomi S, Rahmanifar F. Hydroalcoholic extract of flaxseed improves polycystic ovary syndrome in a rat model. *Iran J Basic Med Sci.* 2018;21(6):645.

95. Hossein KJ, Leila KJ, koukhdan Ebrahim T, Nazanin SJ, Farzad P, Elham R. The effect of pomegranate juice extract on hormonal changes of female Wistar rats caused by polycystic ovarian syndrome. *Biomed Pharmacol J.* 2015;8(2):971-977.

96. Wang JG, Anderson RA, Graham GM III, et al. The effect of cinnamon extract on insulin resistance parameters in polycystic ovary syndrome: a pilot study. *Fertil Steril.* 2007;88(1):240-243.

97. Demirel MA, Ilhan M, Suntar I, Keles H, Akkol EK. Activity of *Corylus avellana* seed oil in letrozole-induced polycystic ovary syndrome model in rats. *Rev Bras Farmacognosia.* 2016;26:83-88.

98. Kalgaonkar S, Almario RU, Gurusinghe D, et al. Differential effects of walnuts vs almonds on improving metabolic and endocrine parameters in PCOS. *Eur J Clin Nutr.* 2011;65(3):386-393.

23

Evidence-Based Recommendations for Clinical Practice (Future Directions: Research and Practice)

RAHAT NAJAM QURESHI

Introduction

Polycystic ovary syndrome (PCOS) is a prevalent disorder among females.[1] The diagnosis of PCOS has changed to allow for better recognition of the phenotype,[2] which changes in the different stages of a female's life. The phenotype is underpinned by a complex interplay of genetics, hormones, and lifestyle, partly because of the scarcity of literature, particularly from low- and middle-income countries (LMICs).[3] These countries hold a combined population of 6.5 billion[4] and share some common characteristics. In several settings where many adolescent females enter the active reproductive period every year, there is a high fertility rate in the population and weak health systems.[5] The link between PCOS and noncommunicable disease (NCD) is known.[6] Approximately 41 million deaths occur annually because of NCD and 85% of these deaths occur in LMICs, where 15 million people between the ages of 30 and 69 die prematurely.[7] Equally challenging is the high proportion of NCDs such as cardiovascular disease (CVD), diabetes mellitus (DM), respiratory diseases, cancers, and mental disorders.[6,7]

The International Evidence-Based Guidelines for the assessment and management of PCOS include an extensive review of the literature and published guidelines.[8] This review has identified many facets of PCOS, for which evidence is lacking in adolescents and patients with PCOS.[8] The lack of evidence underscores the need for further knowledge generation and fact-finding, especially with regards to social determinants, genetic factors, lifestyle factors that interact with different social factors, and geography across diverse populations with different racial and ethnic backgrounds (because there is some indication that prevalence is higher in specific populations). Strengthening the global knowledge base for PCOS has implications for building contextual and practical approaches in screening, early intervention, and improved long-term outcomes for PCOS.

The primary objective of this chapter is to raise some key research questions to inform further scientific inquiry within this health area. Because this area is constantly evolving, this is not an exhaustive list of concerns to be explored. Researchers and public health implementers should be motivated to find and lead investigations into the many key research questions that these questions contain within themselves.

Questions for Investigating and Establishing Quality Standards for the Diagnosis of PCOS

1. What is the most effective way to measure hyperandrogenism (HA) when diagnosing PCOS? What levels of androgens are considered abnormal in the different life stages of a female who has the phenotype of PCOS?[9]
2. What is the role of ultrasound imaging in the diagnosis of PCOS? Will the improved resolution of ultrasound imaging review the criteria for PCOS diagnoses?[10,11]
3. How can anti-Müllerian hormone (AMH) be used to improve the diagnosis of PCOS? (Further related inquiry: How feasible is this approach in LMICs?)[12]

Questions for Understanding What Works for Improving Treatments and Interventions for PCOS

1. What are the adverse outcomes of patients with PCOS who become pregnant? What interventions can improve outcomes in these people?[13]
2. In patients with PCOS, are lifestyle interventions (compared with usual care) effective for improving weight loss, metabolic, reproductive, fertility, quality of life (QoL), and

emotional wellbeing outcomes? (Further related inquiry: How can behavioral changes be designed to promote a healthy lifestyle in adolescents and adult females?)[14]

3. How can we use social media and electronic health platforms to raise awareness to facilitate behavioral changes in lifestyle for general populations where the risk for PCOS and associated comorbidities are high? (Further related inquiry: In populations with a high risk for CVD, what level of intervention in the PCOS group would be acceptable and at what stage of life?)[15,16]

4. Which progestogen in the combined oral contraceptive pill (COCP) is effective for managing hormonal and clinical PCOS features in adolescents and adults with PCOS? (Further related inquiry: What is the acceptability of COCP use in different age groups in different cultures?)[17]

5. What interventions are effective (compared with usual care) for managing obesity in females and adolescents affected by PCOS? (Further related inquiries: Is metformin alone, or in combination, effective for the management of hormonal and clinical PCOS features and weight in adolescents and adults with PCOS?[17] What is the role of drugs used for reducing obesity in improving hormonal and clinical features of PCOS? Is inositol alone or in combination with other therapies effective for managing hormonal and clinical PCOS features and weight in adolescents and adults with PCOS?[18] What is the role of antiobesity drugs in improving fertility in patients with PCOS?)

6. What interventions effectively address concerns related to infertility among patients with PCOS?[19] (Further related inquiries: What are the long-term risks of PCOS undergoing treatment with different kinds of ovulation induction treatment? Can we design a low-risk-standardized low-dose gonadotropin dosage for PCOS infertile females living in LMICs? Will bariatric surgery improve fertility and pregnancy outcomes in patients with PCOS? What is the role of ultrasound-guided transvaginal ovarian needle drilling for drug-resistant PCOS in subfertile females?)[20]

Questions for Identifying the Mental and Physical Health Comorbidity Associated With PCOS

1. What are the risk factors in patients with PCOS that can predict CVD development in the future? (Further related inquiry: What is the risk of developing a physical or mental health comorbidity with PCOS in adolescents and adults?)

2. Which test would have the highest specificity for diagnosing type 2 DM in patients with PCOS?

3. How should postmenopausal females with PCOS be monitored to detect endometrial cancer? (Further related inquiries: What is the risk of cancer among females diagnosed with PCOS at various ages? How can early

screening of risk factors be integrated into routine gynecologic practice to introduce early intervention for cancer among patients with PCOS? How effective are early intervention approaches to mitigate the onset of cancers in postmenopausal and premenopausal women with PCOS?)[21,22]

4. How can integrated care protect adolescents and adults with PCOS against mental health comorbidities? (Further related inquiry: After diagnosing PCOS, what is the level of anxiety and depression in adolescent and adult females?)

Questions for Exploring the Contextual and Social Factors Related to PCOS Outcomes

1. What are the ethnic and geographic variations for PCOS in different populations? Can we have uniformity in data collection across countries to compare groups and identify any differences or similarities?

2. How should postmenopausal females with PCOS be monitored to detect endometrial cancer?

3. How should we screen and prevent the early detrimental effects of PCOS on QoL for adolescents and adults with PCOS? (Further related inquiries: How does PCOS affect QoL for adolescents and adults diagnosed with PCOS? Does improving QoL contribute to better treatment outcomes for PCOS?)

4. What is the level of psychosexual dysfunction in adolescents and adults diagnosed with PCOS? (Further related inquiries: How does PCOS affect social outcomes for adolescent and adult females in LMICs? What approaches effectively reduce psychosexual dysfunction in adolescent and adult females diagnosed with PCOS?)

5. After diagnosing PCOS, what tools can be used to screen patients for negative body image (commonly associated with multiple physical side effects)?

6. After a diagnosis of PCOS, what tools can be used to screen patients for the presence and severity of eating disorders?

Questions for Strengthening Capacity Building and Organizational Readiness for Health Systems Responsive to the Needs of Populations With or at Risk for PCOS

1. What are the different models of care present in different parts of the world, and what is the success of these models in terms of patient satisfaction, fertility, and HA? How is the access to culturally and linguistically diverse appropriate care?

2. What training programs are required for community workers and lay health workers to allow them to influence communities at high risk for CVD and PCOS? (Further related inquiry: How can we adapt these to

their current training and use technology to reinforce the message?)

3. How can health policy be influenced to strengthen the detection, treatment, and long-term support of populations affected by PCOS in low-resource settings?

4. What are the implications of integrating a complex care package for populations affected by PCOS into health-care settings and community settings? (Further related inquiry: What are the challenges for system-level PCOS programming in low-resource or rural areas?)

Concluding Remarks

Studies of PCOS have shown an association between genetics and lifestyle. Cases within families are seen commonly, reinforcing the association between genetic contributions. Genome-wide association studies have identified several PCOS catalogs of gene loci, and an investigation is needed to identify the causal variants and their importance to the underlying pathophysiology of PCOS.[23]

The reviews of the brain and the neuroendocrine changes in animal models show how the hypothalamic-pituitary axis and its functioning can contribute to the etiology of the adult phenotype of PCOS. We need findings in PCOS females to better understand this phenomenon.[24]

Are we aware of any similarity between obesity and ensuing physical, mental, and psychological issues between adolescent males and females? We have manifestations in females (i.e., PCOS), but are there any manifestations in males?

References

1. March WA, Moore VM, Willson KJ, Phillips DI, Norman RJ, Davies MJ. The prevalence of polycystic ovary syndrome in a community sample assessed under contrasting diagnostic criteria. *Hum Reprod.* 2010;25(2):544-551.

2. Rotterdam ESHRE/ASRM-Sponsored PCOS Consensus Workshop Group. Revised 2003 consensus on diagnostic criteria and long-term health risks related to polycystic ovary syndrome. *Fertil Steril.* 2004;81(1):19-25.

3. Bozdag G, Mumusoglu S, Zengin D, Karabulut E, Yildiz BO. The prevalence and phenotypic features of polycystic ovary syndrome: a systematic review and meta-analysis. *Hum Reprod.* 2016;31(12):2841-2855.

4. Sexton C, Snyder HM, Chandrasekaran L, Worley S, Carrillo MC. Expanding representation of low and middle income countries in global dementia research: commentary from the Alzheimer's Association. *Front Neurol.* 2021;12:633777.

5. Mills A. Health care systems in low-and middle-income countries. *N Engl J Med.* 2014;370(6):552-557.

6. Tosatti JA, Sóter MO, Ferreira CN, et al. The hallmark of pro-and anti-inflammatory cytokine ratios in women with polycystic ovary syndrome. *Cytokine.* 2020;134:155187.

7. Cooney LG, Dokras A. Beyond fertility: polycystic ovary syndrome and long-term health. *Fertil Steril.* 2018;110(5):794-809.

8. Teede H, Misso M, Costello MF, et al. *International Evidence-Based Guideline for the Assessment and Management of Polycystic Ovary Syndrome 2018.* National Health and Medical Research Council (NHMRC), Monash University; 2018:1-198.

9. Rosenfield RL, Ehrmann DA. The pathogenesis of polycystic ovary syndrome (PCOS): the hypothesis of PCOS as functional ovarian hyperandrogenism revisited. *Endocr Rev.* 2016;37(5):467-520.

10. Rackow BW, Brink HV, Hammers L, Flannery CA, Lujan ME, Burgert TS. Ovarian morphology by transabdominal ultrasound correlates with reproductive and metabolic disturbance in adolescents with PCOS. *J Adolesc Health.* 2018;62(3):288-293.

11. Teede HJ, Misso ML, Boyle JA, et al. Translation and implementation of the Australian-led PCOS guideline: clinical summary and translation resources from the international evidence-based guideline for the assessment and management of polycystic ovary syndrome. *Med J Aust.* 2018;209:S3-S8.

12. Teede H, Misso M, Tassone EC, et al. Anti-müllerian hormone in PCOS: a review informing international guidelines. *Trends Endocrinol Metab.* 2019;30(7):467-478.

13. Artini PG, Obino MER, Sergiampietri C, et al. PCOS and pregnancy: a review of available therapies to improve the outcome of pregnancy in women with polycystic ovary syndrome. *Expert Rev Endocrinol Metab.* 2018;13(2):87-98.

14. Lim S, Wright B, Savaglio M, Goodwin D, Pirotta S, Moran L. An analysis on the implementation of the evidence-based PCOS lifestyle guideline: recommendations from women with PCOS. Paper presented at the *Semin Reprod Med.* 2021;39(3-4):153-160.

15. Abroms LC. Public health in the era of social media. *Am J Public Health Assoc.* 2019;109:S130-S131.

16. Stellefson M, Paige SR, Chaney BH, Chaney JD. Evolving role of social media in health promotion: updated responsibilities for health education specialists. *Int J Environ Res Public Health.* 2020;17(4):1153.

17. Fraison E, Kostova E, Moran LJ, et al. Metformin versus the combined oral contraceptive pill for hirsutism, acne, and menstrual pattern in polycystic ovary syndrome. *Cochrane Database Syst Rev.* 2020;8(8):CD005552.

18. Pundir J, Psaroudakis D, Savnur P, et al. Inositol treatment of anovulation in women with polycystic ovary syndrome: a meta-analysis of randomised trials. *BJOG.* 2018;125(3):299-308.

19. Cena H, Chiovato L, Nappi RE. Obesity, polycystic ovary syndrome, and infertility: a new avenue for glp-1 receptor agonists. *J Clin Endocrinol Metab.* 2020;105(8):e2695-e2709.

20. Zhang J, Tang L, Kong L, et al. Ultrasound-guided transvaginal ovarian needle drilling for clomiphene-resistant polycystic ovarian syndrome in subfertile women. *Cochrane Database Syst Rev.* 2019;7(7):CD008583.

21. Glueck CJ, Goldenberg N. Characteristics of obesity in polycystic ovary syndrome: etiology, treatment, and genetics. *Metabolism.* 2019;92:108-120.

22. Saboor Aftab S, Kumar S, Barber T. The role of obesity and type 2 diabetes mellitus in the development of male obesity-associated secondary hypogonadism. *Clin Endocrinol.* 2013;78(3):330-337.

23. Hiam D, Moreno-Asso A, Teede HJ, et al. The genetics of polycystic ovary syndrome: an overview of candidate gene systematic reviews and genome-wide association studies. *J Clin Med.* 2019;8(10):1606.

24. Coutinho EA, Kauffman AS. The role of the brain in the pathogenesis and physiology of polycystic ovary syndrome (PCOS). *Med Sci.* 2019;7(8):84.

24

Polycystic Ovary Syndrome in South Asians

OUMA PILLAY, KIMMEE KHAN, AND KAMAL OJHA

Polycystic ovary syndrome (PCOS) is the most common endocrinologic condition and affects 4% to 25% of females in the reproductive age group, depending on the diagnostic criteria used.[1-3] Features of PCOS include oligomenorrhea, amenorrhea/anovulation, signs of hyperandrogenism (HA) such as acne and hirsutism, and changes to the ovary visible on ultrasound. The 2003 Rotterdam criteria is the most commonly used criteria for clinical and research purposes.[4] PCOS has an estimated prevalence of obesity of 50%, which is higher than the background population rate.[5] It also has a metabolic component, predominantly insulin resistance (IR), which may affect future morbidity.

South Asian is a collective term that refers to the population originating from India, Pakistan, Sri Lanka, Bangladesh, and Nepal. These countries are densely populated and, like many regions of the world, have people who suffer from PCOS. People originating from the South Asian region account for 20% of the global population.[2] In real terms, 1.6 million United States (US) residents were South Asians (0.7%) in 2000.[6] Similarly, 1 million Canadian residents were South Asian in 2011, and another 1 million South Asians resided in Australia (1.3%).[7] In the United Kingdom (UK), 5.7% of the residents consider themselves Asian or Asian-British.[9] This made South Asians the largest ethnic minority group in the UK in 2001, constituting 4% of the country's population.[10] Considering the large number of people suffering from PCOS globally, it is essential to further understand this condition and its effects on patients and to match treatment to the patients' needs.

Different regions of the world display ethnic variations in the expression of PCOS (Fig. 24.1); however, much of what is known about PCOS is based on evidence obtained in studies involving predominantly European females. In the UK, in a community-based study, Caucasian females were found to have a lower prevalence of polycystic ovaries (PCO) (22%) compared with their South Asian counterparts (52%).[11] A Sri Lankan community-based study identified the prevalence of PCOS to be 6.3%.[12] Additionally, South Asians have a higher prevalence of IR and type 2 diabetes mellitus (DM). This may worsen the future morbidity for patients suffering concomitantly from PCOS (Table 24.1).[13]

Genetics of PCOS in the South Asian Population

There is little doubt that PCOS is a genetic condition; however, a candidate gene or genes have yet to be identified. Additionally, the mode of inheritance is disputed and evidence is still lacking.

Like many previous studies in siblings of patients with PCOS aiming to establish a genetic link, Kaushal et al. found that the brothers of South Asian females with PCOS had an increased risk of DM, endothelial cell dysfunction, and premature male pattern balding.[14]

Siddamalla et al. studied the single nucleotide polymorphisms (SNPs) of the tumor suppressor gene phosphate and tensin homolog (PTEN) in South Indian females, looking for a correlation with the acquisition of PCOS. PTEN is an important controller of cell proliferation, migration, and death. PTEN genes *rs1903858A/G*, *rs185262832G/A*, and *rs10490920T/C*, and gene polymorphisms correlated with PCOS, which means these genes are inheritable risk factors in South Indian females.[15]

Furthermore, Tumu et al. noted an interleukin-6 (IL-6) gene promoter polymorphism that was significantly higher in South Asian females with PCOS.[16] They later found mitochondrial DNA copy number and displacement loop alteration in a further study within the Sri Lankan population.[17]

A gene of interest is the *FTO* (fat mass and obesity–associated) gene, which may play a part in regulation of body weight because it is present in multiple organs including the adipose tissue, brain, and muscle. It is located within chromosome 16, and there has been research into multiple SNPs. The most extensively studied variant, *rs9939609,* is

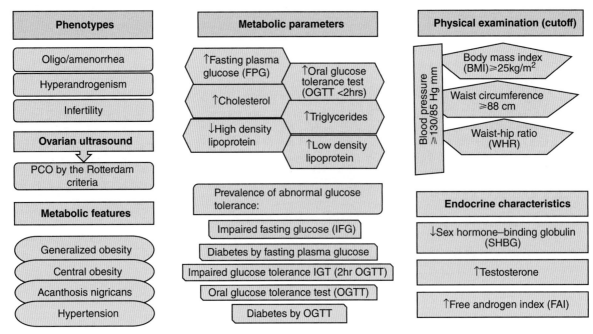

• **Fig. 24.1** Heterogeneous Manifestations of Polycystic Ovary Syndrome *(PCOS)* Observed in South Asian Females With PCOS (Phenotype, Physical Examination, and Impairments in Metabolic Profile).

found in the first FTO intron made up of two alleles (A and T). The A allele has been associated with an increased risk of obesity and type 2 DM.[18]

Branavan et al. investigated the *FTO* (*rs9939609*) polymorphism and found it associated with metabolic disorder and high testosterone levels in young Sri Lankan females with PCOS. The FTO gene variant *rs9939609* was associated both with physical signs of metabolic disease and HA, as well as raised hormonal markers, including kisspeptin and testosterone, all of which are features of PCOS.[18]

A further inheritable risk factor in South Indian females is the VEGF +405G/C polymorphism identified by Guruvajah et al.[19]

Follistatin is a single-chain glycoprotein expressed in a number of tissues, including the ovary, and its primary function is to antagonize the activity of activin, resulting in some characteristic features of PCOS. These include reduced serum follicle-stimulating hormone (FSH), impaired ovarian follicle development, and increased ovarian androgen production.[20,21] Because of its functional significance and the strong linkage pattern observed, the *FST* gene was considered a suitable candidate for PCOS. There have been a limited number of studies that attempted to identify sequence variants within this gene and their association with PCOS, and results are not all conclusive. A large-scale study was conducted among 150 families to test for evidence of linkage or association of 37 candidate genes with PCOS, and the strongest evidence of linkage was reported in the follistatin (FST) gene region.[22] Nevertheless, Dasgupta et al. found no exonic variants near the follistatin genes in the South Asian population studied. They concluded that gene expression vary based on the ethnic populations being studied.[23]

Metabolic Disorders and Other Medical Conditions in South Asians With PCOS

Metabolic syndrome (MetS) is a collection of metabolic irregularities encompassing conditions that lead to atherosclerosis and endothelial dysfunction, such as hyperlipidemia, hypertension, and DM/prediabetes.

MetS has been reported to be 4.6 times higher in the South Asian population in the UK, compared with the Caucasian population (in patients with body mass index [BMI] over 25). Nevertheless, this was found to be even higher in obese South Asian females with PCOS.

PCOS varies in presentation and symptoms across differing ethnic groups. Apridonidze et al. looked at females aged 30 to 39 years old and found that when they were matched for BMI, those with PCOS had almost double the rates of MetS compared with those without PCOS (43% vs. 24%).[25] These rates of MetS in patients with PCOS were similar in other studies (33%–46%).[26] Even though there is still some controversy in some of the findings, there is a difference depending on race and ethnicity in the prevalence of MetS in patients with PCOS and its features, including fasting serum glucose, fasting serum triglyceride, waist circumference, high-density lipoprotein, and hypertension.

Kudesia at al. performed a cross-sectional analysis of infertility patients, including 52 South Asian and 52 Caucasian females. The South Asian cohort had similar BMI to the Caucasian cohort and on the whole were not obese. Nevertheless, the South Asian cohort had increased rates of metabolic disease (IR, DM, and dyslipidemia), and endometrial disease (endometrial hyperplasia and polyps). On the whole, the South Asians were younger and had a higher incidence of PCOS, as well as metabolic and endometrial abnormalities.[27]

These findings were further reinforced by Chahal et al. in a cross-sectional study of multiple ethnic groups, in which East and South Asian females (in the 25–30 and >30 age groups) had elevated 2-hour insulin levels compared with Caucasian females. The subjects were matched for BMI and age.[26]

In a study of different phenotypes of PCOS in Sri Lankan females of reproductive age, Wijeyaratne et al. compared females with PCOS and MetS with those with PCOS alone. Both groups were found to have similar testosterone concentrations. Nevertheless, those with PCOS and MetS had higher BMI, blood pressure (BP), fasting plasma glucose, insulin, and triglycerides and lower high-density lipoprotein (HDL) and sex hormone–binding globulin (SHBG).[12] They also found that obesity was more common in the patients with oligomenorrhea with PCOS and compared with the PCOS and control group, acanthosis nigricans (AN), a strong marker of IR, was more prevalent in the patients exhibiting both PCOS and MetS. In fact, they performed a multivariate logistic regression on patients with PCOS, which suggested that factors such as age 35 years or older, BMI 25 kg/m^2 or greater, and AN can be used as predictors of having MetS. Furthermore, other predictors that resulted in a higher risk of having MetS were found using case-control comparison. These included a high waist circumference, high diastolic BP, deranged fasting lipids, high fasting insulin, and increased testosterone levels.[12]

Sundararaman et al. investigated South Indian females with PCOS, looking at their glucose/insulin ratio and carotid artery intimal media thickness as markers of vascular disease. The remit was the assumption of South Asians having a predisposition to IR and MetS at an early age. They found that South Indian females with PCOS have greater IR and intimal medial thickness, and hence a higher risk of atherosclerosis.[28]

PCOS in South Asians has been positively associated with nonalcoholic fatty liver disease (NAFLD), which was particularly worse in patients with a high BMI and HA.[29] This was further supported by studies where IR and HA were independent risk factors in predicting the development of NAFLD in South Asian females with PCOS.[30] This has been used as proof to recommend screening in this particular group of females to improve early detection and instigate treatment.

There is also a significant finding of vitamin D deficiency in South Asian females with PCOS. Azhar et al. found a prevalence of vitamin D deficiency as high as 85% in this particular group of females.[31] This was supported in another study where the incidence of MetS in South Asian females with PCOS was associated with low vitamin D levels.[32]

Romitti et al. conducted a systematic review and meta-analysis to look at the association between PCOS and autoimmune thyroid disease (AITD).[33] They found that up to 40% of patients with PCOS were also diagnosed with AITD, with the risk being higher in Asian females with PCOS compared with other ethnicities.

South Asian patients would benefit from screening and subsequent counseling considering the increased risk of cardiometabolic disease within this population.

PCOS Fertility and Pregnancy

Subfertility is a well-recognized sequelae of PCOS because one key component of PCOS is oligo-ovulation/anovulation. Females with anovulatory infertility make up a large number of the patients who go to fertility clinics, and PCOS is the most common cause. It can be deduced from this that that a significant proportion of people receiving assisted reproductive techniques (ART) suffer from the condition.

This also applies to females of South Asian ethnic background. Compared with Caucasian females, those of South Asian origins have lower live birth rates after in vitro fertilization. Additionally, they see healthcare professionals earlier for reproductive difficulties and have worse symptoms of hirsutism, infertility, and acne.[34] In fact, fertility issues tend to manifest themselves at an earlier age compared with other ethnicities with worse outcomes after ART (reports showing 2.5 times lower success rates than their Caucasian counterparts).[35]

In addition, South Asian females with PCOS also have riskier pregnancies. They are at increased risk for cervical insufficiency and gestational DM (GDM) in pregnancy. Feigenbaum at el. performed a retrospective cohort study in which 2.9% of patients with PCOS had cervical insufficiency. Of that cohort of PCOS patients with cervical insufficiency, they demonstrated that South Asian and Black females were overrepresented, although the sample size was small.[36]

The higher risk profile in this group of females remains in the postnatal period, as found by Wijeyaratne et al. In a case control study of 274 Sri Lankan females with PCOS, the risk of developing MetS 3 years postpartum was significantly higher if the patient had GDM during their pregnancy.[37] The relationship between PCOS and GDM was further supported by Kousta et al. when they investigated PCO and irregular menstrual cycle in females who previously had been diagnosed with GDM.[38]

In the UK, females are stratified according to their preexisting risk and family history before being referred to a prenatal counseling clinic or even to have a glucose tolerance test.[39] Being of South Asian descent and having PCOS does not feature in that list. It may be time to review this and change the way these females are managed before pregnancy, during pregnancy, and in the postnatal period to improve their outcomes and long-term morbidity.

Physical Characteristics of PCOS in South Asian Females With PCOS and the Impact on Quality of Life

Health-related quality of life (HRQoL) and emotional and sexual well-being are important parameters to consider when assessing patients holistically. Unfortunately, PCOS can result in symptoms that affect these aspects of patients' lives, and they are difficult to measure objectively. It is a well-documented fact that patients with PCOS suffer more emotional distress than their counterparts who suffer from other chronic conditions, such as asthma, arthritis, or heart disease.[2] The actual changes associated with the syndrome, such as hirsutism, obesity, and acne, along with irregular cycles and infertility, are felt to cause more psychological distress. It is somewhat difficult to measure those parameters accurately.

South Asian females seem to demonstrate some slight differences where the physical characteristics of PCOS are concerned, compared with Caucasian females with PCOS. They are more likely to be hirsute with a higher Ferriman-Gallwey score and to display worse degrees of AN and acne.[40]

Interestingly, South Asian females were less perturbed by obesity and more distressed by hirsutism than Caucasian females.[41] This attitude toward obesity may be explained by cultural differences. South Asians have a different way of dressing, and their outlook on physical appearance and central obesity may be different from the Western world.

Nevertheless, Jones et al. demonstrated that South Asian females living in the UK had developed similar distress about their weight, pointing toward a shift in cultural beliefs when living in Western society.[2]

The negative side of not being concerned about central obesity, however, is that South Asian females have poor compliance with weight reduction strategies and physical exercise.[41] Obesity is a known factor in the development of MetS and is also linked to worse long-term morbidity. This should be a key area for education and change in this group of patients.

The genetics of PCOS is a complex subject with large gaps still existing in candidate genes. It is becoming apparent that ethnic variations will also be shown to demonstrate different gene expression as is becoming apparent in the South Asian population. The difference is wider than just genetics, however. This group of females seem to demonstrate worst features of PCOS that put them at risk for worse long-term morbidity and mortality. It is time that our guidelines in the UK and worldwide reflect this fact and incorporate measures to significantly reduce the risk for these patients.

TABLE 24.1   A comparison of the Prevalence of Polycystic Ovary Syndrome (PCOS) in Females of Reproductive Age Globally

Authors	Study Population	Prevalence
Kumarapeli et al. ©	South Asian women	6.3% (Rotterdam criteria)
Ding et al. ©	Chinese women	5.6% (Rotterdam criteria)
Chen et al. ©	Women in Southern China	2.2% (National Institutes of Health [NIH] criteria)
Moran et al. ©	Women in Mexico City, Mexico	6.0% (NIH criteria) 6.6% (Rotterdam criteria)
Goodarzi et al. ©	Mexican-American women	13%
Knochenhauer et al. ©	Caucasian women in Southeastern United States	4.7% (NIH criteria)
Knochenhauer et al. ©	Black women in Southeastern United States	3.4% (NIH criteria)
Vaduneme KO®	Nigerian women, Africa	5-10% (Rotterdam criteria)
Gabrielli L Ĝ	Brazilian women	8.5% (Rotterdam criteria)
Sarah C Hillman and Jeremy Dale Ą	Women in Great Britain	2.27% (Rotterdam criteria)
Richard Scott Lucidi, Medscape	Women in USA	4-12%

From Wolf WM, Wattick RA, Kinkade ON, Olfert MD. Geographical prevalence of polycystic ovary syndrome as determined by region and race/ethnicity. *Int J Environ Res Public Health*. 2018;15[11]:2589.

References

1. Hart R, Hickey M, Franks S. Definitions, prevalence and symptoms of polycystic ovaries and polycystic ovary syndrome. *Best Pract Res Clin Obstet Gynaecol*. 2004;18:671-683. Available at: https://doi.org/10.1016/j.bpobgyn.2004.05.001.
2. Jones GL, Palep-Singh M, Ledger WL, et al. Do South Asian women with PCOS have poorer health-related quality of life than Caucasian women with PCOS? A comparative cross-sectional study. *Health Qual Life Outcomes*. 2010;8:149. Available at: https://doi.org/10.1186/1477-7525-8-149.
3. Homburg R. Choices in the treatment of anovulatory PCOS. In: Balen A, Franks S, Homburg R, Kehoe S, eds. *Current Management of Polycystic Ovary Syndrome*. Cambridge, UK: Cambridge University Press; 2010:143-152.
4. Fauser BCJM, Tarlatzis, Fauser, et al. Revised 2003 consensus on diagnostic criteria and long-term health risks related to polycystic ovary syndrome. *Hum Reprod*. 2004;19:41-47. Available at: https://doi.org/10.1093/humrep/deh098.
5. Gambineri A, Pelusi C, Vicennati V, Pagotto U, Pasquali R. Obesity and the Polycystic Ovary Syndrome. *Int J Obes*. 2002;26:883-896. Available at: https://doi.org/10.1038/sj.ijo.0801994.

6. Reeves TJ, Bennett CE, Sweeney J, et al. We the People: Asians in the United States, Census 2000 Special Reports, Issued 2004. U.S. Census Bureau. Available at: https://www.scirp.org/(S(351jmbntvnsjt1aadkposzje))/journal/paperinformation.aspx?paperid=16896

7. Tran K, Kaddatz J, Allard P. *South Asians in Canada: Unity Through Diversity.* n.d. Available at: https://www150.statcan.gc.ca/n1/en/catalogue/11-008-X20050028455

8. Deleted in review.

9. Home - Office for National Statistics. *Coronavirus (COVID-19).* n.d. Available at: https://www.ons.gov.uk/. Accessed December 4, 2021.

10. *Ethnic Group, National Identity and Religion.* Office for National Statistics; n.d. Available at: https://www.ons.gov.uk/methodology/classificationsandstandards/measuringequality/ethnicgroupnationalidentityandreligion. Accessed December 4, 2021.

11. Rodin DA, Bano G, Bland JM, Taylor K, Nussey SS. Polycystic ovaries and associated metabolic abnormalities in Indian subcontinent Asian women. *Clin Endocrinol (Oxf).* 1998;49:91-99. Available at: https://doi.org/10.1046/j.1365-2265.1998.00492.x.

12. Wijeyaratne CN, Balen AH, Barth JH, Belchetz PE. Clinical manifestations and insulin resistance (IR) in polycystic ovary syndrome (PCOS) among South Asians and Caucasians: is there a difference? *Clin Endocrinol (Oxf).* 2002;57:343-350. Available at: https://doi.org/10.1046/j.1365-2265.2002.01603.x.

13. Wild S, Roglic G, Green A, Sicree R, King H. Global prevalence of diabetes: estimates for the year 2000 and projections for 2030. *Diabetes Care.* 2004;27:1047-1053. Available at: https://doi.org/10.2337/diacare.27.5.1047.

14. Kaushal R, Parchure N, Bano G, Kaski JC, Nussey SS. Insulin resistance and endothelial dysfunction in the brothers of Indian subcontinent Asian women with polycystic ovaries. *Clin Endocrinol (Oxf).* 2004;60:322-328. Available at: https://doi.org/10.1111/j.1365-2265.2004.01981.x.

15. Siddamalla S, Govatati S, Venu VK, et al. Association of genetic variations in phosphatase and tensin homolog (PTEN) gene with polycystic ovary syndrome in South Indian women: a case control study. *Arch Gynecol Obstet.* 2020;302:1033-1040. Available at: https://doi.org/10.1007/s00404-020-05658-4.

16. Tumu VR, Govatati S, Guruvaiah P, Deenadayal M, Shivaji S, Bhanoori M. An interleukin-6 gene promoter polymorphism is associated with polycystic ovary syndrome in South Indian women. *J Assist Reprod Genet.* 2013;30:1541-1546. Available at: https://doi.org/10.1007/s10815-013-0111-1.

17. Reddy TV, Govatati S, Deenadayal M, Sisinthy S, Bhanoori M. Impact of mitochondrial DNA copy number and displacement loop alterations on polycystic ovary syndrome risk in south Indian women. *Mitochondrion.* 2019;44:35-40. Available at: https://doi.org/10.1016/j.mito.2017.12.010.

18. Branavan U, Wijesundera S, Chandrasekaran V, Arambepola C, Wijeyaratne C. In depth analysis of the association of FTO SNP (rs9939609) with the expression of classical phenotype of PCOS: A Sri Lankan study. *BMC Med Genet.* 2020;21:30. Available at: https://doi.org/10.1186/s12881-020-0961-1.

19. Guruvaiah P, Govatati S, Reddy TV, et al. The VEGF +405 G>C 5' untranslated region polymorphism and risk of PCOS: a study in the South Indian Women. *J Assist Reprod Genet.* 2014;31:1383-1389. Available at: https://doi.org/10.1007/s10815-014-0310-4.

20. Guo Q, Kumar TR, Woodruff T, Hadsell LA, DeMayo FJ, Matzuk MM. Overexpression of mouse follistatin causes reproductive defects in transgenic mice. *Mol Endocrinol.* 1998;12:96-106. Available at: https://doi.org/10.1210/mend.12.1.0053.

21. Mather JP, Moore A, Li RH. Activins, inhibins, and follistatins: further thoughts on a growing family of regulators. *Exp Biol Med.* 1997;215:209-222. Available at: https://doi.org/10.3181/00379727-215-44130.

22. Urbanek M. The genetics of the polycystic ovary syndrome. *Nat Clin Pract Endocrinol Metab.* 2007;3:103-111. Available at: https://doi.org/10.1038/ncpendmet0400.

23. Dasgupta S, Pisapati SVS, Kudugunti N, Godi S, Kathragadda A, Reddy MM. Does follistatin gene have any direct role in the manifestation of polycystic ovary syndrome in Indian women. *J Postgrad Med.* 2012;58:190-193. Available at: https://doi.org/10.4103/0022-3859.101386.

24. Deleted in review.

25. Apridonidze T, Essah PA, Iuorno MJ, Nester JE. Prevalence and characteristics of the metabolic syndrome in women with polycystic ovary syndrome. *J Clin Endocrinol Metab.* 2005;90(4):1929-1935. Available at: https://doi.org/10.1210/jc.2004-1045.

26. Chahal N, Quinn M, Jaswa EA, Kao CN, Cedars MI, Huddleston HG. Comparison of metabolic syndrome elements in White and Asian women with polycystic ovary syndrome: results of a regional, American cross-sectional study. *F S Rep.* 2020;1:305-313. Available at: https://doi.org/10.1016/j.xfre.2020.09.008.

27. Kudesia R, Illions EH, Lieman HJ. Elevated prevalence of polycystic ovary syndrome and cardiometabolic disease in South Asian infertility patients. *J Immigr Minor Heal.* 2017;19:1338-1342. Available at: https://doi.org/10.1007/s10903-016-0454-7.

28. Sundararaman PG, Manomani R, Sridhar GR, Sridhar V, Sundaravalli A, Umachander M. Risk of atherosclerosis in women with polycystic ovary syndrome: a study from South India. *Metab Syndr Relat Disord.* 2003;1:271-275. Available at: https://doi.org/10.1089/1540419031361435.

29. Shengir M, Krishnamurthy S, Ghali P, et al. Prevalence and predictors of nonalcoholic fatty liver disease in South Asian women with polycystic ovary syndrome. *World J Gastroenterol.* 2020;26:7046-7060. Available at: https://doi.org/10.3748/wjg.v26.i44.7046.

30. Harsha Varma S, Tirupati S, Pradeep TVS, Sarathi V, Kumar D. Insulin resistance and hyperandrogenemia independently predict nonalcoholic fatty liver disease in women with polycystic ovary syndrome. *Diabetes Metab Syndr Clin Res Rev.* 2019;13:1065-1069. Available at: https://doi.org/10.1016/j.dsx.2018.12.020.

31. Azhar A, Abid F, Rehman R. Polycystic ovary syndrome, subfertility and vitamin D deficiency. *J Coll Physicians Surg Pak.* 2020;30:545-546. Available at: https://doi.org/10.29271/jcpsp.2020.05.545.

32. Tuz F, Aalpona Z Association of Vitamin D Status with Metabolic Syndrome and its Components in Polycystic Ovary Syndrome. *Mymensingh Med J.* 2019;28(3):547-552.

33. Romitti M, Fabris VC, Ziegelmann PK, Maia AL, Spritzer PM. Association between PCOS and autoimmune thyroid disease: a systematic review and meta-analysis. *Endocr Connect.* 2018;7:1158-1167. Available at: https://doi.org/10.1530/EC-18-0309.

34. Mehta J, Kamdar V, Dumesic D. Phenotypic expression of polycystic ovary syndrome in South Asian women. *Obstet Gynecol Surv.* 2013;68:228-234. Available at: https://doi.org/10.1097/OGX.0b013e318280a30f.

35. Palep-Singh M, Picton HM, Yates ZR, Barth J, Balen AH. Polycystic ovary syndrome and the single nucleotide polymorphisms of methylenetetrahydrofolate reductase: a pilot observational study. *Hum Fertil.* 2007;10:33-41. Available at: https://doi.org/10.1080/14647270600950157.

36. Feigenbaum SL, Crites Y, Hararah MK, Yamamoto MP, Yang J, Lo JC. Prevalence of cervical insufficiency in polycystic ovarian syndrome. *Hum Reprod.* 2012;27:2837-2842. Available at: https://doi.org/10.1093/humrep/des193.

37. Wijeyaratne CN, Waduge R, Arandara D, et al. Metabolic and polycystic ovary syndromes in indigenous South Asian women with previous gestational diabetes mellitus. *BJOG*. 2006;113:1182-1187. Available at: https://doi.org/10.1111/j.1471-0528.2006.01046.x.

38. Kousta E, Cela E, Lawrence N, et al. The prevalence of polycystic ovaries in women with a history of gestational diabetes. *Clin Endocrinol (Oxf)*. 2000;53:501-507. Available at: https://doi. org/10.1046/j.1365-2265.2000.01123.x.

39. NICE. Overview | Diabetes in Pregnancy: Management from Preconception to the Postnatal Period. NICE - National Institute for Health and Care and Excellence. n.d. Available at: https:// www.nice.org.uk/guidance/ng3.

40. Afifi L, Saeed L, Pasch LA, et al. Association of ethnicity, Fitzpatrick skin type, and hirsutism: a retrospective cross-sectional study of women with polycystic ovarian syndrome. *Int J Womens Dermatol*. 2017;3:37-43. Available at: https://doi.org/10.1016/j. ijwd.2017.01.006.

41. Kumarapeli VL, De A Seneviratne R, Wijeyaratne CN. Health-related quality of life and psychological distress in polycystic ovary syndrome: a hidden facet in South Asian women. *BJOG*. 2011;118:319-328. Available at: https://doi.org/10.1111/j.1471-0528.2010.02799.x.

25

Situation Analysis of Polycystic Ovary Syndrome in Central and East Asia

REHANA REHMAN, FAIZA ALAM, AND RAKHSHAAN KHAN

Asia has the largest area, covering approximately one-third of the total land area of Earth, and the population as of 2021 is around 4.68 billion.[1] There are five main regions of Asia: Central Asia, East Asia, South Asia, Southeast Asia, and Western Asia. North Asia is now being defined to include Siberia and the northeastern parts. The countries included in these five regions have different demographics, ethnicities, cultures, and prevalence and pattern of diseases.

Understanding Polycystic Ovary Syndrome in the Region

Polycystic ovary syndrome (PCOS) affects almost 6% to 10% of reproductive-age females globally, with reproductive and metabolic dysfunction such as obesity, impaired glucose tolerance, acne, hirsutism, and anovulatory cycles all occurring simultaneously.[2] One well-established cause for PCOS is genetics, but the phenotypic manifestations cannot be neglected. When considering various ethnicities globally, East Asian females have a lower prevalence of PCOS compared with Caucasian females. The ethnic groups also respond differently to treatment regimens.[3]

Prevalence

The prevalence of PCOS is established on the basis of the diagnostic criteria used for a particular set of population. Choice of diagnostic criteria may affect the prevalence from 1.6% to 18% in the similar population under study, which shows that a number of patients are unaware and ultimately untreated because of this ambiguity.[4]

Factors Influencing the Prevalence, Diagnosis, and Management of PCOS

The social and physical conditions prevalent in the environment show a vital role in fabricating the health, disease, and injury patterns in a given population. The factors that directly or indirectly affect the prevalence, diagnosis, and management of PCOS include ethnicity, the healthcare system, the types of prevalent health medicines, the health-seeking behaviors (HSBs) of the population, food culture and habits, the accessibility and affordability of services, lifestyle patterns, and the prevalence of the disease itself.

Ethnicity

Genome-wide association studies are carried out to assess the association of a risk factor involved in the development of PCOS. Similar risk factors may be present in two different groups presenting with the same complaints. Generally, hirsutism is a less predominant feature in East Asians, and the cutoff score used for diagnosis is lesser than that for Caucasians, whereas the feature of irregular menstrual cycles is a usual presentation in East Asians but not in Caucasians. A higher measure of insulin resistance (IR) is a cross-cutting feature across all ethnicities. East Asian females showed a lower prevalence of body mass index (BMI) and metabolic errors; however, the incidence of diabetes mellitus (DM) suggested metabolic complications.[5]

The prevalence of PCOS is lower in certain East Asian groups (e.g., Korean, Chinese and Thai females) (about 5%) compared with Caucasian females (11%–20%). Ethnic differences should be considered in treatment plans because different ethnic groups respond differently.[3]

Lifestyle Behavior and Food Habits of PCOS Patients

Lifestyles often reflect diet and exercise. Both these factors lead to increased fat content in the body and instigate IR. The pathogenesis of PCOS is very much dependent on the oxidative milieu in the body leading to the manifestation of these factors. Dietary preferences are specific to every society. For example, fish is a much beloved staple diet of some ethnic groups; other groups, however, like to consume more rice or fatty food traditionally. Similarly, in some societies, fancy drinks and fast food are considered the custom. A diet made up of high fiber antiinflammatory components and less refined carbohydrates and trans fats will have less oxidative stress in the body and will imprint its effect on corrections in the hormonal profile of PCOS patients. Polycystic patients have frequently been diagnosed with heart disease, impaired glucose tolerance, and metabolic syndrome (MetS). Quite a large number express obesity, which is either because of genetic make-up or because of lifestyle and environmental factors. The levels of oxidative stress in a specific society might reflect their cultural consumption of certain dietary factors and thus might show a prominent association with certain diseases like obesity and cardiovascular disease.[6]

Central Asia

Central Asia is the most neglected region of Asia and remained under the influence of the Soviet Union until 1991. There are five countries in this region: Tajikistan, Uzbekistan, Kazakhstan, Turkmenistan, and Kyrgyzstan.

The Healthcare System in Central Asia

Since independence, the countries in Central Asia have confronted unfavorable political and economic conditions to pull themselves out of the centralized Soviet health system model. Strategies to improve standards and quality of care are being implemented in each country. So far, there is little documentation of female health in this region.[7] Demographic details are given in Table 25.1.

Health-Seeking Behaviors

Since 1990, each country has developed its own health sector reforms that are still struck up because of budget constraints, lack of training of health personnel, and resources for services. In an evaluation conducted in different countries, the raised mortality and morbidity figures are because of self-medication and the cost of treatment. There is remarkably little published research on patterns of health and its determinants in the region (EN: Healthcare).[8]

Prevalence of PCOS and Women's Health

Women's health, with reference to maternal and neonatal health indicators, has received attention in the last two decades. Research publications on women's health are found on issues other than PCOS. The prevalence of PCOS in Central Asia, according to 16 reviewed research papers, is 14.24%.[9] The "Global Burden of Disease Study" in 2016 revealed a prevalence of 42% in Kazakhstan.

Lifestyle Behaviors

The lifestyle habits of the Central Asian "nomads" are evident from their environmental conditions, local economy, and by the rituals and religious views regarding what may be consumed. They raise their livestock and their diet is mostly made up of milk, milk products, and meat. In addition to fruits and vegetables, dry fruits are also richly consumed.

Impact of Culture on Health-Seeking Behavior

Data on the HSBs among the population subgroups in Central Asia are scanty. Because of various political, geographic, and economic instabilities, more than one-half of the people opt for self-medication, believing that health problems will subside on their own. The cost of treatment is also beyond affordability, and the health facilities are either closed, too far, or unable to provide quality service.[8,10]

Psychological Impact

Access to "quality healthcare services for all" is a challenge to policy makers in this region. This is important not only from the perspective of human development but also from the perspective of human rights because the development prospects of the republics of Central Asia rest on their human, social, and intellectual capital.

East Asia

East Asia is spread over an area of 4,571,092 square miles and the inhabitants number more than 1.641 billion. There are eight countries included in the region of East Asia: People's Republic of China (ROC), Japan, Mongolia, North Korea, South Korea, Hong Kong, Macau, and Taiwan. The latter three are Chinese autonomous regions that have their own political system and economy (Table 25.2).

TABLE 25.1	Health Profile of Countries Included in Central Asia						
	CPR	EmOC Facility	ANC %	SBA %	CS %	IMR (as of 2020)	MMR (Ratio)
Kazakhstan	53 (2018)	245	99 (2015)	100 (2018)	11.5	9	9 (2015)
Kyrgyzstan	39 (2018)	71	100 (2018)	100 (2018)	58.36	16	30 (2016)
Tajikistan	29 (2017)	88	92 (2017)	95 (2017)	2.8	28	7 (2016)
Turkmenistan	50 (2019)	59	100 (2019)	100 (2016)	4	36	3 (2015)
Uzbekistan	65 (2006)	2775	99 (2015)	100 (2018)	6.3	13	18 (2016)

ANC, Antenatal care; *CPR*, contraceptive prevalence rate; *CS*, Cesarean section; *EmOC*, emergency obstetric care; *IMR*, Infant mortality rate (per 1000 live births); *MMR*, maternal mortality ratio (per 1000 live births); *SBA*, skilled birth attendance.

Rehman, R., Alam, F. and Khan, R., 2022. *World Bank Open Data | Data*. [online] Data.worldbank.org. Available at: <https://data.worldbank.org/> [Accessed 7 October 2022].

TABLE 25.2	Health Profile of Countries included in East Asia						
	Crude death rate (as of 2020)	IMR (as of 2020)	Neo MR (as of 2020)	≤5 MR (as of 2020)	ANC %	SBA%	MMR (Ratio)
China	7	6	4	7	100 (2018)	100 (2016)	27 (2013)
Hong Kong	7	NA	NA	NA	NA	100 (2005)	NA
Japan	11	2	0.84	3	100	100 (2018)	4 (2014)
Macau	4	NA	NA	NA	NA	100 (2004)	NA
Mongolia	6	13	8.14	15	99 (2018)	99 (2018)	49 (2016)
North Korea	9	12	2	17	100 (2017)	100 (2017)	8 (2016)
South Korea	6	3	NA	3	98.1	100 (2015)	11 (2016)
Taiwan	7.89	3.42	NA	4.33	NA	NA	NA

IMR, Infant mortality rate (per 1000 live births); *Neonate MR*, neonate mortality rate; *≤5 MR*, under 5 mortality rate; *ANC*, antenatal care; *SBA*, skilled birth attendance; *MMR*, maternal mortality ratio (per 100,000 live births); *NA*, not available

Rehman, R., Alam, F. and Khan, R., 2022. *World Bank Open Data | Data*. [online] Data.worldbank.org. Available at: <https://data.worldbank.org/> [Accessed 7 October 2022].

China

The population of China is around 1.37 billion, which equals 18.47% of the world population (2021) (http://srv1.worldometers.info/world-population). The human development index (HDI) ranking for China is medium (HDRO).[11]

Factors influencing the Prevalence, Diagnosis, and Management of PCOS in China

The factors that directly or indirectly affect the prevalence, diagnosis, and management of PCOS in China include ethnicity, health systems, types of healthcare, and health beliefs.

Ethnicity

China is a large united multinational state and includes 56 ethnic groups. Of these, 91.59% are Han Chinese.[12] Evidence-based research has shown the effects of ethnicity on the clinical features of PCOS.

Health Systems

More than one-half of the Chinese population resides in mountainous areas of China that have limited health resources and access to the primary healthcare system. There were many gaps in the Western health system that have been addressed by the 2009 reforms, improving many indexes on maternal and neonatal care.

Types of Healthcare

China provides two types of healthcare: the public system, which uses Western medicine, and the private system, which uses both Western and traditional Chinese medicine (TCM). People in China have the right to select the type of care they prefer (Fig. 25.1).
- The *Western healthcare system* provides services to almost 95% of the population in both public and private medical centers and hospitals. The "Healthy China 2020" initiative aims to include the older cohort of people suffering from chronic diseases. The use of services, however, depends on the HSB of the population.
- *TCM*, accompanied with a variety of allied practices, recommends lifestyle changes, electroacupuncture, herbs, and acupuncture treatments to bypass the use of harmful pharmaceutical drugs or invasive surgery. TCM practitioners prescribe herbal medicine to balance the energies of the body. Herbology, along with diagnostics, makes up the bulk of TCM.
- *Traditional Chinese healing* includes acupuncture, massage, therapies based on the theories of vital energies, and diet. Massage carried out by a "Tui na" practitioner aims to stimulate acupressure points.

Chinese Health Beliefs and Their Impact on Healthcare

Chinese believe that "yin and yang" are two environment forces that control people's health and energy balance.[13] They believe that TCM is more compatible with these forces than Western medicine. These beliefs favor self-medication or consultation with a TCM practitioner and limit the use of public health services.

Health Beliefs That Have Impacted the Minds of Health Educators

Research has shown that the perceptions of nurse educators in regards to acquiring or maintaining good health are subject to their cultural health beliefs and affect their teachings and practices.[14]

Health-Seeking Behaviors of the Older Cohort of the Chinese Population and How They Impact the Health Behaviors of Families

Various sociocultural factors affect HSBs that are different for each country in East Asia.[15] As of 2018, 17.9% of the

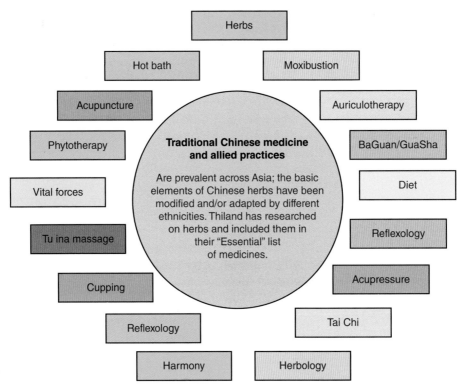

• **Fig. 25.1** Traditional/Classical Chinese Medicine and Allied Practices Prevalent Across Asia, Also Used for Polycystic Ovary Syndrome (PCOS).

Chinese population was 60 years of age or older.[16] According to Chinese culture, this cohort is the ruler of the house and determines the HSB of the family. They themselves have a firm belief in self-medication and may opt for TCM, considering it spirituality. This is part of why primary healthcare services are underutilized.

Health Risk Behaviors of the Older Cohort

The older cohort is a big challenge for China to organize a "Healthy Aging" model for the construction of "Healthy China." Evidence-based results showed that, in the event of sickness, almost half of the rural population did not seek medical care. The decision-making elders in the house did not feel the need to visit a health center and preferred self-medication. There is a need for awareness sessions to change the opinions of older people.[17] Older adults are involved in behaviors that may present a personal risk to their health, such as smoking, physical inactivity, unhealthy dietary behaviors, and sleep disorders. Approximately 77.2% of these behaviors show the tendency to be "modified."[18] Only 10% of the youth was involved in eHealth behaviors, primarily to look for health information.[19]

Food Culture

Diet is a tool in Chinese medicine that is believed to be crucial to treat PCOS. In Asian culture, PCOS is considered a "cold and damp" disease because it causes problems in the spleen. Soup is therefore preferred over smoothies, juice, or yogurt for breakfast to keep the gut warm. There are a number of recommendations for treating PCOS through food.

Foods to be Avoided in PCOS. Foods to be avoided in PCOS include dairy (even yogurt), soy, white wheat flour, sugar, white potatoes, fried foods, sweeteners of any kind, cold beverages (e.g., ice water, iced coffee), smoothies, juices, and frequent/daily use of salads.

Foods Recommended to Prevent Disease, Especially in PCOS. In the Chinese culture, the consumption of root vegetables, steamed vegetables, soups, bone broth, cooked protein, warmer temperature beverages, and whole grains is believed to boost health and cure diseases such as PCOS.

Prevalence of PCOS in China

Evidence-based results suggest that in a single topographic area the occurrence and presentations of PCOS may vary among races and origins.[20]

Using the Rotterdam criteria, 5.6% of Chinese females were found to have PCOS[21] in contrast to 15% of females in the Western populations.[22] Even Southern Chinese females had the same prevalence rate of 5.6%,[21] Thai females were at 5.7%,[23] Sri Lankan females at 6.3%,[24] and Iranian females at 14.3%.[25]

Using the Rotterdam criteria, therefore, Chinese females had the lowest prevalence across all continents at 5.6%.[26]

PCOS Features in Chinese Females

PCOS and Hirsutism

When comparing different groups, Asian females were found to be less hirsute than Caucasians.[3]

PCOS Phenotypes

A large group showed a 5.6% prevalence of PCOS in Han Chinese females. Younger females were more likely to have PCOS and to present with menstrual irregularities, hyperandrogenism (HA), polycystic ovarian (PCO) features on ultrasound, and infertility. Obese females also showed an increased risk of MetS and IR increasing with age.[21] Females in Southern China showed a 2.2% prevalence according to the 1990 National Institutes of Health (NIH) criteria.[27]

Pooled Prevalence Rates in China

The pooled prevalence rates of PCOS in China ranged from 0.45% to 35.14% and a combined conversion rate of 10.01%. Regional analysis revealed that the west had 13.35% prevalence, the east had 7.82%, the central region had 24%, and northeast China had 8.68% prevalence. The prevalence in infertile patients was 13.69%.[9]

Ethnic Comparisons

In a few Asian countries, the comparative PCOS prevalence figures ranged from 2% to 7.5% in China and 6.3% in Sri Lanka (nhp.gov.in).

Chinese females with PCOS in East Asia showed a reduced prevalence of impaired glucose tolerance and IR compared with Caucasian females.[28]

Trend of Prevalence Decreasing With Age

In a community-based cross-sectional survey using all three criteria, the trend in prevalence decreased with age, suggesting that PCOS is a temporary condition that decreases with age.[29]

PCOS With a History of Previous Gestational Diabetes Mellitus, Obesity, and Lipids

Using the revised ultrasound criterion, the prevalence of PCOS was higher in females with a previous history of DM during pregnancy. These patients also showed a risk of developing obesity and DM with raised fasting sugar and lipid profile levels.[30]

PCOS and High Risk of Diabetes

Females with PCOS had a higher risk of developing cardiac problems and DM 10 years earlier than non-PCOS women.[31]

PCOS and Obesity

An analysis of clinical and metabolic characteristics in obese Chinese females showed a higher lipid profile and a positive relation to IR.[32]

PCOS and Hyperandrogenism

The risk of having unfavorable pregnancy outcomes (delivery before term and hypertension) were twice as high in Chinese females with HA.[33]

Association of PCOS With Diabetes and Hypertension During Pregnancy and Preterm Delivery

Mothers with spontaneous and singleton pregnancies from the 32 provinces in China were assessed. PCOS females were at an increased risk for developing DM, hypertension, and preterm delivery.[34]

Taiwan

Taiwan has a population of approximately 24 million over an area of about 36,000 km^2. The native inhabitants are Han Chinese settlers who emigrated from Southeast Asia. The culture is therefore a mix of aboriginal, Taiwanese, and Chinese culture and is also heavily influenced by the modern culture of the West. The literacy rate is 98.2%. Taiwan, like Hong Kong, ranks high on the HDI.

Health Systems in Taiwan

Hong Kong, the Republic of Korea, and Taiwan are called the "Asian Tigers." The recent reforms developed by these countries have resulted in comparable standards in health statistics and provide valuable lessons to the remaining four countries in East Asia. Reforms in these regions include benefit packages, the approach to rate-setting for insured services, careful cost control, "rational" prescribing, and "cost-savings concessions to providers."[35]

Types of Healthcare

Both Western medicine and TCM are practiced in Taiwan. TCM is based on the same philosophy as in China. Traditional doctors define illness in terms of dynamic forces of the body, and weather conditions define a patient's emotional state. Doctors suggest a mix of herbal preparations and allied practices, such as acupuncture, to deal with illnesses.

Taiwanese Health Beliefs and Their Impact on Healthcare

The healthcare system in Taiwan provides high-quality care to 99% of its population. Nevertheless, religious beliefs also prevail and affect the HSB of the community. The prevalent belief is that illness is punishment for wrongdoing, and therefore an individual is often hesitant to let anyone know about their disease.

Cultural/Religious Beliefs Prevalent in Taiwan

The Taiwanese are superstitious about misfortunes on a few lunar dates; as such, they do not plan elective surgeries on the seventh lunar month of each year, which is known as the "Ghost Month." Similarly, no elective surgeries or emergent surgeries can fall on the eve of the Chinese New Year festival.[36]

PCOS: Prevalence and Features in Taiwanese Females

There are no national prevalence figures for PCOS. Research has been conducted in different geographic locations, hospitals, ethnic groups, and age groups.

PCOS and Depression

The Taiwanese database shows that younger females with PCOS (15–29 years) are at an increased risk for depression.[37]

Polycystic Ovary Morphology
PCO morphology (PCOM) on ultrasound is the most prominent feature of PCOS in Taiwanese females.[38]

PCOS and Hirsutism
Only 28% to 35% of Taiwanese females present with hirsutism.[38]

PCOS With Obesity, Body Mass Index, and Acne
A significantly notable relationship between BMI and serum total testosterone was observed in obese females. The features of acne were also less pronounced in overweight females compared with those who were not overweight.[39]

Obesity and Follicle-Stimulating Hormone to Luteinizing Hormone Ratios
Obese females with PCOS showed significantly lower luteinizing hormone (LH) to follicle-stimulating hormone (FSH) ratios compared with nonobese females. Similarly, a raised BMI was related to lower LH levels in females with PCOS.[40]

Hong Kong

Hong Kong is a small country with a size of 1110 km² and a population of over 7 million. A majority (93.6%) of residents are ethnic Chinese. The HDI of Hong Kong is high.

Healthcare System in Hong Kong
Hong Kong is one of the "Asian Tigers," who have set high standards of medical practice and have been accredited by the Royal College of Physicians and Surgeons of Canada. The healthcare system offers both public and private healthcare care. Public healthcare is free of charge or for a small fee.

Use of Traditional Chinese Medicine in Hong Kong
A survey in 2002 exploring the HSB of the Hong Kong population highlighted the need for TCM. The government has formulated a holistic Chinese medicine (CM) policy and incorporated CM as an integral part of the healthcare system in Hong Kong.

Prevalence of PCOS in Hong Kong
PCOS Features
Using the Rotterdam criteria for PCOS, the most prevalent features of PCOS identified in Hong Kong women were anovulation and hyperandrogenism (with other endocrine causes excluded), polycystic ovarian features on ultrasonography, luteinising hormone predominance, obesity, and insulin resistance (IR).

PCOS and Metabolic Syndrome
Chinese females with PCOS showed that MetS was prevalent in Hong Kong, and even when age and BMI were controlled, the risk for metabolic errors increased fivefold.[41]

PCOS and Risk of Diabetes
Hong Kong females with PCOS have a younger onset of DM, and the risk of developing type 2 DM is four times higher compared with those without PCOS.

Japan

In 2021, the population of Japan[1] was 125,932,148 and the area covered 364,555 km². All multiethnic background groups are considered to be Japanese in the population census of Japan. Japan occupies a high rank in the HDI.

Healthcare System in Japan
The life expectancy of Japanese citizens is longer than any other nation, possibly because of the focus of healthcare on preventative services. The food habits, composition of diet, and access to quality healthcare contribute to the longevity of population. Every individual in the Japanese medical system has direct access to a specialist. Japan is among four Asian countries whose health systems match the quality level of the health systems of the Western world.

Religious Options for Healthcare
Religious options for healthcare may involve visiting a priest to remove bad spells and requesting spell removers for special prayers.

Folk Remedies
Some folk remedies include hot sauna baths and herbal preparations and products, which are available at pharmacies without prescription. Traditional healing services and assistance are offered by herbalists and skilled providers of acupuncture and massage therapy.

Cultural Influences
TCM is also a part of Japanese culture. Chinese-style herbalists receive proper training in Japan to practice as licensed medical doctors in Japan.

Health Beliefs and Their Impact on Nurse Educators
The beliefs of clinical and academic nurses were assessed and showed that nurses were passing health information received from others to patients without any scientific evidence.[42]

Ethnicity
HA is not a predominant feature of Japanese females with PCOS, and thus it is not a part of the Japanese diagnostic criteria.[43] Instead, estimation of LH is considered.

Japanese Food Culture
According to the United Nations Population Division,[44] the life expectancy of Japanese females is the longest at 87 years. In Japanese culture, people do not overeat above 70% to 80% fullness. Additionally, their diet is simple and made up

of rice, noodles, or pasta with soup and fish. The Japanese are otherwise physically very active and drink plenty of water and tea. Japanese people have the lowest obesity rate (3%) among developed countries (Medscape).

The Prevalence of PCOS and Associated Features in Japanese Females

Prevalence

The prevalence of PCOS in Japanese females is 3% to 5%.[45]

PCOS and Obesity and Hirsutism

Although PCOS patients in Japan have lower rates of obesity and hirsutism, rates of androgen excess and IR are still comparable to the United States and Italy.[46]

PCOM and Type 1 Diabetes Mellitus

The presence of PCO features on ultrasound, higher levels of the androgen dehydroepiandrosterone sulfate (DHEA-S), and menstrual irregularities were higher in females with type 1 DM.[47]

Liver Enzymes and Body Mass Index as Risk Factors for PCOS

BMI and liver enzymes were significantly higher in PCOS patients.[47]

PCOS and Miscarriages

There was no evidence of any connection between PCOS and miscarriages in Japanese females who had two consecutive first trimester miscarriages.[48]

PCOS and Infertility Management With Metformin

Ovulation rates in clomiphene citrate (CC)–resistant infertile Japanese females with PCOS can be improved with the addition of a low-dose combination of metformin in three cycles of the CC regimen.[49]

North Korea

The population of North Korea is estimated to be 25,917,513.[1]

The natives are primarily Koreans. The health indicators are given in Table 25.2.

Healthcare System in North Korea

The free Western health system from farms to hospitals collapsed during the famine, and unregistered healing practices and practices in private hospitals blossomed. Herbal plants and traditional remedies became a common resort for those who had financial barriers to access either formal or informal healthcare personnel.

Women's Health Issues

Because of the political isolation of North Korea, the status of women is unclear. The government, however, claims that women have equal rights with men.

Ethnicity

The majority are native Koreans, with a few minor Chinese and Japanese groups.

North Korean Food

The staples tend to be rice or noodle dishes accompanied by kimchi (vegetables with every meal), bulgogi (when meat is available), and, of course, soju (soup). Recently North Korean beers have also become a part of North Korean culture. Korean ginseng tea is popular across the world as an antioxidant.

PCOS: Prevalence in North Korean Females

PCOS With Glucose Intolerance, Body Mass Index, and Lipid Profile in Korean Females

PCOS patients had 28 times greater glucose intolerance than general females. Similarly, skinny PCOS patients had 9.8 times higher glucose intolerance compared with age-matched Korean females without PCOS.[50]

South Korea

South Korea has a population of 51,323,965 and covers an area of 38,502 square miles. The country has a heterogeneous ethnicity with migrants from China, North America, Vietnam, Russia, the Philippines, and Uzbekistan.

Healthcare in South Korea

The healthcare in South Korea was rated as the second most efficient healthcare system in the world, providing free healthcare across the nation. Treatment is mostly more curative than preventive with more urban localization of health professionals. With an increase in the elderly population, there is a corresponding increase in health burden because of chronic degenerative diseases.

Ethnic Groups

Other than native Koreans, a minor group of Chinese also inhabit the country.

South Korean Food Culture

The main bulk of the South Korean diet, also known as the K-diet, is made up of large amounts of vegetables, legumes, and fish, consumed with rice.[51] Consumption of raw vegetables, such as lettuce, peppers, carrots, and cucumbers, is also very common.

PCOS: Prevalence and Features in South Korean Females

Prevalence of PCOS Subgroups in South Korean Females

Korean females with PCOS were found to have a lower BMI and serum sex hormone–binding globulin (SHBG) levels compared with Caucasian females. HA was also not a predominant feature, suggesting that Korean females could be at a lower risk for metabolic disorder compared with other ethnicities.[52]

Prevalence of PCOS in Youth

A 4.9% prevalence of PCOS was observed in students. The features of obesity and hirsutism were not common.[53]

PCOS and Inappropriate Gonadotropin Secretion

A negative correlation of inappropriate gonadotropin secretion with BMI was observed in PCOS patients.[54]

The Association of Diet With Depression in Korean Females With PCOS

The use of animal proteins was linked to mental health symptoms in Korean females.[55]

Dyslipidemia in Korean Females With PCOS

An association of adiponectin gene polymorphism with PCOS was responsible for dyslipidemia.[56]

Macau (Chinese Special Administrative Region)

Macau is a densely populated country with a blend of Eastern and Western culture. TCM is very popular, and the government has developed strategies to integrate international experience to develop TCM.

Healthcare in Macau

Healthcare in Macau has no international healthcare accreditation. There is one major public hospital, one private hospital, a university hospital, and a minor hospital in Macau. Basic care is provided through health centers that are free for residents. TCM is also available at these health centers.

Women's Health

No literature is available on women's health in Macau.

Conclusion

Central Asia, ever since its independence in 1991, is still in the process of implementing new health reforms and improving basic indicators like maternal and neonatal morbidities and mortalities. With the strengthening of the health system in the region, academic and research institutions will have the opportunity to explain the pattern of prevalent diseases such as PCOS.

Research in East Asia has identified the role of ethnicity, lifestyle patterns, cultural and religious beliefs, and the HSBs of the community as key health determinants in the area. The identification of PCOS, early diagnosis, and proper management can prevent the development of complications like infertility that add a huge cost to the health budget. With the prevalence of different types of healthcare, compliance to management often gets compromised; hence awareness of the problem coupled with health education and individual counseling is still a gray area that needs looking into.

References

1. Saharan T, Pfeffer K, Baud I Urban livelihoods in slums of Chennai: Developing a relational understanding. *Eur J Dev Res.* 2018;30(2):276–296.
2. Laven JS, Imani B, Eijkemans MJ, Fauser BC. New approaches to PCOS and other forms of anovulatory infertility. *Obstet Gynecol Surv.* 2002;57(11):755-767.
3. Huang Z, Yong EL. Ethnic differences: is there an Asian phenotype for polycystic ovarian syndrome? *Best Pract Res Clin Obstet Gynaecol.* 2016;37:46-55.
4. Amato MC, Galluzzo A, Finocchiaro S, Criscimanna A, Giordano CJ. The evaluation of metabolic parameters and insulin sensitivity for a more robust diagnosis of the polycystic ovary syndrome. *Clin Endocrinol.* 2008;69(1):52-60.
5. Kim JJ, Choi YM. Phenotype and genotype of polycystic ovary syndrome in Asia: ethnic differences. *J Obstet Gynaecol Res.* 2019;45(12):2330-2337.
6. Liepa GU, Sengupta A, Karsies D. Polycystic ovary syndrome (PCOS) and other androgen excess–related conditions: can changes in dietary intake make a difference? *Nutr Clin Pract.* 2008;23(1):63-71.
7. UNFPA. *A Review of Progress in Maternal Health in Eastern Europe and Central Asia (unfpa.org).* UNFPA; 2019.
8. McKee M, Healy J, Falkingham J. *Health Care in Central Asia.* London UK: Open University Press; 2002.
9. Wu Q, Gao J, Bai D, Yang Z, Liao Q. The prevalence of polycystic ovarian syndrome in Chinese women: a meta-analysis. *Ann Palliat Med.* 2021;10(1):74-87.
10. Omaleki V, Reed E. *The role of gender in health outcomes among women in Central Asia: a narrative review of the literature.* Paper presented at the Women's Studies International Forum; 2019.
11. Malik K. *Human Development Report 2014: Sustaining Human Progress: Reducing Vulnerabilities and Building Resilience.* New York: United Nations Development Programme; 2014.
12. Communiqué on Major Figures of the 2000 Population Census (No. 1). *National Bureau of Statistics of China.* 2002-04-23. Archived from the original on 2021-05-16. Retrieved 2021-05-16.
13. Capell J, Veenstra G, Dean EJ. Cultural competence in healthcare: critical analysis of the construct, its assessment and implications. *J Theory Constr Test.* 2007;11(1):30-37.
14. Cao R, Stone T, Petrini M, & Turale S. Nurses' perceptions of health beliefs and impact on teaching and practice: a Q-sort study. *Int Nurs Rev.* 2018;65(1):131-144.
15. Gupta VB. Impact of culture on healthcare seeking behavior of Asian Indians. *J Cult Divers.* 2010;17(1):13-19.
16. Ministry of Ecology and Environment of the People's Republic of China. *Regular Press Conference (September) September 29, 2018.* Paper presented at the 2018 Press Conference Records of Ministry of Ecology and Environment, the People's Republic of China. Springer; 2021.
17. Fang P, Han S, Zhao L, Fang Z, Zhang Y, Zou X. What limits the utilization of health services among the rural population in the Dabie Mountains-evidence from Hubei province, China? *BMC Health Serv Res.* 2014;14(1):1-7.
18. Yang Y, Wang S, Chen L, et al. Socioeconomic status, social capital, health risk behaviors, and health-related quality of life among Chinese older adults. *Health Qual Life Outcomes.* 2020;18(1):291.
19. Hong YA, Zhou Z. A profile of eHealth behaviors in China: results from a national survey show a low of usage and significant digital divide. *Front Public Health.* 2018;6:274.

20. Chang AY, Oshiro J, Ayers C, Auchus RJ. Influence of race/ethnicity on cardiovascular risk factors in polycystic ovary syndrome, the Dallas Heart Study. *Clin Endocrinol.* 2016;85(1):92-99.

21. Li R, Zhang Q, Yang D, et al. Prevalence of polycystic ovary syndrome in women in China: a large community-based study. *Hum Reprod.* 2013;28(9):2562-2569.

22. Fauser BC, Tarlatzis BC, Rebar RW, et al. Consensus on women's health aspects of polycystic ovary syndrome (PCOS): the Amsterdam ESHRE/ASRM-Sponsored 3rd PCOS Consensus Workshop Group. *Fertil Steril.* 2012;97(1):28-38.e25.

23. Vutyavanich T, Khaniyao V, Wongtra-ngan S, Sreshthaputra O, Sreshthaputra R, Piromlertamorn W. Clinical, endocrine and ultrasonographic features of polycystic ovary syndrome in Thai women. *J Obstet Gynaecol Res.* 2007;33(5):677-680.

24. Kumarapeli V, Seneviratne Rde A, Wijeyaratne CN, Yapa RM, Dodampahala SH. A simple screening approach for assessing community prevalence and phenotype of polycystic ovary syndrome in a semi-urban population in Sri Lanka. *Am J Epidemiol.* 2008;168(3):321-328.

25. Tehrani FR, Simbar M, Tohidi M, Hosseinpanah F, Azizi F. The prevalence of polycystic ovary syndrome in a community sample of Iranian population: Iranian PCOS prevalence study. *Reprod Biol Endocrinol.* 2011;9(1):1-7.

26. Ding T, Hardiman PJ, Petersen I, Wang FF, Qu F, Baio GJ. The prevalence of polycystic ovary syndrome in reproductive-aged women of different ethnicity: a systematic review and meta-analysis. *Oncotarget.* 2017;8(56):96351-96358.

27. Chen X, Yang D, Mo Y, et al. Prevalence of polycystic ovary syndrome in unselected women from southern China. *Eur J Obstet Gynecol Reprod Biol.* 2008;139(1):59-64.

28. Wei HJ, Young R, Kuo IL, Liaw CM, Chiang HS, Yeh CY. Prevalence of insulin resistance and determination of risk factors for glucose intolerance in polycystic ovary syndrome: a cross-sectional study of Chinese infertility patients. *Fertil Steril.* 2009;91(5):1864-1868.

29. Zhuang J, Liu Y, Xu L, et al. Prevalence of the polycystic ovary syndrome in female residents of Chengdu, China. *Gynecol Obstet Invest.* 2014;77(4):217-223.

30. Chan CC, Ng EH, Tang OS, Lee CP, Ho PC. The prevalence of polycystic ovaries in Chinese women with a history of gestational diabetes mellitus. *Gynecol Endocrinol.* 2006;22(9):516-520.

31. Ng NYH, Jiang G, Cheung LP, et al. Progression of glucose intolerance and cardiometabolic risk factors over a decade in Chinese women with polycystic ovary syndrome: a case-control study. *PLoS Med.* 2019;16(10):e1002953.

32. Shi Y, Guo M, Yan J, et al. Analysis of clinical characteristics in large-scale Chinese women with polycystic ovary syndrome. *Neuro Endocrinol Lett.* 2007;28(6):807-810.

33. Naver KV, Grinsted J, Larsen S, et al. Increased risk of preterm delivery and pre-eclampsia in women with polycystic ovary syndrome and hyperandrogenaemia. *BJOG.* 2014;121(5):575-581.

34. Li Y, Ruan X, Wang H, et al. Comparing the risk of adverse pregnancy outcomes of Chinese patients with polycystic ovary syndrome with and without antiandrogenic pretreatment. *Fertil Steril.* 2018;109(4):720-727.

35. Wagstaff A. Health systems in East Asia: what can developing countries learn from Japan and the Asian Tigers? *Health Econ.* 2007;16(5):441-456.

36. Chiu SL, Gee MJ, Muo CH, Chu CL, Lan SJ, Chen CL. The sociocultural effects on orthopedic surgeries in Taiwan. *PLoS One.* 2018;13(3):e0195183.

37. Harnod T, Chen W, Wang JH, Lin SZ, Ding DC. Association between depression risk and polycystic ovarian syndrome in young women: a retrospective nationwide population-based cohort study (1998-2013). *Hum Reprod.* 2019;34(9):1830-1837.

38. Hsu MI, Liou TH, Chou SY, Chang CY, Hsu CS. Diagnostic criteria for polycystic ovary syndrome in Taiwanese Chinese women: comparison between Rotterdam 2003 and NIH 1990. *Fertil Steril.* 2007;88(3):727-729.

39. Yang JH, Weng SL, Lee CY, Chou SY, Hsu CS, Hsu MI. A comparative study of cutaneous manifestations of hyperandrogenism in obese and non-obese Taiwanese women. *Arch Gynecol Obstet.* 2010;282(3):327-333.

40. Hsu MI. Clinical characteristics in Taiwanese women with polycystic ovary syndrome. *Clin Exp Reprod Med.* 2015;42(3):86-93.

41. Cheung L, Ma R, Lam P, et al. Cardiovascular risks and metabolic syndrome in Hong Kong Chinese women with polycystic ovary syndrome. *Hum Reprod.* 2008;23(6):1431-1438.

42. Stone TE, Kang SJ, Cha C, Turale S, Murakami K, Shimizu A. Health beliefs and their sources in Korean and Japanese nurses: a Q-methodology pilot study. *Nurse Educ Today.* 2016;36:214-220.

43. Sugimoto O. The Committee for Reproductive and Endocrine in Japan Society of Obstetrics and Gynecology. Annual report (1991-1992) for the determination of diagnostic criteria for polycystic ovary syndrome. *Acta Obstet Gynaecol Jpn.* 1993;45:1359-1367.

44. United Nations. Department of Economic, Social Affairs, Population Division. World Population Ageing. 2015;2015:1–164.

45. Baba T, Endo T, Ikeda K, et al. Distinctive features of female-to-male transsexualism and prevalence of gender identity disorder in Japan. *J Sex Med.* 2011;8(6):1686-1693.

46. Zhao Y, Qiao J. Ethnic differences in the phenotypic expression of polycystic ovary syndrome. *Steroids.* 2013;78(8):755-760.

47. Miyoshi A, Nagai S, Takeda M, et al. Ovarian morphology and prevalence of polycystic ovary syndrome in Japanese women with type 1 diabetes mellitus. *J Diabetes Investig.* 2013;4(3):326-329.

48. Sugiura-Ogasawara M, Sato T, Suzumori N, Kitaori T, Kumagai K, Ozaki YJ. The polycystic ovary syndrome does not predict further miscarriage in Japanese couples experiencing recurrent miscarriages. *Am J Reprod Immunol.* 2009;61(1):62-67.

49. Kurabayashi T, Suzuki M, Kashima K, et al. Effects of low-dose metformin in Japanese women with clomiphene-resistant polycystic ovary syndrome. *Reprod Med Biol.* 2004;3(1):19-26.

50. Lee H, Oh JY, Sung YA, Chung H, Cho WY. The prevalence and risk factors for glucose intolerance in young Korean women with polycystic ovary syndrome. *Endocrine.* 2009;36(2):326-332.

51. Kim SH, Kim MS, Lee MS, et al. Korean diet: characteristics and historical background. *J Ethnic Foods.* 2016;3(1):26-31.

52. Chae SJ, Kim JJ, Choi YM, et al. Clinical and characteristics of polycystic ovary syndrome in Korean women. *Hum Reprod.* 2008;23(8):1924-1931.

53. Byun EK, Kim IIJ, Oh JY, Hong YS, Sung YA. The prevalence of polycystic ovary syndrome in college students from Seoul. *J Korean Endocr Soc.* 2005;20(2):120-126.

54. Shim AR, Im Hwang Y, Lim KJ, et al. Inappropriate gonadotropin secretion in polycystic ovary syndrome: the relationship with clinical, hormonal and metabolic characteristics. *Korean J Obstet Gynecol.* 2011;54(11):659-665.

55. Kim SH, Kim HS, Park SH, Hwang JY, Chung HW, Chang NS. Dietary intake, dietary habits, and depression in Korean women with polycystic ovary syndrome. *J Nutr Health.* 2012;45(3):229-239.

56. Lee H, Byun EK, Park HR, et al. Adiponectin and ghrelin polymorphism in Korean women with polycystic ovary syndrome. *J Korean Endocr Soc.* 2006;21(5):394-401.

26

Situational Analysis of Polycystic Ovary Syndrome in Southeast Asia

RAKHSHAAN KHAN, FAIZA ALAM, AND REHANA REHMAN

Brunei

Also called Brunei Darussalam, Brunei has an area of 5765 km^2. It gained independence from the British Empire in 1984 and is a high-income country with vast petroleum and natural gas reservoirs. It is ranked second highest by the Human Development Index (HDI) among the Southeast Asian nations (Table 26.1).

Health Systems in Brunei

Brunei has a well-established public healthcare system, free of cost for nationals. Primary healthcare services are provided by the government and private hospitals and community health centers. Distinctive services are provided in the rural areas, and citizens are also sent abroad (https://www.everyculture.com/Bo-Co/Brunei-Darussalam.html).

Health-Seeking Behaviors

Health service utilization rates are reflected in terms of health indicators as shown in Fig. 26.1. The use of healthcare services by males, however, is less because it is considered a way of displaying masculinity.[1]

Women's Health

Women can share their health experiences in "Brunei Hive," a web portal aimed at improving the health and well-being of women. A "Primary Care Clinical Guide" is also available on women's health. There are subsidized packages of routine "women health screening services" for the three most common cancers among females in Brunei (breast, bowel, and cervical cancer), which are available in hospitals. Screening for polycystic ovary syndrome (PCOS) has been done on a yearly basis and was again restarted in 2020, out of a belief that it can lead to cancers.

Cambodia

Cambodia has an area of 181,035 km^2 and a population of 16,718,965. The Khmer are the largest of the ethnic groups in Cambodia, making up approximately 90% of the total population. Vietnamese and Chinese are other ethnic groups in Cambodia.

Health Systems in Cambodia

The Ministry of Health oversees health service delivery through a series of tiers from the primary to hospital levels. Health centers provide preventative and basic therapeutic services. Services are funded by the government and are supported by donor funding. Health reforms are being initiated to improve the mortality rates and to increase the life expectancy, tackle undernutrition, and prevent prevalent communicable diseases and emerging noncommunicable diseases.[2]

Maternal Health

Reforms are being initiated with donor support to improve maternal health indicators of mortality and morbidity. Statistics on the prevalence of PCOS are difficult to obtain.

East Timor (Timor-Leste)

East Timor is a lower-income country that has an area of 14,874 km^2 and a population of 1267,974. The Timorese are a racially mixed people that have both Melanesian and Malay genetic elements.

Health Systems in Timor-Leste

Independence-related violence destroyed and damaged health centers and hospitals in the public and private sectors.

TABLE 26.1	Key Health Indicators in Southeast Asian Countries						
Country	Pop (Millions) Ĝ	Crude β death rate	IMR β	Neo MR β	≤5 MR β	SBA % β	MMR (Ratio) β
Brunei	0.449	4.7	10	6	12	100	31
Indonesia	275.5	7	20	12	23	95	282
Cambodia	16.77	6	22	13	26	89	184
Philippines	115.6	6	21	13	26	84	206
Laos	7.5	6	35	22	44	64	217
Malaysia	33.9	5	7	5	9	100	23
Myanmar	54.2	8	35	22	45	60	244
Singapore	6.0	5	2	1	2	100	4
Thailand	71.7	8	7	5	9	99	24
Vietnam	98.2	6	17	9	21	94	42
Timor-Leste	1.3	6	37	19	42	57	129

IMR, Infant mortality rate; *MMR*, maternal mortality rate; *MR*, mortality rate; *SBA*, skilled birth attendant;
β https://data.worldbank.org/ 2020
Ĝ South-Eastern Asia Population 2022 (Demographics, Maps, Graphs) (worldpopulationreview.com)

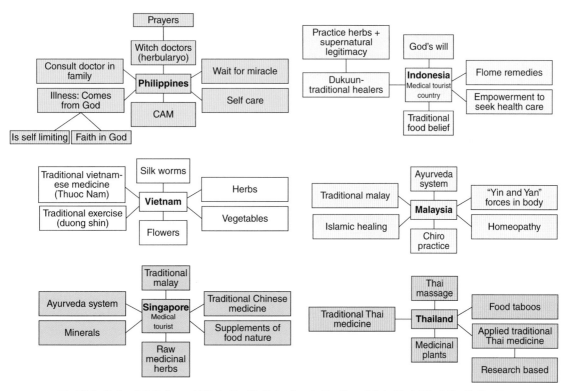

• **Fig. 26.1** Cultural Belief's and Ethnic Health Behaviors in Southeast Asia That Affect Health Seeking Behavior and Treatment. *CAM*, Complementary Alternative Medicine.

A majority of the health workers and medical professionals, who were Indonesian nationals, also left the country in 1999. In 2003, Cuba and Timor-Leste entered an agreement whereby hundreds of medical students in Timor-Leste studied medicine in Cuba on scholarships. Cuba also organized the placement of Cuban doctors in Timor-Leste to run the health facilities in the interim period. The World Health Organization (WHO), the United Nations Population Fund (UNFPA), UNICEF, and many international organizations are contributing to the development of health system infrastructure in Timor-Leste, as well as human resource training for delivery services.

Women's Health

The indicators related to women's health are given in Fig. 26.1. Because the country is struggling when it comes to even basic healthcare needs, no information on PCOS could be found from health desks.

Indonesia

Indonesia has an area of 1,904,569 km². The national census of 2020 revealed a population of 270.20 million, predominantly in Java.

Health Systems in Indonesia

Indonesia's community health system is organized into three tiers. A Puskesmas (public healthcare center) is the primary unit of function where trained nurses provide the most essential services, such as vaccinations, antenatal care, and wound care. The number of fully equipped public and private hospitals in 2019 was almost 2813, and they provide a wide range of services, including diagnosis and management of PCOS.

Prevalence of Polycystic Ovary Syndrome in Indonesia

PCOS is an endocrine problem related to reproductive-age females. PCOS is one of the causes of infertility in Indonesia, and the hospitals are equipped to deal with the situation. Prevalence of PCOS in Indonesia is estimated to be 5% to 10%.[3]

Polycystic Ovary Syndrome and Factors Affecting the Incidence of PCOS

PCOS often receives little attention because of unrecognized risk factors. The results of a study identified irregular menstrual cycles as the variable most related to the incidence of PCOS.[4]

Polycystic Ovary Syndrome and Infertility Management

A combination therapy using metformin and clomiphene citrate was used to treat PCOS patients, which improved the condition by decreasing the homeostatic model assessment for insulin resistance (HOMA-IR) and estradiol levels and the diameter of follicles in females with PCOS.[3]

Laos

Laos has an area of 236,800 km². The current population of Laos is 7,404,929 based on projections of the latest United Nations (UN) data, with 80% of the population living in rural areas.

Health Systems in Laos

Laos achieved political stability in 1975 at the end of a civil war. The healthcare system in Laos is still inadequate and unevenly distributed with a shortage of trained staff, scanty infrastructure/equipment, and few drug resources. Laos is dependent on global aid for immunization, training for medical and allied staff, and strengthening of maternal and child health (https://www.pacificbridgemedical.com/publication/healthcare-in-laos/). Laos still has the highest under-5 child mortality rate in Southeast Asia (https://www.unicef.org/eap/what-we-do/health).

Women's Health in Laos

Maternal and child health indicators are given in Fig. 26.1. No evidence-based research was found for PCOS in Laos.

Malaysia

The area of Malaysia is 329,847 km², and the size of the population in 2020 was 32,365,999. There are multiple ethnic groups that inhabit the country. Malaysia's HDI value for 2019 was very high and falls in the category of high-income countries.

Healthcare in Malaysia

Malaysia generally has an efficient and widespread two-tier system of healthcare: a public universal healthcare system running parallel with a private healthcare system. Although the services are free in the public healthcare system, with access to specialist services, a long waiting time may be an issue. Malays, Chinese, and Indians are the main ethnic groups in Malaysia.

Healthcare-Seeking Behavior in Malaysia (Research Studies)

Results of a survey revealed that Malaysians were the highest group who called on treatment for government health facilities. The Chinese sought more treatment from private hospitals. Educational status also affected healthcare-seeking behaviors. Those with less education preferred government facilities, and others opted for private clinics.[5] High self-medication was reported.[6]

Women's Health

A wide range of comprehensive women health screening services are available in the leading hospitals for different age groups. Additionally, there are exclusive women's clinics that offer a variety of women health services. Screening and management of PCOS are also available in hospitals in urban areas. Teleconsultation facilities are also functional and manned by a doctor or a senior healthcare provider.

Prevalence of Polycystic Ovary Syndrome in Malaysia

The prevalence of PCOS in Malaysia was obtained as 12.6%.[7]

Polycystic Ovary Syndrome and Dietary Supplements

The findings of one article recommended the use of vitamin D supplements in females with PCOS to decrease the chronic inflammation associated with PCOS. Studies have also shown improvement in PCOS symptoms with exposure to healthy gut bacteria, suggesting the use of prebiotics and probiotics as part of the treatment for PCOS.[8]

Polycystic Ovary Syndrome and Specific Phenotypes among Malaysian Female University Staff

The prevalence of PCOS was reported to be 12.6% in Malaysian employees, and they exhibited hyperandrogenism (HA) and polycystic ovaries; anovulation was confirmed in one patient. The diagnosis correlated with increased body mass index (BMI) and waist circumference, features of hirsutism and amenorrhea. This study showed dominance of explicit phenotypes of PCOS in these females.[7]

Prevalence of Metabolic Syndrome in Polycystic Ovary Syndrome

It was detected in 43.4% of females, who were predisposed to age and a family history of diabetes.[9]

Polycystic Ovary Syndrome and the Prevalence of Metabolic Syndrome and Hypertriglyceridemic-waist

The prevalence of hypertriglyceridemic-waist was 19.7% in PCOS subjects. Based on the International Diabetes Federation criteria, 97.5% participants with hypertriglyceridemic-waist suffered from metabolic syndrome (MetS).[10]

Polycystic Ovary Syndrome and Sexual Dysfunction

Sixty-two percent of patients had sexual disorders concerned with arousal and lubrication. Sexual dysfunction was also greater in patients with symptoms of depression, anxiety, and stress.[11]

Polycystic Ovary Syndrome and a Review of the Treatments

This systematic review revealed that lifestyle modifications and metformin treatment may result in improvements in insulin sensitivity and improve the outcome of the prevention strategies.[12]

Myanmar

The area of Myanmar is 676,578 km^2, and the population in 2021 was 54,903,837. Myanmar transitioned to a civilian government in March of 2011. The country has 135 ethnic groups recognized by the government.

Healthcare in Myanmar

Myanmar has one of the worst healthcare systems in the world, and the need for improvement in the system is paramount. The country is facing a shortage of medical professionals, and health allocations are not sufficient. International donors are coming in to strengthen the health system (https://borgenproject.org/healthcare-in-myanmar/). Maternal and neonatal health indicators are given in Fig. 26.1.

Philippines

The area of the Philippines is 300,000 km^2, and the 2020 population was 109,581,078. The culture of the Philippines is a combination of cultures of the East and West. According to the WHO, about 90% of Filipino males are circumcised, one of the world's highest circumcision rates.

Healthcare in the Philippines

Healthcare in the Philippines involves private, public, and barangay health centers. Only 30% of public sector health professionals cater to all the health requirements. Consequently, the national burden of healthcare is taken up by the expensive private health providers. Indicators for maternal and infant health are poor, as given in Fig. 26.1.

Prevalence of Polycystic Ovary Syndrome in the Philippines

There are little local data on the prevalence of PCOS in the Philippines. A study on Filipino females diagnosed with Endometrial Cancer showed a higher incidence of PCOS in these patients (https://seud.org/wp-content/uploads/2017/07/2-2548.pdf).

Polycystic Ovary Syndrome and Hirsutism

An association of biochemical HA with a modified Ferriman-Gallwey (mFG) score was observed in Filipino PCOS females; hirsute females had a higher mFG score of 7 or greater. Free testosterone was also found to be significantly related with hirsutism[13]

Singapore

The area of Singapore is 719.2 km^2, and the population was 5,925,000 in 2021. Singapore ranks high on the HDI with three medical schools and three types of hospitals.

Healthcare in Singapore

Singapore is famous for its exemplary healthcare standard, ranking among the best systems in Asia. The healthcare is supervised by the health ministry of Singapore. There are general hospitals, community hospitals, and specialist hospitals or institutions that provide the fullest range of PCOS diagnostic and treatment services. Private and public sector services are accessible to all citizens. Teleconsulting facilities are also available. A women's forum is available for advisory services. Traditional Chinese medicine (TCM), acupuncture, homeopathy, naturopathy, osteopathy, and complementary medicine are all provided by registered practitioners.

Prevalence of Polycystic Ovary Syndrome in Singapore

In fact, up to 10% of females in Singapore may have PCOS (https://www.womensweekly.com.sg/gallery/beauty-and-health/living-with-pcos-symptoms-polycystic-ovarian-syndrome/). In Singapore, PCOS is most commonly managed and followed up annually by gynecologists because there are some associated risks with PCOS, such as diabetes and heart disease.

Effect of Body Mass Index on Phenotypic Features of Polycystic Ovary Syndrome

Singapore PCOS patients had a higher BMI, increased hair growth, and higher mean differences in mFG scores, which explains the effect of BMI and PCOS on the free androgen index.[14]

Polycystic Ovary Syndrome and Lifestyle Management Practices

A study analyzed the importance of lifestyle modifications for PCOS in Singapore, in accordance with recent national and worldwide evidence-based guidelines.[15]

Thailand

Also known as "The Kingdom of Thailand," it has an area of 513,120 km², and the 2021 population was 69,799,978. The country's diverse geography, tourist-attracting landscape, and welcoming people are represented in the slogan "land of a thousand smiles." Buddhism is practiced in Thailand.

Healthcare in Thailand

Thailand has had "a long and successful history of health development."[16] Long-lasting, noncommunicable diseases and infectious diseases such as malaria and tuberculosis are some public health issues. Overseen by the Ministry of Public Health, the network of public hospitals provide universal healthcare to all in urban areas, although some rural areas lag far behind. Most doctors in Thailand are multilingual specialists and general practitioners are very few. Hospitals are equipped with the facilities of diagnosis and management of PCOS.

Other Types of Healthcare and Public Health Research

The public health perspective of Thai healthcare is reflected in research work carried out to evaluate public health initiatives.

Thai Traditional Medicine

People may opt for Thai traditional medicine (TTM), which, after research, is now successfully implemented in many modern hospitals in Thailand and known as applied TTM (ATTM).[17]

Medicinal Plants

The collaboration of the Ministry of Public Health, with other organizations in the "Medicinal Plants and Primary Health Care Project," adds medicinal plants to the National List of Essential Medicines.[18,19]

Health-Seeking Behaviors of the Community

Self-medication was observed to be the root cause of perceived minor illness.[20] Evaluation of health-seeking behaviors among healthcare providers in influenza-like illness revealed positive healthcare practices among health providers.[21]

Prevalence of Polycystic Ovary Syndrome in Thailand

In one study, the prevalence of PCOS in Thai adolescents was found to be 5.29%. Moderate acne was the strongest associated risk factor, although mild acne and oligo/amenorrhea also showed significant association.[22]

Polycystic Ovary Syndrome and Hyperandrogenism

Another study on PCOS patients in Thailand evaluated the relationship between clinical HA and biochemical HA (hyperandrogenemia). The majority were found to be presented with oligomenorrhea or amenorrhea and acne (56.6%). Two-fifths of the participants had high concentrations of serum-free testosterone (FT). A statistically significant correlation was observed between hirsutism and FT; hirsutism and total testosterone (TT); and acne and TT. Others had little or no correlations.[23]

Vietnam

The area of Vietnam is 331,210 km², and the 2020 population was 97,141,003. The Vietnamese culture is one of the oldest in Southeast Asia and is heavily influenced by

Chinese culture. Superstition is a part of the tradition and customs in Vietnam.

Healthcare in Vietnam

Healthcare in Vietnam is a combination of Eastern and Western medicine. Both public and private hospitals are located in big cities that are well equipped to provide quality services and are accessible. The public healthcare system is partially underfunded. Private hospitals charge more but provide quality services. Diagnostic and management services for PCOS are available in these hospitals. The healthcare system in Vietnam is presently oriented to a universal healthcare system. Today most residents in Vietnam have to pay for medical services themselves. Traditional Vietnamese medicine is also practiced, which is very similar to TCM.

Prevalence of Polycystic Ovary Syndrome in Vietnam

Polycystic Ovary Syndrome and Phenotype

The PCOS patients in Vietnam have a characteristic lean physique, hirsutism excluding the face, polycystic ovaries with anovulation, and characteristic PCOS serum hormone markers with low risk factors for MetS. Nonclassical phenotypes for PCOS were found to be significantly more frequent than the classic phenotype.[24]

Polycystic Ovary Syndrome: Awareness and Compliance

Countries like India, China, and Vietnam have started increased awareness campaigns focused on evidence-based recommendations for the management of PCOS and models for clinical care and screening with directed interventions.[25]

Polycystic Ovary Syndrome and Infertility Management

Research was carried out to induce ovulation using a low-dose step-up protocol along with recombinant follicle-stimulating hormone in Vietnamese patients with PCOS. It was observed that an initiation dose of 25 IU/day was safe for Vietnamese PCOS patients presenting with anovulation and low or normal BMI. This regimen proved to have high clinical and ongoing pregnancy rates.[26]

Conclusion

According to a WHO report published in 2000,[27] women's health issues in Southeast Asia need attention. Based on the report, donor agencies support the health systems to strengthen countries where gender issues and women's reproductive health need additional assistance. A paper published in 2018 reveals that the situation of women is still at a lower level.[28] An in-depth analysis of issues such as PCOS and their timely and appropriate management can reduce the burden on the health budget.

References

1. Idris DR, Hassan NS, Sofian N. Masculinity, ill health, health help-seeking behavior and health maintenance of diabetic male patients: preliminary findings from brunei darussalam. *Belitung Nurs J.* 2019;5(3):123-129.
2. Annear PL, Grundy J, Ir P, et al., World Health Organization. The Kingdom of Cambodia Health System Review. *Health Syst Transit.* 2015;5(2). https://apps.who.int/iris/handle/10665/208213.
3. Dzykryanka SM, Yulistani Y, Santoso BJ. Analysis of homa-IR, follicle size, and estradiol after combination therapy of metformin and clomiphene citrate in polycystic ovary syndrome's patient. *Folia Medica Indonesiana.* 2015;51(3):162-167.
4. Okta PP. *Faktor-Faktor Yang Mempengaruhi Kejadian Sindrom Ovarium Polikistik di RSUP Dr. M. Djamil Padang Tahun 2015-2019.* Diploma Thesis: Univeritas Andalas; 2020.
5. Amal N, Paramesarvathy R, Tee G, Gurpreet K, Karuthan C. Prevalence of chronic illness and health seeking behaviour in Malaysian population: results from the Third National Health Morbidity Survey (NHMS III) 2006. *Med J Malaysia.* 2011;66(1):36-41.
6. Dawood OT, Hassali MA, Saleem F, Ibrahim IR, Abdulameer AH, Jasim HH. Assessment of health seeking behaviour and self-medication among general public in the state of Penang, Malaysia. *Pharm Pract (Granada).* 2017;15(3):991.
7. Dashti S, Abdul Hamid H, Mohamad Saini S, et al. Prevalence of polycystic ovary syndrome among Malaysian female university staff. *J Midwifery Womens Health.* 2019;7(1):1560-1568.
8. Mohammed SB, Nayak B. Polycystic ovarian syndrome trend in a nutshell. *Int J Womens Health Reprod Sci.* 2017;5(3):153-157.
9. Ishak A, Kadir AA, Hussain NHN, Ismail SB. Prevalence and characteristics of metabolic syndrome among polycystic ovarian syndrome patients in Malaysia. *Int J Collab Res Intern Med Public Health.* 2012;4(8):1577-1588.
10. Bee Jr YT, Haresh KK, Rajibans S. Prevalence of metabolic syndrome among Malaysians using the International Diabetes Federation, National Education Program and modified World Health Organization definitions. *Malays J Nutr.* 2008;14(1):65-77.
11. Dashti S, Latiff LA, Hamid HA, et al. Sexual dysfunction in patients with polycystic ovary syndrome in Malaysia. *Asian Pac J Cancer Prev.* 2016;17(8):3747-3751.
12. Dashti S, Latiff LA, Zulkefli NAB, et al. A review on the assessment of the efficacy of common treatments in polycystic ovarian syndrome on prevention of diabetes mellitus. *J Family Reprod Health.* 2017;11(2):56-66.
13. Ilagan MKCC, Paz-Pacheco E, Totesora DZ, Clemente-Chua LR, Jalique JRK. The modified Ferriman-Gallwey score and hirsutism among Filipino women. *Endocrinol Metab (Seoul).* 2019;34(4):374-381.
14. Neubronner SA, Indran IR, Chan YH, Thu AWP, Yong EL. Effect of body mass index (BMI) on phenotypic features of polycystic ovary syndrome (PCOS) in Singapore women: a prospective cross-sectional study. *BMC Womens Health.* 2021;21(1):1-12.
15. Ko H, Teede H, Moran L. Analysis of the barriers and enablers to implementing lifestyle management practices for women with PCOS in Singapore. *BMC Res Notes.* 2016;9(1):1-11.
16. Wibulpolprasert S, Fleck F. Thailand's health ambitions pay off. *Bull World Health Organ.* 2014;92(7):472-473.
17. Fakkham S, Sirithanawutichi T, Jarupoonpol V, Homjumpa P, Bunalesnirunltr M. The integration of the applied Thai traditional medicine into hospitals of the current health delivery system: the development of an administrative/management model. *J Med Assoc Thai.* 2012;95(2):257.

18. Andrade C, Gomes NG, Duangsrisai S, Andrade PB, Pereira DM, Valentao P. Medicinal plants utilized in Thai Traditional Medicine for diabetes treatment: ethnobotanical surveys, scientific evidence and phytochemicals. *J Ethnopharmacol.* 2020;263: 113177.

19. Chotchoungchatchai S, Saralamp P, Jenjittikul T, Pornsiripongse S, Prathanturarug S. Medicinal plants used with Thai Traditional Medicine in modern healthcare services: a case study in Kabchoeng Hospital, Surin Province, Thailand. *J Ethnopharmacol.* 2012; 141(1):193-205.

20. Sangngern L, Kanchanakhan N, Somrongthong RJ. Health status and health seeking behaviours among the elderly in the Donmuang slum community, Bangkok, Thailand. *J Health Res.* 2014;28(3):205-210.

21. Chaipung B, Chapman RS. Health seeking behaviors in influenza-like illness among healthcare providers in angthong province, Thailand. *J Health Res.* 2014;28(2):127-134.

22. Kaewnin J, Vallibhakara O, Arj-Ong Vallibhakara S, et al. Prevalence of polycystic ovary syndrome in Thai University adolescents. *Gynecol Endocrinol.* 2018;34(6):476-480.

23. Leerasiri P, Wongwananuruk T, Indhavivadhana S, Techatraisak K, Rattanachaiyanont M, Angsuwathana S. Correlation of clinical and biochemical hyperandrogenism in Thai women with polycystic ovary syndrome. *J Obstet Gynaecol Res.* 2016;42(6):678-683.

24. Cao NT, Le MT, Nguyen VQH, et al. Defining polycystic ovary syndrome phenotype in Vietnamese women. *J Obstet Gynaecol Res.* 2019;45(11):2209-2219.

25. Garad RM, Teede H Polycystic ovary syndrome: improving policies, awareness, and clinical care. *Curr Opin Endocr Metab Res.* 2020;12:112-118.

26. Lan VTN, Norman RJ, Nhu GH, Tuan PH, Tuong HM. Ovulation induction using low-dose step-up rFSH in Vietnamese women with polycystic ovary syndrome. *Reprod Biomed Online.* 2009;18(4):516-521.

27. Kumar S. WHO draws attention to women's health in south-east Asia. *Lancet.* 2000;356(9233):922.

28. Feng C, Lai Y, Li R, et al. Reproductive health in Southeast Asian women: current situation and the influence factors. *Midwifery.* 2018;2(1):32-41.

27

Situation Analysis of Polycystic Ovary Syndrome in Western Asia

RAKHSHAAN KHAN, REHANA REHMAN, AND FAIZA ALAM

The population of Western Asia is dispersed into three belts or stretches. First, the Fertile Crescent is made up of nine countries: Iran, Iraq, Turkey, Syria, Lebanon, Israel, Palestine, Cyprus, and Jordan. Second, the north part of West Asia includes Georgia, Armenia, and Azerbaijan. Finally, the Arabian Peninsula includes Yemen, Oman, the United Arab Emirates, Bahrain, Qatar, Kuwait, and Saudi Arabia. Turkey is the most overcrowded country in Western Asia, whereas Cyprus is the least populous. The health situation in each country is given in Table 27.1.

Countries in the Northern Region of Western Asia

Republic of Armenia

Armenia has a population[1] of 2,969,323 and has an area of 28,470 km². The modern Republic of Armenia is a developing country that gained its freedom from the Soviet Union in 1991 and is 98% Armenian by ethnicity. Armenia is a nuclear weapon country that continues to make advancements in the fields of science, technology, and education.

Health Services Delivery System

The World Bank is providing advisory and financial support to improve health service delivery in Armenia. The health indicators are given in Table 27.1. As of 2018, there are 102 hospitals operating in Armenia, located in major cities, in addition to medical centers spread throughout the country. Rural centers have limited access to health. There are five Western and one traditional medical university in Armenia. Continuum of education is recommended for both doctors and nurses in the new health policy.

Women's Health

The new health policy has research initiatives to assess the gaps in indicators of maternal and neonatal health. Scholarly articles on women's health are available on a few topics prevalent in the country, but there is nothing on polycystic ovary syndrome

(PCOS). Nevertheless, diagnosis and management of PCOS are available in big hospitals in urban areas.

Azerbaijan

Azerbaijan has a population[1] of 10,244,502 with an area of 82,658 km². Liberated from the Soviet Union in 1991, Azerbaijan is facing economic difficulties in terms of managing finances.

Health Services Delivery System

Healthcare is the responsibility of the state. Services are provided in Azerbaijan through both public and private health facilities. International organizations (e.g., the United States Agency for International Development [USAID], the United Nations International Children's Emergency Fund [UNICEF], the World Health Organization [WHO], the World Bank) are providing support to improve health indicators. Nevertheless, the healthcare system in Azerbaijan still requires attention. Health indicators are given in Table 27.1.

Women's Health

Donor-driven research initiatives on indicators of maternal and neonatal health are available. Scholarly articles on women's health, especially PCOS, are not currently available.

Georgia

Georgia has a population[1] of 3,977,281 and an area of 69,490 km². It borders on Europe and is a member of many European organizations. It has a high-ranked medical school with an affiliated research institute that publishes scholarly articles in its journal.

Health Services Delivery System

Health is provided by the government through a comprehensive program to improve access to all citizens. Since May 2015, significant steps have been taken to strengthen the maternal and newborn healthcare system and to improve

TABLE 27.1   **Demographic and Health Profile of Countries Included in West Asia**

Country	Pop (Millions) ©	Crude death rate €	IMR €	Neo MR €	≤5 MR €	SBA % €	MMR (Ratio) €
Armenia	2.96	10	10	6	11	100	7 (2017)
Azerbaijan	10.3	8	17	10	19	99	12 (2017)
Bahrain	1.5	2	6	3	7	100	9 (2014)
Cyprus	1.2	7	2	2	3	98	0 (2016)
Egypt	111	6	17	10	20	92	15 (2015)
Georgia	3.7	13	8	5	9	99	14 (2018)
Iraq	44.5	5	21	14	25	96	60 (2013)
Iran	88.5	5	11	8	13	99	7 (2015)
Israel	9	5	3	2	4	99	2 (2017)
Kuwait	4.2	3	8	5	9	100	2 (2012)
Lebanon	5.4	5	6	4	7	98	46 (2018)
Oman	4.5	2	10	5	11	99	23 (2018)
Palestine	5.2	NA	NA	NA	NA	NA	NA
Qatar	2.69	1	5	4	6	100	0 (2016)
Saudi Arab	36.4	4	6	4	7	99	25 (1998)
Turkey	85.3	5	8	5	10	98	16 (2018)
UAE	9.4	2	6	4	7	100	2 (2009)
Yemen	33.7	6	46	28	60	45	137 (2013)

©Source: World Population Review (2022). https://worldpopulationreview.com/;
€Source: World Bank Open Data (2022). https://data.worldbank.org/
Crude death rate (per 1,000 live births); *IMR*: Infant mortality rate (/1000 live births); *Neo MR*: Neonatal mortality rate (/1000 live births); *≤5 MR*: Under-5 mortality rate (/1000 live births); *SBA*: Skilled birth attendance (%); *MMR*: Maternal mortality ratio (/100,000 live births –national estimates – year of estimate)

the health indicators. Doctors receive academic and clinical education at Georgia's medical school.

Women's Health

Various research initiatives focus on maternal and neonatal health indicators. Scholarly articles on women's health, especially PCOS, are not currently available.

Countries in the Fertile Crescent of Western Asia

Iraq

Iraq has a population[1] of 41,423,242 and an area of 434,320 km². The majority of people (three-fourth of the population) are ethnically Iraqi. The life expectancy is 74.9 years. The people of Iraq are mostly Arabs; Kurds and Turkmen are fewer in number.

Healthcare Delivery System

Healthcare in Iraq is central, with free healthcare provided to the population. Since the gulf crises, and because of poor attention on the part of the government toward the system, Iraq is struggling again to rebuild the health system, with financial and technical support being provided by the WHO.

Women's Health

Matters on the health of females (other than basic maternal indicators) have received due attention, and research has been conducted to understand the pattern of many diseases so as to provide appropriate diagnostic services and management.

PCOS: Prevalence and Features in Iraq

Prevalence in Infertile Couples

A case control study carried out in an infertility clinic in a teaching hospital in Iraq revealed that the incidence of infertility because of PCOS is about 12%.[2]

Iran

The country has a population[1] of 85,286,927 and an area of 1,628,550 km². The inhabitants are mainly Iranians, with a minority mix of refugees from Afghanistan and Iraq. Iran produces medical graduates through a system of schools.

Healthcare Delivery System

Iran has a well-established system of providing healthcare that reaches the deeper grassroot levels of the population. Doctors receive medical education and training in both public and private hospitals in the country. In rural areas, primary services are provided through midwives who are in charge of maternal care services (skilled birth attendance). In bigger cities, hospitals meet international standards with well-trained medical staff and are fully equipped to identify, diagnose, and manage PCOS patients.

Public Health Initiatives and Research Culture of Iranian Healthcare System

Iran has a continuum of medical education program, and the graduates and postgraduates undertake research assignments that are published in local and international medical journals. PCOS is under the agenda of this research, and so far, Iran has contributed a total of 176 articles on the disease pattern and management of PCOS. Iran is among one of the six countries of West Asia that have collaborated in global research for PCOS by contributing 17 articles (Fig. 27.1).[3]

PCOS: Prevalence and Features in Iran

Prevalence

Estimated prevalence was 7% by National Institutes of Health (NIH) criteria, 15.2% by Rotterdam criteria, and 7.92% as per Androgen Excess Society (AES) criteria.[4]

The *prevalence* of the syndrome in another subset of population was between 7.1% and 14.6%. The features that affected people in a descending order included hirsutism, infertility, and menstrual irregularity.[5]

PCOS and Presenting Features

The occurrence of idiopathic hirsutism was 10.9%; oligo/anovulation (OA) was 8.3%; and polycystic ovarian morphology (PCOM) was 8%. The prevalence of PCOS in the community using different diagnostic criteria was 7.1% (NIH), 11.7% (AES), and 14.6% (Rotterdam).[6]

Biochemical and Hormonal Disturbances and PCOS

PCOS interrelated disorders such as hirsutism, infertility, and menstrual problems affect quality of life (QoL).[5]

PCOS and Health-Related Quality of Life

An in-depth understanding of health-related QoL (HRQoL) revealed a negative physical, sexual, and psychological impact on QoL.[7]

PCOS and Quality of Life

The features that influenced a patient's life in descending order were hirsutism, body mass index (BMI), menstrual disturbances, and failure to conceive.[8]

Quality of Modified PCOS HRQoL Questionnaire

Both discriminant and convergent validity showed a constructive relationship between calibrations of the instrument.[9]

Quality of PCOS HRQoL Questionnaire

The quantitative and qualitative validity and reliability of the questionnaire showed satisfactory results for internal consistency and intraclass correlation coefficients.[10]

PCOS Questionnaire-50 (PCOSQ-50)

A new 50-item questionnaire (The PCOSQ-50) was declared as valid and reliable in assessing quality-related health indicators.

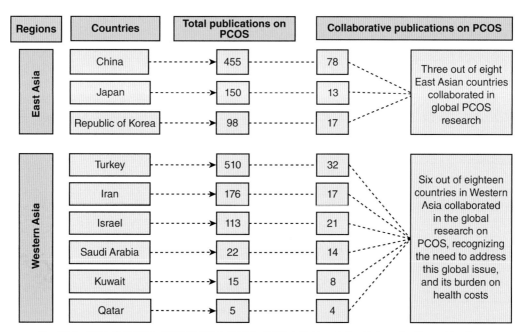

• **Fig. 27.1** Asian Countries That Collaborated in Global Research for Polycystic Ovary Syndrome *(PCOS).* Total publications reflect each country's public health initiatives. (From Brüggmann D, Berges L, Klingelhöfer D, et al. Polycystic ovary syndrome: analysis of the global research architecture using density equalizing mapping. *Reprod Biomed Online.* 2017;34[6]:627-638.)

The new tool was designed to include those aspects that were missed in the previous HRQoL questionnaires.[11]

PCOS and Vitamin D

Vitamin D levels are found to affect the oxidative status (OS) of PCOS. Supplementation of vitamin D improved the defense mechanism in patients with PCOS in Iran.[12] Similar associations of subfertility and Vitamin D were observed in the same geographic belt.[13]

Palestine

Palestine has a population[1] of 5,253,580 and an area of 6020 km². The largest ethnic groups are the Arabs, whereas Jews are more in the occupied areas. The literacy rate is 96.9%.

Healthcare in Palestine

According to the WHO report, until 2016, Palestine had a high level of coverage and commitment to universal health coverage through donor funding. Since the Israeli occupation and because of continuous violations, the demands for health services and the rebuilding of infrastructure have led to a financial crisis regarding purchasing essential medications and preventing epidemics. Specialized workforce and qualified health personnel are also migrating. Teaching hospitals affiliated with universities are currently more focused on emergency situations.

Women's Health in Palestine

The women's health programs in Palestine are donor-funded working groups in their respective areas to improve maternal health and neonatal care.

Cyprus

Cyprus is an island that has a population[1] of 1,217,746 and an area of 9240 km². The largest ethnic group in Cyprus is the Greek Cypriots. Other residents include mostly Turks and a few Russians.

System of Healthcare

Public healthcare in Cyprus is subsidized by the Ministry of Health and is quite cheap compared with private healthcare. There are 42 primary healthcare centers in rural areas. Hospitals are located both in rural and urban areas that have specialized staff for delivery of services. Traditional healers are also frequently consulted.

Women's Health Issues in Cyprus

These are usually limited to the wider term of maternal healthcare, childbirth, and communicable diseases. Data on health conditions of women's health and related comorbidities are deficient, although the country has a high level of diagnostic and management care for infertility. There are multiple infertility centers that attract expatriates because of the relatively low healthcare costs.

Republic of Turkey

Turkey has a population[1] of 85,235,532 and an area of 769,630 km². The population is made up of 75% Turkish people and 18% Kurdish people. The literacy rate is 95.6%.

Healthcare of Turkey

In 2003, a form of universal healthcare called "Genel Sağlık Sigortas" was introduced in Turkey to strengthen the health system and improve the quality of services through evidence-based research initiatives. Both public and private doctors provide services through their respective institutions.

Public Health Initiatives and Research Culture in Turkey

Turkey is a research-oriented country that invests in the field of public health initiatives to improve the quality standards of the health system. Turkey has contributed 510 research articles toward understand the pattern of disease and management of PCOS. Turkey is one of six countries in Western Asia who have collaborated in the global research program on PCOS by contributing 32 articles.[3]

PCOS: Prevalence and Features

Phenotypes

Turkish females who presented with hirsutism and OA had all three phenotypes with similar clinical or biochemical characteristics.[14]

Phenotypes Linked to Obesity

The features of phenotype 1 (OA + hyperandrogenism [HA] + PCO) were present in 47.1% of PCOS females with disturbed luteinizing hormone (LH)/follicle-stimulating hormone (FSH) ratios. An increase in BMI was associated with lipid profile, fasting insulin, and the homeostatic model assessment for insulin resistance (HOMA-IR), suggesting that obesity plays the main role in metabolic disruptions in PCOS patients.[15]

Prevalence as Per Criteria

The prevalence in Turkish females was 6.1% (NIH), 19.9% (Rotterdam), and 15.3% (AES) depending on the criteria used.[16]

Risk for Metabolic Syndrome

Irrespective of the diagnostic criteria, the risk of developing metabolic errors was twofold higher in Turkish patients with PCOS.[16]

Prevalence in Central European Turkey

The prevalence in Central European Turkey was estimated to be 11.4%.[17]

PCOS and Uterine Anomalies

In Southeastern Turkey, 8% of patients with PCOS who sought infertility treatment had uterine anomalies.[18]

Lebanon

Lebanon is a middle-income country that has a population[1] of 6,761,926 and an area of 10,230 km². Lebanon includes 1.5 million Syrians, 470,000 Palestinians, and 5700 Iraqis. The life expectancy is approximately 77.8 years of age.

Healthcare in Lebanon

Healthcare in Lebanon is made up of the basic primary healthcare (PHC) infrastructure. Successive crises and political instability have affected the implementation of health policies, although multiple nongovernmental organizations are supporting health and social welfare. Bilateral agencies are providing funds and technical assistance to uplift the PHC system (WHO-EM/PHC/141/E).

Women's Health

Currently, women's health information is limited to maternity and infant care.

Syria

Syria has a population[1] of 18,439,007, including Iraqi and Palestinians refugees. Approximately 60% of the population is in need of humanitarian aid. The area of Syria is 183,630 km².

Health Situation in Syria

Since the crisis, the health infrastructure in Syria has collapsed. The public hospitals and health centers that were once meant for primary and preventive care are being used for first aid and emergency care. Funding from the Qatar Fund for Development (QFFD) and the Qatar Charity has supported the establishment of four primary healthcare centers in Syria.

Women's Health

Currently, women's health is not a priority.

Israel

Israel has a population[1] of 8,824,544, and the area is 21,640 km². Israel has a very high ranking on the Human Development Index (HDI). The ethnicity is mainly Jews.

Healthcare in Israel

Israel provides coverage to the entire population, although they have to pay some part of it through insurance programs. The strategies are innovative, improving to establish quality standards. The system was ranked the "third most efficient" in the world in 2020, offering both preventive and curative care as well as initiation of research activities.

Women's Health

A lot of work has been done in the field of women's health in Israel. Research has contributed almost 103 scientific papers on the subject of PCOS. Of these, 21 research papers were collaborative publications for the Global Strategy on PCOS.[3]

Jordan

Jordan has a population[1] of 10,292,771 including refugees from Iraq, Syria, Turkey, and Iran, and the area is 88,780 km².

Health Situation in Jordan

Jordan's vision of healthcare and health planning has made the health system of Jordan comparable to many developed countries. Both the public and private sectors are well established. There is a total of 106 hospitals in Jordan equipped with diagnostic and operative facilities. Jordan has been considered malaria-free since 2001.

Women's Health and PCOS

Other than the focus on maternal and newborn health indicators, Jordan has a vision to improve the quality of women's health. A few initiatives include studies to understand the pattern and impact of PCOS.

PCOS and Anxiety Disorders

PCOS patients in Syria and Jordan were educated to improve lifestyle behaviors, such as compliance with treatment, breathing, and other exercises along with diet recommendations to lower stress levels.[19]

Countries Situated in the Arab Peninsula

Kingdom of Saudi Arabia

The Kingdom of Saudi Arabia (KSA) has a population[1] of 35,476,659 and an area of 2,149,690 km². The country ranks high on the HDI. Medical schools are affiliated with research institutes, and health information is disseminated through medical journals.

Healthcare in Saudi Arabia

Healthcare in KSA is supported by a private sector with a ranking for high-quality healthcare services. Hospitals are furnished with the latest diagnostic equipment and treatment facilities. A database of all health records is maintained and used for research purposes. Hospital care matches international standards.

Women's Health Issues

Cancer, obesity, and vitamin D deficiency are very common in Saudi females. Obesity in females is a public health concern because it is a risk factor for many metabolic issues and PCOS. All hospitals are equipped with the diagnostics and treatment facilities to deal with issues like PCOS. A change in lifestyle behavior and weight reduction is particularly important from the perspective of public health. The Annals of Saudi medicine publish articles on the patterns of PCOS, risks, identification, and management in reputed medical journals.

Public Health Initiatives, Research Institutions, and Publications

There are 220 hospitals affiliated with five medical schools in KSA. A functional referral system links all hospitals with primary healthcare services. Evidence-based research to assess the pattern and management of PCOS is disseminated through Saudi medical journals and through other international journals. Research on PCOS in Saudi Arabia shares 22 publications; of these, 14 are collaborative publications (Fig. 27.1).[3]

PCOS: Prevalence and Features in the Population of KSA

Prevalence of PCOS

Self-reporting of PCOS in Madinah was 32.5%.[20]

PCOS Features

PCOM was seen in 53.7% of young unmarried Saudi females who also presented with menstrual irregularities and dermatologic manifestations.[20]

PCOS and Obesity

Self-reported PCOS cases were 16% higher in overweight and obese females, indicating a positive association between obesity and PCOS.[21]

PCOS and Risk of Obesity

Obesity was identified as a risk factor associated with PCOS.[20]

PCOS and Hirsutism

In total, 82% of Saudi females with PCOS presented with hirsutism.[22]

PCOS and Infertility Management

A combination of clomiphene citrate (CC) and metformin has been successful in regulating menstrual cycles and enhancing fertility in patients with BMI greater than 25.[23]

PCOS Link with BMI and LH/FSH Ratios

No meaningful correlation could be identified between PCOS and BMI and levels of circulating hormones (LH/FSH ratio, prolactin, or thyroid-stimulating hormone [TSH]).[24]

PCOS and Psychosomatic Symptoms

The odds of developing stress were the highest in university educated young females (26–35 years) who presented with disturbed cycles, hirsutism, acne, and infertility. Depression and anxiety were also present but to a lesser extent.[25]

PCOS and Glucose Metabolism

Prevalence of aberrant glucose metabolism was high in Saudi females.[26]

Awareness of PCOS

The level of awareness regarding PCOS was found to be high among Saudi females. The main source of information was the internet. Scoring was higher among graduates and medical graduates. There was more awareness of symptoms than of complications.[27]

PCOS and Levels of Reproductive Hormones

It was observed that that irrespective of age and weight factors, levels of LH/FSH and serum total testosterone were higher in Saudi females. On the other hand, serum FSH, sex hormone–binding globulin (SHBG), and progesterone were lesser than in controls.[28]

United Arab Emirates

The kingdom of United Arab Emirates (UAE) is made up of a confederation of seven states: Abu Dhabi, Ajman, Dubai, Fujairah, Ras Al Khaimah, Sharjah, and Umm Al Quwain.

UAE has a population[1] of 10,017,129 covering a land area of 83,600 km². The population is concentrated more in Abu Dhabi, Dubai, and Sharjah. A majority of the UAE population is made up of expatriates that fall in the young age bracket.

Healthcare in UAE

Healthcare for the population is funded by the government. Each emirate has its own healthcare system run by a health ministry and supervised by a separate health authority that overlooks the functions. Females have equal access to healthcare, where services are provided by females. Hospitals match international quality standards.

Health Concerns Regarding the Increasing Incidence of PCOS

In the words of a senior gynecologist, the incidence of PCOS is increasing in UAE, yet no measures have been taken to create awareness for prevention. In the UAE, its prevalence is considerably high because of the comfortable, overindulgent, and inactive lifestyle in the region. Females of Gulf Arab ethnicity in a fertility hospital in Sharjah showed a PCOS prevalence of 39.38%. Almost 80.9% of these patients had insulin resistance (IR) compared with 50% to 70% in world literature (Khaleej times: health news).[28a]

PCOS: Prevalence and Features in UAE

PCOS and Dyslipidemia in UAE

Diabetes and IR were related to PCOS but not dyslipidemia in UAE. The lipid profile suggested the possibility of subclinical atherosclerosis.[29]

Prevalence

The prevalence of PCOS among medical students between 18 and 24 years of age was 27.6%. Obesity was the associated risk factor present in almost half of the PCOS participants. Menstrual irregularities and hirsutism were prevalent presenting complaints.[30]

Structured Health Education Program for PCOS

The results of a planned program aimed at creating awareness and imparting health education showed a significant increase in the knowledge and management of PCOS assessed through pre and posthoc tests.[31]

Risk Factors for PCOS

It was disclosed that females who had history of PCOS in the family, who consumed more fast food, and who were obese had a greater risk of developing PCOS.[30]

PCOS and Associated Factors in Sharjah

The prevalence was revealed as 20% with a family history of PCOS in 22% of the patients.[32]

Pooled Prevalence of PCOS

Using the NIH criteria, PCOS pooled prevalence was 8.9% in UAE and 18.8% in Gulf Arab states.[33]

Perceptions Regarding Reproductive Health and PCOS

Gaps were identified in the understanding of PCOS patients to develop structured health education and promotion campaigns to promote healthy lifestyle and prevent infertility and related problems.[34]

Bahrain

Bahrain has a population[1] of 1,760,392 and has an area of 760 km². The ethnic profile of the population is Bahraini. Asians, Arabs, and other immigrants make up about 52.6% of the overall population.

Healthcare Delivery System

The government of Bahrain provides free healthcare to all Bahraini citizens and subsidized care for non-Bahrainis. The medical facilities in the hospitals of Bahrain are world-class, the health professionals are highly qualified, and medical treatments are easily accessible to all. A research trend is also observed in medical health universities.

PCOS: Prevalence and Features in the Population of Bahrain

Identifying Appropriate Endocrine Markers

Insulin and LH/FSH ratios are best identified with the free androgen index (FAI), whereas IR, inappropriate gonadotrophin secretion, and HA are estimated by sex hormone–binding capacity.[35]

DENND1A Gene Variants in Bahraini Arab Females

No association has been observed between DENND1A gene variants and PCOS, as were observed in Asians and Bahraini Arab females.[36]

Ovarian Drilling and Pregnancy Outcomes

Despite glucose derangements and hypertension in pregnant PCOS patients, no observable differences were seen in neonatal outcomes or premature delivery.[37]

C-Reactive Protein/Albumin Ratio as a Biomarker

PCOS patients were found to have raised C-reactive protein/albumin levels that could be used as a biomarker.[38]

Sultanate of Oman

The sultanate of Oman has a population[1] of 5,255,727 and has an area of 309,500 km². The population is mostly made up of expatriates from different races and ethnicities. The government has a vision to improve the standards of the Omani population.

Health Service Delivery System

The health ministry owns the responsibility of the healthcare of the people. Hospitals are fully equipped with all kind of services. Health education is the government's priority, and the medical school affiliated with the university offers graduate and diploma course programs. The continuation of education in the short term and a refresher course facility are also available.

PCOS: Prevalence and Features in the Sultanate of Oman

Prevalence

The hospital-based prevalence of PCOS in Oman was found to be 7% among females in the 25- to 34-year age group.[39]

PCOS and Emotional Disturbances

Females with PCOS presented with an increased risk of emotional disturbances; however, no statistical difference was noted between stress, anxiety, and depression.[40]

PCOS and Risk of Oxidative Stress

The role of OS has been signified in the pathogenesis of PCOS and can be used to identify high-risk groups.[40]

Prevalence and Features in the Buraimi Region of Oman

The prevalence of PCOS in Oman was found to be 7% and the common presentations included menstrual irregularities, infertility, abnormal uterine bleeding, and hirsutism.[41]

Qatar

The population of Qatar[1] is 2,944,736 covering an area of 11,610 km². Ethnically, a majority are natives of the Arab peninsula, although a few are from Oman. Qatar is a rich country that invests resources into strengthening the community.

Health Service Delivery System

The ministry of public health is responsible for the healthcare of the people of Qatar. The quality standards of healthcare are ranked among one of the top five in the world. Hospitals are fully equipped with all kind of services. Continuation of education and research is also seen.

Public Health Initiatives and Publications

Evidence-based research has been published in many journals. Qatar has shared five publications on PCOS; of these, four are collaborative publications involving global strategy for PCOS (Fig. 27.1).[3]

PCOS: Prevalence and Features in Qatar

Metabolic Features of PCOS

Qatari females in the 18- to 40-year age group who presented with menstrual irregularities were found to have a 12.1% prevalence of PCOS. These women had a 4.5 times higher FAI and a high metabolic profile.[42]

Metabolic Comparison: Ethnic Qatari and UK Females

BMI, waist and hip measurements, systolic and diastolic blood pressure, and triglycerides were higher in the UK cohort, whereas testosterone, high density lipoprotein (HDL), and C-reactive protein were higher in Qatari females.[43]

Risk of Diabetes With PCOS

Qatari PCOS patients were more susceptible to develop diabetes, but had an opposing cardiovascular risk profile.[44]

Kuwait

The population of Kuwait[1] is 4,352,157 covering an area of 17,820 km². Kuwaitis constitute 28% to 32% of the total population, and the remaining part of the population is made up of expatriates.

Health Services Delivery System

Kuwait has a state-funded healthcare system for Kuwaiti nationals. Nonnationals have access to insurance at subsidized costs. Kuwait has a vision to improve the quality and standards of healthcare.

Public Health Initiatives and Publications

Kuwait public health initiatives include research publications on women's health issues, such as PCOS. Qatar has shared 15 publications on PCOS; of these, eight publications are collaborative to global research (Fig. 27.1).[3]

PCOS: Prevalence and Features in Kuwait

Prevalence

The percentage of females with PCOS in Kuwait is 37%. These patients are overweight but not obese.[45]

Infertility and PCOS

One of the major causes of infertility in Kuwait is PCOS.

Laparoscopic Ovarian Drilling and Anti-Müllerian Hormone Levels

Anti-Müllerian hormone levels and indices of Doppler flow before and after the drilling procedure have a significant relationship with PCOS.[46]

PCOS and Obesity

In infertile PCOS females, obesity compromised infertility treatment plans with a reduction in clinical pregnancy rates.[47]

References

1. World population review, 2022. https://worldpopulationreview.com/.
2. Mousa BA. The Prevalence of PCOS in Infertile Women According to Clinical Features and its Associated Hormonal Changes in Al-Hilla City, Iraq. *Indian J Public Health Res Dev.* 2019;10(10).
3. Brüggmann D, Berges L, Klingelhöfer D, et al. Polycystic ovary syndrome: analysis of the global research architecture using density equalizing mapping. *Reprod Biomed Online.* 2017;34(6):627-638.
4. Mehrabian F, Khani B, Kelishadi R, Ghanbari E. The prevalence of polycystic ovary syndrome in Iranian women based on different diagnostic criteria. *Endokrynol Pol.* 2011;62(3):238-242.
5. Behboodi Moghadam Z, Fereidooni B, Saffari M, Montazeri A. Polycystic ovary syndrome and its impact on Iranian women's quality of life: a population-based study. *BMC Womens Health.* 2018;18(1):1-8.
6. Tehrani FR, Simbar M, Tohidi M, Hosseinpanah F, Azizi F. The prevalence of polycystic ovary syndrome in a community sample of Iranian population: Iranian PCOS prevalence study. *Reprod Biol Endocrinol.* 2011;9(1):1-7.
7. Taghavi SA, Bazarganipour F, Hugh-Jones S, Hosseini N. Health-related quality of life in Iranian women with polycystic ovary syndrome: a qualitative study. *BMC Womens Health.* 2015;15(1):1-8.
8. Khomami MB, Tehrani FR, Hashemi S, Farahmand M, Azizi F. Of PCOS symptoms, hirsutism has the most significant impact on the quality of life of Iranian women. *PLoS One.* 2015;10(4):e0123608.
9. Bazarganipour F, Ziaei S, Montazeri A, Foroozanfard F, Faghihzadeh S. Iranian version of modified polycystic ovary syndrome health-related quality of Life questionnaire: discriminant and convergent validity. *Iran J Reprod Med.* 2013;11(9):753.
10. Bazarganipour F, Ziaei S, Montazeri A, Faghihzadeh S, Frozanfard F. Psychometric properties of the Iranian version of modified polycystic ovary syndrome health-related quality-of-life questionnaire. *Hum Reprod.* 2012;27(9):2729-2736.
11. Nasiri-Amiri F, Tehrani FR, Simbar M, Montazeri A, Mohammadpour RA. Health-related quality of life questionnaire for polycystic ovary syndrome (PCOSQ-50): development and psychometric properties. *Qual Life Res.* 2016;25(7): 1791-1801.
12. Masjedi F, Keshtgar S, Agah F, Karbalaei N. Association between sex steroids and oxidative status with vitamin D levels in follicular fluid of non-obese PCOS and healthy women. *J Reprod Infertil.* 2019;20(3):132.
13. Azhar A, Abid F, Rehman R. Polycystic ovary syndrome, subfertility and vitamin D deficiency. *J Coll Physicians Surg Pak.* 2020;30(5):545-546.
14. Hassa H, Tanir H, Yildiz Z. Comparison of clinical and laboratory characteristics of cases with polycystic ovarian syndrome based on Rotterdam's criteria and women whose only clinical signs are oligo/anovulation or hirsutism. *Arch Gynecol Obstet.* 2006;274(4):227-232.
15. Ates S, Sevket O, Sudolmus S, et al. Different phenotypes of polycystic ovary syndrome in Turkish women: clinical and endocrine characteristics. *Gynecol Endocrinol.* 2013;29(10):931-935.
16. Yildiz BO, Bozdag G, Yapici Z, Esinler I, Yarali H. Prevalence, phenotype and cardiometabolic risk of polycystic ovary syndrome under different diagnostic criteria. *Hum Reprod.* 2012;27(10):3067-3073.
17. Miazgowski T, Martopullo I, Widecka J, Miazgowski B, Brodowska A. National and regional trends in the prevalence

of polycystic ovary syndrome since 1990 within Europe: the modeled estimates from the Global Burden of Disease Study 2016. *Arch Med Sci.* 2021;17(2):343.

18. Ege S, Peker N, Bademkıran MH. The prevalence of uterine anomalies in infertile patients with polycystic ovary syndrome: a retrospective study in a tertiary center in Southeastern Turkey. *Turk J Obstet Gynecol.* 2019;16(4):224.

19. Lai L, Flower A, Moore M, Prescott P, Lewith G. Polycystic ovary syndrome: a randomised feasibility and pilot study using Chinese Herbal medicine to explore Impact on Dysfunction (OR-CHID)—study protocol. *Eur J Integr Med.* 2014;6(3):392-399.

20. Guraya SS. Prevalence and ultrasound features of polycystic ovaries in young unmarried Saudi females. *J Microsc Ultrastruct.* 2013;1(1-2):30-34.

21. Aldossary K, Alotaibi A, Alkhaldi K, Alharbi R. Prevalence of polycystic ovary syndrome, and relationship with obesity/over-weight: cross-sectional study in Saudi Arabia. *J Adv Pharm Educ Res.* 2020;10(1):187.

22. Al-Ruhaily AD, Malabu UH, Sulimani RA. Hirsutism in Saudi females of reproductive age: a hospital-based study. *Ann Saudi Med.* 2008;28(1):28-32.

23. Ayaz A, Alwan Y, Farooq MU. Metformin—clomiphene citrate vs. clomiphene citrate alone: polycystic ovarian syndrome. *J Hum Reprod Sci.* 2013;6(1):15.

24. Saadia Z. Follicle stimulating hormone (LH: FSH) ratio in polycystic ovary syndrome (PCOS)-obese vs. non-obese women. *Med Arch.* 2020;74(4):289.

25. Asdaq SMB, Yasmin F. Risk of psychological burden in polycystic ovary syndrome: a case control study in Riyadh, Saudi Arabia. *J Affect Disord.* 2020;274:205-209.

26. Abdel-Rahman MY, Abdellah AH, Ahmad SR, Ismail SA, Frasure H, Hurd WW. Prevalence of abnormal glucose metabolism in a cohort of Arab women with polycystic ovary syndrome. *Int J Gynecol Obstet.* 2011;114(3):288-289.

27. Alessa A, Aleid D, Almutairi S, et al. Awareness of polycystic ovarian syndrome among Saudi females. *Int J Med Sci Public Health.* 2017;6(6):1013-1020.

28. Fakhoury H, Tamim H, Ferwana M, Siddiqui IA, Adham M, Tamimi W. Age and BMI adjusted comparison of reproductive hormones in PCOS. *J Family Med Prim Care.* 2012;1(2):132.

28a. Asma Alizain (2015). *Polycystic Ovarian Syndrome on 'staggering' rise in UAE.* Home/Health, Khaleej Times. Published 25th May, 2014. Available at: https://www.khaleejtimes.com/health/polycystic-ovarian-syndrome-on-staggering-rise-in-uae

29. Al Mulla A, El Sokkary A, Ekladiou S, Khamis AH. Prevalence of dyslipidemia among women with polycystic ovary syndrome based on body mass index. W J Gynecol Women's Health. 2020;4(1). doi:WJGWH.MS.ID.000580.

30. Saidunnisa B, Atiqulla S, Ayman G. Prevalence of polycystic ovarian syndrome among students of RAK Medical and Health Sciences University United Arab Emirates. *IJMPS.* 2016;109:118.

31. Shariff A, Begum GS, Ayman G, Mohammad B, Housam R, Khaled N. An interventional study on effectiveness of structured education programme in improving the knowledge of polycystic ovarian syndrome among female students of Ras Al Khaimah Medical & Health Sciences University, UAE. *IJSR.* 2016;5(1):1659-1663.

32. Attlee A, Nusralla A, Eqbal R, Said H, Hashim M, Obaid RS. Polycystic ovary syndrome in university students: occurrence and associated factors. *Int J Fertil Steril.* 2014;8(3):261.

33. Mousa M, Al-Jefout M, Alsafar H, et al. Prevalence of common gynecological conditions in the Middle East: systematic review and meta-analysis. *Front Reprod Health.* 2021;3:7.

34. Pramodh S. Exploration of lifestyle choices, reproductive health knowledge, and polycystic ovary syndrome (PCOS) awareness among female Emirati University students. *Int J Womens Health.* 2020;12:927.

35. Golbahar J, Al-Ayadhi M, Das NM, Gumaa K. Sensitive and specific markers for insulin resistance, hyperandrogenemia, and inappropriate gonadotropin secretion in women with polycystic ovary syndrome: a case-control study from Bahrain. *Int J Womens Health.* 2012;4:201.

36. Gammoh E, Arekat MR, Saldhana FL, Madan S, Ebrahim BH, Almawi WY. DENND1A gene variants in Bahraini Arab women with polycystic ovary syndrome. *Gene.* 2015;560(1):30-33.

37. Al-Ojaimi EH. Pregnancy outcomes after laparoscopic ovarian drilling in women with polycystic ovarian syndrome. *Saudi Med J.* 2006;27(4):519.

38. Kalyan S, Goshtesabi A, Sarray S, Joannou A, Almawi WY. Assessing C reactive protein/albumin ratio as a new biomarker for polycystic ovary syndrome: a case–control study of women from Bahraini medical clinics. *BMJ Open.* 2018;8(10):e021860.

39. Al Khaduri M, Al Farsi Y, Al Najjar TAA, Gowri V. Hospital-based prevalence of polycystic ovarian syndrome among Omani women. *Middle East Fertil Soc J.* 2014;19(2):135-138.

40. Sulaiman MA, Al-Farsi YM, Al-Khaduri MM, Saleh J, Waly MI. Polycystic ovarian syndrome is linked to increased oxidative stress in Omani women. *Int J Womens Health.* 2018;10:763.

41. Varghese U, Varughese S. Prevalence of polycystic ovarian syndrome in the Buraimi region of Oman. *Brunei Int Med J.* 2012;8(5):248-252.

42. Dargham SR, Ahmed L, Kilpatrick ES, Atkin SL. The prevalence and metabolic characteristics of polycystic ovary syndrome in the Qatari population. *PLoS One.* 2017;12(7):e0181467.

43. Butler AE, Abouseif A, Dargham SR, Sathyapalan T, Atkin SL. Metabolic comparison of polycystic ovarian syndrome and control women in Middle Eastern and UK Caucasian populations. *Sci Rep.* 2020;10(1):1-5.

44. Dargham SR, El Shewehy A, Dakroury Y, Kilpatrick ES, Atkin SL. Prediabetes and diabetes in a cohort of Qatari women screened for polycystic ovary syndrome. *Sci Rep.* 2018;8(1):1-6.

45. Ching H, Burke V, Stuckey B. Quality of life and psychological morbidity in women with polycystic ovary syndrome: body mass index, age and the provision of patient information are significant modifiers. *Clin Endocrinol.* 2007;66(3):373-379.

46. Elmashad AI. Impact of laparoscopic ovarian drilling on anti-Müllerian hormone levels and ovarian stromal blood flow using three-dimensional power Doppler in women with anovulatory polycystic ovary syndrome. *Fertil Steril.* 2011;95(7):2342-2346.

47. Al-Azemi M, Omu FE, Omu AE. The effect of obesity on the outcome of infertility management in women with polycystic ovary syndrome. *Arch Gynecol Obstet.* 2004;270(4):205-210.

28

Situation Analysis, Cultural Beliefs, Lifestyle, and the Psychological Impact of Polycystic Ovary Syndrome in Europe

HAFIZ SOHAIL KAMRAN AND TAMAR SAEED

Background

The prevalence of polycystic ovary syndrome (PCOS) is between 5% and 10% in females of childbearing age. The hallmark of PCOS is long-term anovulation, which ultimately leads to menstrual problems and a higher rate of infertility. The syndrome can also manifest as excessive facial hair and pimples.

Certain endocrine abnormalities in the form of serum insulin, glucose levels, the homeostatic model assessment of insulin resistance (IR), high body mass index (BMI), and high systolic and diastolic blood pressures (SBP and DBP, respectively) are reported in patients with PCOS. Noticeable differences have been recorded in patients from different ethnicities and backgrounds. The distribution of PCOS varies across geography, ethnicity, and race. Studies negate the deep impact of genotypic buildup, being the sole contributor to the numbers/presentations of PCOS patients. That is why environmental factors are regarded as the other major stake holders, that play a major role in the presentation/Numbers of patients with PCOS. As research shows more and more evidence about the role of environmental factors on the variability in presentation, about the effects of lifestyles changes, about noticeable variations in people from different backgrounds, and about the importance of raising awareness of individual groups that are at greater risk, this will lead to superior treatment for metabolic and fertility dysfunction.

Situation in Europe

The rate of PCOS varies in different regions in Europe, which is highly suggestive of the association between environmental/genetic factors and PCOS.

A study done in 2016 showed the highest number of PCOS cases in the Czech Republic and the lowest in Sweden. In addition, the study also revealed that age plays an important role in the distribution of PCOS because numbers were higher in certain age groups. Overall, across all three European regions, the numbers showed a gradual increase with age with the highest rates in females aged 35 to 39 and 40 to 44 years; the trend almost remained the same in Eastern Europe (EE) and Central Europe (CE) from age 20 years on. In fact, in the youngest age group (15–19 years), very few females developed this condition. In this age group, in the period from 1990 to 2016, the number of PCOS prevalent cases increased in EE by 0.73% (95% uncertainty interval [UI]: from –0.18 to 1.83) and CE by 1.87% (95% UI: 0.42–3.68), whereas it decreased in Western Europe (WE; by 1.30%; 95% UI: from 4.65–2.64)[1] (Table 28.1).

Cultural Beliefs and Implication of Lifestyle in Patients With PCOS

Data have confirmed the link between environmental and genetic factors with regard to PCOS. One of the key environmental factors that has been identified as a major contributor to PCOS is low socioeconomic status; people with such a background do not have enough knowledge, which leads to less adaptation of healthy lifestyles and manifests in the form of weight gain, disturbances in hormonal levels, and increased susceptibility to PCOS.

Low socioeconomic status may mean that such people have less access to healthcare facilities and less awareness and knowledge about PCOS, thus increasing the burden of PCOS in the community. Managing such patients is always

Table 28.1   Numbers and Trends of Polycystic Ovary Syndrome in 2016 for European Countries and Regions for Females Aged 15 to 49 Years

Country	Prevalent cases per 100,000	Lower bound	Upper bound	Percent of total prevalent cases	Lower bound	Upper bound
Albania	373.94	280.2	498.4	0.38	0.29	0.51
Andorra	119.88	90.26	158.8	0.12	0.09	0.16
Austria	211.74	167.5	266.2	0.22	0.17	0.27
Belarus	430.98	325.2	561.7	0.44	0.33	0.58
Belgium	131.70	95.97	172.5	0.13	0.10	0.18
Bosnia and Herzegovina	420.45	315.8	553.1	0.43	0.32	0.56
Bulgaria	435.76	329.3	571.4	0.44	0.37	0.58
Croatia	415.90	312.2	546.1	0.43	0.32	0.56
Czech Republic	460.60	346.2	602.1	0.47	0.35	0.62
Denmark	117.43	88.24	157.5	0.12	0.09	0.16
Estonia	432.44	326.2	567.4	0.44	0.34	0.56
Finland	121.62	91.37	162.2	0.12	0.09	0.17
France	120.68	90.61	160.1	0.12	0.09	0.16
Germany	114.96	87.70	147.7	0.12	0.84	0.15
Greece	136.07	100.1	177.9	0.14	0.10	0.18
Hungary	428.72	322.5	561.4	0.44	0.30	0.57
Iceland	120.65	90.51	161.6	0.12	0.09	0.16
Ireland	127.61	98.13	168.0	0.13	0.10	0.17
Italy	138.11	106.8	178.9	0.14	0.11	0.18
Kazakhstan	417.23	311.2	546.9	0.42	0.31	0.53
Latvia	427.92	321.8	563.2	0.41	0.31	0.54
Lithuania	406.38	304.8	535.4	0.41	0.31	0.54
Luxembourg	123.65	92.91	163.8	0.12	0.09	0.17
North Macedonia	411.45	309.4	543.2	0.42	0.32	0.56
Malta	123.51	92.99	164.1	0.13	0.09	0.17
Moldova	435.78	325.8	578.6	0.44	0.33	0.59
Montenegro	410.91	309.2	542.4	0.42	0.32	0.56
Netherlands	117.50	88.29	156.3	0.12	0.09	0.16
Norway	106.55	80.62	137.9	0.11	0.08	0.14
Poland	447.22	336.3	588.9	0.46	0.34	0.6
Portugal	126.00	94.98	165.7	0.13	0.10	0.17
Romania	409.06	307.1	534.8	0.42	0.31	0 55
Russia	443.14	333.9	583.2	0.45	0.34	0.59
Serbia	409.00	308.6	536.5	0.42	0.32	0.55
Slovakia	437.15	328.6	573.7	0.45	0.34	0.59
Slovenia	402.66	302.6	528.0	0.41	0.31	0.54
Spain	132.35	97.34	178.6	0.13	0.10	0.18
Sweden	34.10	24.59	45.77	0.04	0.03	0.05

Table 28.1	Numbers and Trends of Polycystic Ovary Syndrome in 2016 for European Countries and Regions for Females Aged 15 to 49 Years—cont'd					
Country	Prevalent cases per 100,000	Lower bound	Upper bound	Percent of total prevalent cases	Lower bound	Upper bound
Switzerland	121.31	91.03	160.7	0.12	0.09	0.16
Turkey	258.52	195.3	333.2	0.26	0.20	0.34
Ukraine	428.91	321.5	565.7	0.44	0.33	0.57
United Kingdom	117.40	87.36	155.3	0.12	0.09	0.16
All countries	276.35	207.8	363.2	0.28	0.23	0.37
Western Europe	123.42	93.04	162.3	0.13	0.13	0.17
Central Europe	408.68	307.4	536.7	0.42	0.32	0.55
Eastern Europe	427.79	321.3	562.8	0.43	0.33	0.56

Miazgowski, et al. (2021). National and regional trends in the prevalence of polycystic ovary syndrome since 1990 within Europe: the modeled estimates from the Global Burden of Disease Study 2016. Arch Med Sci, 17 (2): 343-351.

a challenge because managing PCOS requires a multidisciplinary approach. Research suggest that right from the start, babies of mothers from low socioeconomic backgrounds are small for gestational age because of poor nutrition and not eating the right food during pregnancy, which has been established as a key factor that contributes to PCOS in later life.

Between 1990 and 2016, the rates in WE, EE, and CE countries were almost unchanged, but there was remarkable variation when specific regions were compared; the differences can be attributed to the unequal distribution of health facilities, which resulted from less resource allocation for this disorder because it requires a multidisciplinary approach and many of the countries were not able to precisely calculate the economic burden it would cause.

Because of variability in the clinical presentation (i.e., because of the involvement of different body systems), patients tend to present to different specialists, such as the gynecologist, the general practitioner, or the endocrinologist. In all these patients, there is always a chance for each specialty to add on to the management. One key factor in the management of patients with PCOS is to provide them with knowledge and awareness because most of the problems can be solved if simple lifestyle interventions are made. That is why patients internationally report that they have been provided with less information to manage their symptoms. The other major factor is the communication barrier. In Europe, there are people from different backgrounds/regions (Immigrants) and many of them do not understand the native / official language that is being spoken in that particular country, they are being residing in, specially if they are new immgirants. So, if that particular language is the only medium a clinician can communicate in, it will ultimately affect the information being given to the patients. Because of the wide presentation of PCOS and its psychosocial impact, it is of prime importance to create awareness in populations from lower economic backgrounds because the level of understanding is very different in people who are from higher economic backgrounds and those who are

not. Education can help the family of patients understand the issues a patient faces and how badly it can affect mental health. In PCOS, it is important to not only address the physical, underlying hormonal changes (i.e., weight gain and infertility) but to also see mental wellbeing as important. Awareness can be created by arranging for education sessions, which should address the individual concerns of the patients and should address patients from every background, keeping their level of previous understanding in mind. Many patients with PCOS remain undiagnosed because of lack of knowledge. A dietitian can play a major role in addressing patients with PCOS because the right food choice can help them lose weight and minimize the effects of IR.

Studies have established a connection between barriers, enablers, and satisfaction when it comes to both patients and health professionals and have revealed the benefits of information and socioemotional support. PCOS patients need individual and personalized support because it is a long-term condition. Inadequate information can result in frustration for the patient.

One study asked PCOS patients about their experience with PCOS, especially about the responses they had received from healthcare professionals, the obstacles they had faced in receiving a timely diagnosis of PCOS, and the level of acceptability of their condition across different ethnicities and cultures. The responses indicated that often females presented their issues to the healthcare provider, but their symptoms were either ignored or, if diagnosed, less information was provided than needed. Respondents reported poor communication on behalf of the healthcare providers. On various occasions, education was not individualized and families were not involved, which led to frustration. Many gaps were reported in care, and patients had to search online for resources, but much of the information they found online was commercialized. All the aforementioned factors led to poor quality of life in patients with PCOS. It was suggested that proper courses and individual education should be provided to target specific patients, and patients should be given a choice on how to manage their condition by giving them sufficient information. Often, mental wellbeing was ignored and the healthcare provider focused solely on treating physical features (i.e., acne, weight, and infertility). Thus there is a need for a more comprehensive approach. Because PCOS is a chronic condition, educating patients will help them feel more confident in managing their symptoms and making correct choices for themselves. Patient information leaflets, the use of electronic and paper media, and PCOS discussion groups were all suggested as ways to create awareness in patients. All these need support from the government and from charities.

It has been reported that sometimes addressing the patient alone does not solve the issue. That is why it is important to address the family as a whole and keep them in the loop during discussions, ultimately creating awareness among the families who then understand the needs of the patients. Data have revealed that the higher prevalence of PCOS in Europe has partially been caused by less acceptance of the PCOS diagnosis by families, less education, cultural barriers (such as not seeing a male physician), and not considering weight gain as the cause for PCOS.

Psychological Impact

It has been suggested that patients with PCOS should be screened for depression and anxiety because a high prevalence of such symptoms has been reported in these patients and is usually ignored. If identified, depression and anxiety should be dealt with accordingly. Nevertheless, overdiagnosis should be avoided.

Some patients with PCOS have reported mental health issues with psychosexual origins based in cognition, body image, and depression. The prevalence of psychosexual dysfunction varies from 13.3% to 62.5% in PCOS.[2-5] Studies have shown the relation between PCOS and psychosexual dysfunction and how PCOS can contribute to negative self-esteem, negative body image, a less feminine identity, and less sexual satisfaction.

A recent systematic review by the Guidelines Development Group (GDG) identified 18 relevant studies using validated sexual function questionnaires and visual-analog scales (VAS). Small yet significant differences were detected in sexual function subscales, and arousal, lubrication, satisfaction, and orgasm were all impaired in PCOS compared with females without PCOS. Large effects were seen when it came to the impact of body hair, the social impact of appearance, and sexual attractiveness. Satisfaction with sex life was impaired, whereas the importance of sex was similar to that of non-PCOS females. Physical PCOS symptoms, such as hirsutism, obesity, menstrual irregularity, and infertility, may cause loss of feminine identity and a feeling of being unattractive, which may affect sexuality.[6-8]

Therapy should be targeted, if needed, based on the presentation of symptoms and may involve drugs or psychological therapy for mental wellbeing. It warrents the need for updating the existing guidlines on regular basis for managing PCOS patients as per their needs, keeping different aspects in mind, as research continues to reveale more and more insight in to the symptoms of PCOS.

PCOS is a diagnosis that affects quality of life in a number of ways because of high BMI, negative cultural beliefs, poor quality of care, less understanding of the issues with PCOS, and the length of consultation needed with healthcare professionals.

PCOS poses a high risk for eating disorders; therefore consideration should be given for screening these disorder in PCOS patients, so that they are not overlooked or underdiagnosed.

Screening for obstructive sleep apnea (OSA) has been suggested in PCOS patients because excessive weight puts these patients at high risk for developing OSA and its complications. Although routine screening for endometrial carcinoma is not suggested in all patients with PCOS, it is recommended for those with increased endometrial thickening, which can result from overexposure to estrogen, increased body weight, and abnormal vaginal bleeding. Screening can be done through different imaging modalities.

References

1. Miazgowski T, Martopullo I, Widecka J, Miazgowski B, Brodowska A. National and regional trends in the prevalence of polycystic ovary syndrome since 1990 within Europe: the modeled estimates from the Global Burden of Disease Study 2016. *Arch Med Sci.* 2019;17(2):343-351.
2. Dashti S, Latiff LA, Hamid HA, et al. Sexual dysfunction in patients with polycystic ovary syndrome in Malaysia. *Asian Pac J Cancer Prev.* 2016;17(8):3747-3751.
3. Eftekhar T, Sohrabvand F, Zabandan N, et al. Sexual dysfunction in patients with polycystic ovary syndrome and its affected domains. *Iran J Reprod Med.* 2014;12(8):539-546.
4. Ercan CM, Coksuer H, Aydogan U, et al. Sexual dysfunction assessment and hormonal correlations in patients with polycystic ovary syndrome. *Int J Impot Res.* 2013;25(4):127-132.
5. Veras AB, Bruno RV, de Avila MA, Nardi AE. Sexual dysfunction in patients with polycystic ovary syndrome: clinical and hormonal correlations. *Compr Psychiatry.* 2011;52(5):486-489.
6. Hahn S, Janssen OE, Tan S, et al. Clinical and psychological correlates of quality-of-life in polycystic ovary syndrome. *Eur J Endocrinol.* 2005;153(6):853-860.
7. Elsenbruch S, Hahn S, Kowalsky D, et al. Quality of life, psychosocial well-being, and sexual satisfaction in women with polycystic ovary syndrome. *J Clin Endocrinol Metab.* 2003;88(12):5801-5807.
8. Janssen O, Hahn S, Tan S, et al. Mood and sexual function in polycystic ovary syndrome. *Semin Reprod Med.* 2008;26(1):45-52.

29

Global Approach to Polycystic Ovary Syndrome in Africa

SAIRA BANU MOHAMED RASHID SOKWALA AND RAJ DODIA

Introduction

Polycystic ovary syndrome (PCOS) is a complex, genetic, multisystem chronic disorder associated with reproductive, metabolic, and psychosocial comorbidities. These patients are predisposed to further health complications such as higher rates of infertility, cardiovascular disease (CVD) risk, and endometrial/ovarian malignancies.[1] Such important and far-reaching health effects make PCOS worth understanding better. It has been noted that both genetic and environmental factors (sedentary lifestyles and westernized dietary habits) contribute to the overall pathophysiology of PCOS through dysregulated androgen synthesis and insulin resistance.[2,3] This complex interaction of genetic and environmental factors further contributes to the various phenotypic presentations of PCOS and variations in ethnicities/races and global regions, hence the need to start exploring the genotype-environment correlations of such disorders.[4] Because of the varied environments that humans live in all over the world, the nuances of such disorders need to be scrutinized to appropriately guide management principles.

Africa is the second-largest and second-most populous continent in the world, with a population of over 1.3 billion.[5] Nevertheless, it remains the world's poorest and least developed continent. This is most evident in the sub-Saharan regions, where about 50% of the population live below the poverty line.[6] The prevalence of PCOS is increasing globally, and Africa is no exception.

The dynamics of PCOS phenotypic recognition, diagnostics, and management are variable globally. They depend on factors such as awareness, cost, accessibility to healthcare, stakeholder involvement, availability of clinical guidelines, and health-seeking behaviors (HSBs). With the increase of these factors in many parts of Africa, it has been noted that noncommunicable diseases (NCDs) are quickly catching up with the bulk of ailments (infectious and malnutrition-associated conditions), likely because of the changing lifestyles with the increased adoption of Western diets and sedentary habits.[7]

With an upsurge and escalating awareness of PCOS as a significant cause of female morbidity, research on PCOS is gradually increasing from the African continent, albeit at a slower pace than required.[8] Culture and tradition form a significant part of African life, and over 85% of Africans seek traditional medicine for their ailments,[9] further complicating allopathic research goals. Thus there remains a paucity of data on most spheres of PCOS in Africa.

This chapter aims at highlighting the various aspects of PCOS on the African continent and discusses the prevalence, unique clinical features, diagnostic and treatment options, HSBs, and challenges of PCOS in Africa.

Prevalence of Polycystic Ovary Syndrome in Africa

As a syndrome, PCOS is identified by a collection of symptoms. The diagnosis is made once clinical conditions with similar signs and symptoms are ruled out. This inherently makes the prevalence of such a syndrome complex. This is because of the phenotypic types of PCOS that would present to the clinical care provider. It has been noted that the clinical features of PCOS in medically referred patients are much more severe than in those of a medically unbiased group of people. The clinically referred (hence medically biased) individuals more frequently showed the more complete PCOS phenotype (phenotype A), with more hirsutism, higher serum androgen levels, and more obesity compared with individuals identified in the unselected cohort.[10] A systematic review and meta-analysis confirmed these findings of referral bias and concluded that the referred PCOS patients were overall more obese and showed more severe symptoms.[11] Referral bias automatically confounds prevalence studies. Data would be more readily available for those clinical conditions that do not have silent features or have symptoms that require medical attention more readily, rather than those that present with PCOS for example.[12] It is less likely for a female who has sprouted a hair on the chin or chest to present to a medical care provider than to have that patient seek medical advice for breaking a leg after a fall. This complicates prevalence studies for clinical conditions such as PCOS.

An overwhelming majority (if not all) of studies of PCOS prevalence are from populations in North America, Europe, the Middle East, southern Asia, and Australia.[13] There are no significant data from South America, Russia, the island countries of Oceania (Melanesia, Micronesia, and Polynesia), or Africa. Africa being the home of the Black female, there is a vacuum of studies regarding PCOS prevalence in Africa, with available studies only showing prevalence among Black females on other continents.[14-16] This is despite a meta-analysis showing that Black females are more at risk for developing PCOS,[12] and evidence to show that Black females with PCOS have an increased risk for metabolic syndrome (MetS).[17]

Overall, the available data suggest that well-controlled epidemiologic studies of unselected (medically unbiased) populations are required worldwide to define the true prevalence and phenotype of the disorder in the regions studied. The impact of differences in race and/or ethnicity, environment, socioeconomics, and nutrition on the development, complications, phenotype, and prevalence of PCOS will be clearer with such studies. Such research is also essential for determining the relationship between genotype and phenotype, encouraging an improved understanding of the molecular mechanisms underlying the disorder. Well-conducted epidemiologic studies may also provide clues to the evolutionary history of the disorder, which may potentially identify the core elements of PCOS. Understanding the public health and economic implications of PCOS in a region may help facilitate the development of effective public health and prevention policies once identified.

Clinical Picture of Polycystic Ovary Syndrome in Africans

Typically, PCOS presents with signs and symptoms related to androgen excess and ovulatory dysfunction, disrupting the hypothalamic-pituitary-ovarian (HPO) axis. Classic clinical features include irregular menses, longstanding anovulation, hirsutism, infertility/subfertility, and/or polycystic ovarian morphology.[18] Depending on the presentation and observable characteristics, there are different phenotypes of PCOS as per the 2012 National Institutes of Health-Sponsored Evidence-Based Methodology PCOS Workshop[19] (Table 29.1). In addition, PCOS is associated

with metabolic abnormalities, including impaired glucose tolerance (IGT)/impaired fasting glucose, type 2 diabetes mellitus (DM), MetS, overweight/obesity, atherogenic dyslipidemia, systemic inflammation, nonalcoholic fatty liver disease (NAFLD), hypertension, and coagulation disorders.[20] PCOS also carries significant psychological implications,[21-23] which will be discussed in detail later.

Ethnic variations exist in the various phenotypes of PCOS (Table 29.2). Black Americans with PCOS had a higher prevalence of MetS compared with White Americans.[17] Nevertheless, comparing Hispanic females with non-Hispanic Black and White American females, Engmann et al. found that Hispanic females have the most severe phenotype of PCOS in terms of both hyperandrogenism (HA) and metabolic parameters.[24] In their study, they found that non-Hispanic Black females had a milder phenotype than Hispanics and, in some elements, than non-Hispanic White females. Of the studies in Africa, a Nigerian study on infertile females found that 16.7% had PCOS and these patients had a statistically higher occurrence of hirsutism, anovulatory cycle with oligomenorrhoea, and serum testosterone levels compared with infertile females with normal ovaries.[25] A similar study on infertile females conducted in Tanzania in a gynecology outpatient department found a higher prevalence of PCOS (32%) with over three-quarters (78%) having polycystic ovaries, 75% having oligo/anovulation, and over half (56%) presenting with hirsutism. Nevertheless, even among those without PCOS, 10.3% had polycystic ovaries.[26] Among 131 females with oligomenorrhoea and amenorrhoea attending a gynecology clinic at a tertiary referral hospital in Kenya, about 1 in 3 (37.4%) had PCOS as defined by the Rotterdam Criteria.[27] Mean ovarian size was larger and total testosterone levels were higher in the PCOS patients compared with those without PCOS.[28]

It is thus evident that although many of the features of PCOS cut across borders, ethnicity, and cultures, there are ethnoracial variations in the clinical presentation and clinical impact of PCOS, dependent on genetic and environmental factors.

Psychosocial and Cultural Aspects of PCOS in Africa

PCOS is a chronic condition that impacts feminine identity and is thus associated with significant psychological comorbidity presenting in various ways (Table 29.3). Female sex, obesity, and infertility are independent risk factors for both anxiety and depression. Females with a combination of these features in PCOS are at a higher risk for psychological disturbances.[30] Because of hirsutism and negative body image self-perception, body dissatisfaction is more frequent among PCOS patients. Of note is that psychological illness might go undetected in PCOS patients, and this eventually affects their quality of life.[31] Hence there is a requirement for awareness of the psychosocial aspects of PCOS management, especially among healthcare providers.

TABLE 29.1 Phenotypes of Polycystic Ovary Syndrome

Phenotype	Features
A	Hyperandrogenism, ovulatory dysfunction, and polycystic ovary morphology
B	Hyperandrogenism and ovulatory dysfunction
C	Hyperandrogenism and polycystic ovary morphology
D	Ovulatory dysfunction and polycystic ovary morphology

TABLE 29.2 Ethnic Specific Polycystic Ovarian Syndrome Variations[29]

Ethnic group/geographic region	Key phenotypic variations
African Origin	
American black	More obese than whites; more hypertension than T2DM; central obesity, IR, elevated TG; MetS 26% (less than Asians and Hispanics); community prevalence similar to white Europeans
Asian	
East Asian	• **Japanese:** low BMI (<25 kg/m^2); less hirsute; • **Chinese** -age 25 years; BMI 22 kg/m^2; FG = 3; PCO 96%; MetS 22-28% • **Taiwanese** -age 26 years; BMI 28 kg/m^2; acanthosis 31%; AGT 42%.
South Asian (Sri Lankan, Indian, Pakistani)	Mean BMI 26 kg/m^2; higher central obesity; greater risk of diabetes; Severe symptoms at younger age (25 years) than white Europeans; lower SHBG; greater IR than Caucasians; MetS 30%; similar prevalence of MetS among phenotypes; Acanthosis nigricans ++; family history of T2DM common; **Pakistanis** more hirsute than Sri Lankans/south Indians; **Sri Lankan** -community prevalence 6.3% (Rotterdam)
Southeast Asian (Thai, Singaporean, Malay)	Mean BMI ~27 kg/m^2; mean age 27 years; MetS 35%; AGT in 42%; Acanthosis nigricans important predictor; Thai -community prevalence 5% (Rotterdam)
White European (Caucasian)	
Hispanic:	MetS 31% (USA)
-Caribbean	Higher IR than non-Hispanic blacks and whites; PCOS has an additive effect
-Mexican	Higher IR 73 vs 44% in whites
-American	Greater prevalence (13%) -(selected population)
North European:	Mean BMI 35 kg/m^2; mean age 32 years; less insulin resistant; SHBG higher
-UK, Dutch, Icelandic	PCO prevalence 20-33%; PCOS (Rotterdam) ~8%
-USA (non-Hispanic)	Caucasians taller; Icelandics less hirsute
Mediterranean:	MetS and AGT ~20-24%
-Greek, Turkish	Prevalence 6.8% (NIH criteria)
South European:	BMI 30-35 kg/m^2, AGT 25%; hirsutism FG = 8 (71%); MetS
-Italian, Spanish	Prevalence 6.5% (NIH criteria)
East European:	Hirsutism not marked; MetS less prevalent
-Chez	IGT in 12%; higher CVD risk than matched controls
South American Brazilian	MetS in 31%; indicators of central obesity (waist circumference and waist-to-height ratio) were accurate predictors of MetS; frequency of MetS similar in the phenotypes
Middle Eastern (Caucasian)	
Arab	Overweight/obesity in 79%; BMI >30 kg/m^2 in 51%
-Iranian, Saudi Arabian	Similar prevalence of MetS among phenotypes
-Migrants (Canada and Austria)	High insulin response to glucose; infertility, rather than their obesity, affecting QoL

AGT, abnormal glucose tolerance (includes impaired glucose tolerance (IGT), impaired fasting glucose (IFG), frank diabetes; *BMI,* body Mass Index; *CVD,* cardiovascular diseases; *IR,* insulin Resistance (calculated by valid mathematical forumulae using plasma glucose and insulin); *FBS,* fasting blood glucose; *MetS,* Metabolic Syndrome; *NIH,* National Institute of Health; *PCO,* polysystic ovaries; *QoL,* quality of life; *SBP,* systolic blood pressure; *SHBG,* sex hormone binding globulin; *T2DM,* type 2 diabetes mellitus; *TG,* triglycerides.

TABLE 29.3	Psychological Comorbidity in Polycystic Ovary Syndrome
Psychological Disturbances in Polycystic Ovary Syndrome (PCOS)[23]	
Anxiety: 29%–50% compared with 18% in females without PCOS[32,33]	
Depression: 57% compared with 7% in females without PCOS[32]	
Helplessness[34]	
Increased risk of social phobia and difficulties in social skills and daily life[34]	
Painful chronic emotional stress[34]	
Elevated dysphoric feelings[34]	
Suicidal ideation[34]	
Bipolar disorder[34,35]	
Attention-deficit/hyperactivity disorder[36]	

It is pertinent to note that most communities within the African continent pay high tribute to physical appearance and a variation in the norm can significantly affect the individual and family living with it. A study conducted in the United States comparing adolescent females with PCOS and those without found that those with PCOS had a significantly higher prevalence of anxiety, depression, and attention-deficit/hyperactivity disorder compared with those without PCOS. In addition, Black females with PCOS in the study had less psychological impact than their White counterparts, possibly because of differences in the diagnosis of psychological disorders or increased barriers to accessing mental healthcare in racial/ethnically diverse populations.[23] African females with PCOS thus have a stigma associated with its physical presentation of acne, hirsutism, menstrual irregularities, obesity, and infertility,[21] which affects their cultural integration and existence within community-based social life.

Fertility is held in high esteem and considered mandatory in traditional African society. It is both a marker of normalcy and wealth in many parts of Africa, and subfertility is thus considered a taboo. A Nigerian study found that females with infertility have significantly more psychiatric morbidity than those without. This was significantly associated with discrimination, absence of family support, and history of induced abortion.[37] Among 100 females with infertility in Ghana, almost two-thirds (62%) had depression, which was significantly associated with lower socioeconomic status.[38] Additionally, a survey on infertile couples in Rwanda found that union dissolutions, sexual dysfunction, and domestic violence were significantly more frequently reported among infertile versus fertile couples.[39] These studies show how the presentation of PCOS patients with fertility issues may be marginalized, hence contributing to psychological morbidity.

Although there are limited studies to look at the racial/ethnic variations in PCOS from the African continent, by extrapolating from studies conducted from other global regions and in females presenting with individual features similar to those of PCOS, we can conclude that PCOS has a significant clinical, psychosocial, and cultural impact on African females and their families. It would thus be imperative to not only focus on the physical involvement but also ensure even the psychosocial and cultural aspects have been evaluated during the management of the condition.

Health-Seeking Behaviors for PCOS in Africans

There are many reasons why a person may not seek medical care. Factors that would prevent someone from seeking healthcare include language,[40] affordability, availability/accessibility, and acceptability.[41] Poverty, stigma, and inadequate knowledge or misinformation are likely to be strong cultural and socioeconomic factors affecting medical care seekers in Africa[42] (Fig. 29.1).

Diagnosing PCOS and the pitfalls associated with understanding the clinical presentation of this condition further compounds HSB. With more than half of PCOS sufferers seeing three or more doctors before diagnosis confirmation, less than one-quarter satisfied with PCOS-related information given at diagnosis about lifestyle management and medical therapy, and with over 50% not receiving any information about long-term PCOS complications or emotional support and counseling, it is not surprising that most PCOS sufferers are unlikely to continue turning up for costly medical care when there are other, more demanding activities that require their energy.[43] This would be more so in Africa, a continent plagued by poverty and traditional practices including religious prayer/practices to curb spirit-borne diseases such as tuberculosis. The cultural factors within households that pertain to power struggles between married/housed couples may also determine HSB, with usually the male dictating whether or not the female should seek care.[42] With 85% of Africans living on less than $5.50 per day,[44] it would be understandable why a patient with irregular menses and some hair on the chin may not consider paying for medical care.

With factors such as poverty, the stigma of attending allopathic medical clinics, and inadequate knowledge about the clinical presentations of PCOS as being abnormal, females in Africa may not have ideal HSB where PCOS is concerned.

With the concept of online access to information and recognition of the physical abnormalities brought about by PCOS and its contrast to the near-perfect skin and other physical characteristics of online avatars of many females, more and more younger females within the urban centers are reporting to their medical care providers, searching for remedies to ensure they look better. With this broad spectrum of seekers, it would be folly to generalize how African females seek care for something that may, or may not, bother their daily grind (see Fig. 29.1).

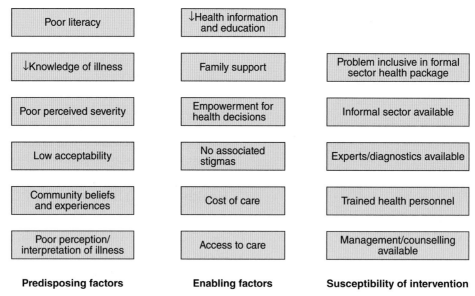

Predisposing factors	Enabling factors	Susceptibility of intervention
Poor literacy	↓Health information and education	
↓Knowledge of illness	Family support	Problem inclusive in formal sector health package
Poor perceived severity	Empowerment for health decisions	Informal sector available
Low acceptability	No associated stigmas	Experts/diagnostics available
Community beliefs and experiences	Cost of care	Trained health personnel
Poor perception/ interpretation of illness	Access to care	Management/counselling available

• **Fig. 29.1** Factors Affecting the Health-Seeking Behavior of the Community: A Challenge to Managing Polycystic Ovary Syndrome in Africa.

Treatment Modalities for PCOS in Africa

Because of the inherent challenges facing PCOS sufferers in Africa, it can be difficult to determine what treatment modalities are most used for alleviating their suffering. As previously alluded to, diseases such as tuberculosis are thought to be caused by spirits and therefore cured by spiritual rites and rituals or religious prayers.[42] The relative dearth of medical specialists in Africa further amplifies the limitations for PCOS patients. Practitioners such as clinical endocrinologists, clinical geneticists, physiologists, cytotherapeutic practitioners, dedicated reproductive endocrinologists, and gynecologists with a special interest in endocrinology are few and far between on the continent. The general gynecologists that do practice in the same geographic location as the authors of this chapter very rarely comanage PCOS patients with endocrinologists and prefer to manage their patients individually. These factors overall limit the available modalities used to combat PCOS in Africa.

PCOS Challenges in Africa

Having understood that PCOS is a multisystem disorder associated with significant clinical and psychosocial implications, it is crucial to recognize that its awareness, acceptance, and treatment grossly vary across the different global regions. Specific challenges of PCOS in Africa have been summarized in Table 29.4.

In Africa, a continent already hit hard by communicable diseases, there has been limited focus on NCDs overall. As the burden of NCDs is increasing and there is heightened awareness of the same globally, there is growing research from the African continent,[13] although at a much slower pace than required. There is thus paucity of data, particularly from resource-scarce sub-Saharan African countries

relating to the epidemiology, diagnosis, and management of PCOS.

Although limited studies are assessing HSB for PCOS from the African continent, the HSB for chronic NCDs in most parts of Africa is curative rather than preventive, implying that patients present late into the disease and have poor follow-up patterns. Idriss et al., in a study in Sierra Leone, found that although there was adequate basic knowledge on common NCDs among community members and leaders both in urban and rural regions, there was a heightened response only to severe symptoms. They also found that care-seeking is influenced by previous experiences, personal beliefs, and community beliefs on the appropriateness of methods, proximity to and cost of health facilities, and disease-specific factors, such as an acute presentation.[45]

Stigma related to features of PCOS (e.g., subfertility), particularly in low socioeconomic settings, could further influence HSB in Africa.[39] A Nigerian study on civil servants found high levels of appropriate HSB. Among the lower socioeconomic cadre, however, lack of health insurance and low level of education were associated with poorer health-seeking.

Another challenge for PCOS faced in Africa is lack of knowledge, expertise, and support by relevant stakeholders. Endocrinology/reproductive endocrinology is a limited specialty in most African countries, particularly in the sub-Saharan region, and a vast majority of patients with PCOS are thus managed primarily by obstetricians/gynecologists rather than by multidisciplinary teams. The focus of management thus leans toward the reproductive aspects of PCOS, with limited attention to the metabolic and psychosocial elements. Additionally, minimal funding and focus are provided for research and public health awareness of PCOS in the public health sector, which forms the bulk of healthcare requirements in the majority of African countries.

TABLE 29.4 Challenges of Polycystic Ovary Syndrome in Africa

Challenge	Discussion
Focus on communicable diseases	Less focus on noncommunicable diseases (NCDs), including polycystic ovary syndrome (PCOS)
Paucity of data on PCOS	Limited studies because of poor funding and awareness
Health-seeking behavior	Presentation with acute/severe symptoms rather than preventive, chronic care seeking. Thus PCOS patients present late and with complications/comorbidities
Stigma and beliefs	Features of PCOS are associated with stigma and false beliefs/myths
Lack of knowledge	Poor knowledge of PCOS among stakeholders including governments, healthcare providers, and public
Limited expertise	Few trained specialists and subspecialists
Specialized healthcare distribution	Most specialist facilities and subspecialty practitioners located in major towns
Cost of care	Limited health insurance and mostly out-of-pocket cost of healthcare, hormonal assays, and management of PCOS is expensive
Lack of guidelines	Most African countries do not have guidelines for PCOS diagnosis and management
Limited laboratory infrastructure and personnel	Poor quality assurance of hormonal assays, few laboratories providing specialist services and at distance from regional centers.
International funding	Most funding is directed to communicable diseases and limited NCDs; PCOS is not a priority
Specialist/subspecialist distribution	Few specialists/subspecialists in the countries, most in big towns/cities or recruited by funded programs

The specific diagnostic and management challenges of PCOS in Africa are detailed next.

Diagnostic Challenges of PCOS in Africa

Subfertility is recognized as a major health problem in African countries, and there are limited clinical guidelines for PCOS as an entity; thus it is not part of most minimum health packages.[46] Lack of guidelines translates to diagnostic challenges; thus many patients have delayed or no diagnosis. This then increases the risk of developing complications/associations of PCOS, including subfertility, dysfunctional uterine bleeding, endometrial cancer, and metabolic, cardiovascular, and psychosocial comorbidities.

In any resource-poor setting, the standard of care of PCOS could be challenging because of the limited laboratory infrastructure and appropriate personnel. The 2003 Rotterdam Criteria are the most commonly used for PCOS diagnosis and include at least two out of three features (clinical and/or biochemical HA, chronic oligo/anovulation, and polycystic ovarian morphology) after the exclusion of other disorders (hyperprolactinemia, thyroid disease, late-onset congenital adrenal hyperplasia, or androgen-secreting tumors).[27] For PCOS suspects, this requires a minimum evaluation including testosterone levels, dehydroepiandrosterone (DHEA) sulfate, thyroid-stimulating hormone (TSH), prolactin, 17-hydroxyprogesterone (17-HP), transvaginal ultrasound (evaluation for polycystic and endometrial morphology), and an endometrial biopsy as needed.[47]

Metabolic evaluation also forms part of the PCOS diagnostics armamentarium, which includes glucose assessment (preferably with the 75 g oral glucose tolerance test), insulin levels, and a lipid profile. These assessments require good laboratory support for PCOS detection, control, management, and surveillance. In low- and middle-income countries, there is limited access to quality-assured laboratory services, thus leading to late and inaccurate diagnosis, with ineffective treatment and impact on the safety of the patient.[48] Most of the laboratory services are concentrated in major cities/towns and are run privately or in the central referral facilities,[49] thus limiting the vast majority of public, general, and regional referral hospitals from conducting hormonal assays.[46] In addition, distance to such care points and poverty contribute to inequality and lack of equity in PCOS care in the continent. Significant funding is available for low- to middle-income countries (LMIC; e.g., from United Nations agencies and not-for-profit organizations), but this does not include PCOS recognition, diagnosis, and management.[46] This further reduces access to equitable healthcare for Africans.

Many LMICs have severe shortages of trained medical personnel, leading to less knowledgeable nonspecialists like clinical officers and nonspecialist doctors/physicians handling complex conditions such as PCOS.[49] This leads to inappropriate and missed diagnoses because of the wide variability in PCOS presentation and lack of adequate knowledge of the providers. Furthermore, the few trained specialist and subspecialist healthcare providers are either concentrated in major cities or recruited by nongovernmental organization programs, leading to regional shortages.

Management Challenges

Other than the limited accessibility to specialists, the African PCOS population has other challenges when it comes to the management of the condition. Lack of awareness, both within the society at large and within the medical community (primarily because of lack of structured education and dedicated specialists), hampers effective treatment exploration. Poverty in itself is a major hindrance to searching out appropriate healthcare, and other, more acute, medical conditions are likely to take priority over chronic medical conditions that may not present as emergencies. Lack of access to appropriate medical facilities manned by medical practitioners is another hurdle. Because countries such as Finland have maternal mortality rates of 3 per 100,000 live births stable from 2014 to 2017,[50] countries such as Kenya have to wonder why its rates are well over 300, with 1% yearly declines over the same years of 2014 to 2017.[51] It begs the question of whether Finland is over a hundred times better when it comes to maternal care. It is interesting to understand and view this from a zoom-out lens, which takes us to the period of 1900 to 1904, where Finland's maternal mortality ratio was 240 per 100,000 live births.[52] That is still below the maternal mortality rates for the year 2017 of Angola, Djibouti, Rwanda, Myanmar, Gabon, Comoros, Mozambique, Sudan, Equatorial Guinea, Ghana, Senegal, Burkina Faso, Madagascar, Kenya, Malawi, Uganda, Congo, Togo, Benin, Ethiopia, Eswatini, Zimbabwe, the Democratic Republic of the Congo, Eritrea, Haiti, Niger, Tanzania, Cameroon, Lesotho, Burundi, Mali, Guinea, Gambia, Côte d'Ivoire, Afghanistan, Liberia, Guinea-Bissau, Mauritania, Central African Republic, Somalia, Nigeria, Sierra Leone, Chad, and South Sudan.[53] Only two countries in this list are not within the territory of Africa. Between the years 2001 and 2003, in a certain rural location within the coast province of Kenya, East Africa, only 5.4% of births occurred within a health facility.[54] When such vital allopathic medical care provision (care to mothers giving birth) can be such a problem, perhaps it is asking for too much to have PCOS management in Africa be in the spotlight.

Recommendations and Conclusions

PCOS, with its spectrum of clinical and biochemical presentation, can now be classed as a recognized condition with most medical care providers being aware of its existence. The Rotterdam Criteria are the most used in diagnosing the disease. With the standardization of evaluation criteria and therefore definition of the malady, it would be much easier to identify subclinical disease presentation and make it easier for healthcare providers to recognize the affliction.

As this chapter is written, there is no Africa-wide body responsible for PCOS education (for health professionals or patients). Education, in this case, could be diagnosis and management guidelines for professionals, for example. Such an establishment could help produce literature specific to the African continent and help spread more information about PCOS in stakeholder circles, including providing content that may inform government policy. With the advent of the Internet and urged on by COVID-19, geographic restriction is a poor excuse for not getting enough information out there. Health education can also be directed toward the patients, who should be given further information regarding the ailment, as well as how best to seek help and take care of themselves. Support groups are a big positive step toward helping those with PCOS, and they help provide evidence-based information, provide peer support, raise awareness, and help advocate for female-centered care.[55] Many support groups worldwide have partnerships with healthcare providers and researchers, making substantial contributions to advocacy and raising awareness of conditions. Such partnerships represent an opportunity for collaboration, leading to the availability of evidence-based information for both other professional groups and for those they support. Robust, continent-wide policy groups may also have the power to guide local curriculum inclusion of PCOS education. As more healthcare workers are sensitized to PCOS, early recognition is likely to occur. This helps increase the quality of life for these patients sooner, allowing them to live with less suffering. PCOS awareness in medical circles will undoubtedly lead to more professionals specializing in PCOS care, allowing the formation of multidisciplinary teams (MDTs) that help support groups of patients. Policy or support groups are in an ideally leveraged position to identify and strengthen streamlined referral systems, allowing a vast number of PCOS patients to take advantage of specialized care provider groups working in a multidisciplinary format.

Another advantage of sensitization would be an increase in the diagnostic requests for helping to rule out other disorders as the healthcare practitioners work toward a diagnosis of PCOS. Such an increase in laboratory requests may lead to a surge of centers that provide such services, allowing decentralization of laboratory infrastructure/expertise and providing an opportunity for regional collection point pathology networks. Increased diagnosis and management of PCOS sufferers are likely to attract interest from health insurance providers, and here is another opportunity to elevate equitable access to healthcare on the continent.

With all the dearth of information regarding PCOS in Africa, various opportunities and scopes for improvement can be identified in ensuring early diagnosis and appropriate management for PCOS sufferers. Well designed research can assist in filling existing knowledge gaps to further guide improved diagnosis and management for women living with PCOS.

References

1. El Hayek S, Bitar L, Hamdar LH, Mirza FG, Daoud G. Polycystic ovarian syndrome: an updated overview. *Front Physiol.* 2016;7:124. doi:10.3389/FPHYS.2016.00124.

2. Charifson MA, Trumble BC. Evolutionary origins of polycystic ovary syndrome: an environmental mismatch disorder. *Evol Med Public Health.* 2019;2019:50-63. doi:10.1093/emph/eoz011.

3. Unluturk U, Harmanci A, Kocaefe C, Yildiz BO. The genetic basis of the polycystic ovary syndrome: a literature review including discussion of PPAR-γ. *PPAR Res.* 2007;2007:49109. doi:10.1155/2007/49109.

4. *Genotype Environment Interaction - An Overview.* ScienceDirect Topics; 2021. Available at: https://www.sciencedirect.com/topics/medicine-and-dentistry/genotype-environment-interaction.

5. United Nations Department of Economics and Social Affairs *The World Population Prospects: 2015 Revision.* United Nations; 2015. https://www.un.org/en/development/desa/publications/world-population-prospects-2015-revision.html#:~:text=The%20current%20world%20population%20of,2015%20Revision%E2%80%9D%2C%20launched%20today.

6. United Nations. Economic Commission for Africa (2004). Unlocking Africa's trade potential in the global economy : policy paper. [Addis Ababa] :. © UN.ECA,. https://hdl.handle.net/10855/5506"

7. World Health Organization, 2016. *Report on the Status of Major Health Risk Factors for Noncommunicable Diseases: WHO African Region, 2015* [Online]. Available at: https://www.afro.who.int/publications/report-status-major-health-risk-factors-noncommunicable-diseases-who-african-region-0.

8. Ntumy M, Maya E, Lizneva D, Adanu R, Azziz R. The pressing need for standardization in epidemiologic studies of PCOS across the globe. *Gynecol Endocrinol.* 2019;35(1):1-3. doi:10.1080/09513590.2018.1488958.

9. Kofi-Tsekpo M. Institutionalization of African traditional medicine in health care systems in Africa. *Afr J Health Sc.* 2004;11(1-2):i-ii. doi:10.4314/AJHS.V11I1.30772.

10. Ezeh U, Yildiz BO, Azziz R. Referral bias in defining the phenotype and prevalence of obesity in polycystic ovary syndrome. *J Clin Endocrinol Metab.* 2013;98(6):E1088-E1096. doi:10.1210/JC.2013-1295.

11. Lizneva D, Kirubakaran R, Mykhalchenko K, et al. Phenotypes and body mass in women with polycystic ovary syndrome identified in referral versus unselected populations: systematic review and meta-analysis. *Fertil Steril.* 2016;106(6):1510-1520.e2. doi:10.1016/J.FERTNSTERT.2016.07.1121.

12. Ding T, Hardiman PJ, Petersen I, et al. The prevalence of polycystic ovary syndrome in reproductive-aged women of different ethnicity: a systematic review and meta-analysis. *Oncotarget.* 2017;8(56):96351-96358. doi:10.18632/ONCOTARGET.19180.

13. Maya ET, Guure CB, Adanu RMK, et al. Why we need epidemiologic studies of polycystic ovary syndrome in Africa. *Int J Gynecol Obstet.* 2018;143(2):251-254. doi:10.1002/IJGO.12642.

14. Alur-Gupta S, Lee I, Chemerinski A, et al. Racial differences in anxiety, depression, and quality of life in women with polycystic ovary syndrome. *F S Rep.* 2021;2(2):230-237. doi:10.1016/J.XFRE.2021.03.003.

15. Azziz R, Woods KS, Reyna R, Key TJ, Knochenhauer ES, Yildiz BO. The prevalence and features of the polycystic ovary syndrome in an unselected population. *J Clin Endocrinol Metab.* 2004;89(6):2745-2749. doi:10.1210/JC.2003-032046.

16. Knochenhauer ES, Key TJ, Kahsar-Miller M, Waggoner W, Boots LR, Azziz R. Prevalence of the polycystic ovary syndrome in unselected black and white women of the southeastern United States: a prospective study. *J Clin Endocrinol Metab.* 1998;83(9):3078-3082. doi:10.1210/JCEM.83.9.5090.

17. Hillman JK, Johnson LNC, Limaye M, Feldman RA, Sammel M, Dokras A. Black women with polycystic ovary syndrome (PCOS) have increased risk for metabolic syndrome and cardiovascular disease compared with white women with PCOS. *Fertil Steril.* 2014;101(2):530-535. doi:10.1016/J.FERTNSTERT.2013.10.055.

18. Witchel SF, Oberfield SE, Peña AS. Polycystic ovary syndrome: pathophysiology, presentation, and treatment with emphasis on adolescent girls. *J Endocr Soc.* 2019;3(8):1545-1573. doi:10.1210/JS.2019-00078.

19. Johnson TRB, Kaplan LK, Ouyang P, Rizza RA, National Institutes of Health Evidence-based methodology workshop on polycystic ovary syndrome. Bethesda, Maryland: National Institutes of Health; 2012. https://prevention.nih.gov/sites/default/files/2018-06/FinalReport.pdf.

20. Anagnostis P, Tarlatzis BC, Kauffman RP. Polycystic ovarian syndrome (PCOS): long-term metabolic consequences. *Metabolism.* 2018;86:33-43. doi:10.1016/J.METABOL.2017.09.016.

21. Hadjiconstantinou M, Mani H, Patel N, et al. Understanding and supporting women with polycystic ovary syndrome: a qualitative study in an ethnically diverse UK sample. *Endocr Connect.* 2017;6(5):323. doi:10.1530/EC-17-0053.

22. Moulana M. Persistent risk: psychological comorbidity in polycystic ovary syndrome. *Endocrinol Metab Int J.* 2020;8(6):139-141. doi:10.15406/EMIJ.2020.08.00297.

23. Moulana M, Lim CS, Sukumaran AP. High risk of psychological disorders: anxiety and depression in adolescent girls with polycystic ovary syndrome. *Endocrinol Metab Int J.* 2020;8(3):73-77. doi:10.15406/emij.2020.08.00282.

24. Engmann L, Jin S, Sun F, et al. Racial and ethnic differences in the polycystic ovary syndrome (PCOS) metabolic phenotype. *Am J Obstet Gynecol.* 2017;216(5):493.e1. doi:10.1016/J.AJOG.2017.01.003.

25. Oriji VK. Prevalence of polycystic ovary syndrome (PCOS) among infertile women attending fertility clinic at a university teaching hospital in Nigeria. *J Gynecol Womens Health.* 2019;15(5):555922. doi:10.19080/JGWH.2019.15.555922.

26. Pembe AB, Abeid AM. Polycystic ovaries and associated clinical and biochemical features among women with infertility in a tertiary hospital in Tanzania. *Tanzan J Health Res.* 2009;11(4):175-180.

27. The Rotterdam ESHRE/ASRM-Sponsored PCOS Consensus Workshop Group. Revised 2003 consensus on diagnostic criteria and long-term health risks related to polycystic ovary syndrome. *Hum Reprod.* 2004;19:41-47. Available at: https://doi.org/10.1093/humrep/deh098.

28. Odera FO. (2019). *Prevalence of Polycystic Ovary Syndrome Among Women Presenting with Amenorrhea and Oligomenorrhea at the Kenyatta National Hospital* [Online]. Available at: http://erepository.uonbi.ac.ke/bitstream/handle/11295/108179/Odera_Prevalence%20of%20polycystic%20ovary%20syndrome%20among%20women%20presenting%20with%20amenorrhea%20and%20oligomenorrhea%20at%20the%20kenyatta%20national%20hospital.pdf?sequence=1&isAllowed=y.

29. Wijeyaratne CN, Dilini Udayangani SA, Balen AH. Ethnic-specific PCOS. *Expert Rev Endocrinol Metab.* 2013;8(1):71-79.

30. Kocełak P, Chudek J, Naworska B, et al. Psychological disturbances and quality of life in obese and infertile women and men. *Int J Endocrinol.* 2012;2012:236217. doi:10.1155/2012/236217.

31. Elsenbruch S, Benson S, Hahn S, et al. Determinants of emotional distress in women with polycystic ovary syndrome. *Hum Reprod.* 2006;21(4):1092-1099. doi:10.1093/HUMREP/DEI409.

32. Deeks AA, Gibson-Helm ME, Teede HJ. Anxiety and depression in polycystic ovary syndrome: a comprehensive investigation. *Fertil Steril.* 2010;93(7):2421-2423. doi:10.1016/J.FERTNSTERT.2009.09.018.

33. Benson S, Hahn S, Tan S, et al. Prevalence and implications of anxiety in polycystic ovary syndrome: results of an internet-based survey in Germany. *Hum Reprod.* 2009;24(6):1446-1451. doi:10.1093/HUMREP/DEP031.

34. Scaruffi E, Gambineri A, Cattaneo S, Turra J, Vettor R, Mioni R. Personality and psychiatric disorders in women affected by polycystic ovary syndrome. *Front Endocrinol.* 2014;5:185. doi:10.3389/FENDO.2014.00185.

35. Klipstein KG, Goldberg JF. Screening for bipolar disorder in women with polycystic ovary syndrome: a pilot study. *J Affect Disord.* 2006;91(2-3):205-209. doi:10.1016/J.JAD.2006.01.011.

36. Hergüner S, Harmancı H, Toy H. Attention deficit-hyperactivity disorder symptoms in women with polycystic ovary syndrome. *Int J Psychiatry Med.* 2015;50(3):317-325. doi:10.1177/0091217415610311.

37. Makanjuola AB, Elegbede AO, Abiodun OA. Predictive factors for psychiatric morbidity among women with infertility attending a gynaecology clinic in Nigeria. *Afr J Psychiatry (South Africa).* 2010; 13(1):36-42.

38. Alhassan A, Ziblim AR, Muntaka S. A survey on depression among infertile women in Ghana. *BMC Womens Health.* 2014;14(1):42. doi:10.1186/1472-6874-14-42.

39. Dhont N, van de Wijgert J, Coene G, Gasarabwe A, Temmerman M. 'Mama and papa nothing': living with infertility among an urban population in Kigali, Rwanda. *Hum Reprod.* 2011;26(3): 623-629. doi:10.1093/HUMREP/DEQ373.

40. Al Shamsi H, Almutairi AG, Al Mashrafi S, Al Kalbani T. Implications of language barriers for healthcare: a systematic review. *Oman Med J.* 2020;35(2):e122. doi:10.5001/OMJ.2020.40.

41. Goudge J, Gilson L, Russell S, Gumede T, Mills A. Affordability, availability and acceptability barriers to health care for the chronically ill: longitudinal case studies from South Africa. *BMC Health Serv Res.* 2009;9:75. Available at: https://doi.org/10.1186/1472-6963-9-75.

42. Msoka EF, Orina F, Sanga ES, et al. Qualitative assessment of the impact of socioeconomic and cultural barriers on uptake and utilisation of tuberculosis diagnostic and treatment tools in East Africa: a cross-sectional study. *BMJ Open.* 2021;11(7):e050911. doi:10.1136/BMJOPEN-2021-050911.

43. Gibson-Helm M, Teede H, Dunaif A, Dokras A. Delayed diagnosis and a lack of information associated with dissatisfaction in women with polycystic ovary syndrome. *J Clin Endocrinol Metab.* 2017;102(2):604-612. doi:10.1210/JC.2016-2963.

44. World Bank Blogs. *85% of Africans Live on Less than $5.50 Per Day.* 2019. Available at: https://blogs.worldbank.org/opendata/85-africans-live-less-550-day.

45. Idriss A, Diaconu K, Zou G, Senesi RG, Wurie H, Witter S. Rural–urban health-seeking behaviours for non-communicable diseases in Sierra Leone. *BMJ Global Health.* 2020;5(2):e002024. doi:10.1136/BMJGH-2019-002024.

46. Pebolo FP, Grace AA, Gasthony A. Polycystic ovarian syndrome: diagnostic challenges in resource-poor settings, Ugandan perspectives. *PAMJ Clin Med.* 2021;5:41. Available at: https://doi.org/10.11604/PAMJ-CM.2021.5.41.26386.

47. Azziz R, Marin C, Hoq L, Badamgarav E, Song P. Health care-related economic burden of the polycystic ovary syndrome during the reproductive life span. *J Clin Endocrinol Metab.* 2005;90(8):4650-4658. doi:10.1210/JC.2005-0628.

48. Nkengasong JN, Yao K, Onyebujoh P. Laboratory medicine in low-income and middle-income countries: progress and challenges. *Lancet (London, England).* 2018;391(10133):1873-1875. doi:10.1016/S0140-6736(18)30308-8.

49. Benediktsson H, Whitelaw J, Roy I. Pathology services in developing countries a challenge. *Arch Pathol Lab Med.* 2007;131:1636-1639.

50. *Finland Maternal Mortality Rate 2000-2021.* MacroTrends; 2021. Available at: https://www.macrotrends.net/countries/FIN/finland/maternal-mortality-rate.

51. *Kenya Maternal Mortality Rate 2000-2021.* MacroTrends; 2021. Available at: https://www.macrotrends.net/countries/KEN/kenya/maternal-mortality-rate.

52. Högberg U. The decline in maternal mortality in Sweden: the role of community midwifery. *Am J Public Health.* 2004;94(8): 1312-1320. doi:10.2105/AJPH.94.8.1312.

53. *Maternal Mortality Rates and Statistics.* Unicef Data; 2017. Available at: https://data.unicef.org/topic/maternal-health/maternal-mortality/.

54. Cotter K, Hawken M, Temmerman M. Low use of skilled attendants' delivery services in rural Kenya. *J Health Popul Nutr.* 2006;24(4):467. Available at: https://www.ncbi.nlm.nih.gov/pmc/articles/PMC3001150/.

55. Avery J, Ottey S, Morman R, Cree-Green M, Gibson-Helm M. Polycystic ovary syndrome support groups and their role in awareness, advocacy and peer support: a systematic search and narrative review. *Curr Opin Endocr Metab Res.* 2020;12:98-104. doi:10.1016/J.COEMR.2020.04.008.

30

Polycystic Ovary Syndrome in North America

MAHEEN SHAHID AND MUNEELA WAJID

North America

North America (NA), covering an area of 24,230,000 km^2, is the third largest of the world's continents and is home to less than 10% of the world's population.[1] It has grown to become one of the world's most economically developed regions.[1] The continent has not only the highest income per person but also the highest food intake,[1] leading to a higher prevalence of overweight and obese people in NA.[2]

Definition

Polycystic ovary syndrome (PCOS) may present with a spectrum of metabolic, dermatologic, and gynecologic signs and symptoms together forming a disorder with variable presentation ranging from mildly symptomatic to severe disease.[3] The American Society of Reproductive Medicine (ASRM) defines PCOS as having at least two of the three following features: hyperandrogenism (HA; clinical or biochemical), oligoanovulation, and polycystic ovaries.[4] It is the most frequent endocrinopathy seen in females of childbearing age in the United States, affecting approximately 7%.[3] In the United States, PCOS contributes significantly to the healthcare economic burden with about 4 billion dollars being spent per year on PCOS and its related comorbidities.[5]

Polycystic Ovary Syndrome–Associated Disorders in Females in the United States

Dermatologic Disorders

Hirsutism and Acne

Almost 70% of females with hirsutism have PCOS in the United States, making it a frequent presenting complaint.[6] It is defined as male-pattern distribution of terminal hair growth in areas such as the upper lip, chin, areola, chest, back, and lower abdomen.[7] A study conducted by the University of Alabama reports that 74% of females with hirsutism have PCOS

in the United States.[7] HA also manifests physically as acne. Its distribution is the same as that of hirsutism, extending mainly to the neck, chest, lower face, and upper abdomen.[8] Acne that is resistant to treatment or extends to adulthood should raise clinical suspicion and the need for further evaluation.[9]

Hair Loss

PCOS was reported to be the most prevalent endocrine disorder in patients presenting with hair loss complaints in the United States.[10] A study conducted by Mount Sinai School of Medicine reported that 38.5% of females presenting with alopecia also had HA.[10]

Ovulatory Dysfunction/Menstrual Irregularity

Ovulatory dysfunction is clinically defined as a menstrual cycle lasting less than 26 or more than 35 days in length or a history of having less than 9 cycles per year.[11] A prospective study on reproductive-age females in Alabama undergoing a preemployment medical examination reported a 22.8% prevalence of menstrual dysfunction.[12] Among Black females, the prevalence rate of menstrual disturbance was 25.1%; it was 20.5% in White females.[12] Hartz et al. conducted a study on American females aged 20 to 39 and observed that those with a greater waist to hip ratio were at an increased risk for developing menstrual irregularities.[13] It has also been noted that PCOS patients with normal cycles exhibit less derangement of their metabolic profile.[11]

Metabolic Syndrome

According to The National Cholesterol Education Program Adult Treatment Panel (NCEP ATP III), the presence of at least three of the five following abnormalities is defined as metabolic syndrome (MetS): waist circumference in females greater than 88 cm, fasting blood sugar (FBS) up to 110 mg/dL, fasting serum triglyceride up to 150 mg/dL, serum high-density lipoprotein (HDL) less than 50 mg/dL, and blood pressure (BP) of at least

130/85 mm Hg.[14] The prevalence of MetS in American females with PCOS is reported to be 43%, which is much higher than the 24% prevalence found in non-PCOS females of the region.[14,15] Its prevalence is found to be even lower in other parts of the world such as Italy where 8.2% of females with PCOS report MetS.[16] Dietary habits in the United States and the obesity epidemic may be factors contributing to these statistics, hence proving the profound effect of lifestyle on MetS and PCOS. It has been observed that American females with PCOS and MetS together exhibit more severe HA and related symptomatology than those with PCOS alone.[14] Low HDL is the most frequently observed finding and is present in up to 68% of PCOS patients in the United States, followed by elevated body mass index (BMI) in 67%, hypertension in 45%, hypertriglyceridemia in 35%, and abnormal FBS in 4%. The risk for developing type 2 diabetes mellitus (DM)[14] and cardiovascular complications is increased in patients with MetS.[14]

Insulin Resistance and Hyperinsulinemia

Hyperinsulinemia is an important extrinsic factor that further exacerbates the HA observed in PCOS patients.[17] It is known to occur even in the absence of obesity, and hence the diseases of insulin resistance (IR), such as DM, are commonly associated with PCOS.[18] Legro et al. reported 31.1% prevalence of impaired glucose tolerance (IGT) in American females with PCOS and 7.8% in age- and BMI-matched controls.[18] Another study reports higher IR in Hispanic females with PCOS than non-Hispanic White females with PCOS.[19]

Dyslipidemia

Dyslipidemia, characterized by high triglyceride and low HDL, is a commonly observed finding in PCOS patients in the United States.[20] A study conducted to compare dietary habits in the American and Italian population reported twice as much consumption of saturated fat by American females compared with Italians even though total calorific intake was similar between both groups.[20] Because of changes in diet and lifestyle, abnormal lipid profile is a feature observed in 70% to 90% PCOS patients in the United States.[21] The University of Pittsburg conducted a large cohort of PCOS females in the United States and reported that dyslipidemia occurs earlier in life there, at younger than 45 years in many patients.[22]

Diabetes Mellitus

In the United States, prevalence of DM in PCOS females is reported to be 7.5% compared with 0.7% in healthy young females.[23] A large cohort of young females in the United States found that those with PCOS in their 20s are at a greater for developing DM and lipid disorder by their 50s; this increased risk is independent of their BMI.[17]

Cancer

Breast Cancer

Higher circulating sex steroids are known to increase the risk for breast cancer.[24] A large case control study was conducted on breast cancer patients between the ages of 50 and 75 from Wisconsin, Massachusetts, and New Hampshire and showed increased risk of breast cancer with androgen excess disorders such as PCOS.[25]

Ovarian Cancer

Ovarian cancer in the United States is the fourth most frequent cause of cancer death among females.[26] Ovarian cancer has also been linked to increased androgen exposure as seen in PCOS.[27] In the United States, obesity, which is a frequently observed finding in PCOS patients, has been positively linked to ovarian cancer.[26]

Endometrial Cancer

Chronic anovulation results in higher estrogen levels that are unopposed by progesterone secretion. As a consequence, endometrium is chronically exposed to higher estrogen levels, which results in endometrial hyperplasia and an increased risk for endometrial carcinoma.[28] Obesity, hyperinsulinemia, increased androgen, and increased insulin-like growth factor 1 secretion as seen in PCOS are also known risk factors for endometrial carcinoma.[29] A large cohort study conducted on American females with endometrial cancer reported that 39% of them had a history of irregular menses, 33% had a history of DM, and 56% of them were obese. These set of symptoms are frequently seen to be associated with PCOS.[28]

Fertility in Polycystic Ovary Syndrome

Anovulation secondary to PCOS often leads to infertility and is the most common cause of subfertility seen in American females.[30] The ASRM reported a 70% to 80% rate of infertility in patients with PCOS.[31] Therefore the ASRM recommends initiating infertility workup 6 months after unsuccessful attempts at conception in patients with PCOS.[31]

Pregnancy Loss in Polycystic Ovary Syndrome

Unopposed estrogen, androgen, and insulin influence the endometrium, resulting in a greater risk of pregnancy loss observed in PCOS patients.[32] Pregnancy loss is reported to be 30% to 40% in PCOS patients in the United States, which is much higher than the 10% to 15% in females without PCOS.[33] In addition to the hormonal and metabolic abnormalities observed, gestation and PCOS both are procoagulant states; all these factors cumulatively pose an increased risk to pregnancy.

Venous Thromboembolism

Both deep vein thrombosis (DVT) and pulmonary embolism (PE) are included in venous thromboembolism

(VTE). The hyperinsulinemia observed in PCOS causes an elevation of plasminogen activator inhibitor 1, which has an important role in the inhibition of fibrinolysis.[34] A case control study conducted on PCOS females reported higher VTE prevalence in patients with PCOS than in patients without it.[34] Moreover, the use of oral contraceptive pills (OCPs) among PCOS patients was found to be protective.

Cardiovascular Disease

The hyperinsulinemia observed in PCOS promotes the transport of cholesterol into arterial smooth muscles in addition to increasing cholesterol synthesis in these cells. This predisposes patients to a greater risk of cardiovascular disease (CVD) and cerebrovascular disease.[35] The HA in PCOS also contributes to the greater CVD risk seen in patients.[36] The University of Pittsburg conducted a case control study on American females with 125 PCOS patients and 142 controls to assess intima-media thickness (IMT) using carotid ultrasonography. The study reported significantly greater IMT in females with PCOS than in those without.[37]

The American Heart Association (AHA) puts females with PCOS into the "at risk for PCOS–associated CVD" and "high risk for PCOS–associated CVD" categories.

- At-risk females are defined as having abdominal obesity, hypertension, a deranged lipid profile, IGT, positive family history of CVD, subclinical vasculopathy, and smoking.
- High-risk females are defined as having type 2 DM, MetS, and the presence of renal and vascular disease.[38]

PCOS puts patients at a greater risk for developing CVD and cerebrovascular disease, and there is need for aggressive symptom control along with increased screening and surveillance for the disease.[39]

Gastrointestinal and Liver Issues

IR and compensatory hyperinsulinemia increase lipolysis in adipose tissue and de novo lipogenesis in liver, which both cause an increase flow of free fatty acids (FFA) to the liver and consequently contribute to hepatic fat accumulation, causing the nonalcoholic fatty liver disease (NAFLD) observed in many PCOS patients.[40] In a study conducted in California, aminotransferase, a surrogate marker for NAFLD, was seen to be elevated in 30% of females with PCOS.[41] Another study in North Carolina reported that 15% of PCOS patients had abnormal aminotransferases along with biopsy evidence of NASH.[42] A retrospective disease conducted on American females having PCOS demonstrated 55% of them as having fatty liver; it is important to note that of these 55% females, almost 40% were lean.[43] NAFLD puts patients at risk for progressive liver disease.[42] Carmina et al. proposed the need for liver assessment in patients with PCOS; NAFLD female patients should also be evaluated for the presence of PCOS.[44]

Sleep Disorder

IR is strongly associated with obstructive sleep apnea (OSA) and excessive daytime sleepiness (EDS) independent of obesity.[45] The prevalence of OSA is seen to be significantly higher in patients with PCOS (obese and nonobese) compared with healthy controls.[45] Vgontzas et al. concluded that females with PCOS are 30 times more likely to develop OSA than healthy controls; in addition, 80% of PCOS females (obese and nonobese) report EDS compared with 25% of controls.[45] PCOS patients are also frequently seen to report difficulty in falling asleep, which can be attributed to stress system activation.[46] PCOS patients with OSA also report a greater derangement of metabolic profile than PCOS patients without OSA.[47] The University of Chicago conducted a study on PCOS females and reported the prevalence to be 56% among patients compared with 19% in controls.[48]

Mood Disorders

High androgen production and low sex hormone–binding globulin (SHBG) together contribute to the augmented free testosterone levels observed in PCOS patients.[49] Weiner et al. in his study conducted on American females reported that females with abnormal testosterone levels were noted to be more depressed.[49] This supports the argument that physical symptoms alone are not responsible for the deteriorating mental wellbeing observed in PCOS patients. Mental health disorders, especially mood disorders, are seen to be highly prevalent in PCOS females.[50] The disease is well known to reduce the quality of health because its symptoms increases patients' distress regarding their menstrual cycle, cosmetic problems, fertility concerns, and risk of developing complications in the future. All these contribute to overall reduced mental, physical, and sexual wellbeing.[51]

Depression

Females with PCOS are at a significantly greater risk for developing depression.[52] A longitudinal prospective study in the United States reports 35% prevalence of depression in PCOS females compared with 10% in healthy controls.[52] Even independent of obesity and fertility problems, American females possess a greater risk for developing depressive disorder.[53] These statistics warrant the need for aggressive screening for depression in patients with PCOS.

Anxiety

A prevalence of 15% for anxiety is reported in PCOS females in the United States.[52] Concerns regarding weight gain and inability to lose weight were reported to cause greater anxiety in the study population in the United States than hirsutism.[52] This may be associated with access and availability to advanced dermatologic services like laser hair removal in the high-income world.

Eating Disorders

Females with PCOS are at greater risk for developing eating disorders than healthy controls.[52] A study conducted in the United States reports a 14% risk of developing eating disorder in females with PCOS.[52] Clinical manifestations of PCOS are negatively affected by obesity,[52] making weight loss a frequent recommendation provided to patients with PCOS. Females with eating disorder are often seen to struggle with weight reduction, which further poorly impacts their mental and physical health.

Diagnosis

The ASRM recommends using history, physical examination, blood tests, and ultrasonography together to aid in the diagnosis of PCOS.

Healthcare providers should look for physical and biochemical evidence of HA, which manifests as hirsutism in PCOS females. Menstrual irregularity is also a frequent complaint encountered during history taking of PCOS patients; this may present as amenorrhea, which is defined as a cycle of greater than 199 days or oligomenorrhea with a cycle length of more than 35 to 199 days.[54] Ultrasound examination is used to evaluate polycystic ovaries; up to 61% of American PCOS patients have ultrasound or laparoscopic evidence of polycystic ovaries.[55] Obesity is defined as BMI greater than 30 to 40 and extreme obesity as BMI greater than 40. It is also commonly noted in PCOS patients, especially in the United States where the prevalence of obesity in a large study was reported to be 45% and extreme obesity was 31%.[55] According to a recommendation by the American College of Obstetrics and Gynecology, each patient's BP must be evaluated at every visit, in addition to an oral glucose tolerance test to screen for type 2 DM and testing serum lipids at the time of diagnosis.[3]

A study conducted in the United States found high variability in the clinical approach of healthcare providers to PCOS in NA. For the initial test for diagnosis, 87% of physicians were noted to order thyroid-stimulating hormone (TSH) tests and 78% ordered serum prolactin. For the evaluation of metabolic features, 61% ordered lipid profile and 60% ordered serum glucose, 41% assessed fasting insulin, and 25% ordered serum Hb A_{1c}.[56]

Treatment (According to Recommendations Made by the ASRM)

A holistic approach toward patient care in PCOS is needed, where a patient's physical and emotional symptoms are both addressed.

Lifestyle Modification

Counseling regarding weight reduction, exercise, and alcohol and smoking cessation should be advised along with pharmacologic interventions.[54]

Metabolic

Metformin is frequently used in the treatment of PCOS. It not only improves insulin sensitivity but also has a positive effect menstrual irregularity.[57,58]

Dermatologic

Hormone Suppression

Inhibition of sex steroid production is usually the emphasis of treatment of dermatologic conditions associated with PCOS because they mostly stem from high circulating androgen levels. This goal is frequently achieved with the use of combined oral contraceptive pills (COCP).[59]

Peripheral Androgen Blockade

Blockade of peripheral androgen is achieved via androgen blocking agents such as spironolactone, finasteride, and flutamide.[59]

Cosmetic Treatments

Laser therapy is a mechanical solution to the problem of hirsutism.

Menstrual Irregularity

OCPs are frequently used for improvement of menstrual irregularity and hormonal profile in PCOS patients.[3]

PCOS and Fertility

First-line therapy in obese PCOS females seeking infertility treatment is weight loss. Clomiphene citrate is the first choice for ovulation induction; failure to respond to clomiphene is usually followed by gonadotropin administration. An alternative to gonadotropin therapy is laparoscopic ovarian surgery, which is considered in patients resistant to treatment with clomiphene citrate. In case of failure, IVF is also considered.[60]

Community-Based Trials

A randomized trial in the United States reported improved quality of life, reduced depressive symptoms, and better weight loss when patients were provided with community-based trials and lifestyle change compared with when only lifestyle modification was offered.[61]

Comorbidities and Ethnicity

Because NA is a place where multiple ethnic groups reside, it is important to consider ethnicities and their predisposition to develop certain PCOS comorbidities. Increased prevalence of hirsutism is observed among females of Middle Eastern or Mediterranean descent. Abnormal glucose tolerance is more commonly observed in South Asian and Hispanic females compared with Southern or Eastern Europeans. Those more prone to obesity and metabolic problems are Black and Hispanic females. CVD is more commonly observed in Black females. Type 2 DM and MetS is seen to be greater in Hispanic females.[54] This may be attributed to genetic predisposition or changes in diet and lifestyle.

Polycystic Ovary Syndrome in Adolescence in the United States

PCOS is frequently studied and treated in the adult population; however, it is also seen in adolescent females. Childhood obesity may increase the risk for developing PCOS because obesity is associated with higher IR along with HA caused by increased androgen production and suppression of SHBG.[62] In the United States, PCOS is known to be the most common cause of endocrine obesity syndrome in adolescent females.[9] The prevalence of obesity in PCOS adolescent females was reported to be 60% compared with 18% of healthy controls.[63]

Identifying PCOS in this population is especially challenging because of overlapping findings observed in normal pubertal development and PCOS. Findings such as menstrual irregularity, an anovulatory cycle, multiple ovarian follicles, and higher than normal androgen concentrations are frequently observed, making early disease identification a challenge for most physicians.[64] In addition, evaluation of HA through physical examination is also difficult because of different Tanner stages of pubertal development.[64]

Although acne is common in this age group, persistence of acne in adulthood and resistance to treatment warrants the need for further evaluation.[9]

Irregular menstruation in the first-year post menarche is having a cycle of longer than 90 days. In the second to third year post menarche, it is defined as having a cycle of less than 21 or more than 45 days, and more than 3 years post menarche a cycle of less than 21 days or more than 35 days is considered irregular.[65] Nevertheless, only 40% of females complaining of menstrual irregularity have PCOS.[54]

Hirsutism is observed in more than half of adolescent females with HA; however, it may not be fully developed in early adolescence.[9]

Baumann et al. recommends having a higher index of clinical suspicion for PCOS in adolescent girls presenting with obesity, hirsutism, acne, and complaints of hair loss or menstrual irregularity because they may be the only features presenting of the disease.[9] Also, a positive diagnosis means an enhanced risk of CVD, dyslipidemia, and type 2 DM.[64] Lewy et al. conducted a study on adolescent American females and reported 50% reduction in peripheral insulin sensitivity in HA females, putting them at much greater risk for developing type 2 DM.[66]

Diagnosis of Adolescent PCOS in USA

A study conducted by John Hopkins University studied the approach of physicians in the USA toward adolescent PCOS. It was observed that majority of physicians would initiate workup in adolescent girls presenting with menstrual irregularity within 1 to 2 years of menarche. Blood serum studies commonly ordered would include luteinizing hormone (LH), follicle-stimulating hormone (FSH), testosterone levels, prolactin, progesterone, dehydroepiandrosterone (DHEA), and glucose.[67]

Treatment of Adolescent Polycystic Ovary Syndrome in the United States

Recommended treatment options in adolescent PCOS patients are similar to those in adults, which include lifestyle modification, insulin sensitizers, and COCP.[67] For treatment, most healthcare providers in the United States were reported to use metformin, along with a combination of estrogen and progesterone.[67] Another study was conducted to assess the approach of physicians in NA to adolescent PCOS; it was observed that 98% prescribe OCPs and 90% recommend lifestyle modifications, such as diet and exercise.[56] A small pilot study on American adolescent females with PCOS reported a greater reduction in weight and mood disorder in patients going for cognitive behavioral therapy.[68]

Polycystic Ovary Syndrome and Obesity in North America

Obesity in North America

Obesity affects more than one-third of adults[69] and 20% of females in the reproductive-age group in America.[70] Research has shown that when increased food portion size is offered to people, they tend to consume more; the consumption is seen to increase up to 30%.[71] A study conducted by Nestle and Young reports a two to five times increase in portion size in the United States.[72] In America, fast food portion sizes are bigger than those in Europe.[73] Portion sizes in the United States have continued to grow in proportion with the increasing body weight of its population from 1970, contributing to the growing overweight and obese population.[72]

Pathophysiology of Polycystic Ovary Syndrome in Obese Females

A history of weight gain is frequently seen to precede symptoms of anovulation and HA, suggesting a connection between obesity and PCOS.[74] Obesity has various effects on the female reproductive system, and the increasing prevalence is a challenge for physicians providing fertility care to these individuals.[75] Adipose tissue secretes adipokines such as leptin, ghrelin, adiponectin, and resistin; these are known to influence gonadal function.[75] Leptin, the most researched adipokine, influences gonadal function by inhibiting the development of the ovarian follicle, stimulating the hypothalamic-pituitary axis,[76] and regulating early embryo development.[77] It is known to reduce insulin-induced steroidogenesis in theca and granulosa cells by acting on follicular cell receptors.[78] In addition, it limits granulosa cells to produce estradiol by causing an inhibition of LH. All these contribute to the reduced reproductive potential and altered function observed in obese females.[76] In obese females, adiponectin levels are seen to be decreased and are negatively associated with insulin.[79] This may be an important contributor to the IR and HA observed in obese females.

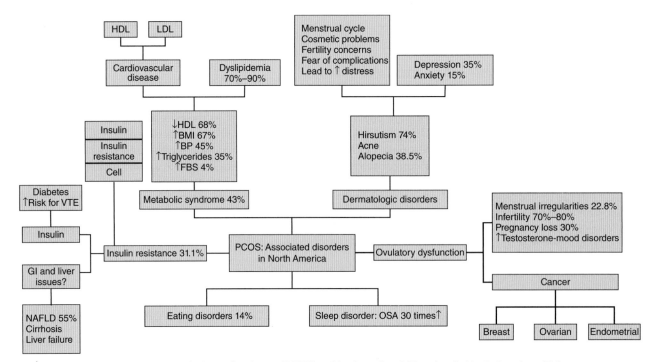

• **Fig. 30.1** Polycystic Ovary Syndrome *(PCOS)* and Its Associated Disorders in North America. *BMI*, Body mass index; *BP*, blood pressure; *FBS*, fasting blood sugar; *GI*, Gastrointestinal; *HDL*, high-density lipoprotein; *LDL*, low-density lipoprotein; *NAFLD*, nonalcoholic fatty liver disease; *OSA*, obstructive sleep apnea; *VTE*, venous thromboembolism.

In summary, HA and hyperinsulinemia are the key consequences of obesity. HA, through granulosa cell apoptosis, causes anovulation.[80] A higher prevalence of HA is reported in obese adolescent females, putting them at risk for developing PCOS.

Impact of Obesity on Females
In a large cohort study conducted of more than 7000 American females, it was observed that overweight and obese females show reduced fertility even with the presence of a normal menstrual cycle compared with females with optimal BMIs.[81] Some obese populations have a prevalence of PCOS as high as 30%, although a causative role is yet to be established.[82] Exacerbation of the symptoms of PCOS can be seen in obese females with a greater derangement of the metabolic and reproductive profile[83] (Fig. 30.1).

REFERENCE

1. Schaetzl RJ, Zelinsky W, Hoffman PF, Watson JW. North America. Encyclopedia Britannica. 2022. https://www.britannica.com/place/North-America
2. James PT, Leach R, Kalamara E, Shayeghi M. The worldwide obesity epidemic. *Obes Res.* 2001;9(suppl 11):228S-233S.
3. Williams T, Mortada R, Porter S. Diagnosis and treatment of polycystic ovary syndrome. *Am Fam Physician.* 2016;94(2):106-113.
4. Cırık DA, Dilbaz B. What do we know about metabolic syndrome in adolescents with PCOS? *J Turk Ger Gynecol Assoc.* 2014;15(1):49.
5. Azziz R, Marin C, Hoq L, Badamgarav E, Song P. Health care-related economic burden of the polycystic ovary syndrome during the reproductive life span. *J Clin Endocrinol Metab.* 2005;90(8):4650-4658.
6. Archer JS, Chang RJ. Hirsutism and acne in polycystic ovary syndrome. *Best Pract Res Clin Obstet Gynaecol.* 2004;18(5):737-754.
7. Azziz R. The evaluation and management of hirsutism. *Obstet Gynecol.* 2003;101(5):995-1007.
8. Housman E, Reynolds RV. Polycystic ovary syndrome: a review for dermatologists: part I. Diagnosis and manifestations. *J Am Acad Dermatol.* 2014;71(5):847.e1-847.e10.
9. Baumann EE, Rosenfield RL. Polycystic ovary syndrome in adolescence. *Endocrinologist.* 2002;12(4):333-348.
10. Futterweit W, Dunaif A, Yeh HC, Kingsley P. The prevalence of hyperandrogenism in 109 consecutive female patients with diffuse alopecia. *J Am Acad Dermatol.* 1988;19(5):831-836.
11. Strowitzki T, Capp E, von Eye Corleta H. The degree of cycle irregularity correlates with the grade of endocrine and metabolic disorders in PCOS patients. *Eur J Obstet Gynecol Reprod Biol.* 2010;149(2):178-181.
12. Azziz R, Woods KS, Reyna R, Key TJ, Knochenhauer ES, Yildiz BO. The prevalence and features of the polycystic ovary syndrome in an unselected population. *J Clin Endocrinol Metab.* 2004;89(6):2745-2749.
13. Hartz AJ, Rupley DC, Rimm AA. The association of girth measurements with disease in 32,856 women. *Am J Epidemiol.* 1984;119(1):71-80.
14. Apridonidze T, Essah PA, Iuorno MJ, Nestler JE. Prevalence and characteristics of the metabolic syndrome in women with polycystic ovary syndrome. *J Clin Endocrinol Metab.* 2005;90(4):1929-1935.
15. Ford ES, Giles WH, Dietz WH. Prevalence of the metabolic syndrome among US adults: findings from the third National Health and Nutrition Examination Survey. *JAMA.* 2002;287(3):356-359.

16. Carmina E, Napoli N, Longo RA, Rini GB, Lobo RA. Metabolic syndrome in polycystic ovary syndrome (PCOS): lower prevalence in southern Italy than in the USA and the influence of criteria for the diagnosis of PCOS. *Eur J Endocrinol.* 2006;154(1):141-145.

17. Wang ET, Calderon-Margalit R, Cedars MI, et al. Polycystic ovary syndrome and risk for long-term diabetes and dyslipidemia. *Obstet Gynecol.* 2011;117(1):6.

18. Legro RS, Kunselman AR, Dodson WC, Dunaif A. Prevalence and predictors of risk for type 2 diabetes mellitus and impaired glucose tolerance in polycystic ovary syndrome: a prospective, controlled study in 254 affected women. *J Clin Endocrinol Metab.* 1999;84(1):165-169.

19. Kauffman RP, Baker VM, DiMarino P, Gimpel T, Castracane VD. Polycystic ovarian syndrome and insulin resistance in white and Mexican American women: a comparison of two distinct populations. *Am J Obstet Gynecol.* 2002;187(5):1362-1369.

20. Carmina E, Legro RS, Stamets K, Lowell J, Lobo RA. Difference in body weight between American and Italian women with polycystic ovary syndrome: influence of the diet. *Hum Reprod.* 2003;18(11):2289-2293.

21. Berneis K, Rizzo M, Lazzaroni V, Fruzzetti F, Carmina E. Atherogenic lipoprotein phenotype and low-density lipoproteins size and subclasses in women with polycystic ovary syndrome. *J Clin Endocrinol Metab.* 2007;92(1):186-189.

22. Talbott EO, Guzick DS, Sutton-Tyrrell K, et al. Evidence for association between polycystic ovary syndrome and premature carotid atherosclerosis in middle-aged women. *Arterioscler Thromb Vasc Biol.* 2000;20(11):2414-2421.

23. Ehrmann DA, Barnes RB, Rosenfield RL, Cavaghan MK, Imperial J. Prevalence of impaired glucose tolerance and diabetes in women with polycystic ovary syndrome. *Diabetes Care.* 1999;22(1):141-146.

24. Hankinson SE, Eliassen AH. Endogenous estrogen, testosterone and progesterone levels in relation to breast cancer risk. *J Steroid Biochem Mol Biol.* 2007;106(1-5):24-30.

25. Baron JA, Weiderpass E, Newcomb PA, et al. Metabolic disorders and breast cancer risk (United States). *Cancer Causes Control.* 2001;12(10):875-880.

26. Risch HA. Hormonal etiology of epithelial ovarian cancer, with a hypothesis concerning the role of androgens and progesterone. *J Natl Cancer Inst.* 1998;90(23):1774-1786.

27. Kuper H, Cramer DW, Titus-Ernstoff L. Risk of ovarian cancer in the United States in relation to anthropometric measures: does the association depend on menopausal status? *Cancer Causes Control.* 2002;13(5):455-463.

28. Soliman PT, Oh JC, Schmeler KM, et al. Risk factors for young premenopausal women with endometrial cancer. *Obstet Gynecol.* 2005;105(3):575-580.

29. Giudice LC. Endometrium in PCOS: implantation and predisposition to endocrine CA. *Best Pract Res Clin Endocrinol Metab.* 2006;20(2):235-244.

30. Laven JS, Imani B, Eijkemans MJ, Fauser BC. New approach to polycystic ovary syndrome and other forms of anovulatory infertility. *Obstet Gynecol Surv.* 2002;57(11):755-767.

31. Practice Committee of the American Society for Reproductive Medicine. Definitions of infertility and recurrent pregnancy loss: a committee opinion. *Fertil Steril.* 2013;99(1):63.

32. Lentscher JA, Slocum B, Torrealday S. Polycystic ovarian syndrome and fertility. *Clin Obstet Gynecol.* 2021;64(1):65-75.

33. Jakubowicz DJ, Iuorno MJ, Jakubowicz S, Roberts KA, Nestler JE. Effects of metformin on early pregnancy loss in the polycystic ovary syndrome. *J Clin Endocrinol Metab.* 2002;87(2):524-529.

34. Okoroh EM, Hooper WC, Atrash HK, Yusuf HR, Boulet SL. Is polycystic ovary syndrome another risk factor for venous thromboembolism? United States, 2003–2008. *Am J Obstet Gynecol.* 2012;207(5):377.e1-377.e8.

35. Defronzo RA, Ferrannini E. Insulin resistance, a multifaceted syndrome responsible for NIDDM, obesity, hypertension, dyslipidemia, and atherosclerotic cardiovascular disease. *Diabetes Care.* 1991;14:173-194.

36. Cobin RH. Cardiovascular and metabolic risks associated with PCOS. *Intern Emerg Med.* 2013;8(1):61-64.

37. Talbott EO, Guzick DS, Sutton-Tyrrell K, et al. Evidence for association between polycystic ovary syndrome and premature carotid atherosclerosis in middle-aged women. *Arterioscler Thromb Vasc Biolo.* 2000;20(11):2414-2421.

38. Mosca L. Guidelines for prevention of cardiovascular disease in women: a summary of recommendations. *Prev Cardiol.* 2007;10:19-25.

39. Wild S, Pierpoint T, McKeigue P, Jacobs H. Cardiovascular disease in women with PCOS at long-term follow-up: a retrospective cohort study. *Clin Endocrinol.* 2000;522:595-600.

40. Utzschneider KM, Kahn SE. The role of insulin resistance in nonalcoholic fatty liver disease. *J Clin Endocrinol Metab.* 2006;91(12):4753-4761.

41. Schwimmer JB, Khorram O, Chiu V, Schwimmer WB. Abnormal aminotransferase activity in women with polycystic ovary syndrome. *Fertil Steril.* 2005;83(2):494-497.

42. Setji TL, Holland ND, Sanders LL, Pereira KC, Diehl AM, Brown AJ. Nonalcoholic steatohepatitis and nonalcoholic fatty liver disease in young women with polycystic ovary syndrome. *J Clin Endocrinol Metab.* 2006;91(5):1741-1747.

43. Gambarin–Gelwan M, Kinkhabwala SV, Schiano TD, Bodian C, Yeh HC, Futterweit W. Prevalence of nonalcoholic fatty liver disease in women with polycystic ovary syndrome. *Clin Gastroenterol Hepatol.* 2007;5(4):496-501.

44. Carmina E. Need for liver evaluation in polycystic ovary syndrome. *J Hepatol.* 2007;47(3):313-315.

45. Vgontzas AN, Legro RS, Bixler EO, Grayev A, Kales A, Chrousos GP. Polycystic ovary syndrome is associated with obstructive sleep apnea and daytime sleepiness: role of insulin resistance. *J Clin Endocrinol Metab.* 2001;86(2):517-520.

46. Chrousos GP. The role of stress and the hypothalamic–pituitary–adrenal axis in the pathogenesis of the metabolic syndrome: neuro-endocrine and target tissue-related causes. *Int J Obes.* 2000;24(2):S50-S55.

47. Sam S, Ehrmann DA. Pathogenesis and consequences of disordered sleep in PCOS. *Clin Med Insights Reprod Health.* 2019;13:1179558119871269.

48. Tasali E, Van Cauter E, Hoffman L, Ehrmann DA. Impact of obstructive sleep apnea on insulin resistance and glucose tolerance in women with polycystic ovary syndrome. *J Clin Endocrinol Metab.* 2008;93(10):3878-3884.

49. Weiner CL, Primeau M, Ehrmann DA. Androgens and mood dysfunction in women: comparison of women with polycystic ovarian syndrome to healthy controls. *Psychosom Med.* 2004;66:356-362.

50. Himelein MJ, Thatcher SS. Polycystic ovary syndrome and mental health: a review. *Obstet Gynecol Surv.* 2006;61:723-732.

51. Hahn S, Janssen OE, Tan S, et al. Clinical and psychological correlates of quality-of-life in polycystic ovary syndrome. *Eur J Endocrinol.* 2005;153:853-860.

52. Kerchner A, Lester W, Stuart SP, Dokras A. Risk of depression and other mental health disorders in women with polycystic

ovary syndrome: a longitudinal study. *Fertil Steril.* 2009;91(1): 207-212.

53. Hollinrake E, Abreu A, Maifeld M, Van Voorhis BJ, Dokras A. Increased risk of depressive disorders in women with polycystic ovary syndrome. *Fertil Steril.* 2007;87(6):1369-1376.

54. Fauser BC, Tarlatzis BC, Rebar RW, et al. Consensus on women's health aspects of polycystic ovary syndrome (PCOS): the Amsterdam ESHRE/ASRM-Sponsored 3rd PCOS Consensus Workshop Group. *Fertil Steril.* 2012;97(1):28-38.

55. Glueck CJ, Dharashivkar S, Wang P, et al. Obesity and extreme obesity, manifest by ages 20–24 years, continuing through 32–41 years in women, should alert physicians to the diagnostic likelihood of polycystic ovary syndrome as a reversible underlying endocrinopathy. *Eur J Obstet Gynecol Reprod Biol.* 2005;122(2): 206-212.

56. Bonny AE, Appelbaum H, Connor EL, et al. Clinical variability in approaches to polycystic ovary syndrome. *J Pediatr Adolesc Gynecol.* 2012;25(4):259-261.

57. Romualdi D, De Cicco S, Tagliaferri V, Proto C, Lanzone A, Guido M. The metabolic status modulates the effect of metformin on the antimullerian hormone-androgens-insulin interplay in obese women with polycystic ovary syndrome. *J Clin Endocrinol Metab.* 2011;96(5):E821-E824.

58. Moghetti P, Castello R, Negri C, et al. Metformin effects on clinical features, endocrine and metabolic profiles, and insulin sensitivity in polycystic ovary syndrome: a randomized, double-blind, placebo-controlled 6-month trial, followed by open, long-term clinical evaluation. *J Clin Endocrinol Metab.* 2000;85(1):139-146.

59. Archer JS, Chang RJ. Hirsutism and acne in polycystic ovary syndrome. *Best Pract Res Clin Obstet Gynaecol.* 2004;18(5): 737-754.

60. Thessaloniki ESHRE/ASRM-Sponsored PCOS Consensus Workshop Group. Consensus on infertility treatment related to polycystic ovary syndrome. *Hum Reprod.* 2008;23(3):462-477.

61. Rofey DL, Szigethy EM, Noll RB, Dahl RE, Lobst E, Arslanian SA. Cognitive–behavioral therapy for physical and emotional disturbances in adolescents with polycystic ovary syndrome: a pilot study. *J Pediatr Psychol.* 2009;34(2):156-163.

62. Anderson AD, Solorzano CMB, McCartney CR. Childhood obesity and its impact on the development of adolescent PCOS. *Semin Reprod Med.* 2014;32(3):202-213.

63. Roe AH, Prochaska E, Smith M, Sammel M, Dokras A. Using the Androgen Excess–PCOS Society criteria to diagnose polycystic ovary syndrome and the risk of metabolic syndrome in adolescents. *J Pediatr.* 2013;162(5):937-941.

64. Warren-Ulanch J, Arslanian S. Treatment of PCOS in adolescence. *Best Pract Res Clin Endocrinol Metab.* 2006;20(2):311-330.

65. Peña AS, Witchel SF, Hoeger KM, et al. Adolescent polycystic ovary syndrome according to the international evidence-based guideline. *BMC Med.* 2020;18(1):1-16.

66. Lewy VD, Danadian K, Witchel SF, Arslanian S. Early metabolic abnormalities in adolescent girls with polycystic ovarian syndrome. *J Pediatr.* 2001;138(1):38-44.

67. Guttmann-Bauman I. Approach to adolescent polycystic ovary syndrome (PCOS) in the pediatric endocrine community in the USA. *J Pediatr Endocrinol Metab.* 2005;18(5):499-506.

68. Rofey DL, Szigethy EM, Noll RB, Dahl RE, Lobst E, Arslanian SA. Cognitive–behavioral therapy for physical and emotional disturbances in adolescents with polycystic ovary syndrome: a pilot study. *J Pediatr Psychol.* 2009;34(2):156-163.

69. US Department of Health and Human Services. *Overweight and Obesity Statistics.* National Institute of Diabetes and Digestive and Kidney Diseases; 2015.

70. Broughton DE, Moley KH. Obesity and female infertility: potential mediators of obesity's impact. *Fertil Steril.* 2017;107(4):840-847.

71. Steenhuis IH, Leeuwis FH, Vermeer WM. Small, medium, large or supersize: trends in food portion sizes in The Netherlands. *Public Health Nutr.* 2010;13(6):852-857.

72. Young LR, Nestle M. The contribution of expanding portion sizes to the US obesity epidemic. *Am J Public Health.* 2002;92(2): 246-249.

73. Young LR, Nestle M. Portion sizes and obesity: responses of fast-food companies. *J Public Health Policy.* 2007;28(2):238-248.

74. Littlejohn EE, Weiss RE, Deplewski D, Edidin DV, Rosenfield R. Intractable early childhood obesity as the initial sign of insulin resistant hyperinsulinism and precursor of polycystic ovary syndrome. *J Pediatr Endocrinol Metab.* 2007;20(1):41-52.

75. Metwally M, Li TC, Ledger WL. The impact of obesity on female reproductive function. *Obes Rev.* 2007;8(6):515-523.

76. Moschos S, Chan JL, Mantzoros CS. Leptin and reproduction: a review. *Fertil Steril.* 2002;77:433-444.

77. Brannian JD, Hansen KA. Leptin and ovarian folliculogenesis: implications for ovulation induction and ART outcomes. *Semin Reprod Med.* 2002;20:103-112.

78. Spicer LJ. Leptin: a possible metabolic signal affecting reproduction. *Domest Anim Endocrinol.* 2001;21:251-270.

79. Gil-Campos M, Canete RR, Gil A. Adiponectin, the missing link in insulin resistance and obesity. *Clin Nutr.* 2004;23:963-974.

80. Billig H, Chun SY, Eisenhauer K, Hsueh AJ. Gonadal cell apoptosis: hormone-regulated cell demise. *Hum Reprod Update.* 1996;2: 103-117.

81. Gesink Law DC, Maclehose RF, Longnecker MP. Obesity and time to pregnancy. *Hum Reprod.* 2007;22(2):414-420.

82. Alvarez-Blasco F, Botella-Carretero JI, San Millán JL, Escobar-Morreale HF. Prevalence and characteristics of the polycystic ovary syndrome in overweight and obese women. *Arch Intern Med.* 2006;166(19):2081-2086.

83. Broughton DE, Moley KH. Obesity and female infertility: potential mediators of obesity's impact. *Fertil Steril.* 2017;107(4): 840-847.

Index

Note: Page numbers followed by *f*, *t*, or *b* indicate figures, tables, or boxes, respectively.